Wilkins'
Clinical Assessment in Respiratory Care

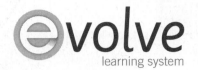
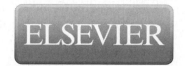
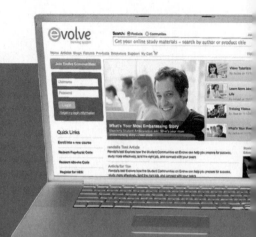

Seventh Edition

Wilkins'
Clinical Assessment
in Respiratory Care

Albert J. Heuer, PhD, MBA, RRT, RPFT
Program Director, Masters in Health Care Management &
Associate Professor, Respiratory Care Program-North
School of Health Related Professions
University of Medicine and Dentistry of New Jersey
Newark, New Jersey

Craig L. Scanlan, EdD, RRT, FAARC
Professor Emeritus
School of Health Related Professions
University of Medicine and Dentistry of New Jersey
Newark, New Jersey

3251 Riverport Lane
Maryland Heights, Missouri 63043

WILKINS' CLINICAL ASSESSMENT IN RESPIRATORY CARE   ISBN: 978-0-323-10029-8

Notice

Knowledge and best practice in this field are constantly changing. As new research and experience broaden our knowledge, changes in practice, treatment, and drug therapy may become necessary or appropriate. Readers are advised to check the most current information provided (i) on procedures featured or (ii) by the manufacturer of each product to be administered, to verify the recommended dose or formula, the method and duration of administration, and contraindications. It is the responsibility of the practitioners, relying on their own experience and knowledge of the patient, to make diagnoses, to determine dosages and the best treatment for each individual patient, and to take all appropriate safety precautions. To the fullest extent of the law, neither the Publisher nor the Editors/Authors assume any liability for any injury and/or damage to persons or property arising out of or related to any use of the material contained in this book.

The Publisher

Library of Congress Cataloging-in-Publication Data
Wilkins' clinical assessment in respiratory care / [edited by] Albert J. Heuer, Craig L. Scanlan. – 7th ed.
    p. ; cm.
  Clinical assessment in respiratory care
  Rev. ed. of: Clinical assessment in respiratory care / Robert L. Wilkins, James R. Dexter ; consulting editor, Albert J. Heuer. 6th ed.
c2010.
  Includes bibliographical references and index.
  ISBN 978-0-323-10029-8 (pbk. : alk. paper)
  I. Heuer, Albert J. II. Scanlan, Craig L., 1947- III. Wilkins, Robert L. Clinical assessment in respiratory care.
IV. Title: Clinical assessment in respiratory care.
  [DNLM: 1. Diagnostic Techniques, Respiratory System. 2. Physical Examination.
3. Respiratory Therapy–methods. WF 141]
  617'.075—dc23   2012045666

Content Strategy Director: Jeanne Olson
Content Manager: Billi Sharp
Senior Content Development Specialist: Kathleen Sartori
Publishing Services Manager: Gayle May
Project Manager: Deepthi Unni
Design Direction: Maggie Reid

Printed in the United States of America

Last digit is the print number: 9 8 7 6 5 4 3 2 1

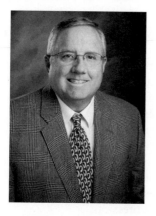

Through the leadership and scholarly commitment of Dr. Robert L. Wilkins, PhD, RRT, this text has become a cornerstone resource in respiratory patient assessment and is used by a majority of respiratory programs worldwide. This accomplishment can be attributed directly to the significant and sustained efforts of Dr. Wilkins, through the many editions of this text for which he has been senior editor. *Simply stated*, this book is current, thorough, concise, and clearly written. As a result of his untimely death, Dr. Wilkins' presence in preparing this edition was greatly missed, and maintaining his high standard was a challenge. However, both editors for this seventh edition, Dr. Craig Scanlan and I, had worked with Bob on other projects, including prior editions of this and other texts. In addition, we assembled a team of returning and new contributors. These factors, coupled with the appropriate retention of content written by Dr. Wilkins for prior editions, have resulted in what we believe is worthy of the standard and style set by Dr. Wilkins. In recognition and appreciation of his contributions to this text and to respiratory therapy education, this text has been renamed *Wilkins' Clinical Assessment in Respiratory Care*. Dr. Wilkins is deeply missed by me on a personal and professional level, and his absence from our profession will be felt for some time. However, his legacy will live on in the memory of his family, friends, and colleagues, as well as the pages of this text.

Warmly, Al Heuer

To Dr. Robert L. Wilkins and Dr. Craig L. Scanlan for their unwavering mentorship, to my lovely wife Laurel for her patience and support, and to the students, faculty, and my fellow respiratory therapists, who are constant sources of inspiration.
AJH

To Mom and Dad who believed in me;
to Barrie and Craig Patrick, in whom I believe.
CLS

Douglas D. Deming, MD
Professor of Pediatrics
Loma Linda University
Medical Director of Neonatal Respiratory Care
Medical Director of ECMO
Loma Linda University Children's Hospital
Loma Linda, California

De De Gardner, MSHP, RRT, FAARC
Associate Professor and Chair
Department of Respiratory Care
School of Health Professions
University of Texas Health Science Center at San Antonio
San Antonio, Texas

Susan L. McInturff, RCP, RRT
Clinical Director
Farrell's Home Health
Bremerton, Washington

S. Gregory Marshall, PhD, RRT, RPSGT, RST
Associate Professor/Chair
Department of Respiratory Care
College of Health Professions
Texas State University—San Marcos
San Marcos, Texas

James A. Peters, MD, DrPH, MPH, RD, RRT, FACPM
Attending Physician, Preventive Medicine
Department of Internal Medicine and Center for Health
St. Helena Hospital and Health Center;
Physician and Owner
Nutrition and Lifestyle Medical Clinic
St. Helena, California

Helen M. Sorenson, MA, RRT, FAARC
Assistant Professor
Department of Respiratory Care
School of Health Professions
University of Texas Health Science Center at San Antonio
San Antonio, Texas

Cheryl Thomas Peters, DCN, RD
Clinical Manager St. Helena Center for Health
St. Helena, California

Richard Wettstein, BS, RRT
Assistant Professor
Department of Respiratory Care
School of Health Professions
University of Texas Health Science Center at San Antonio
San Antonio, Texas

Contributors

Robert F. Allen, III, MA, RPSGT
Manager, Sleep Wake Disorder Lab
St. Mary's Medical Center
Langhorne, Pennsylvania

Zaza Cohen, MD, FCCP
Assistant Professor
Fellowship Program Director
Division of Pulmonary and Critical Care Medicine
University of Medicine and Dentistry of New Jersey
Newark, New Jersey

Cara DeNunzio, MPH, RRT, CTTS
Adjunct Assistant Professor
Respiratory Care Program—North
School of Health Related Professions
University of Medicine and Dentistry of New Jersey
Newark, New Jersey

Nadine A. Fydryszewski, PhD, MLS
Associate Professor
School of Health Related Professions
University of Medicine and Dentistry of New Jersey
Newark, New Jersey

David A. Gourley, RRT, MHA, FAARC
Executive Director of Regulatory Affairs
Chilton Hospital
Pompton Plains, New Jersey

Elaine M. Keohane, PhD, MLS
Professor and Chairman
Department of Clinical Laboratory Sciences
University of Medicine and Dentistry of New Jersey
Newark, New Jersey

Kenneth Miller, MEd, RRT-NPS, AE-C
Educational Coordinator, Dean of Wellness
Respiratory Care Services
Lehigh Valley Health Network
Allentown, Pennsylvania

Ruben D. Restrepo, MD, RRT, FAARC
Professor
Director, Bachelor's Completion Program
School of Health Professions
Department of Respiratory Care
University of Texas Health Science Center
San Antonio, Texas

Narciso Rodriguez, BS, RRT-NPS, RPFT, AE-C
Assistant Professor and Program Director
Respiratory Care Program
University of Medicine and Dentistry of New Jersey
School of Health Related Professions
Newark, New Jersey

David L. Vines, MHS, RRT, FAARC
Chair and Program Director
Department of Respiratory Care
Rush University
Chicago, Illinois

Jane E. Ziegler, MD, DCN, RD, LDN
Assistant Professor
Graduate Programs in Clinical Nutrition
School of Health Related Professions
University of Medicine and Dentistry of New Jersey
Newark, New Jersey

Reviewers

Georgine Bills, MBA/HAS, RRT
Program Director, Respiratory Therapy
Dixie State College of Utah
St. George, Utah

Craig P. Black, PhD, RRT-NPS, FAARC
Director, Respiratory Care Program
The University of Toledo
Toledo, Ohio

Helen Schaar Corning, AS, RCP, RRT
Shands Jacksonville Medical Center
Jacksonville, Florida

Erin Ellis Davis, MS, MEd, RRT-NPS, CPFT
Director of Clinical Education-Clinical Coordinator
Our Lady of Holy Cross College/Ochsner Health System
New Orleans, Louisiana

Dale Bruce Dearing, RCP, RRT, MSc
Respiratory Therapy Program Assessment Coordinator
San Joaquin Valley College
Visalia, California

Lindsay Fox, MEd, RRRT-NPS
Respiratory Care Program Coordinator
Southwestern Illinois College/St. Elizabeth Hospital
Belleville, Illinois

Laurie A. Freshwater, MA, RCP, RRT, RPFT
Health Sciences Division Director
Carteret Community College
Morehead City, North Carolina

Christine A. Hamilton, DHSc, RRT, AE-C
Assistant Professor, Director of Clinical Education
Cardio-Respiratory Care Sciences Program
Tennessee State University
Nashville, Tennessee

Sharon L. Hatfield, PhD, RRT, RPFT, AE-C, COPD-C
Chair of Community Health Sciences, Associate Professor
of Respiratory Therapy and Healthcare Management
Jefferson College of Health Sciences
Roanoke, Virginia

Robert L. Joyner, PhD, RRT, FAARC
Associate Dean and Director, Respiratory Therapy
Program
Henson School of Science & Technology
Salisbury University
Salisbury, Maryland

Chris Kallus, MEd, RRT
Professor and Program Director
Victoria College Respiratory Care Program
Victoria, Texas

Kevin Shane Keene, DHSc, RRT-NPS, CPFT, RPSGT
Program Director
Respiratory Care
University of Cincinnati
Cincinnati, OH

Tammy Kurszewski, MEd, RRT
Director of Clinical Education, Respiratory Care
Midwestern State University
Wichita Falls, Texas

J. Kenneth LeJeune, MS, RRT, CPFT
Program Director Respiratory Education
University of Arkansas Community College at Hope
Hope, Arkansas

Stacy Lewis-Sells, EdM, RRT-NPS, CPFT, AE-C
Program Director for Respiratory Care
Southeastern Community College
West Burlington, Iowa

Cory E. Martin, EdS, RRT
Program Director, Associate Professor
Volunteer State Community College
Gallatin, Tennessee

Michael McLeland, MEd, RPSGT, RST
Program Director
Sanford-Brown College
Fenton, Missouri

Harley R. Metcalfe, BS, RRT
Adjunct Professor. Respiratory Care Program
Johnson County Community College;
Vice President
PM Sleep Lab LLC
Overland Park, Kansas

Michell Oki, MPAcc, RRT RPFT, RPSGT
Assistant Professor
Weber State University Respiratory Therapy
Ogden, Utah

Timothy Op't Holt, EdD, RRT, AE-C, FAARC
Professor
University of South Alabama
Mobile, Alabama

Sara Parker, BHS-RT, RRT-NPS, AE-C
Clinical Instructor
University of Missouri School of Health Professions
Columbia, Missouri

José D. Rojas, PhD, RRT
Associate Professor
University of Texas Medical Branch
Galveston, Texas

Paula Denise Silver, BS Biology, PharmD
Medical Instructor
ECPI University
Newport News, Virginia

Helen M. Sorenson, MA, RRT, FAARC
Associate Professor Department of Respiratory Care
UT Health Science Center
San Antonio, Texas

Shawna L. Strickland, PhD, RRT-NPS, AE-C, FAARC
Clinical Associate Professor
University of Missouri
Columbia, Missouri

Cam Twarog, RRT-NPS, BSRT, MBA
Director of Clinical Education
Respiratory Care Practitioner Program
Wheeling Jesuit University
Wheeling, West Virginia

Michael D. Werner, MS, RRT, CPFT
Respiratory Therapy Program Director
Concorde Career College North Hollywood
Los Angeles, California

Ancillary Authors

Craig P. Black, PhD, RRT-NPS, FAARC
Director, Respiratory Care Program
The University of Toledo
Toledo, Ohio

Jill H. Sand, MEd, RRT
Program Chair Respiratory Care
Southeast Community College
Lincoln, Nebraska

Preface

The primary purpose of the seventh edition is the same as the previous ones: to provide relevant information related to the knowledge and skills needed for respiratory therapists (RTs) to be competent and to trust in their patient assessment skills. The seventh edition is based on the assumption that every patient is an interactive, complex being who is more than a collection of his or her parts. The health status of patients depends on many internal and external environmental interactions. These interactions occur within their physical environments and include what they eat, drink, and breathe; how they sleep; and if and when they exercise. External or social environments also affect their health status and include what kind of activity and work they participate in and where they live. Other factors, such as when, why, and how often patients seek health care, can also affect their overall well-being.

Although the language of this text continues to be aimed primarily at students, experienced therapists or other health care clinicians may benefit from its content as well. We hope that this book helps students and clinicians gain important insight into the value, purpose, and skills associated with patient assessment. The important tools provided in these pages can assist you to inspect and examine the patient's body. However, learning to listen to the patient's explanation of what is wrong and right is often the most valuable practice in meeting a patient's health needs.

Assisting physicians in assessing patients for the treatment needed, the complications that may arise, and when treatment regimen should be changed or discontinued is a competency expected of almost all health care professionals.

We have seen firsthand the difference in patient care when clinicians are competent at patient assessment. Identifying the early signs of atelectasis through the use of a stethoscope and evaluation of breathing pattern, identifying the potential misplacement of an endotracheal tube through the use of a stethoscope and the chest radiograph, and recognizing serious abnormalities based on the arterial blood gas are all scenarios in which you could find yourself.

Application of such skills can favorably affect the outcomes experienced by patients both in and outside the hospital. On the other hand, those clinicians who lack good assessment skills generally are relegated to following the orders of others, which is not always the best way to serve the patient. Although we believe that high-tech equipment can be smart and sophisticated, it can never replace the well-honed bedside assessment skills of the experienced clinician. We hope that the knowledge in this book will help develop and refine your clinical skills and inspire you to develop a passion for patient assessment.

New to This Edition

The seventh edition retains the strengths of the first six editions: a clear, approachable writing style; an attractive and user-friendly format; and the inclusion of relevant clinical case studies and helpful hints for practice. However, this new edition ushers in many significant changes:

- With the passing of the author, Robert Wilkins, in September 2010, two highly experienced respiratory care textbook editors have now assumed primary responsibility for the book, which now bears his name.
  - Albert J. Heuer is a long-time respiratory educator and is Associate Professor for the Respiratory Care Program at the University of Medicine and Dentistry in Newark, New Jersey. Dr. Heuer served as contributor and consulting editor on the sixth edition and is a coeditor of *Egan's Fundamentals of Respiratory Care*, 10th edition. Dr. Heuer is a practicing respiratory therapist who continues to work regularly in acute care at a major medical center in New Jersey. It was because of his expertise as a respiratory educator, scholar, and clinician, coupled with their professional relationship, that Robert Wilkins requested to have Dr. Heuer succeed him as lead editor for this project. Dr. Heuer is continuing Wilkins' legacy in maintaining the high standards of this text set into motion six editions ago.
  - Craig L. Scanlan is the new coeditor of this project. Dr. Scanlan is a Professor Emeritus at the University of Medicine and Dentistry with over 40 years of experience in respiratory care. He was a coeditor for four editions of *Egan's Fundamentals of Respiratory Care*, two in collaboration with Dr. Wilkins.
- Each chapter has been carefully updated to reflect the latest standards of practice and credentialing exam content.
- All chapters also have been peer reviewed, and the content is reflective of reviewer input and expertise.
- Revised chapter organization reflects a more logical progression of assessment.
- A greater emphasis on infection control throughout the text highlights its continued importance across health care.
- Enhanced chapters include Preparing for the Patient Encounter, Fundamentals of Physical Assessment, Clinical Laboratory Studies, Cardiac Output Measurement, Bronchoscopy, Respiratory Monitoring in Critical Care, and Sleep and Breathing Assessment.

Features

We continue to use learning features to help guide the student to mastery of the content. This edition features the following:

- Chapter outlines introduce students to chapter content and progression to enhance note taking.
- Measurable chapter learning objectives help with mastery of information.
- Key terms are bolded and defined within the text to enhance terminology comprehension.
- "Simply Stated" boxes are scattered throughout each chapter to succinctly summarize and highlight key points within the text.
- Bulleted "Key Points" at the end of each chapter emphasize the topics identified in the learning objectives and provide the student with an overview of chapter content for easy review.
- Select chapters include "Case Studies," which feature realistic clinical scenarios for student practice and/or classroom discussion.
- "Questions to Ask" boxes are also included in select chapters. They provide lists of questions that practitioners should ask when confronted with certain pathologies.
- "Assessment Questions" conclude each chapter to easily assess understanding.

Learning Aids

Evolve Resources— http://evolve.elsevier.com/Heuer/Wilkins
Evolve is an interactive learning environment designed to work in coordination with this text. Instructors may use Evolve to provide an Internet-based course component that reinforces and expands the concepts presented in class. Evolve may be used to publish the class syllabus, outlines, and lecture notes; set up "virtual office hours" and e-mail communication; share important dates and information through the online class calendar; and encourage student participation through chat rooms and discussion boards. Evolve allows instructors to post examinations and manage their grade books online.

For the Instructor

Evolve offers valuable resources to help instructors prepare their courses, including:

- A test bank of approximately 1000 questions in ExamView
- An image collection of the figures from the book Comprehensive PowerPoint presentations for each chapter
- NBRC CRT/RRT Summary Content Outline Correlation Guide mapping the text to the content outlines

For Students

Evolve offers valuable resources to help students succeed in their courses, including:

- Student Lecture Notes in PowerPoint format for students to print and take to lecture for enhanced note taking
- NBRC CRT/RRT Summary Content Outline Correlation Guide mapping the text to the content outlines
  For more information, visit http://evolve.elsevier.com/Heuer/Wilkins/ or contact an Elsevier sales representative.

Acknowledgments

We wish to thank the previous editor, Dr. James Dexter, for his many years of devotion to earlier editions of this project. Without him, this book would not have become the cornerstone text in respiratory patient assessment. We also thank the new and returning contributors to the chapters in this text. Their expertise, as well as their willingness and ability to share it, is most important to the value of this text. Finally, we would like to thank the peer reviewers, who provided invaluable and practical feedback for all chapters, which has been appropriately reflected in this edition.

Contents

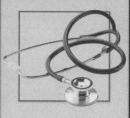

Chapter 1

Preparing for the Patient Encounter

CRAIG L. SCANLAN*

CHAPTER OUTLINE

Individualized Care
    Providing Empathetic Two-Way Communication
    Respecting Patient Needs and Preferences
    Assuring Privacy and Confidentiality
    Being Sensitive to Cultural Values
Patient Involvement
    Assessing Learning Needs and Providing Patient
      Education

Sharing Goal-Setting and Decision-Making
    Responsibilities
Encouraging Patient and Family Participation in
    Care and Safety
Provider Collaboration
    Enhancing Interprofessional Communication
    Coordinating Patient Care
    Sharing Responsibility

LEARNING OBJECTIVES

After reading this chapter, you will be able to:
1. Define patient-centered care and identify its key elements.
2. Identify the major factors affecting communication between the patient and clinician.
3. Differentiate among the stages of the clinical encounter and the communication strategies appropriate to each stage.
4. Incorporate patients' needs and preferences into your assessment and care planning.
5. Apply concepts of personal space and territoriality to support patients' privacy needs.
6. Employ basic rules to assure the confidentiality and security of all patient health information.
7. Identify the key abilities required for culturally competent communication with patients.
8. Specify ways to involve patients and their families in the provision of heath care.
9. Identify the steps in assessing a patient's learning needs, including how to overcome any documented barriers to learning.
10. Explain the use of patient action plans in facilitating goal setting and patient self-care.
11. Specify steps the patient and family can take to enhance safety and reduce medical errors.
12. Identify standard infection control procedures needed during patient encounters.
13. Outline ways to assure effective communication with other providers when receiving orders and reporting on your patient's clinical status.
14. Specify how to coordinate your patient's care with that provided by others, as well as when transferring responsibilities to others and planning for patient discharge.
15. Identify examples of how respiratory therapists can participate effectively as a team member to enhance outcomes in caring for patient with both acute and chronic cardiopulmonary disorders.

KEY TERMS

action plan
culturally competent
   communication
intimate space
nonverbal communication
patient-centered care

personal space
Protected Health Information
   (PHI)
return demonstration
social space
SBAR

Speak Up initiative
standard precautions
teach-back method
territoriality

---

*Dr. Robert Wilkins, PhD, RRT, contributed much of the content for this chapter as the coeditor of the prior edition of this text.

During the past decade, numerous governmental agencies and private provider groups have concluded that meaningful improvements in health care require a renewed focus on the interaction between patient and provider. This new focus is termed **patient-centered care**.

Figure 1-1 depicts the three main elements underlying patient-centered care: individualized care, patient involvement, and provider collaboration. Patient-centered care is founded on a two-way partnership between providers and patients (and their families) designed to ensure that (1) the care given is consistent with each individual's values, needs, and preferences, and (2) patients become active participants in their own care. By improving communication and creating more positive relationships between patients and providers, patient-centered care can improve adherence to treatment plans and thus help achieve higher-quality outcomes. In addition, patient-centered care can help minimize medical errors and contribute to enhanced patient safety.

The patient-provider encounter is at the heart of effective patient-centered care. Such encounters are so commonplace in the daily routine of the respiratory therapist (RT) that we often forget how important these short interactions can be in determining the effectiveness of the care we provide. To that end, this chapter focuses on how RTs can use these encounters to promote high-quality care that is attentive to the needs and expectations of each individual patient.

Individualized Care

Individualized care requires empathetic, two-way communication; respect for each patient's values and privacy; and sensitivity to cultural values.

Providing Empathetic Two-Way Communication

Underlying patient-centered communication is empathetic and effective communication. Communication is a two-way process that involves both sending and receiving meaningful messages. *If the receiver does not fully understand the message, effective communication has not occurred.* As indicated in Figure 1-2, multiple personal and environmental factors influence the effectiveness of communication during clinical encounters. Attending to how each of these components may affect communication can make the difference between an effective and ineffective clinical encounter.

Each party to a clinical encounter brings attitudes and values developed by prior experiences, cultural heritage, religious beliefs, level of education, and self-concept. These personal factors affect the way a message is sent as well as how it is interpreted and received. Messages can be sent in a variety of ways and at times without awareness. Body movement, facial expression, touch, and eye movement are all types of **nonverbal communication**. Combined with voice tone, nonverbal cues frequently say more than words. Because one of the purposes of the encounter is to establish a trusting relationship with the patient, the clinician must make a conscious effort to send signals of genuine concern, that is, to exhibit compassion and empathize with the patient's circumstances. Techniques useful for this purpose are facing the patient squarely, using appropriate eye contact, maintaining an open posture, using touch, and actively listening. It also may be helpful to act according to what you would expect from health care team members were you in the patient's situation (the "golden rule" of bedside care).

One of the most common mistakes made by clinicians during patient encounters is failing to listen carefully to the patient. Good listening skills require concentration on the task at hand. Active listening also calls for replying to the patient's comments and questions with appropriate responses. Patients are quick to identify the clinician who is not listening and will often interpret this as a lack of empathy or concern. If the patient says something you do not understand, it is best to ask the patient to clarify what was said rather than replying with the response you think is right. Asking for clarification tells the patient that you want to make sure you get it right.

Messages are also altered by feelings, language differences, listening habits, comfort with the situation, and preoccupation. Patients experiencing pain or difficulty breathing will have a hard time concentrating on what you are communicating until their comfort is restored. The temperature, lighting, noise, and privacy of the environment also may contribute to comfort. Patients may communicate their discomfort nonverbally using cues such as sighing, restlessness, looking into space, and avoiding eye contact.

Your use of communication techniques may differ according to the stage of interaction with a patient. Generally, a patient encounter begins with a chart review and then progresses through four additional stages: introductory, initial assessment, treatment and monitoring, and follow-up. Table 1-1 outlines the purpose of these stages and provides example strategies to help ensure effective communication during each major aspect of the patient encounter.

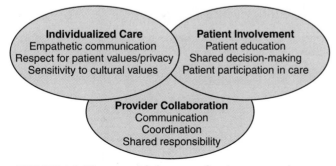

FIGURE 1-1 The essential elements of patient-centered care.

Respecting Patient Needs and Preferences

In addition to effective communication, individualized care requires that providers respect each patient's needs, preferences, and privacy. Within this framework, we do not, for example, treat "the COPD patient in room 345," but a *patient with COPD,* whose ability to cope with its full range of physical and psychosocial consequences is unique. Indeed, effective therapy requires that the individual patient's response to disease be ascertained as part of the initial patient encounter and, for those with chronic afflictions, be regularly assessed and incorporated into care plans.

Whenever possible, care plans also should reflect each individual patient's preferences as determined during initial assessment and treatment. For example, after their urgent situation is resolved, patients with asthma should be allowed to participate in deciding which aerosol drug delivery system is best for them. Likewise, a patient with cystic fibrosis should be allowed to participate in selecting from a variety of equally effective positive-pressure devices to assist in airway clearance. Accommodating an individual's needs *during* treatment also involves modifying the therapy based on the patient's response.

Assuring Privacy and Confidentiality

Anyone who has been hospitalized understands the need for privacy. We address privacy concerns in part by respecting personal space. Respecting patients' privacy rights is both a legal and a moral obligation for health care professionals.

To respect patients' personal space, one needs to understand both the general and cultural implications of proximity and direct contact. Figure 1-3 depicts the three zones of space commonly associated with the bedside patient encounter.

The **social space** (4 to 12 feet) is used primarily in the introductory stage of the encounter during which you begin to establish rapport. At this distance, you can see the "big picture" and gain an appreciation for the whole patient and the patient's environment. Vocalizations are limited to the more formal issues, and personal questions in this space are to be avoided because others in the room may overhear the conversation.

The **personal space** (18 inches to 4 feet) is used primarily during the interview component of the initial assessment, usually after establishing rapport with the patient. This enhanced proximity is generally needed to garner sensitive patient information, such as questions about daily sputum production or smoking habits. To better assure privacy in this space, pulling the bedside curtain may help the patient feel more comfortable about sharing personal information. Most patients also feel more comfortable and confident when your appearance is neat, clean, and professional. Patient trust can be enhanced by assuring appropriate eye contact while in the patient's personal space.

Intimate space (0 to 18 inches) is reserved primarily for the physical examination component of the initial assessment and the treatment and monitoring stage of the encounter. Generally, moving into such proximity and touching the patient should be done only after establishing rapport and being given permission to do so. Such permission often is obtained by simply requesting consent to listen to breath sounds or check vital signs. Asking permission to move into the intimate space communicates both your respect for patient privacy and your willingness to share responsibility for decision making. *Minimal eye contact is used in this space.* Verbal communication with the patient should be limited to simple questions or brief commands, such as, "Please take a deep breath."

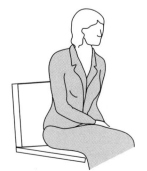

INTERNAL FACTORS

Previous experiences
Attitudes, values
Cultural heritage
Religious beliefs
Self-concept
Listening habits
Preoccupations, feelings

SENSORY/EMOTIONAL FACTORS

Fear
Stress, anxiety
Pain
Mental acuity, brain damage, hypoxia
Sight, hearing, speech impairment

ENVIRONMENTAL FACTORS

Lighting
Noise
Privacy
Distance
Temperature

VERBAL EXPRESSION

Language barrier
Jargon
Choice of words/questions
Feedback, voice tone

NONVERBAL EXPRESSION

Body movement
Facial expression
Dress, professionalism
Warmth, interest

INTERNAL FACTORS

Previous experiences
Attitudes, values
Cultural heritage
Religious beliefs
Self-concept
Listening habits
Preoccupations, feelings
Illness

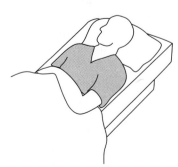

FIGURE 1-2 Factors influencing the effectiveness of communication during clinical encounters.

TABLE 1-1

Stages of the Clinical Encounter

Stage	Purpose	Communication Strategies
Chart review (preinteraction)	Identifying key patient information	Apply this information in the introductory and initial assessment stages
Introductory	Introducing oneself Confirming patient identity Clarifying purpose/your role Acknowledging family presence Building rapport Inspecting the patient (initial)	Look and act in professional manner Refer to patient using formal last name Avoid encroaching on personal space Pay attention to nonverbal cues Identify patient emotions Express support and empathy (compassion) React in nonjudgmental way
Initial assessment	Determining patient's status (interview and physical examination) Determining learning needs Assessing cultural differences Determining appropriateness of orders (new Rx)	Use active listening: · Avoid interrupting the patient · Use body position to indicate interest · Avoid writing while patient is talking · Make eye contact but do not stare · Encourage open expression Reflect what the patient shares Summarize/request feedback Make facilitative responses, e.g., nodding
Treatment and monitoring	Demonstrating/teaching treatment technique Implementing and modifying treatment based on patient's preferences, monitored responses	Explain therapy in understandable terms Invite questions about the treatment Confirm acceptance of the treatment Assess patient's concerns, expectations Attend to patient discomfort
Follow-up	Confirming patient response Developing shared goals Assuring follow-up Restoring environment	Invite questions from patient and family Determine information preferences Check the patient's ability to follow the plan Discuss follow-up (e.g., treatment schedule, what to do if symptoms worsen)

Be aware that some patients may respond poorly to encroachment into their space. Gender, age, race, physical appearance, health status, and cultural background are among the many factors that may influence a patient's comfort level when you enter the intimate space. Should the patient's words or nonverbal responses indicate hesitancy with your actions, be prepared to move more slowly and communicate your intent very carefully.

Related to the concept of proximity is that of **territoriality**. Most patients "lay claim" to all items within a certain boundary around their bed. For patients in a private room, the boundary extends to the walls of the room. Removing items from the patient's "territory" should occur only after permission has been obtained. For example, when borrowing a chair from the bedside of Mr. Jones for use at the bedside of Mr. Smith, you should ask Mr. Jones for permission. Likewise, at the end of the patient encounter, be sure to replace any items temporarily removed from the patient's territory, such as the over-the-bed table and its essential contents.

SIMPLY STATED

The social space (4 to 12 feet) is for introductions, the personal space (18 inches to 4 feet) is for interviewing, and the intimate space (0 to 18 inches) is for physical examination.

In regard to maintaining confidentiality, all health professionals become privy to sensitive patient information. For example, your chart review may reveal that a patient under your care has a history of drug abuse or has been diagnosed with a sexually transmitted disease. This information is private and not for public knowledge. You have both a legal and a moral obligation to keep this information in strictest confidence and share it only with other health professionals who have a need to know, such as the patient's nurse or attending physician. Most often, violations of patient confidentiality occur in public spaces when a clinician discusses a certain patient with other caregivers while being overheard by visitors. A good basic rule to follow is to *discuss your patient's health status only with other members of the health care team who need to know such information and only in a private area where visitors are not allowed.*

Family members and visitors often ask questions about the patient's diagnosis but always should be referred to the attending physician. This should be done in a way that does not alarm or offend those asking the questions. Most people will appreciate an honest response in which you tell them that privacy rights prevent you from discussing the patient's diagnosis with others.

Your legal obligations regarding patient information are specified under the privacy and security rules of the Health Insurance Portability and Accountability Act (HIPAA). These rules establish regulations for the use

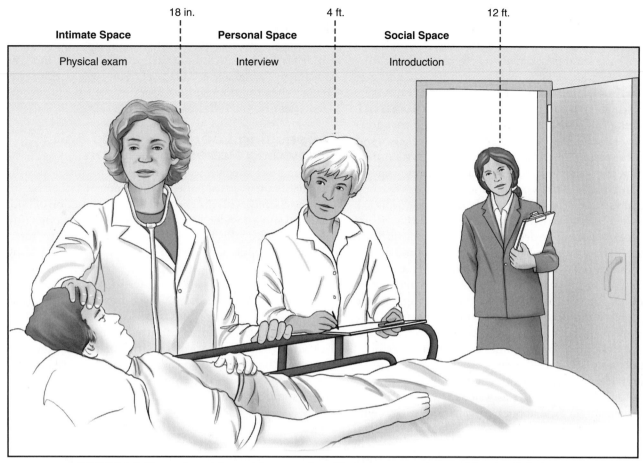

Intimate Space	Personal Space	Social Space
Physical exam	Interview	Introduction

18 in.   4 ft.   12 ft.

FIGURE 1-3 Illustration of the social, personal, and intimate spaces characterizing the clinical encounter.

and disclosure of **Protected Health Information (PHI)**. PHI is any information about health status, provision of health care, or payment for health care services that can be linked to an individual. Examples of PHI include names and addresses, phone numbers, e-mail addresses, Social Security and medical record numbers, and health insurance information. Under the law, patients control access to their PHI. For this reason, use or disclosure of PHI for purposes *other than* treatment, payment, health care operations, or public health requires patient permission. Table 1-2 provides summary guidance on key privacy and security considerations under HIPAA.

Being Sensitive to Cultural Values

As already mentioned, individualized care requires that clinicians be sensitive to their patients' cultural values and expectations. To achieve a full partnership with your patient, you'll need to identify and respond appropriately to the many cultural cues that can affect the clinical encounter and thus the success of therapy. Failure to do so can result in patient dissatisfaction, poor adherence to treatment regimens, and unsatisfactory health outcomes.

In the past, clinicians were expected to learn about the cultural norms of each and every ethnic group they would likely encounter. Certainly some knowledge about specific cultural issues is helpful and tends to grow with

TABLE 1-2	
HIPAA-Related Privacy and Security Considerations	
Do's	**Don'ts**
Do access only that information needed to perform your job	Don't discuss a patient's PHI with people with no need to know
Do keep voices low when discussing patient issues in joint treatment areas	Don't share your computer passwords and log-on information
Do provide only the minimal needed information on request	Don't leave a computer unattended without logging off
Do position workstations so that the screens are not visible to prying eyes	Don't discuss a patient's PHI in public settings where you can be overheard
Do keep patient information on whiteboards to a minimum	Don't communicate PHI by methods that the patient has not approved
Do place fax machines used to receive PHI in secure locations	Don't leave a patient's paper records open and available for prying eyes

experience. One should over time aim to achieve at least a basic understanding of various cultures' beliefs. Realistically however, the growing diversity of the U.S. population makes it impossible to master all the nuances characterizing the many cultures now represented. Instead, one needs to develop culturally competent communication skills.

Culturally competent communication is founded on the same basic strategies underlying empathetic and caring patient interaction, that is, active listening, attending to individual needs, eliciting patient concerns, and expressing genuine concern. Ideally, the RT should apply these strategies during the initial assessment stage of the encounter to briefly explore the patient's key cultural beliefs, especially those related to gender and family roles, responses to authority, personal space, religious values, and concepts of health and disease. For example, in some cultures it is normal to always defer to the authority of a doctor or health care professional when deciding what is best so that efforts to involve the patient in decision making may be difficult. Likewise, patients who believe that fate determines disease outcomes may be reluctant to participate in their own care. Reflecting on what the patient shares in a nonjudgmental way can help further the development of rapport and enhance one's ability to adapt to cultural differences.

Complementing the use of general communication skills are three additional abilities that can enhance one's cultural competence: self-awareness, situational awareness, and adaptability. Self-awareness involves knowledge of one's own cultural beliefs as well as any potential stereotypes one might hold about particular groups. By being self-aware, you can recognize in advance possible cultural prejudices or emotions you might have toward certain patients and thus negate their impact on the care you provide. Situational awareness is the ability to recognize misunderstandings associated with patient-provider cultural differences as they occur during a patient encounter. For example, a woman who is constantly looking toward her husband for approval during a clinical interaction may be signaling a cultural tendency to defer to the man for all major decision making. Once such cues are recognized, the culturally competent clinician should be able to adapt to the specific situation by individualizing the communication approach in a manner consistent with the patient's (and family's) values and beliefs. In this case, one might consider reorienting the encounter by making the husband a major partner into the conversation.

> **SIMPLY STATED**
>
> During the assessment component of the clinical encounter, you should explore your patient's key cultural beliefs and use this knowledge to adapt your communication to the patient's and family's values and beliefs.

Patient Involvement

Patient-centered care is a two-way street. As such, tailoring care to the individual is not enough. To be successful, patient-centered care must involve the patient and family as partners in setting goals, making decisions, participating in the treatment regimen, providing appropriate self-care, and helping assure safety. To meet these expectations, patients—especially those with chronic conditions—must understand the basics about their disease process and how to effectively manage it. This level of involvement can only occur when the clinician incorporates needed educational activities into each clinical encounter.

Assessing Learning Needs and Providing Patient Education

Patient and caregiver education aims to foster healthy behaviors and increase patients' involvement in their health care and safety, with the end goal being satisfaction of both patient and provider with the outcomes. Although full achievement of this goal requires a comprehensive, interdisciplinary approach, RTs can play a key role in improving outcomes by providing appropriate patient education.

The first step in patient education is to assess the patient's learning needs. In most hospitals, the initial assessment of learning needs is conducted by nursing staff, occurs after the patient is admitted to a care unit, and is documented in the patient's chart. For this reason, during your chart review, you should access and evaluate this record for any important information helpful in planning the respiratory care of your patient.

> **SIMPLY STATED**
>
> Effective respiratory care requires a knowledgeable patient willing and able to participate in treatment, for which patient education is a prerequisite. The first step in patient education is to assess the patient's learning needs.

More often than not, you will need to briefly conduct your own assessment, with a focus on learning needs specific to the patient's disorder and the planned therapy. In general, a learning needs assessment progresses through the following key steps:

1. Identifying and accommodating barriers to patient learning
2. Assessing the patient's preferred learning method
3. Evaluating the patient's readiness to learn
4. Determining the patient's specific learning needs

Table 1-3 identifies several of the barriers to learning commonly encountered by RTs in the clinical setting as well as various ways to accommodate them.

To assess a patient's preferred way of learning, first observe the environment for clues such as the presence of reading materials, use of television, or (for children) use of toys and games. You also should ask the patient about any recent learning efforts. Sometimes, preferred methods of learning can be determined from questions about the patient's work or hobbies.

Evaluating the patient's readiness to learn is the next step in assessing learning needs. Patients' spontaneous questions about their condition, its management, or their

TABLE 1-3

Barriers to Learning and Their Accommodation

Barrier to Learning	Accommodation
Age (young child)	Keep teaching/learning episodes short
	Use fun-and-games approach
	Enlist family assistance
Reduced level of consciousness	Postpone until patient becomes alert
	Apply methods that don't require cooperation
Presence of pain	Recommend analgesia
	Postpone until pain management is effective
Presence of anxiety	Take time to calm the patient and explain your actions
	Postpone until anxiety management is effective
	Enlist family assistance
	Recommend anxiolytic therapy
Physical limitations	Ascertain specific limitations
	Apply methods that circumvent limitation
	Enlist family assistance
Educational level (low)	Emphasize oral (vs. written) instruction
	Adjust language level as appropriate
	Provide written materials at fifth- to eighth-grade level
Potential language barrier	Enlist family assistance
	Secure translator
Cultural or religious factors	Ascertain key factors affecting care
	Modify to accommodate
	Enlist family assistance
Vision difficulty	Have patient wear glasses
	Emphasize sound and touch
	Enlist family assistance
Hearing difficulty	Speak slowly and clearly while facing the patient
	Have patient use hearing aid
	Emphasize visualization and touch
	Enlist family assistance

From Scanlan CL, Heuer AJ, Sinopoli L: *Certified respiratory therapist exam review guide*, Sudbury, MA: Jones & Bartlett Learning; 2009. (www.jblearning.com). Reprinted with permission.

respiratory care indicate a desire to learn, as do expressions of discomfort with their current abilities or situation.

After you have addressed any barriers to learning and confirmed the patient's desire to progress, you should determine what the patient knows about the care you will provide. To do so, you'll need to ask pertinent questions, using terms and language appropriate to the patient's level of understanding. Questions in this phase of the assessment need to address the following patient capabilities:

• Understanding of the current condition or disease process
• Knowledge of prescribed medications
• Familiarity with the procedures you will implement
• Familiarity with the equipment you plan to use

Box 1-1	**Example Questions Assessing a Patient's Knowledge about a Medication**

Which medicine are you currently taking? How often?
Do you know why you are taking this medicine?
Who is responsible for administering the medicine?
Please show me how you take the medicine.
How many times a week do you miss taking the medicine?
What problems have you had taking the medicine (cost, time, lack of need)?
What concerns do you have about your medicine?

Box 1-1 provides example questions focusing on a patient's knowledge about a prescribed medication.

If any of the patient's answers indicates a shortcoming in knowledge, you have identified a specific learning need. In addition to assessing needs, you also should focus on determining "wants," that is, anything the patient wishes to learn more about. Together, these needs and wants can help establish education goals acceptable to both the patient and family.

After conducting any learning activity, you should evaluate the results. To evaluate a desired change in knowledge, have the patients repeat in their own words the information you are trying to get them to understand (the **teach-back method**). On the other hand, to confirm that your patients have learned how to perform a particular skill, have them provide you with a **return demonstration**, that is, going through the motions of the procedure after you have shown it to them.

Sharing Goal-Setting and Decision-Making Responsibilities

Effective patient education is a prerequisite to shared responsibility for goal setting and decision making. All key decisions regarding patient management and the degree to which a patient partners in that process are made by the attending physician. In this regard, good communication between the RT and the patient's physician is essential. Ideally, a knowledgeable physician will give you the latitude needed not only to assess learning needs but also to help the patient set tangible goals related to the care you provide. Such goals may be as simple as achieving a targeted inspiratory capacity after abdominal surgery or as complex as reaching agreement with the patient on an action plan for routine self-care of asthma and proper management of its exacerbations.

Written **action plans** are a particularly useful tool for involving patients in goal-setting and self-care activities. Action plan goals should be *SMART*, that is, *s*pecific, *mea*surable, *a*ction oriented, *r*ealistic, and *t*ime limited. The action plan itself should address the following elements:

• Exactly what is the goal?
• How will the goal be achieved (e.g., how, how much, how often)?
• What barriers might prevent achieving the goal?

Box 1-2	Example Action Plan Developed by a Patient with Asthma

ACTION PLAN

1. **Goals** (something you *want* to do): cut school absences in half

   How: make sure I take my controller medicine as prescribed; avoid my triggers (pet hair and tobacco smoke); monitor my symptoms (cough, wheeze, chest tightness, shortness of breath); take my reliever if symptoms develop/worsen

   Where: administer meds at home (controller) and at home/school if reliever is needed

   What: controller: Pulmicort Flexhaler (b.i.d.); reliever: Proventil canister

   When: Pulmicort: AM/PM; Proventil puffs as needed; monitor symptoms

   Frequency: medications as prescribed; symptom monitoring daily using diary

2. **Barriers**: many friends smoke or have house pets; hate diary keeping

3. **Plans to overcome barriers**: avoid spending time indoors with smokers or pets; use Twitter to keep my diary entries

4. **Conviction**: 7/10 (being pushed by parents!); **confidence**: 9 (I'm stubborn)

5. **Follow-up**: track absences for the coming semester (goal is less than 5)

Box 1-3	Speak Up: Help Prevent Errors in Your Care

Everyone has a role in making health care safe. The joint Commission's Speak Up™ program gives simple advice on how you can help make health care a good experience. Research shows that patients who take part in decisions about their own health care are more likely to get better faster. To help prevent health care mistakes, patients are urged to "Speak Up."

S | Speak up if you have questions or concerns. If you still don't understand, ask again. It's your body and you have a right to know.

P | Pay attention to the care you get. Always make sure you're getting the right treatments and medicines by the right health care professionals. Don't assume anything.

E | Educate yourself about your illness. Learn about the medical tests you get, and your treatment plan.

A | Ask a trusted family member or friend to be your advocate (advisor or supporter).

K | Know what medicines you take and why you take them. medicine errors are the most common health care mistakes.

U | Use a hospital, clinic, surgery center, or other type of health care organization that has been carefully checked out. For example, The Joint Commission visits hospitals to see if they are meeting The Joint Commission's quality standards.

P | Participate in all decisions about your treatment. You are the center of the health care team.

The Joint Commission, Oakbrook Terrace, III., www.jointcommission.org/speakup.aspx

---

- How can the anticipated barriers be overcome?
- By what mechanism will follow-up occur?
- How much confidence does the patient have in achieving the goal?

Box 1-2 provides an example of a simple action plan for an adolescent with moderate asthma who has a recent history of exacerbations causing frequent absences from school.

Encouraging Patient and Family Participation in Care and Safety

Joint goal setting provides the basis for greater patient and family involvement in treatment regimens and, for those with chronic conditions, ongoing self-care. Given that the effectiveness of most respiratory care treatments requires patient cooperation and follow-through, you need to constantly reiterate how better participation can result in better outcomes. A case in point is the daily tracking of symptoms that the patient with asthma included in her action plan (see Box 1-2). A good example for an acute care patient with cystic fibrosis would be monitoring sputum production after self-administered positive airway pressure therapy. Regarding involving the family, there is no better illustration than preparing a patient requiring long-term mechanical ventilation for discharge to home.

Involvement of the patient and family in care delivery also has been shown to enhance safety and reduce medical

errors. The joint Commission's "Speak Up" initiative provides excellent guidance in this regard. Box 1-3 provides a summary of the key guidance this initiative provides to patients, using the "Speak Up" acronym. Although most hospitals orient patients upon admission to their role in helping assure safety, respiratory therapists should use the clinical encounter to reinforce this important role.

To further promote infection control, you should instruct all patients, family members, and visitors with signs or symptoms of a respiratory infection to follow the Centers for Disease Control and Prevention (CDC) guidance on respiratory hygiene and cough etiquette:

- Covering the nose and mouth when coughing or sneezing
- Using tissues to contain respiratory secretions
- Disposing of tissues in the nearest hands-free waste receptacle after use

---

SIMPLY STATED

Involvement of the patient and family in care delivery enhances safety and reduces medical errors. Respiratory therapists should orient patients and their families to their role in helping assure safety using strategies like The Joint Commission *Speak Up* initiative and sharing the CDC guidance on respiratory hygiene and cough etiquette.

Box 1-4	CDC Standard Precautions

HAND HYGIENE

Always perform hand hygiene in the following situations:
- Before touching a patient, even if gloves will be worn
- After contact with a patient and before leaving the patient care area
- After contact with blood, body fluids, excretions, or wound dressings
- Before performing an aseptic task (e.g., accessing a vascular port)
- Whenever hands move from a contaminated body area to a clean area
- After glove removal

GLOVES

Wear gloves when there is potential contact with blood, body fluids, mucous membranes, nonintact skin, or contaminated equipment
- Wear gloves that fit appropriately (select gloves according to hand size)
- Do not wear the same pair of gloves for the care of more than one patient
- Do not wash gloves for the purpose of reuse
- Perform hand hygiene before and immediately after removing gloves

GOWNS

Wear a gown to protect skin and clothing during procedures or activities in which contact with blood or body fluids is anticipated.
- Do not wear the same gown for the care of more than one patient
- Remove gown and perform hand hygiene before leaving the patient's environment (e.g., examination room)

FACEMASKS, EYE PROTECTION, RESPIRATORS

Use a facemask during patient care activities likely to generate splashes or sprays of blood, body fluids, or secretions—especially during airway suctioning (using a standard catheter), endotracheal intubation, catheter insertion, and encounters with any patient under droplet precautions.

    Personal eyeglasses and contact lenses do not provide adequate eye protection
    Use goggles with facemasks, or face shield alone, to protect the mouth, nose, and eyes
    Wear an N95 or higher respirator when there is potential exposure to infectious agents transmitted by the airborne route (e.g., tuberculosis)

SOILED PATIENT CARE EQUIPMENT

Handle in a manner to prevent contact with skin or mucous membranes and to prevent contamination of clothing or the environment.
- Wear gloves if equipment is visibly contaminated
- Perform hand hygiene after handling

NEEDLES AND OTHER SHARPS
- Do not recap, bend, break, or hand-manipulate used needles
- If recapping is required, use a one-handed scoop technique only
- Use safety features when available
- Place used sharps in puncture-resistant container

PATIENT RESUSCITATION
- Use mouthpiece with one-way valve, resuscitation bag, other ventilation devices to prevent contact with mouth and oral secretions (Centers for Disease Control and Prevention. http://cdc.gov.)

- Performing hand hygiene after contacting secretions or contaminated objects

Safety demands that clinicians themselves also implement infection control procedures before, during, and after all patient encounters. At a minimum, this involves application of **standard precautions**, as outlined in Box 1-4. Good hand hygiene is the single most important element in preventing spread of infection. Alcohol-based rubs are the preferred method, except when either one's hands become visibly soiled with dirt, blood, or body fluids, or when caring for patients with infectious diarrhea (e.g., *Clostridium difficile*, norovirus). In these cases, one should proceed with a vigorous soap and water handwashing for at least 15 seconds.

Provider Collaboration

During the course of a hospital stay, a patient may interact with dozens of health care providers. Quality patient-centered care requires that these providers work together as a team. When health care professionals fail to collaborate effectively, patient safety is put at risk. Ineffective provider collaboration also can result in increased length of stay, wasted resources, and less than optimal patient outcomes.

Collaboration occurs when health care providers assume complementary roles and cooperatively work together, sharing responsibility for patient care. Unfortunately, many RTs function more as "lone rangers" than as integral players on the health care team. To maximize their impact on patient outcomes, RTs must better integrate their services with those of other providers. To do so requires enhanced interprofessional communication, interdisciplinary coordination, and better sharing of responsibilities.

Enhancing Interprofessional Communication

The Joint Commission defines effective communication as being timely, accurate, complete, unambiguous, and understood by the recipient. Because good interprofessional communication is essential to quality care, all RTs must exhibit these skills. Such skills are particularly important when receiving orders, coordinating the patient's care, reporting the patient's clinical status, and helping plan for patient discharge.

Often, a clinical encounter begins with receipt of an order from an authorized health care provider, most often a physician, physician's assistant, or nurse practitioner. You cannot accept orders transmitted to you by unauthorized third parties, such as registered nurses. If an order is transmitted to you by a third party, you must verify the order in the patient's chart before proceeding. If the order is transmitted orally and you are authorized to take it, you must avoid communication errors. The following actions should be taken to avoid such errors:

- Record the complete order in the chart as it is being transmitted.
- Read the order back to the originator exactly as written and clarify as needed.
- Have the originator confirm the accuracy of the order as read back.
- Time and date the order with the name and credentials of the originator, specify "read back and confirmed," and provide your signature and credentials.

Regardless of their source or route of transmission, all respiratory care orders must be verified as accurate and complete. Should any element of an order be missing or unclear, you must contact the prescriber for clarification before implementing the request. The same procedure applies if the order falls outside one's institutional standards. For example, if the order specifies an abnormally high drug dosage or includes a ventilator setting not normally applied in similar cases, you should contact the prescriber and request an explanation before proceeding. More detail on standards for order writing and order taking is provided in Chapter 21.

After most patient encounters, you will need to communicate your findings to other members of the health care team. Written documentation in the patient's chart may suffice if the patient is stable after routine treatment. However, whenever a patient's condition changes or a procedure is poorly tolerated, in addition to providing written documentation, you *must* communicate your findings orally to the patient's nurse and physician. In this case, your chart documentation should include not only your findings but also who was notified about the change in the patient's condition.

For example, on entering the room of Mr. Jones to provide treatment for his asthma, you note that he appears much more short of breath than usual. The treatment you give him does not appear to help. It is imperative that you document and communicate your findings. Oral discussion with the patient's nurse is a good place to start. Notifying the patient's physician of the change in Mr. Jones' condition may also be appropriate in such cases. Next, you must document the patient's condition in his chart and note whom you communicated with about the patient and what was said. If there is evidence of deteriorating vital signs, you should call the Medical Emergency or Rapid Response Team and support the patient until the team arrives.

> **SIMPLY STATED**
>
> Whenever you observe a change in a patient's condition, note your observations in the chart, orally report your findings to the patient's nurse, and document in writing whom you notified about the situation.

Coordinating Patient Care

RTs also need to help coordinate their patients' care. To do so, you need to communicate with the patient's nurse or attending physician to schedule therapy at times least likely to conflict with other essential patient activity and most likely to coincide with any relevant drug regimen. For example, you would avoid performing postural drainage on a postoperative patient immediately after a meal but would instead schedule this encounter after administration of pain medication. Likewise, you would communicate with nursing to ensure that before implementing a ventilator weaning trial, all sedatives have been held back from the patient.

Another key aspect related to good communication and coordinating patient care is the patient "hand-off." Common patient hand-offs occur when delivering a patient to or receiving a patient from a care unit or diagnostic facility, when providing patient reports at shift change, or when having a colleague take over in an emergency situation. Ideally, communication during such hand-offs should be short but precise, providing the essential information needed by the recipient. One popular method for standardizing these brief episodes is the **SBAR** format. When using this format, communication about your patient should address the following four essential elements: *s*ituation, *b*ackground, *a*ssessment, *r*ecommendation. The same format also can be used when making recommendations to the patient's physician for a change in therapy or when documenting a patient encounter in the medical record. Chapter 21 provides more detail on the appropriate use of this communication tool, including an example.

Patient care should not end abruptly at hospital discharge. Ideally, an interdisciplinary post-hospitalization care plan should be developed based on each patient's individual needs and consistent with current guidelines for managing the patient's condition. Such plans normally are ordered by the patient's primary care provider and coordinated by a nurse practitioner or case manager. As identified by the American Association for Respiratory Care (AARC), patient discharge plans should include the following:

- A time frame for implementation
- Clearly defined responsibilities of team members for daily care
- Mechanisms for communication among members of the health care team
- Arrangements for patient integration back into the community
- Plans for medication administration
- Strategies for patient self-care as appropriate
- Mechanisms for securing and training caregivers
- Plans for monitoring and responding to changes in the patient's condition
- Alternative emergency and contingency plans
- Plans for use, maintenance, and troubleshooting of equipment
- Methods for ongoing assessment of outcomes
- Specification of follow-up mechanisms

At least for patients with respiratory-related diagnoses, RTs should participate in discharge planning. For example, to help prevent exacerbations and readmission of a patient with asthma, you should help in coordinating plans for aerosol drug therapy (based on assessment of learning needs), developing strategies for patient self-care, participating as appropriate in caregiver training, establishing action plans for responding to changes in the patient's condition, planning for equipment needs, and specifying approaches for assessing patient progress. More detail on the role of the RT in assessing the patient and planning for care at home is provided in Chapter 20.

Sharing Responsibility

Truly integrated care requires that all the clinicians involved in a patient's management share a common set of goals and assume joint responsibility for their achievement. Ideally, each team member should be tasked with addressing a particular patient problem. For example, a RT working in the intensive care unit may be given primary responsibility for implementing a ventilator weaning protocol. However, the team as a whole must coordinate these individual efforts and evaluate their overall success.

Team membership depends on each patient's unique set of problems. As experts on respiratory care, RTs should function as vital members of teams supporting management of patients with both chronic and acute cardiopulmonary disorders. In terms of sharing responsibility for the management of chronic disorders such as chronic obstructive pulmonary disease (COPD), respiratory therapists can and should assume responsibility for providing patient education about the nature of the disease process, training patients in applicable self-care techniques (such as aerosol drug administration), and helping patients develop good action plans to deal with exacerbations. In regard to shared responsibility for management of patients with acute care needs, working as a team member to prevent ventilator-associated pneumonia and weaning a patient from ventilatory support are good examples.

The best-documented approach to sharing responsibility for patients in acute care settings is to combine interdisciplinary intensive care unit rounds with a daily goals form (Fig. 1-4). The form facilitates communication during rounds by requiring team members, including RTs, to state their goals, the tasks needed to achieve them, and how they will communicate with the patient, family, and other caregivers. All members of the team then review the goals during each shift and modify or update them as needed. For example, a RT might set a goal for a newly intubated patient with acute respiratory distress syndrome (ARDS) of reducing the patient's plateau pressure below 30 cm H_2O while maintaining adequate ventilation. Tasks involved might include making incremental adjustments in the tidal volume and rate according to the ARDSNet protocol while monitoring changes in arterial pH. As the patient's status improves, the therapist would recommend new goals, such as reducing the F_1O_2 or positive end-expiratory pressure levels, with the ultimate aim being extubation and removal of ventilatory support. With the therapist no longer a solo player but instead a key contributor to the management team, the full potential of the patient clinical encounter can be realized.

DAILY GOALS			
Room Number:	Date:		
Attending initials:	Initial as Goals Are Reviewed		
Goals+	0700-1500	1500-2300	2300-0700
What needs to be done to discharge the patient from the ICU?			
What is this patient's greatest safety risk? How can we reduce that risk?			
Pain management/sedation			
Cardiac/volume status			
Pulmonary/ventilator (PP, VAP bundle)			
Mobilization			
Infectious disease, cultures, drug levels			
GI/nutrition			
Medication changes (can any be discontinued?)			
Tests/procedures			
Review scheduled labs; morning labs and CXR			
Consultations			
Communication with primary service			
Family communication			
Can catheters/tubes be removed?			
Is this patient receiving DVT/PUD prophylaxis?			
+PP, plateau pressure; HOB, head of bed; GI, gastrointestinal; labs, laboratory tests; CXR, Chest radiograph; DVT, deep venous thrombosis; PUD, peptic ulcer disease			

FIGURE 1-4 Daily goals form. (Adapted from Pronovost P, Berenholtz S, Dorman T, et al: Improving communication in the ICU using daily goals. *J Crit Care* 2003; **18**(2):71–75.)

KEY POINTS

▶ Patient-centered care involves three key elements: individualized care, patient involvement and provider collaboration.

▶ Communication during a clinical encounter is affected by the attitudes and values of the clinician and patient, one's choice of words, nonverbal expressions, and environmental factors.

▶ A patient encounter generally begins with a chart review and then progresses through four stages: introductory, initial assessment, treatment and monitoring, and follow-up; communication strategies vary according to the purpose of each stage.

▶ Whenever possible, respiratory care plans should reflect each patient's preferences, as determined during initial assessment and treatment.

▶ Use the social space (4 to 12 feet) during the introductory stage of the clinical encounter to establish rapport, the personal space (18 inches to 4 feet) for the interview, and the intimate space (0 to 18 inches) to conduct the physical examination and apply and monitor therapy; enter the intimate space only after gaining patient permission.

▶ Discuss your patient's health status only with other members of the health care team who need to know such information and only in locations where others cannot overhear; always refer questions about your patient's diagnosis to the attending physician.

▶ The culturally competent clinician is a good communicator who is aware of his or her own cultural beliefs and can recognize and adapt to differences in values and beliefs during the clinical encounter.

KEY POINTS—cont'd

▶ Patients and their families should be engaged as partners in setting health care goals, making decisions, participating in the treatment regimen, providing appropriate self-care, and helping assure safety.

▶ To assess a patient's learning needs, (1) identify and accommodate any barriers to learning, (2) assess the patient's preferred learning method, (3) evaluate the patient's readiness to learn, and (4) determine the patient's specific learning needs.

▶ Involve patients in goal-setting and self-care activities using a written action plan that specifies a measurable goal, the actions needed to achieve the goal (including barriers to overcome), and an appropriate follow-up mechanism.

▶ During clinical encounters, orient patients and their families to their role in helping assure safety using strategies like The Joint Commission **Speak Up initiative** and sharing the CDC guidance on respiratory hygiene and cough etiquette.

▶ Good hand hygiene is the single most important element in preventing spread of infection in the hospital.

▶ If any element of a respiratory care order is missing, is unclear, or falls outside institutional standards, you must contact the prescriber for clarification before implementing the request.

▶ To coordinate your patient's care with that provided by others, communicate with the patient's nurse or attending physician to schedule therapy at times least likely to conflict with other essential activity and most likely to coincide with any relevant drug regimen.

KEY POINTS—cont'd

▶ Whenever you observe a change in a patient's condition or judge that a procedure was poorly tolerated, you must communicate your findings orally to the patient's nurse and physician and document in writing whom you notified about the situation; if the change involves deteriorating vital signs, call for the Medical Emergency or Rapid Response Team and support the patient until the team arrives.

▶ To effectively communicate relevant information about your patient during hand-offs to others, use the SBAR format (situation, background, assessment, recommendation).

▶ To enhance outcomes in critical care settings, respiratory therapists should participate in interdisciplinary rounds and be responsible for communicating the essential respiratory-related daily goals and tasks needed to achieve them as well as coordinating these efforts with other members of the team.

ASSESSMENT QUESTIONS

See Appendix for answers.

1. Which of the following are key elements in the provision of patient-centered care?
   1. Patient involvement
   2. Individualized care
   3. Legal representation
   4. Provider collaboration
      a. 1 and 2
      b. 1, 2, and 4
      c. 3 and 4
      d. 1, 2, 3, and 4

2. After a postoperative patient you are interviewing grimaces while holding her abdomen, you note some confusion about her responses. Which of the following factors likely is affecting communication?
   a. Self-concept
   b. Listening habits
   c. Pain and anxiety
   d. Hearing impairment

3. Active listening is most essential during what stage of the clinical encounter?
   a. Introductory stage
   b. Initial assessment stage
   c. Treatment and monitoring stage
   d. Follow-up stage

4. After several attempts to instruct a patient with COPD on the proper use of a metered-dose inhaler, the patient complains of the inability to master the correct technique. Applying patient-centered principles, you should:
   a. Request permission from the patient's doctor to find a more acceptable delivery system
   b. Cease trying to train the patient and recommend discontinuing the therapy
   c. Push the patient to keep practicing until a return demonstration indicates competency
   d. Chart the treatment as not given and return for another try on second rounds

5. In which of the following spaces is patient rapport best established?
   a. Social
   b. Personal
   c. Intimate
   d. Territorial

6. Which of the following violates HIPAA-related privacy and security rules?
   a. Providing the minimal needed patient information on request
   b. Keeping patient information on a whiteboard in the staff room
   c. Discussing a patient's health status with the nurse at the bedside
   d. Leaving a computer unattended without logging off

7. Which of the following cultural beliefs should be explored with your patients during the initial assessment stage of the clinical encounter?
   1. Concepts of health and disease
   2. Responses to authority
   3. Gender and family roles
   4. Religious values
      a. 1 and 2
      b. 3 and 4
      c. 1, 2, and 3
      d. 1, 2, 3, and 4

8. For most respiratory care to succeed, patients need to:
   a. Have at least a high-school education
   b. Actively participate in the treatment regimen
   c. Demonstrate good hand-eye coordination
   d. Be at least somewhat fluent in English

9. During an initial patient encounter, you note that her acute anxiety appears to be affecting your ability to help her learn more about her disease process. To overcome this problem, you would consider all of the following, *except*:
   a. Recommending that the doctor prescribe an analgesic
   b. Enlisting family assistance to calm the patient down
   c. Recommending that the doctor prescribe an anxiolytic
   d. Postponing further efforts until anxiety management is effective

10. A good patient action plan should include which of the following elements?
    1. Actions needed to achieve the goal
    2. Barriers to goal achievement
    3. A specific, measurable goal
    4. A follow-up mechanism
       a. 3 and 4
       b. 1 and 2
       c. 1, 2, and 3
       d. 1, 2, 3, and 4

11. While supervising a respiratory therapy student, you observe that an anxious patient asks her if the aerosol bronchodilator she is about to deliver has any bad effects. The student replies "none to worry about." After the treatment session is over, you should explain to the student that:
    a. Only the patient's doctor should be discussing medication effects with the patient
    b. Her reply was consistent with what the patient needs to know
    c. Patients should be encouraged to ask questions about their medications
    d. Her reply was good—no need to further worry an anxious patient

12. For a clinical encounter with a patient on airborne precautions, you should:
    a. Wear goggles or an eye shield
    b. Wear a properly fitting N95 respirator
    c. Perform a surgical hand scrub
    d. Don sterile gloves

13. A patient responds poorly to a treatment you have given. After assuring that the patient is stable, you should:
    a. Carefully note the patient's response to treatment in the patient's chart
    b. Speak with the patient's nurse, chart the response and whom you notified
    c. Orally notify the patient's nurse of his poor response to treatment
    d. Request that the patient's physician discontinue the therapy

14. In setting up a postural drainage treatment schedule for a postoperative patient, which of the following information would you try to obtain from the patient's nurse?
    1. Patient's medication schedule
    2. Patient's ideal body weight
    3. Patient's meal schedule
        a. 1 only
        b. 1, 2, and 3
        c. 1 and 3
        d. 2 and 3

15. All of the following are appropriate roles for a respiratory therapist serving on a team managing a patient with COPD, *except*:
    a. Helping the patient develop good action plans
    b. Training the patient in self-care techniques
    c. Recommending changes in diet and nutrition
    d. Providing patient education about the disease

Bibliography

Agency for Healthcare Research and Quality. *National healthcare quality report*. Rockville, MD: U.S. Department of Health and Human Services; 2005.

American Association for Respiratory Care. Clinical practice guideline. Discharge planning for the respiratory care patient. *Respir Care* 1995;**40**(12):1308-12.

Betancourt JR. Cultural competence and medical education: many names, many perspectives, one goal. *Acad Med* 2006;**81**(6):499-501.

Bonello RS, Fletcher CE, Becker WK, et al. An intensive care unit quality improvement collaborative in nine Department of Veterans Affairs hospitals: reducing ventilator-associated pneumonia and catheter-related bloodstream infection rates. *Jt Comm J Qual Patient Saf* 2008;**34**(11):639-45.

Engebretson J, Mahoney J, Carlson ED. Cultural competence in the era of evidence-based practice. *J Prof Nurs* 2008;**24**(3):172-8.

Fortin AH, Smith RC, Dwamena FC, Frankel RM. *Patient-centered interviewing: an evidence-based method*. 3rd ed. New York: McGraw-Hill; 2012.

Giger JN, Davidhizar RE. *Transcultural nursing: assessment and iIntervention*. St. Louis: Mosby; 2008.

Golin CE, Thorpe C, DiMatteo MR. Accessing the patient's world patient-physician communication about psychosocial issues. In: Earp JL, French EA, Gilkey MB, editors. *Patient advocacy for health care quality: strategies for achieving patient*. Sudbury, MA: Jones & Bartlett; 2008.

The Joint Commission. *Advancing effective communication, cultural competence, and patient- and family-centered care: a roadmap for hospitals*. Oakbrook Terrace, IL: The Joint Commission; 2010.

Kacmarek RM, Stoller JK, Heuer AJ. *Egan's Fundamentals of Respiratory Care*. 10th ed. St. Louis: Mosby-Elsevier; 2013.

Lein C, Wills CE. Using patient-centered interviewing skills to manage complex patient encounters in primary care. *J Am Acad Nurse Pract* 2007;**19**(5):215-20.

Makoul G. Essential elements of communication in medical encounters: the Kalamazoo consensus statement. *Acad Med* 2001;**76**(4):390-3.

National Research Council. *Envisioning the national health care quality report*. Washington, DC: The National Academies Press; 2001.

Perry AG. *Fundamentals of nursing*. 7th ed. St Louis: Mosby; 2009.

Perry AG, Potter PA, Elkin MK. *Nursing interventions and clinical skills*. 5th ed. St Louis: Mosby; 2012.

Pierson DJ, Wilkins RL. Clinical skills in respiratory care. In: Pierson DJ, Kacmarek RM, editors. *Foundations of respiratory care*. New York: Churchill Livingstone; 1992.

Pronovost P, Berenholtz S, Dorman T, et al. Improving communication in the ICU using daily goals. *J Crit Care* 2003;**18**(2):71-5.

Robinson JH, Callister LC, Berry JA, et al. Patient-centered care and adherence: definitions and applications to improve outcomes. *J Am Acad Nurse Pract* 2008;**20**(12):600-7.

Scanlan CL, Heuer AJ, Sinopoli L. *Certified respiratory therapist exam review guide*. Sudbury, MA: Jones & Bartlett; 2009.

Siegel JD, Rhinehart E, Jackson M, Chiarello L, et al. *Guideline for isolation precautions: preventing transmission of infectious agents in healthcare settings*. Atlanta: Centers for Disease Control and Prevention; 2007.

Teal CR, Street RL. Critical elements of culturally competent communication in the medical encounter: a review and model. *Soc Sci Med* 2009;**68**(3):533-43.

Chapter 2

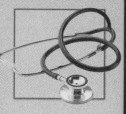

The Medical History and the Interview

ALBERT J. HEUER*

CHAPTER OUTLINE

LEARNING OBJECTIVES

After reading this chapter, you will be able to:
1. Recognize the importance of properly obtaining and recording a patient history.
2. Describe the techniques for structuring the interview.
3. Summarize the techniques used to facilitate conversational interviewing.
4. Identify alternative sources available for the patient history.
5. Define the difference between objective and subjective data and the difference between signs and symptoms.
6. Describe the components of a complete health history and the type of information found in each section of the history.
7. Describe the value in reviewing the following parts of a patient's chart: (1) admission notes, (2) physician orders, (3) progress notes.
8. Summarize what is indicated by a DNR order and label on the patient's chart.

KEY TERMS

do not attempt to resuscitate
    (DNAR)/do not resuscitate
    (DNR)
electronic medical record
    (EMR)

objective data
pack-years
pertinent negatives
pertinent positives
signs

subjective data
symptoms

---

*Dr. Robert Wilkins, PhD, RRT, contributed much of the content for this chapter as the coeditor of the prior edition of this text.

The history is the foundation of comprehensive assessment. It is a written picture of the patient's perception of his or her past and present health status and how health problems have affected both personal and family lifestyle. Properly recorded, it generally provides an organized, unbiased, detailed, and chronologic description of the development of symptoms that caused the patient to seek health care. The history guides the rest of the assessment process: physical examination, x-ray and laboratory studies, and special diagnostic procedures. When skillfully obtained, the history often contributes in a significant way to an accurate diagnosis. It is believed by many clinicians that an accurate diagnosis can often be made after the history has been obtained and before the physical examination begins.

Traditionally, the task of obtaining a patient's complete history has belonged to the physician, and only sections of the history were taken by other members of the health care team. Today, however, complete health histories are taken by nurses and physician assistants. Physical therapists, social workers, dietitians, and respiratory therapists (RTs) obtain medical histories from patients with an emphasis on information pertaining to their specialty.

Regardless of whether a student or clinician is expected to obtain and write a comprehensive history, each must be able to locate and interpret historical information recorded in the patient's medical record. The information is used with other assessment data and provides the foundation for interprofessional communication to enable many medical disciplines to collaboratively develop or alter a plan of care. In addition, identifying the patient's symptoms and changes in those symptoms permits the patient care team to assess the effect of therapeutic interventions and overall progress.

This chapter highlights interviewing principles and describes the types of questions used in history taking and the content of the comprehensive health history, emphasizing specific information needed for assessment of the patient with cardiopulmonary complaints. Chapter 3 discusses the most common cardiopulmonary symptoms.

> **SIMPLY STATED**
>
> The history is the foundation of comprehensive assessment—a written picture of the patient's perception of his or her health status, current problem, and effectiveness of treatment. It comprises subjective data—information that the patient reports, feels, or experiences that cannot be perceived by an observer.

Patient Interview

Principles of Communication

Communication is a process of imparting a meaningful message. The principles and practices of effective communication, which are outlined in Chapter 1, help form the basis for a properly conducted patient interview. Multiple personal and environmental factors affect the way both patients and health care professionals communicate during an interview. As a result, attention to the effects each of these components may have on communication makes the difference between an effective and an ineffective interview.

Structuring the Interview

The ideal interview, whether a 5-minute assessment of therapy or a 50-minute history, is one in which the patient feels secure and free to talk about important personal things. Interviewing is an art that takes time and experience to develop. It is a skill as useful in daily patient care as it is to the person obtaining a comprehensive history. Your ability to project a sense of undivided interest in the patient is the key to a successful interview and patient rapport. As such, it is generally best to review records or new information and prepare equipment and charting materials before entering the room. When practical, the RT or other clinician should know all available details of the patient case before the interview is started.

1. Your introduction establishes your professional role, asks permission to be involved in the patient's care, and conveys your interest in the patient.
   - Dress and groom professionally.
   - Enter with a smile and an unhurried manner.
   - Make immediate eye contact, and if the patient is well enough, introduce yourself with a firm handshake or other appropriate greeting.
   - State your role and the purpose of your visit, and define the patient's involvement in the interaction.
   - Call the patient by name. A person's name is one of the most important things in the world to that person; use it to identify the patient and establish the fact that you are concerned with the patient as an individual. Address adult patients by title—Mr., Mrs., Miss, or Ms.—and their last name. Occasionally, patients will ask to be called by their first name or nickname, but that is the patient's choice and not an assumption to be made by the health care professional. Keep in mind that by using the more formal terms of address, you alert the patient to the importance of the interaction.

2. Professional conduct shows your respect for the patient's beliefs, attitudes, and rights and enhances patient rapport.
   - Be sure the patient is appropriately covered.
   - Position yourself so that eye contact is comfortable for the patient. Ideally, patients should be sitting up with their eye level with or slightly above yours, which suggests that their opinion is important, too. Avoid positions that require the patient to look directly into the light.
   - Avoid standing at the foot of the bed or with your hand on the door while you talk with the patient. This may send the nonverbal message that you do not have time for the patient.

- Ask the patient's permission before moving any personal items or making adjustments in the room (see Chapter 1).
- Remember, the patient's dialogue with you and the patient's medical record are confidential. The patient expects and the law demands that this information be shared only with other professionals directly involved in the patient's care. When a case is discussed for teaching purposes, the patient's identity should be protected.
- Be honest. Never guess at an answer or information you do not know. Remember, too, that you have no right to provide information beyond your scope of practice. Providing new information to the patient is the privilege and responsibility of the attending physician.
- Make no moral judgments about the patient. Set your values for patient care according to the patient's values, beliefs, and priorities. Belittling or laughing at a patient for any reason is unprofessional and unacceptable.
- Be mindful and respectful of cultural, ethnic, religious, and other forms of diversity (see Chapter 1).
- Expect a patient to have an emotional response to illness and the health care environment and accept that response. Listen, then clarify and teach, but never argue. If you are not prepared to explore the issues with the patient, contact someone who is.
- Adjust the time, length, and content of the interaction to your patient's needs. If the patient is in distress, obtain only the information necessary to clarify immediate needs. It may be necessary to repeat some questions later, to schedule several short interviews, or to obtain the information from other sources.

3. A relaxed, conversational style on the part of the health care professional with questions and statements that communicate empathy encourages patients to express their concerns.
   - Expect and accept some periods of silence in a long or first interview. Both you and the patient need short periods to think out the correct responses.
   - Close even the briefest interview by asking if there is anything else the patient needs or wants to discuss and telling the patient when you will return.

SIMPLY STATED

A patient interview, whether a short assessment of therapy or an extended history, must allow the patient to feel secure and free to discuss personal things. Based on the material in this and the preceding chapter, be mindful of the following best practices:
- Dress and act professionally.
- Prepare by reviewing relevant records in advance.
- Project a sense of undivided interest.
- Use a relaxed conversational style.
- Respect your patients' beliefs and attitudes.
- Remember to reassure your patients that their conversation with you as well as their medical record are confidential.

Questions and Statements Used to Facilitate Conversational Interviewing

An interview made up of one direct question followed by an answer and another direct question is mechanical, monotonous, and anxiety producing. Frankly, such an approach can make patients feel as though they are being interrogated. In addition, this type of interview usually takes longer and acquires less pertinent information than a more casual, conversational interview. A rambling discussion is also inefficient and frustrating. Therefore, a conversational style that combines the types of questions and responses as described in the following list encourages open and honest descriptions by the patient, family member, or other historian while giving enough direction to clarify, quantify, and qualify details.

1. Open-ended questions encourage patients to describe events and priorities as they see them and thereby help bring out concerns and attitudes and promote understanding. Questions such as "What prompted you to come to the hospital?" or "What happened next?" encourage conversational flow and rapport while giving patients enough direction to know where to start.
2. Closed questions such as "When did your cough start?" or "How long did the pain last?" focus on specific information and provide clarification.
3. Direct questions can be either open-ended or closed questions and always end in a question mark. Although they are used to obtain specific information, a series of direct questions or frequent use of "Why?" can sound intimidating.
4. Indirect questions are less threatening because they sound like statements: "I gather your doctor told you to monitor your peak expiratory flow rates every day." Inquiries of this type also work well to confront discrepancies in the patient's statements: "If I understood you correctly, it is harder for you to breathe now than it was yesterday."
5. Neutral questions and statements are preferred for all interactions with the patient. "What happened next?" and "Tell me more about . . ." are neutral open-ended questions. A neutral closed question might give a patient a choice of responses while focusing on the type of information desired: "Would you say there was a teaspoon, a tablespoon, or a half-cup?" By contrast, leading questions such as "You didn't cough up blood, did you?" should be avoided because they imply a desired response.
6. Reflecting (echoing) is repeating words, thoughts, or feelings the patient has just stated and is a successful way to clarify and stimulate the patient to elaborate on a particular point. For example, saying to the patient that "So you just said that you could not breathe well and your cough was getting worse for about a week," might encourage the patient to elaborate on these and other symptoms. However, overuse of reflecting can make the interviewer sound like a parrot.

7. Facilitating phrases, such as "yes" or "umm" or "I see," used while establishing eye contact and perhaps nodding your head, show interest and encourage patients to continue their story, but this type of phrase should not be overused.

8. Communicating empathy (support) with statements like "That must have been very hard for you" shows your concern for the patient as a human being. Showing the patient that you really care about how life situations have caused stress, hurt, or unhappiness tells the patient it is safe to risk being honest about real concerns. Other techniques for showing empathy are described in Chapter 1.

Alternative Sources for a Patient History

Various factors affect the patient's ability or willingness to provide an accurate history. Age, alterations in level of consciousness, language and cultural barriers, emotional state, medications, inability to breathe comfortably, and the acuteness of the disease process may alter a patient's ability to communicate. For instance, the patient suffering an acute asthma attack or someone just admitted to an intensive care unit may be unable to give even a brief history. Patients with long-standing chronic disease may have become so accustomed to the accompanying symptoms, or their lives may have changed so gradually, that they may minimize and even deny symptoms. In addition, some aspects of the history may be embarrassing to the patient, such as smoking history or alcohol use. In such cases, family members, friends, work associates, previous physicians, and past medical records often can provide a more accurate picture of the history and progression of symptoms. Keeping these possibilities in mind, most hospital histories begin with a one- or two-sentence description of the current state of the patient, the source of the history, and a statement of the estimated reliability of the historian.

Cardiopulmonary History and Comprehensive Health History

Abnormalities of the respiratory system frequently are manifestations of other systemic disease processes. In addition, alterations in pulmonary function may affect other body systems. Therefore, cardiopulmonary assessment cannot be limited to the chest; a comprehensive evaluation of the patient's entire health status is essential. A detailed discussion of all aspects of obtaining and recording such a health history is beyond the scope of this text but has been well covered by other authors (see the Bibliography). This section provides an overview of the content of complete health histories and discusses specifically (in their classic order) chief complaint, history of present illness, past history, family history, and occupational and environmental history.

Variations in Health Histories

Health (medical) histories vary in length, organization, and content, depending on the preparation and experience of the interviewer, the patient's age, the reason for obtaining the history, and the circumstances surrounding the visit or admission. A history taken for a 60-year-old person complaining of chronic and debilitating symptoms is much more detailed and complex than that obtained for a summer camp application or a school physical examination. Histories recorded in emergency situations are usually limited to describing events surrounding the patient's immediate condition. In such situations, it is often difficult to get a thorough history, unless the patient is accompanied by someone who can speak on their behalf. Nursing histories emphasize the effect of the symptoms on activities of daily living and the identification of the unique care, teaching, and emotional support needs of the patient and family. Histories performed by physicians often focus on making a diagnosis. Since diagnosis and initial treatment may be done before there is time to dictate or record the history, the experienced physician may record data obtained from a combination of the history, physical examination, laboratory tests, and x-ray films rather than the more traditional history outlined in Box 2-1.

General Content of Health Histories

Although variations in recording styles do exist, all histories contain the following same types of information:
- General background information
- Screening information
- Descriptions of present health status or illness

Background Information

Background information tells the interviewer who the patient is and what types of diseases are likely to develop. It also provides a basic understanding of the patient's previous experiences with illness and health care and the patient's current life situation, including the effect of culture, attitudes, relationships, and finances on health. Knowing the level of education, patterns of health-related learning, past health care practices, and reasons for compliance or noncompliance with past courses of therapy gives insight into patients' ability to comprehend their current health status. This may predict their willingness or ability to participate in learning and therapy. From the free discussion used to obtain background information, the interviewer may also get clues about patients' reliability and possible psychosocial implications of their disease.

Screening Information

Screening information is designed to uncover problem areas the patient forgot to mention or omitted. This information is classically obtained by a head-to-toe review of all body systems but may also be obtained by a review of common diseases or from a description of body functions.

Box 2-1	Outline of a Complete Health History

1. Demographic data (usually found on first page of chart): name, address, age, birth date, birthplace, race, nationality, marital status, religion, occupation, source of referral
2. Date and source of history, estimate of historian's reliability ("the patient seems to be a good/fair/poor historian")
3. Brief description of patient's condition at time of history or patient profile
4. Chief complaint: reason for seeking health care
5. History of present illness (chronologic description of each symptom)
   Onset: time, type, source, setting
   Frequency and duration
   Location and radiation
   Severity (quantity)
   Quality (character)
   Aggravating/alleviating factors
   Associated manifestations
6. Past history or past medical history
   Childhood diseases and development
   Hospitalizations, surgeries, injuries, accidents, major illnesses
   Allergies
   Medications
   Immunizations
   General health and sources of previous health care
7. Family history
   Familial disease history
   Family history
   Marital history
   Family relationships
8. Social and environmental history
   Education
   Military experience
   Occupational history
   Religious and social activities
   Living arrangements
   Hobbies, recreation, and travel
   Habits, including smoking
   Alcohol or drug use
   Exposure to friends or family who are ill
   Satisfaction/stress with life situation, finances, relationships
   Recent travel or other event that might affect health
9. Review of systems (see Fig. 2-1)
10. Signature

Description of Present Health Status or Illness

A description of present health status or illness is included in even the briefest histories. Chief Complaint (CC) and History of Present Illness (HPI) are the most commonly used headings, although Reason for Visit and Current Health Status may be seen in some outpatient records. Because this is the information that most concerns the patient, the interview and recording of the history begins with this information.

Review of Systems

Review of systems (ROS) is a recording of past and present information that may be relevant to the present problem but might otherwise have been overlooked. It is grouped by body or physiologic systems to guarantee completeness and to assist the examiner in arriving at a diagnosis. Figure 2-1 is an example of an ROS checklist that may be completed by a patient before an interview or by an examiner. It provides for recording both positive and negative responses so that when the documentation is later reviewed, there is no doubt as to which questions were asked. Negative responses to important questions asked at any time during the interview are termed **pertinent negatives**; affirmative responses are termed **pertinent positives**. For example, if a patient complains of acute coughing but denies any fever, the fever would represent a pertinent negative, whereas the cough is a pertinent positive.

Experienced examiners usually elicit the ROS information in conjunction with the system-by-system physical examination; however, the two must not be confused. The physical examination provides **objective data**, or that which can be seen, felt, smelled, or heard by the examiner, commonly referred to as **signs**. On the other hand, the ROS provides **subjective data**, or that which is evident only to the patient and cannot be perceived by an observer or is no longer present for the observer to see and therefore can only be described by the patient. Subjective manifestations of disease are termed **symptoms**, several of which are detailed in Chapter 3.

Chief Complaint

The CC is a brief notation explaining why the patient sought health care. It is the answer to such open-ended questions as "What caused you to come to the hospital?" or "What is bothering you the most?" Each symptom is recorded separately with its duration or date of initial occurrence. Ideally, symptom descriptions are written in the patient's own words. They should not be diagnostic statements, someone else's opinion, or vague generalities. At times, more directed questions such as "Could you describe what you mean by 'not enough air'?" or "In what ways don't you feel well?" are necessary to clarify the changes in perceptions or body functions experienced by the patient.

Asking the patient to recount the sequence of symptoms and then closing this section of the interview with a question such as "What else is bothering you?" often elicits problems the patient forgot to mention or was too uncomfortable to mention earlier. Now the interviewer is left with two types of problems: (1) those related to the chief complaint and (2) those that are important to the patient but may have little or no relationship to the present illness. The interviewer must now group the problems and decide how to proceed with the interview. Problems not related to the

Have you recently had the following? (Circle "yes" or "no"; if in doubt, leave blank)

General

Tire easily, weakness	yes	no
Marked weight change	yes	no
Night sweats	yes	no
Persistent fever	yes	no
Sensitivity to heat	yes	no
Sensitivity to cold	yes	no

Skin

Eruptions (rash)	yes	no
Change in color	yes	no
Change in hair	yes	no
Change in fingernails	yes	no

Eyes

Trouble seeing	yes	no
Eye pain	yes	no
Inflamed eyes	yes	no
Double vision	yes	no
Wear corrective lenses	yes	no

Ears

Loss of hearing	yes	no
Ringing in ears	yes	no
Discharge	yes	no

Nose

Loss of smell	yes	no
Frequent colds	yes	no
Obstruction	yes	no
Excess drainage	yes	no
Nosebleeds	yes	no

Mouth

Sore gums	yes	no
Soreness of tongue	yes	no
Dental problems	yes	no

Throat

Postnasal drainage	yes	no
Soreness	yes	no
Hoarseness	yes	no

Breasts

Lumps	yes	no
Discharge	yes	no

Cardiorespiratory system

Cough, persistent	yes	no
Sputum (phlegm)	yes	no
Bloody sputum	yes	no
Wheezing	yes	no
Chest pain or discomfort	yes	no
Pain on breathing	yes	no
Shortness of breath	yes	no
Difficulty breathing while lying down	yes	no
Swelling of ankles	yes	no
Bluish fingers or lips	yes	no
High blood pressure	yes	no
Palpitations	yes	no
Vein trouble	yes	no

Digestive system

List average food selection each meal
Breakfast:

Lunch:

Dinner:

Digestive system (cont.)

Change in appetite	yes	no
Difficulty swallowing	yes	no
Heartburn	yes	no
Abdominal distress	yes	no
Belching or excess gas	yes	no
Abdominal enlargement	yes	no
Nausea	yes	no
Vomiting	yes	no
Vomiting of blood	yes	no
Rectal bleeding	yes	no
Tarry stools	yes	no
Dark urine	yes	no
Jaundice	yes	no
Constipation	yes	no
Diarrhea	yes	no
Hemorrhoids	yes	no
Need for laxatives	yes	no

Genitourinary system

Increase in frequency of urination (day)	yes	no
Increase in frequency of urination (night)	yes	no
Feel need to urinate without much urine	yes	no
Unable to hold urine	yes	no
Pain or burning	yes	no
Blood in urine	yes	no
Albuminuria	yes	no
Impotence	yes	no
Lack of sex drive	yes	no
Pain with intercourse	yes	no

Endocrine system

Thyroid trouble	yes	no
Adrenal trouble	yes	no
Cortisone treatment	yes	no
Diabetes	yes	no

Motor system

Muscle cramps	yes	no
Muscle weakness	yes	no
Pain in joints	yes	no
Swollen joints	yes	no
Stiffness	yes	no
Deformity of joints	yes	no

Nervous system

Headache	yes	no
Dizziness	yes	no
Fainting	yes	no
Convulsions or fits	yes	no
Nervousness	yes	no
Sleeplessness	yes	no
Depression	yes	no
Change in sensation	yes	no
Memory loss	yes	no
Poor coordination	yes	no
Weakness or paralysis	yes	no

GYN-OB

Age started menstruating _____
Interval between periods _____
Duration of periods _____
Flow: light   normal   heavy
Pain with periods? _____
Date of last period _____
Pregnancies _____ Births_____
Weight of babies at birth _____

FIGURE 2-1 Review-of-systems form that can be completed by patient or examiner.

illness are usually incorporated with an appropriate section of background data when the history is written.

The symptoms relating to the current illness are listed as the CC and then investigated one by one and described in detail under HPI. Once written, the CC should express the patient's, not the examiner's, priorities; provide a capsule account of the patient's illness; and guide the collection of the HPI.

The symptoms most commonly associated with problems of the cardiopulmonary system include coughing with or without sputum production (expectoration), breathlessness (dyspnea), chest pain, and wheezing, commonly described as chest tightness. Other symptoms associated with cardiopulmonary problems include coughing up blood (hemoptysis), hoarseness, voice changes, dizziness and fainting (syncope), headache, altered mental status, and ankle swelling. These symptoms are discussed in Chapter 3. Some symptoms, such as ankle swelling, can also be seen by the examiner and can therefore be both a sign and a symptom. Common cardiopulmonary signs are also discussed in Chapter 5.

Patients with cardiopulmonary problems may also have any of the so-called constitutional symptoms, which are those commonly occurring with problems in any of the body systems. Constitutional symptoms include chills and fever, excessive sweating, loss of appetite (anorexia), nausea, vomiting, weight loss, fatigue, weakness, exercise intolerance, and altered sleep patterns. Hay fever, allergies, acute sinusitis, postnasal discharge, and frequent bouts of colds or flu are upper respiratory tract symptoms commonly associated with pulmonary disease.

SIMPLY STATED

Cardiopulmonary symptoms are subjective (known only to the patient), so information about symptoms can be obtained only from the patient. Although initial information can be obtained by having the patient complete a questionnaire, a complete history can be obtained only through questioning the patient.

History of Present Illness

The HPI is the narrative portion of the history that describes chronologically and in detail each symptom listed in the CC and its effect on the patient's life. It is the most difficult portion of the history to obtain and record accurately, but it is the information that guides the physical examination and diagnostic testing to follow. All caregivers should be familiar with the HPI for each of their patients.

Encouraging the patient to talk freely about each problem allows maximal information to be obtained. The patient is initially asked to describe the progression of symptoms from the first occurrence to the present. On occasion, patients are unable to recall the first occurrence of the symptom, and the chronologic picture must then be developed by working backward from the most recent event.

Once a rough chronologic picture is outlined, the interviewer obtains a description of each symptom by using

an open-ended approach like "Now tell me about your . . . (cough, chest pain, and so on)." Using silence, nonverbal clues (like leaning forward expectantly), and facilitative expressions such as "Yes," "Hmm," and "Tell me more about . . . ," or restating or summarizing what the patient just said shows interest and encourages the patient to continue talking. When the patient exhausts the spontaneous description of each symptom, directed questions are used to elicit whatever additional information is necessary. Questions that can be answered with "yes" or "no" and leading questions are avoided. For example, "What brings on your cough?" encourages more accurate information than a question like "The only time you cough is when you first get up in the morning, isn't it?" Because most patients want to please the interviewer. They are likely to agree with a leading question rather than report the specific information needed.

SIMPLY STATED

All clinicians who care for patients should be familiar with the history of present illness for each patient treated.

Describing Symptoms

When the patient's descriptions and the interviewer's clarifying questions are complete, it is often appropriate to gather additional information for each symptom. As an example, it is not unusual to ask patients to rate their pain on a scale of 1 to 10 (highest) or to asked nonverbal patients to point to the best visual descriptor, such as a happy or sad face. To accomplish this, the following information should be gathered for each symptom:

1. Description of onset: date, time, and type (sudden or gradual)
2. Setting: cause, circumstance, or activity surrounding onset
3. Location: where on the body the problem is located and whether it radiates
4. Severity: how bad it is and how it affects activities of daily living
5. Quantity: how much, how large an area, or how many
6. Quality: what it is like and character or unique properties, such as color, texture, odor, composition, sharp, viselike, or throbbing
7. Frequency: how often it occurs
8. Duration: how long it lasts and whether it is constant or intermittent
9. Course: is it getting better, worse, or staying the same?
10. Associated symptoms: symptoms from the same body system or other systems that occur before, with, or following the problem
11. Aggravating factors: things that make it worse such as a certain position, weather, temperature, anxiety, exercise, and so on
12. Alleviating factors: things that make it better such as a change in position, hot, cold, rest, and so on

Various listings and mnemonic devices have been suggested to help the novice remember all of the information necessary to fully describe a symptom. One such mnemonic device is PQRST (Box 2-2).

Once all of the information is collected, it is written in narrative form, with a paragraph given to each time division in the chronologic progression of the symptoms. The left-hand margin of the page or the first few words of each paragraph are used to identify the applicable date or the time period (days, weeks, months, or years) prior to admission (PTA).

By the time each symptom is reviewed in detail, even a novice is usually able to assign the majority of the symptoms to one body system. The pertinent points of the ROS, personal history, and family history are reviewed for the applicable body systems. The pertinent negatives, as well as positives, are recorded. Usually, when writing the ROS, the interviewer puts "see HPI" behind the applicable body system rather than restating data previously recorded.

Past History

The past history, also called the past medical history, is a written description of the patient's past medical problems. It may include previous experiences with health care and personal attitudes and habits that may affect both health and compliance with medical treatment plans. Information recorded in the past history includes a chronologic listing of the following:

1. Illnesses and development since birth
2. Surgeries and hospitalizations
3. Injuries and accidents
4. Immunizations
5. Allergies, including a description of the allergic reactions and effective treatment
6. Medications, both prescribed by a physician and over-the-counter (OTC) drugs, vitamins, herbs, and "home remedies"
7. Names of physicians and sources and types of previous health care
8. Habits, including diet, sleep, exercise, and the use of alcohol, coffee, tobacco, and illicit drugs
9. Description of general health

Box 2-2	PQRST Mnemonic

P | Provocative/palliative: What is the cause? What makes it better? What makes it worse?

Q | Quality/quantity: How much is involved? How does it look, feel, sound?

R | Region/radiation: Where is it? Does it spread?

S | Severity scale: Does it interfere with activities? (Rate on scale of 1 to 10)

T | Timing: When did it begin? How often does it occur? Is it sudden or gradual?

Forms (Fig. 2-2) may be used by either the patient or the interviewer to concisely record much of the information just listed. It is important to record the dates of accidents, major illnesses, hospitalizations, and immunizations. If past medical records are needed during the patient's hospitalization, the names and addresses of hospitals and physicians that have provided care to the patient in the past should be recorded.

Disease and Procedure History

For patients with cardiopulmonary complaints, it is important to ask about the frequency and treatment of each of the following diseases: pneumonia, pleurisy, fungal diseases, tuberculosis, colds, sinus infections, bronchiectasis, asthma, allergies, pneumothorax, bronchitis, or emphysema. Because of the close relationship between the heart and the lungs, it is also important to know whether the patient has a history of heart attack, hypertension (high blood pressure), heart failure, or congenital heart disease.

Dates and types of heart or chest surgery and trauma should be recorded. Dates and results of tests that assess pulmonary status, including chest x-ray films, bronchoscopy, pulmonary function tests, and skin tests, should also be documented. This respiratory-specific past history information is summarized in the portion of a pulmonary history questionnaire shown in Figure 2-3. A patient's discussion of previous diseases, tests, and treatments gives a good indication of his or her understanding of the disease process and compliance with medical therapy.

Drug and Smoking History

There is a strong link between the use of illicit drugs and cardiopulmonary problems; however, an honest history of drug abuse is extremely difficult for even the most experienced examiner to obtain. It is often the bedside clinician, such as the RT, who has the first indication that drug abuse may be related to the patient's complaints. The patient should be encouraged to share this information honestly with the primary physician so that the best treatment can be obtained as early as possible. Patients should be reassured of the confidential nature related to such disclosures. In addition, clinicians and students must remember that a breach of this confidentiality is illegal and may result in losing the patient's trust. Also, concluding too quickly that a drug history is the cause of the patient's problem may result in a missed diagnosis and an improper treatment program.

Because of the strong relationship between smoking and chronic pulmonary diseases, respiratory infections, lung cancer, and cardiovascular diseases, a careful and accurate smoking history is important. It is preferable to ask a patient "What types of tobacco have you used or at what age did you begin smoking?" rather than "Do you smoke?" Use of pipes, cigars, marijuana, chewing tobacco,

PERSONAL HISTORY

Birthplace _____ Date _____

Nationality _____ Religion _____

Marital status _____ Health of spouse _____

Occupations _____

_____

Residence past 5 years: _____

Education through _____ grade   Sleep (usual hrs.) _____ Aids to sleep _____

Recreation _____

Exercise _____

Average per day: _____

  Alcohol (type) _____

  Tobacco (type) _____

  Tea, coffee _____

Medicines taken regularly	Reason	Last Dose

PERSONAL PAST HISTORY

Circle "yes" or "no"   Circle "yes" or "no"

Have you ever had:			Year	Operations			Year
Measles	yes	no		Tonsils	yes	no	
Mumps	yes	no		Appendix	yes	no	
Whooping cough	yes	no		Gallbladder	yes	no	
Polio	yes	no		Stomach	yes	no	
Scarlet fever	yes	no		Breast	yes	no	
Diphtheria	yes	no		Uterus and/or ovary	yes	no	
Meningitis	yes	no		Prostate	yes	no	
Infectious mono	yes	no		Hernia	yes	no	
Valley fever	yes	no		Thyroid	yes	no	
Tuberculosis (TB)	yes	no		Varicose veins	yes	no	
Exposure to TB	yes	no		Hemorrhoids	yes	no	
Malaria	yes	no		Heart	yes	no	
Hives	yes	no		Other	yes	no	
Cancer	yes	no		**Injuries**			
Venereal disease	yes	no		Head	yes	no	
Arthritis	yes	no		Chest	yes	no	
Back trouble	yes	no		Abdomen	yes	no	
Bronchitis	yes	no		Broken bones	yes	no	
Pneumonia	yes	no		Back	yes	no	
Pleurisy	yes	no		Other	yes	no	
Asthma	yes	no		**Allergies (are you allergic to)**			
Emphysema	yes	no		Tetanus antitoxin	yes	no	
Rheumatic fever	yes	no		Penicillin	yes	no	
High blood pressure	yes	no		Sulfa	yes	no	
Heart disease	yes	no		Other drugs	yes	no	
Anemia	yes	no		List _____			
Bleeding tendency	yes	no					
Blood transfusion	yes	no					
Hepatitis	yes	no		Foods	yes	no	
(yellow jaundice)				Cosmetics	yes	no	
Ulcer	yes	no		Other	yes	no	
Hemorrhoids	yes	no		**Immunizations**			
Bladder infections	yes	no		Smallpox	yes	no	
Kidney disease	yes	no		Tetanus	yes	no	
Hay fever/sinusitis	yes	no		Polio, shots	yes	no	
Glaucoma	yes	no		Polio, oral	yes	no	
Nosebleeds	yes	no		Other	yes	no	

FIGURE 2-2 Form for recording personal history and personal past history (past medical history).

or snuff is usually recorded in terms of the amount used daily. The consumption of cigarettes should be recorded in pack-years. The term **pack-years** refers to the number of years the patient has smoked times the number of packs smoked each day. It is also important to record the age when the patient began to smoke, variations in smoking habits over the years, the type and length of the cigarettes smoked, the habit of inhaling, the number and success of attempts to stop smoking, and the date when the patient last smoked (see Fig. 2-3). Members of the health care team have a professional responsibility to educate patients and their family about the harmful effects of smoking and guide them to programs designed to help people stop smoking.

SIMPLY STATED

The term *pack-years* is the number of years the patient has smoked multiplied by the number of packs per day. If a patient smoked three packs a day for 10 years, it would be recorded as a 30 pack year smoking history.

Please answer by circling "yes" or "no" and provide the specific information.

PAST MEDICAL HISTORY

Have you ever had the following?			**If "yes" give year/specifics**
Asthma	yes	no	_____
Allergies	yes	no	_____
Frequent colds	yes	no	_____
Sinus infections	yes	no	_____
Chronic bronchitis	yes	no	_____
Emphysema	yes	no	_____
Pleurisy	yes	no	_____
Pneumonia	yes	no	_____
Pneumothorax	yes	no	_____
Tuberculosis	yes	no	_____
Other lung problems	yes	no	_____
Heart trouble of any type	yes	no	_____
Chest trauma	yes	no	_____
Chest, lung, or heart surgery	yes	no	List: _____

Have you ever had any of the following?			**If "yes" give month/year last performed**
Chest x-ray: ever abnormal?	yes	no	_____/_____
TB skin test: ever positive?	yes	no	_____/_____

Have you had any of the following? | | |
--- | --- | --- | ---
Other skin tests | yes | no | _____/_____
Pulmonary function test | yes | no | _____/_____
Bronchoscopy | yes | no | _____/_____
Other pulmonary tests | yes | no | _____/_____

SMOKING HISTORY

Do you currently smoke or use tobacco regularly? yes no
1. How old were you when you started smoking? _____
2. For how many years have you smoked regularly? _____
3. How many cigarettes do you now smoke each day? _____
4. How many cigars do you now smoke each day? _____
5. How much pipe tobacco do you now smoke each week? _____
6. Were there periods when you stopped smoking? _____
7. How long did you stop smoking? _____

Have you ever smoked regularly? yes no
1. How old were you when you started smoking? _____
2. How many years did you smoke regularly? _____
3. When did you quit smoking? (month/year) _____/_____
4. How many cigarettes did you usually smoke per day? _____
5. How many cigars did you usually smoke per day? _____
6. How much pipe tobacco did you smoke per week? _____

Did you smoke anything other than tobacco? yes no
What, how much, how often? _____

Does someone smoke in your home or office? yes no
1. How many years has someone smoked in your home? _____
2. How many years has someone smoked in your office? _____

FIGURE 2-3 Past medical history and smoking sections from a pulmonary history questionnaire.

Family History

The purpose of the family history is to learn about the health status of the patient's blood relatives. This is where the interviewer records the presence of diseases in immediate family members with hereditary tendencies. Sources of physical, emotional, or economic support or stress within the family structure are also documented here when important.

To assess the current health status of the extended family, the patient is asked to describe the present age and state of health of blood relatives for three generations: siblings; parents, aunts and uncles; and grandparents. The resulting information may be recorded in narrative style, drawn schematically as a family tree, or written on a form like the one shown in Figure 2-4. When patients are asked to complete a form before an interview, the responses should be reviewed and notations added as necessary to capture the age and cause of death or current health status for each family member. A notation such as "18 A/W" indicates that the person listed was 18 years old and alive and well on the day the history was recorded.

The health of the current family of a patient who was adopted is important for identification of communicable and environmentally related diseases; however, a history of the patient's true blood relatives is needed to assess genetically transmitted diseases or illnesses with strong familial relationships.

In addition to documenting the current health status of the family members, a review of diseases with strong hereditary or familial tendencies is also performed. Figure 2-4 shows a form that permits either the patient or examiner to record the presence or absence of the most frequently reviewed diseases known to occur in the patient's family (pertinent positives) and those denied by the patient (pertinent negatives).

Patients with cardiopulmonary complaints are asked specifically about the following diseases or problems that have been shown to have a hereditary link with pulmonary disease: chronic allergies, asthma, lung cancer, cystic fibrosis, emphysema, neuromuscular disorders, kyphosis, scoliosis, sleep disturbances and sleep apnea, collagen vascular diseases (e.g., lupus erythematosus), α_1-antitrypsin deficiency, cardiovascular disorders (e.g., hypertension, heart attack, heart failure, and congenital abnormalities), diabetes, and obesity. Because exposure to family and friends with infections can also result in pulmonary symptoms, the patient is asked about contact with or family history of frequent colds, tuberculosis, influenza, pneumonia, and fungal infections.

Occupational and Environmental History

An occupational and environmental history is particularly important in patients with pulmonary symptoms. The purpose is to elicit information concerning exposure to potential disease-producing substances or environments.

Most occupational pulmonary diseases result from workers inhaling particles, dusts, fumes, or gases during the extraction, manufacture, transfer, storage, or disposal of industrial substances (Table 2-1). However, the hazards of an industrial society are not limited to those working directly with the toxic substances. Other employees working in or near an industrial plant, as well as people living in the surrounding areas, are subject to breathing toxic fumes and dusts. Family members come in contact with contaminated clothing, such as asbestos from clothing being laundered, and may develop pulmonary disease years later. Accidental spills of toxic chemicals and gases can endanger and even necessitate evacuation and treatment of large numbers of people.

Although there have been dramatic decreases in exposure to some hazardous materials, exposures to dusts, fumes, and chemicals from indoor and outdoor air pollutants continue to increase. Outbreaks of work-related illnesses in buildings not contaminated by industrial

Has any blood relative had any of the following?	Circle "yes" or "no"		If "yes," what relationship?
Anemia	yes	no	_____
Bleeding tendency	yes	no	_____
Leukemia	yes	no	_____
Repeated infections	yes	no	_____
Crippling infections	yes	no	_____
Heart disease	yes	no	_____
Chronic lung disease	yes	no	_____
Tuberculosis	yes	no	_____
High blood pressure	yes	no	_____
Kidney disease	yes	no	_____
Asthma	yes	no	_____
Severe allergies	yes	no	_____
Mental illness	yes	no	_____
Convulsions or fits	yes	no	_____
Migraine headaches	yes	no	_____
Diabetes	yes	no	_____
Gout	yes	no	_____
Obesity	yes	no	_____
Thyroid trouble	yes	no	_____
Peptic ulcer	yes	no	_____
Chronic diarrhea	yes	no	_____
Cancer	yes	no	_____

	Present Age, or Age at Death	If living, health (good, fair, poor) if deceased, cause of death
Father		
Mother		
Brothers or Sisters		
1.		
2.		
3.		
4.		
5.		
6.		
7.		
Children		
1.		
2.		
3.		
4.		
5.		
6.		
7.		

FIGURE 2-4 Form for recording family history.

TABLE 2-1

Occupational Lung Disease

Inhaled Substance	Occupation or Source	Usual Symptoms and Course	Disease Names
Acute Airway or Lung Reactions			
Irritant Gases			
Chlorine, ammonia, sulfur dioxide	Various industries Accidental exposure	Short exposure Eye and airway irritation, dry cough Prolonged exposure Dyspnea, wheezing, pulmonary edema	
Insoluble Gases and Metal Fumes			
Nitrogen dioxide	Filled silos, closed welding spaces, chemical laboratories	Very little airway irritation Headache, shortness of breath, cough, chest tightness, pulmonary edema	Silo-filler's disease
Phosgene	Chemical warfare, heating metals treated with production chlorine	Acute pulmonary edema, pneumonitis	
Copper, zinc, iron, nickel, tin, antimony, manganese, magnesium	Welders in closed spaces, mining, electroplating	Fever, malaise, nausea, aching muscles, lasting 2-3 days	Metal fume fever Galvanization Polymer fume fever
Cadmium, mercury, beryllium		Above with acute pulmonary edema and pneumonia	
Acute or Subacute Allergic Reactions			
Toluene diisocyanate (TDI)	Plastic and foam production	Immediate or delayed asthma-like reactions usually occur in sensitive persons but may occur in others; fever, chills, malaise, weight loss, nocturnal wheezing, cough, cyanosis, dyspnea at rest	Hypersensitivity pneumonitis
Proteolytic enzymes (detergents)	Industrial accidents Manufacture of detergents		Extrinsic allergic alveolitis Occupational asthma
Droppings/Feathers			
Pigeons, parakeets, chickens, turkeys	Bird handlers	Acute reactions within 4-8 hours Delayed reactions occur at night after leaving work environment In some cases, chronic disease with fibrosis may develop if repeated exposure continues	Bird-fancier's lung, ornithosis Pigeon-breeder's lung
Pituitary Extract/Organic Dusts			
Paprika, fishmeal, coffee bean, weevil-infested flour	Workers with specific products	"Monday fever" Repeated bouts of pneumonia with fever and weight loss	Pituitary snuff-taker's lung Wheat-weevil lung Byssinosis (brown lung)
Cotton, hemp, flax	Textile and farm workers		Farmer's lung
Fungal spores from moldy hay, straw, grains, malt or barley, sugar cane (bagasse), mushroom compost, maple bark, logs, wood pulp (Western red cedar)	Agriculture and farm workers Wood and paper mill workers Lumbering		Malt-worker's lung Bagassosis Mushroom-handler's lung Wood/paper mill–worker's lung Maple bark–stripper's lung
Contaminated water	Air conditioners, humidifiers		Air-conditioner (humidifier) lung
Drugs and chemicals	Antibiotic, pharmaceutical, chemical manufacture		
Chronic Occupational Lung Diseases			
Crystalline-free silica	Sandblasters in enclosed spaces, manufacture of ceramics and abrasive agents, construction, mines, quarries, foundries: gold, copper, lead, zinc, iron, coal, granite	Acute (1-3 years of intense exposure): shortness of breath, fever, frequent pulmonary infections Chronic (20 years or more of exposure): no symptoms to exertional dyspnea, obstructed breathing, productive cough, reduced exercise tolerance, chest pain, weight loss, hemoptysis with fibrosis 40+ years: infection, cor pulmonale	Silicosis Associated in unknown way with rheumatoid arthritis and scleroderma High incidence of associated tuberculosis and bronchogenic cancer

TABLE 2-1

Occupational Lung Disease—cont'd

Inhaled Substance	Occupation or Source	Usual Symptoms and Course	Disease Names
Coal	Coal miners	Simple: asymptomatic, cough with smoking	Coal-worker's pneumoconiosis
		Complicated with fibrosis: as just listed with black sputum	Coal-miner's lung
Asbestos	Manufacture of fireproofing and insulation, shipbuilding, automobile mechanics (clutch and brake), demolition workers, firefighters, living/working near dumps or high-use areas	Exertional dyspnea, clubbing, restricted breathing, crackles at lung bases usually appear before x-ray film changes and cancer symptoms about 20 years after exposure	Asbestosis
Other Mineral Dusts			
Fuller's earth, kaolin (China clay), graphite, tin, iron, mixed dusts, tungsten	Quarrying, mining, milling, drying, bagging, and loading minerals	Vary from asymptomatic with dust retention to same as complicated silicosis	Pneumoconiosis
	Welding and foundries		Stannosis
	Manufacture of industrial precision instruments		Siderosis
Beryllium	Nuclear physics, manufacture of electronics, ceramics, x-ray tube windows (in past: fluorescent lights)	Acute pulmonary edema, pneumonia	Pulmonary granuloma
		Chronic granulomatous disease appears years after exposure	
		Dyspnea, dry cough, weakness, weight loss, skin lesions, crackles	
Paraquat	Agriculture	Inhalation or ingestion may lead to pulmonary fibrosis	

processes can be traced to these pollutants or simply to an inadequate provision of fresh air with no identifiable contaminant. The terms *tight-building syndrome* and *sick-building syndrome* are now used to describe these epidemics in which large numbers of employees complain of symptoms, including runny or stuffy nose, eye irritation, cough, chest tightness, fatigue, headache, and malaise.

Reactions to inhalation of toxic substances can occur within minutes to hours (acute) or may take weeks, months, or years to develop. Inhalation of soluble gases, such as ammonia, chlorine, or sulfur dioxide, causes sufficient upper airway irritation to warn workers of immediate danger. However, metal fumes and insoluble gases, such as phosgene and nitrogen dioxide, are less irritating to the upper airways. Because they may be inhaled for long periods of time with little discomfort, workers are not warned to escape, and more severe pulmonary damage results.

Hypersensitivity reactions may be acute or delayed and often occur in patterns. Shortness of breath, wheezes, or flulike symptoms usually occur within 4 to 8 hours of exposure. However, symptoms may occur only at night and may recur for several nights after a single exposure. In some cases, the most severe symptoms occur at the start of the workweek, and tolerance develops as the week progresses. Such a pattern, often termed *Monday fever*, is commonly seen with inhalation of cotton dust.

More commonly, allergic reactions worsen with reexposure and decrease during days off. In subacute forms of hypersensitivity pneumonitis, symptoms occur insidiously over weeks. Most of the chronic occupational pulmonary diseases (pneumoconioses) take 20 years or more to become symptomatic. Whenever there is a delay in the development of pulmonary symptoms, their relationship to occupational and environmental exposure becomes obscure.

The occupational and environmental history, therefore, must be more than just a chronologic listing of job titles. Questioning may include the occupation of the patient's father and descriptions of childhood residences. Lung disease caused by the inhalation of asbestos fibers (asbestosis) has been seen in people who lived near shipyards or asbestos dump sites as children and in people whose fathers were asbestos workers. The patient should be queried about location of schools, summer jobs, dates and types of military service, and all subsequent full- and part-time jobs. The precise dates, duration, and activities of each job must be delineated. These include materials and processes involved, amount of workspace and type of ventilation, use of protective devices, cleanup practices, and work going on in adjacent areas.

Work or residence near mines, farms, mills, shipyards, or foundries should be clarified. Sources of possible irritants within the home, such as humidifiers, air-conditioning systems, woodpiles, insulation, smoking, paints and glues used for hobbies, and household pets, must also be reviewed.

It is important to review the various places a patient has lived or visited for any period of time. Certain fungal infections that involve the respiratory system have strong geographic relationships. Histoplasmosis is particularly common in Ohio, Maryland, the central Mississippi Valley, and the Appalachian Mountains; blastomycosis is found in the southwestern United States, especially Arizona, Texas, and the San Joaquin Valley in California, as well as sections of South America.

When the pulmonary history is written, occupational and environmental histories are usually given specific headings because of the detail recorded. However, in most routine histories, this information may be found under general headings such as personal history, social history, psychosocial history, or social-environmental history.

Reviewing the Patient's Medical Record

The RT often prepares to visit the patient by first reviewing the patient's medical record. This record may be brief on admission but builds if the patient is admitted for more than a couple of days. It is the RT's responsibility to become familiar with pertinent information recorded in the chart and overall medical record.

In the past, this generally meant reviewing only a hard copy of the patient's chart. However, with the advent of **electronic medical records (EMRs)**, many such records, including admitting information, history and assessment notes, laboratory tests and imaging studies (radiographs and computed tomography scans) are stored in computerized databases. Therefore, it is essential for the RT to confirm the review of both the hard copy and relevant EMR data to ensure a comprehensive review of pertinent records. EMR and overall documentation of the patient assessment and care plan are detailed in Chapter 21. The following information represents aspects of the patient's medical record that are generally most useful.

Admission Note

The admission note is written by the admitting physician and is a narrative description of important facts related to the patient's need to be hospitalized. The physician documents the patient's baseline status on admission in the admission note. The RT should review this important notation before seeing the patient for the initial visit to identify whom the patient is, why the patient was admitted, what the patient's current clinical condition is, and the overall treatment plan.

Physician Orders

The admitting physician lists the treatment plan and monitoring techniques that he or she believes are needed

to best care for the patient. The RT should carefully review all orders related to the treatment and monitoring of cardiopulmonary disorders and specifically review the orders pertaining to respiratory care.

Progress Notes

Each day the attending physician will visit the patient at least once. During this visit the physician will interview and examine the patient to identify the patient's progress and response to treatment. The physician will follow up by documenting progress notes in the patient's chart. RTs should review these notes daily to identify the physician's perception of the patient's progress toward treatment goals.

In addition to the physician, other health care providers will document progress notes in the patient's chart. The nurse, physical therapist, occupational therapist, nutritionist, social worker, and others health care providers may record their findings and treatment plan in a progress note, often using a SOAP (subjective, objective, assessment, plan) format (see Chapter 21).

DNAR/DNR Status

Some patients will have a **do not attempt to resuscitate (DNAR)** or **do not resuscitate (DNR)** label on their chart to alert the patient care team that there is a concurrent physician's order in the chart. In such cases, resuscitation should not be attempted if the patient experiences respiratory or cardiac arrest. DNAR or DNR may be instituted on the basis of an advance directive from a patient or from someone entitled to make decisions on a patient's behalf, such as a health care proxy. In some states, DNAR/DNR can also be instituted on the basis of a physician's own initiative, usually when resuscitation would not alter the ultimate outcome of a disease. This indicates that the family physician, in consultation with the patient and/or family members, has determined that the patient has a terminal illness that is not reversible.

It is important to remember that there are variations of DNAR/DNR orders. One such variation, which prohibits intubation but may allow the administration of certain cardiopulmonary resuscitative medications such as epinephrine or atropine, is known as a do not intubate (DNI) order. It should also be noted that the increasingly popular alternative term for a DNAR is an *allow natural death* (AND) order.

Assessment Standards for Patients with Pulmonary Dysfunction

The beginning student may be confused by the fact that the patient's medical record contains more than one style of history recorded on or about the same date. This occurs in teaching institutions because students and residents, as well as the attending physician, see the patient. It

Box 2-3	American Thoracic Society's Nursing Assessment Guide for Adult Patients with Pulmonary Dysfunction

HISTORY AND SYMPTOMS

*PULMONARY SYMPTOMS**

Dyspnea
Cough
Sputum
Hemoptysis
Wheeze
Chest pain (e.g., pleuritic)

*EXTRAPULMONARY SYMPTOMS**

Night sweats
Headaches on awakening
Weight changes
Fluid retention
Nasal stuffiness, discharge
Fatigue
Orthopnea, paroxysmal nocturnal dyspnea
Snoring, sleep disturbances, daytime drowsiness

Sinus problems

PULMONARY RISK FACTORS

Smoking history and nicotine use
Type (cigarettes, cigar, pipe, or smokeless tobacco)
Amount per day
Duration (years)
Childhood respiratory diseases/symptoms
Family history of respiratory disease
Alcohol and chemical substance abuse (e.g., heroin, marijuana, cocaine)
Environmental exposures
Location (e.g., home, work, region)
Type (e.g., asbestos, silica, gases, aerosols)
Duration
Obesity or nutritional depletion
Compromised immune system function (e.g., immunoglobulin G deficiency, HIV infection, α_1-antitrypsin deficiency)

PREVIOUS HISTORY

Pulmonary problems
Treatments
Number of hospitalizations
Medical diagnoses
Immunizations

SELF-MANAGEMENT CAPACITY

PHYSICAL ABILITY (0 TO 4 SCALE, 0 = INDEPENDENT, 4 = DEPENDENT)

Lower extremity (e.g., walking, stair climbing)

Upper extremity (e.g., shampooing, meal preparation)
Activities of daily living
    Toileting
    Hygiene
    Feeding
    Dressing
Activity pattern during a typical day
Patient statement about management of problems
Sensory-perceptual factors (e.g., vision, hearing)

COGNITIVE ABILITY

Mental age
Memory
Knowledge about diagnosis, end treatment of pulmonary problems, or risk factors of pulmonary disease
Judgment

PSYCHOSOCIAL-CULTURAL FACTORS

Self-concept
Self-esteem
Body image
Roles, changes
Value system (e.g., spiritual and health beliefs)
Coping mechanisms
Displaced anger
Anxiety
Hostility
Dependency
Withdrawal, isolation
Avoidance
Denial
Noncompliance
Acceptance

SOCIOECONOMIC FACTORS

Social support system
Family
Significant others
Friends
Community resources
Government resources
Financial situation/health insurance
Employment/disability

ENVIRONMENTAL FACTORS

Home
Community
Worksite
Health care setting (e.g., hospital, nursing home)

*Consider onset, duration, character, precipitating, aggravating, and relieving factors of symptoms.
Modified from American Thoracic Society Medical Section of the American Lung Association: Standards of nursing care for adult patients with pulmonary dysfunction, *Am Rev Respir Dis* 1991; 144–231.

also occurs because each of the health care professions is responsible for specifying the scope of practice for its practitioners and monitoring the quality of their performance. As a result, there may be patient histories completed by nursing and several allied health professions in addition to those done by physicians. Some hospitals are moving toward what is termed the *patient history*—one history per patient per admission—which is used and augmented by all the allied health professionals involved in the patient's care as well as by physicians.

The American Thoracic Society (ATS) adopted specific standards for assessment of adult patients with actual or potential pulmonary dysfunction. These process and outcome standards are used with assessment, goal setting, intervention, and evaluation to ensure that the patient receives an acceptable level of care. The pulmonary history assessment guide from these standards is shown in Box 2-3. Note that in addition to gathering and analyzing the traditional pulmonary history, this assessment includes additional categories that focus on the patient's response to interferences with normal respiratory function, self-management capacity, resources, and knowledge of respiratory medications and treatments. The student will find this document helpful as a tool to review the multiple variables that affect both the quality of care and quality of life for a patient with pulmonary dysfunction.

KEY POINTS

▶ The medical history of the patient is most often obtained by the patient's physician. RTs often interview the patient to identify changes in the patient's health status in response to therapy.

▶ Interviewing skills require practice to obtain proficiency and are an important part of patient assessment for all health care providers.

▶ Communicating with the patient to obtain information about his or her health status requires the interviewer to be skilled at verbal and nonverbal communication.

▶ Body movement, facial expression, touch, and eye movement are all types of nonverbal communication.

▶ One of the most common mistakes made by the interviewer is failing to listen carefully to the patient's answers and questions.

▶ The ability of the interviewer to project a sense of undivided interest in the patient is the key to a successful interview and the development of good patient rapport.

▶ Open-ended questions encourage patients to describe events and priorities as they see them and thereby help bring out concerns and attitudes and promote understanding.

▶ Closed questions such as "When did your cough start?" or "How long did the pain last?" focus on specific information and provide clarification.

▶ Neutral questions and statements, as opposed to leading questions, are preferred for all interactions with the patient. Leading questions prompt the patient to provide a certain answer and therefore may lead to inaccurate information.

▶ ROS is a recording of past and present information that may be relevant to the present problem but might otherwise have been overlooked.

▶ The CC is a brief notation in the patient's current medical history explaining why he or she sought health care. It is the answer to such open-ended questions as "What brought you to the hospital?"

▶ The HPI is the narrative portion of the history that describes chronologically and in detail each symptom listed in the CC and its effect on the patient's life.

KEY POINTS—cont'd

▶ Because of the strong relationship between smoking and chronic pulmonary diseases, respiratory infections, lung cancer, and cardiovascular diseases, a careful and accurate smoking history is important.

▶ The purpose of the family history is to learn about the health status of the patient's blood relatives. The interviewer records the presence of diseases in immediate family members with hereditary tendencies.

▶ The purpose of the occupational history is to elicit information concerning exposure to potential disease-producing substances or environments. Most occupational pulmonary diseases are the result of workers inhaling particles, dusts, fumes, or gases during the extraction, manufacture, transfer, storage, or disposal of industrial substances.

▶ It is important to document in the history the various places a patient has lived or visited for any period of time. Certain fungal infections that involve the respiratory system have strong geographic relationships.

▶ It is the RT's responsibility to become familiar with pertinent information recorded in the chart before caring for the patient with respiratory illness.

ASSESSMENT QUESTIONS

See Appendix for answers.

1. T/F Proper diagnosis and treatment are determined to a great extent by the accuracy and detail of the patient's history.

2. During the interview, if the therapist responds to the information provided by the patient with appropriate comments, this is evidence of which of the following?
   1. Nonverbal communication
   2. Active listening
   3. Pertinent positives
   4. Reflecting
      a. 1 and 3
      b. 2 and 4
      c. 3 and 4
      d. All of the above

3. Proper introduction of yourself to the patient before the interview is useful for all the following except:
   a. Establishing your role
   b. Asking permission to be involved
   c. Conveying your sincere interest in the patient
   d. Identifying diagnostic information

4. Which of the following would be examples of techniques used in conversational interviewing?
   a. Using questions such as "What happened next?"
   b. Saying things like "You feel better now, don't you?"
   c. Asking for clarification of a symptom
   d. a and c

5. A patient cannot provide a medical history, and it is obtained from a close relative. This is an example of which of the following?
   a. Family history
   b. Background information
   c. Screening information
   d. Alternative source

6. In what section of the patient history can a detailed description of the patient's current symptoms be found?
   a. Chief complaints
   b. History of present illness
   c. Past medical history
   d. Occupational history

7. Information that is evident only to the patient and cannot be perceived by the observer is known as which of the following?
   a. Subjective data
   b. Objective data
   c. Clinical signs
   d. Pertinent negatives

8. In what section of the patient's history would you find information about a possible history of exposure to asbestos?
   a. History of present illness
   b. Family history
   c. Occupational history
   d. Past medical history

9. Your patient has a 50-pack-year smoking history. Which of the following is consistent with this history?
   a. He has smoked 2 packs/day for 25 years
   b. He has smoked 1 pack/day for 50 years
   c. He has smoked 5 packs/day for 10 years
   d. All of the above

10. Subjective manifestations of disease are termed:
    a. Symptoms
    b. Clinical findings
    c. Objective data
    d. Pertinent negatives

11. Your patient has pneumonia and complains of chest pain and cough but denies fever. How would you classify the lack of fever in this case?
    a. Objective data
    b. Pertinent positive
    c. Pertinent negative
    d. Physical examination finding

12. Which of the following is not considered a constitutional symptom?
    a. Nausea
    b. Weakness
    c. Chills and fever
    d. Dyspnea

13. The family history may be helpful in diagnosing a patient with which of the following problems?
    a. Acute bronchitis
    b. Cystic fibrosis
    c. Pneumothorax
    d. Pulmonary edema

14. Which of the following illnesses may be related to visiting or living in certain geographic locations?
    a. Congestive heart failure
    b. Fungal pneumonia
    c. Cystic fibrosis
    d. Emphysema

15. Your patient has a DNR label on his chart and at the head of his bed. This indicates:
    a. The patient is not responsive
    b. The patient is not oriented to time, place, and person
    c. The patient should not be resuscitated if cardiac arrest occurs
    d. The patient has psychiatric problems and needs close supervision

Bibliography

Edwards K, Chiweda D, Oyinka A, et al. Assessing the value of electronic records. *Nurs Times* 2011;**107**:12.

Ferreir-Valente MA, Pais-Rabeiro JL, Jensen MP. Validity of four pain intensity rating scales. *Pain* 2011;**152**:2399.

Heuer AJ, Geisler SL, Kamiensk M, et al. Introducing medical students to the interdisciplinary health care team: piloting a case-based approach. *J Allied Health* 2010;**39**:76.

Jarvis C. *Physical exam and health assessment.* 6th ed. St Louis: Mosby-Elsevier; 2012.

Kacmarek RM, Stoller JK, Heuer AJ. *Egan's fundamentals of respiratory care.* 10th ed. St. Louis: Mosby-Elsevier; 2013.

Seidel HM, Ball J, Dains J, Flynn JA, et al. *Mosby's guide to physical examination.* 7th ed. St. Louis: Mosby-Elsevier; 2011.

Venneman SS, Narnor-Harris P, Perish M, Hamilton M. "Allow natural death" versus "do not resuscitate": three words that can change a life. *J Med Ethics* 2008;**34**:2.

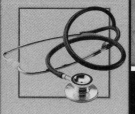

Cardiopulmonary Symptoms

ALBERT J. HEUER*

LEARNING OBJECTIVES

After reading this chapter, you will be able to:
1. Describe the causes and common characteristics of the following symptoms:
    - Cough
    - Sputum production
    - Hemoptysis
    - Dyspnea
    - Chest pain
    - Dizziness and fainting
    - Swelling of the ankles
    - Fever, chills, and night sweats
    - Headache, altered mental status, and personality changes
    - Snoring
    - Gastroesophageal reflux
    - Daytime somnolence (sleepiness)

*Dr. Robert Wilkins, PhD, RRT, and Donna Gardner, MSHP, RRT, contributed much of the content for this chapter as co-editors of the prior edition of the chapter."

KEY TERMS

angina	gastroesophageal reflux	paroxysmal nocturnal dyspnea
cough	disease (GERD)	(PND)
daytime somnolence	hematemesis	phlegm
diaphoresis	hemoptysis	platypnea
dyspnea	night sweats	sleep disordered breathing
edema	obstructive sleep apnea (OSA)	sputum
fetid	orthodeoxia	syncope
fever	orthopnea	tenacious
frothy	orthostatic hypotension	trepopnea

Symptoms are subjective clinical findings generally reported by the patient during or shortly after the initial interview (described in Chapter 2). Clinical signs, on the other hand, are objective and measurable, such as the vital signs and laboratory studies detailed in subsequent chapters of this text. Respiratory therapists (RTs) will encounter patients with a variety of symptoms. The primary symptoms associated with cardiopulmonary disorders are cough, sputum production, hemoptysis, shortness of breath (dyspnea), and chest pain. Other less specific complaints include dizziness and fainting; ankle swelling (peripheral edema); fever, chills, and night sweats; snoring; personality changes; daytime somnolence (sleepiness); and gastric reflux. This chapter defines the terms associated with these symptoms, briefly discusses their causes (etiology), and describes how these symptoms relate to commonly associated diseases. The more familiar RTs are with these symptoms and their characteristics, the better they can ask relevant questions, assist the patient care team in making a correct diagnosis, and help design an appropriate interdisciplinary treatment plan.

SIMPLY STATED

Cardiopulmonary symptoms are assessed to determine the following:
- The seriousness of the patient's problem
- The potential underlying cause of the problem
- The effectiveness of treatment

Cough

Cough is one of the most common, though nonspecific, symptoms seen in patients with pulmonary disease. It is the powerful protective reflex arising from stimulation of receptors located in the pharynx, larynx, trachea, large bronchi, and even the lung and the visceral pleura. Coughing can be caused by inflammatory, mechanical, chemical, or thermal stimulation of cough receptors found anywhere from the oropharynx to the terminal bronchioles or simply by tactile pressure in the ear canal. There are many conditions that can make a patient cough. The key to determining the cause in many cases can be found in a careful review of the history, physical examination, and chest radiograph (Table 3-1).

Impulses generated by stimulation of the cough receptors are carried by afferent pathways of the reflex, primarily the vagus, phrenic, glossopharyngeal, and trigeminal nerves, to the cough center located diffusely in the medulla, separate from the respiratory center. Conduction of the impulses down the efferent pathway of the reflex stimulates the smooth muscles of the larynx and tracheobronchial tree and the diaphragm and other respiratory muscles through the phrenic and other spinal motor nerves. The cough mechanism can be divided into the following three phases:

1. *Inspiratory phase:* reflex opening of the glottis and contraction of the diaphragm, thoracic, and abdominal muscles cause a deep inspiration with a concomitant increase in lung volume accompanied by an increase in the caliber and length of the bronchi.

2. *Compression phase:* closure of the glottis and relaxation of the diaphragm while the expiratory muscles contract against the closed glottis can generate very high intrathoracic pressures and narrowing of the trachea and bronchi.

3. *Expiratory phase:* opening of the glottis, explosive release of trapped intrathoracic air, and vibration of the vocal cords and mucosal lining of the posterior laryngeal wall shake secretions loose from the larynx and move undesired material out of the respiratory tract.

The cough reflex may be voluntary or involuntary and normally occurs in everyone from time to time. The efficiency of the cough (force of the airflow) is determined by the depth of the inspiration and amount of pressure that can be generated in the airways. The effectiveness of a cough is reduced if one or more of the following conditions exist:

1. Weakness of either the inspiratory or expiratory muscles
2. Inability of the glottis to open or close correctly
3. Obstruction, collapsibility, or alteration in shape or contours of the airways
4. Decrease in lung recoil as occurs with emphysema
5. Abnormal quantity or quality of mucus production (e.g., thick sputum)

TABLE 3-1

Possible Causes of Cough Receptor Stimulation

Types of Stimulation	Possible Causes
Inflammatory	Infection, lung abscess, drug reaction, allergy, edema, hyperemia, collagen vascular disease, radiotherapy, pneumoconiosis, tuberculosis
Mechanical	Inhaled dusts, suction catheter, food
Obstructive	Foreign bodies, aspirations of nasal secretions, tumor or granulomas within or around the lung, aortic aneurysm
Airway wall tension	Pulmonary edema, atelectasis, fibrosis, chronic interstitial pneumonitis
Chemical	Inhaled irritant gases, fumes, smoke
Temperature	Inhaled hot or cold air
Ear	Tactile pressure in the ear canal (Arnold nerve response) or from otitis media

Causes and Clinical Presentation

Most patients will have a single cause for their cough; however, in some patients, two or three simultaneous causes (comorbidities) may be present. Cough may be acute (sudden onset, usually severe with a short course, self-limited), chronic (persistent and troublesome for more than 3 weeks), or paroxysmal (periodic, prolonged, and forceful episodes). An acute self-limited cough is usually due to a viral infection involving the upper airway, which usually resolves in a few days. A chronic persistent cough is most commonly caused by postnasal drip syndrome, followed by acute asthma, acute exacerbation of chronic obstructive pulmonary disease (COPD), allergic rhinitis, gastroesophageal reflux disease (GERD), chronic bronchitis, bronchiectasis, and other conditions such as left heart failure, bronchogenic cancer, and sarcoidosis. In smokers, chronic cough is usually due to chronic bronchitis ("smoker's cough"). Still other chronic coughs may result from certain medications, such as angiotensin-converting enzyme (ACE) inhibitors commonly prescribed for congestive heart failure and other cardiac conditions. Though not fully understood, patients taking ACE inhibitors may develop a chronic dry cough, possibly as a result of an increase in cough mediators that accumulate in the upper airway. Hence, the medication history described in Chapter 2 can provide vital clues to the underlying cause. Aggravating, painful, or persistent cough or cough equivalent, such as throat clearing, is not normal and warrants further clinical investigation.

Cough may occur in conjunction with other pulmonary symptoms such as wheezing, stridor, chest pain, and dyspnea. In addition, cough may cause problems. The vigorous muscular activity and high intrathoracic pressures created by forceful coughing may produce a number of complications, such as torn chest muscles, rib fractures, disruption of surgical wounds, pneumothorax or pneumomediastinum, syncope (fainting), arrhythmia, esophageal rupture, and urinary incontinence.

Descriptions

Cough should be described as effective (strong enough to clear the airway) or inadequate (audible but too weak to mobilize the secretions), productive (mucus or other material is expelled by the cough), or dry and nonproductive (moisture or secretions are not produced). Because dry coughs often become productive, a chronologic report of the circumstances surrounding the change and a description of the sputum should be recorded.

The quality, time, and setting in which a cough occurs may also provide some clues to the location and type of disorder (Table 3-2). Barking (like a seal), brassy (harsh, dry), and hoarse coughs, as well as those associated with inspiratory stridor, are usually heard when there is a problem with the larynx (e.g., infection or tumor). Wheezy coughs (accompanied by whistling or sighing sounds) suggest bronchial disorders. Acute, productive coughs are most often seen with allergic asthma as well as bacterial or viral respiratory infections, and chronic productive coughs are generally indicative of significant bronchopulmonary disease (e.g., chronic bronchitis). Hacking (frequent brief periods of coughing or clearing the throat) may be dry and the result of smoking, a viral infection, a nervous habit, or difficult-to-move secretions, which may occur with postnasal drip.

Acute onset or change in a cough is obvious to the patient and family and probably to the interviewer; therefore, an accurate history is very important and easily obtained. However, careful inquiry is often required to identify the characteristics of a chronic cough. Because coughing and sputum production are generally not socially acceptable, patients may deny or minimize the presence of the cough or learn to adapt to the extent that they may even be unaware of coughing chronically. Questioning family members or close friends may provide valuable information about the presence and characteristics of a cough.

QUESTIONS TO ASK

Cough

Ask the patient to describe the cough in his or her own words; if unable to give a description, use suggestions of descriptive words.

- Can you describe your cough? How long have you had the cough?
- When did the cough start? Did the cough start suddenly? What were you doing when the cough started?
- Do you smoke? If so, what do you smoke? How much and for how many years?
- Do you have postnasal drip? Do you wheeze? Do you have heartburn? Do you notice an acid or bitter taste in your mouth?
- Do you cough up sputum or mucus and, if so, what is the amount, color, thickness, and odor?

QUESTIONS TO ASK—cont'd

Cough

- Is your cough better or worse at certain times of the day and does it wake you up?
- Do you cough on most days? Do you cough more during a particular day of the week? A particular season of the year?
- Is the cough worse in any position or when you are in a certain location?
- Is the cough associated with eating, drinking, or medications?
- Are there any other symptoms associated with the cough like chest pain? Wheezing? Fever? Runny nose? Hoarseness? Night sweats? Weight loss? Headache? Dizziness? Loss of consciousness?
- What relieves the cough?
- Have you had the flu or a "cold" with a cough recently?
- Have you ever been exposed to anyone with tuberculosis, the flu or a "cold"?
- Do you have contact with animals? If so, what type, when, and how often?
- Are you taking ACE inhibitors? Have you taken ACE inhibitors in the past?
- Are you under stress?
- Is your cough dry? Do you clear your throat frequently?
- Have you been diagnosed with nasal allergies or allergic rhinitis?
- Do you have chronic bad breath (halitosis)? Do you have facial pain?
- Do you sleep with more than one pillow?
- Do you cough after exercise or physical exertion?
- What is your occupation? Is your cough worse during or immediately after work?

Sputum Production

Sputum is the substance expelled from the tracheobronchial tree, pharynx, mouth, sinuses, and nose by coughing or clearing the throat. The term **phlegm** refers strictly to secretions from the lungs and tracheobronchial tree. These respiratory tract secretions may contain a variety of materials, including mucus, cellular debris, microorganisms, blood, pus, and foreign particles, and should not be confused with saliva. The tracheobronchial tree normally secretes up to 100 mL of sputum each day. Sputum is moved upward by the wavelike motion of the cilia (tiny hairlike structures) lining the larynx, trachea, and bronchi, and it is usually swallowed unnoticed. As previously mentioned, sputum may be difficult or impossible for the patient to describe accurately because of the social stigma and lack of awareness. Thus, collection and inspection of a sputum sample is often necessary to evaluate the patient's pulmonary status.

Causes and Descriptions

Excessive sputum production is most often caused by inflammation of the mucous glands that line the

TABLE 3-2

Terms Used to Describe Cough

Description	Possible Causes
Acute (<3 wk) or recurrent (adults) productive	Postnasal drip, allergies, infections, especially viral URI, bronchitis
Acute or recurrent (adults) and nonproductive	Laryngitis, inhalation of irritant gases
Chronic productive	Bronchiectasis, chronic bronchitis, lung abscess, asthma, fungal infections, bacterial pneumonias, tuberculosis
Chronic (>3 wk) or recurrent (adults) and nonproductive	Postnasal drip, asthma, gastroesophageal reflux, bronchiectasis, COPD, lung tumor, sarcoidosis, ACE inhibitors, left heart failure
Recurrent (children)	Viral bronchitis, asthma, allergies
Dry	Viral infections, inhalation of irritant gases, interstitial lung diseases, pleural effusion, cardiac condition, nervous habit, tumor, radiation therapy, chemotherapy
Dry, progressing to productive	Atypical and mycoplasmal pneumonia, AIDS, legionnaires disease, asthma, silicosis, pulmonary embolus and edema, lung abscess, emphysema (late in disease), smoking
Inadequate, weak	Debility, weakness, oversedation, pain, poor motivation, emphysema
Paroxysmal (especially night)	Aspiration, asthma, left heart failure
Barking	Epiglottal disease, croup, influenza, laryngotracheal bronchitis
Brassy or hoarse	Laryngitis, laryngotracheal bronchitis, laryngeal paralysis, pressure on recurrent laryngeal nerve: mediastinal tumor, aortic aneurysm, left atrial enlargement
Inspiratory stridor	Tracheal or mainstem bronchial obstruction, croup, epiglottitis
Wheezy	Bronchospasm, asthma, bronchitis, cystic fibrosis
Morning	Chronic bronchitis, smoking
Associated with position change or lying down	Bronchiectasis, left heart failure, chronic postnasal drip or sinusitis, gastroesophageal reflux with aspiration
Associated with eating or drinking	Neuromuscular disease of the upper airway, esophageal problems, aspiration

ACE, angiotensin-converting enzyme; AIDS, acquired immunodeficiency syndrome; COPD, chronic obstructive pulmonary disease; TB, tuberculosis; URI, upper respiratory infection (common cold).

tracheobronchial tree. Inflammation of these glands occurs most often with infection, cigarette smoking, and allergies.

Sputum should be described as to the color, consistency, odor, quantity, time of day, and presence of blood or other distinguishing matter. The amount may vary from scanty (a few teaspoons) to copious (as much as a pint or more), as

TABLE 3-3

Presumptive Sputum Analysis

Appearance of Sputum	Possible Cause
Clear, colorless, like egg white	Normal
Black	Smoke or coal dust inhalation
Brownish	Cigarette smoker
Frothy white or pink	Pulmonary edema
Sand or small stone	Aspiration of foreign material, broncholithiasis
Purulent (contains pus)	Infection, pneumonia caused by:
Apple-green, thick	*Haemophilus influenzae*
Pink, thin, blood-streaked	Streptococci or staphylococci
Red currant jelly	*Klebsiella* species
Rusty	Pneumococci
Yellow or green, copious	*Pseudomonas* species pneumonia, advanced chronic bronchitis, bronchiectasis (separates into layers)
Foul odor (fetid)	Lung abscess, aspiration, anaerobic infections, bronchiectasis
Mucoid (white-gray and thick)	Emphysema, pulmonary tuberculosis, early chronic bronchitis, neoplasms, asthma
Grayish	Legionnaires disease
Silicone-like casts	Bronchial asthma
Mucopurulent	As above with infection, pneumonia, cystic fibrosis
Blood-streaked or hemoptysis (frankly bloody)	Bronchogenic carcinoma, tuberculosis, chronic bronchitis, coagulopathy, pulmonary contusion or abscess (see discussion of causes of hemoptysis)

seen in certain chronic bronchial infections and bronchiectasis. These characteristics of the sputum may be highly indicative of the underlying disorder (Table 3-3). Though sputum culture and sensitivity tests described in Chapter 7 provide for a more in depth microbiologic examination of sputum, bedside examination can be helpful as an initial screening tool.

The consistency of sputum may be described as thin, thick, viscous (gelatinous), **tenacious** (extremely sticky), or **frothy**. Color depends on the origin and cause of the sputum production. Descriptions for the color of sputum include mucoid (clear, thin, and may be somewhat viscid as a result of oversecretion of bronchial mucus), mucopurulent (thick, viscous, colored, and often in globs with an offensive odor), and blood-tinged. Copious, foul-smelling **(fetid)** sputum that separates into layers when standing occurs with bronchiectasis and lung abscess when the patient's position is changed.

Morning expectoration implies accumulation of secretions during the night and is commonly seen with bronchitis. Nonpurulent, silicone-like bronchial casts are seen with asthma. Sudden large amounts of sputum production may be indicative of a bronchopleural fistula.

QUESTIONS TO ASK

Sputum

Ask the patient to describe the sputum in his or her own words; if unable to give a description, use suggestions of descriptive words (e.g., green, yellow, white, clear, teaspoon, tablespoon, cup).

- Do you usually bring up phlegm or mucus from your chest first thing in the morning?
- Do you usually bring up phlegm or mucus at other times of the day?
- Can you estimate the amount you bring up? About a cup? About a tablespoon? Has this amount changed?
- What color is it? Does it have a foul odor?
- Has the sputum changed color recently?

SIMPLY STATED

Chronic sputum production is most often related to irritation or disease of the airways (e.g., asthma or chronic bronchitis).

Hemoptysis

Definition

Hemoptysis, expectoration of sputum containing blood, varies in severity from slight streaking to frank bleeding. It can be an alarming symptom that may suggest serious disease and massive hemorrhage. In more severe forms, it is a frightening experience for both the patient and the RT or other member of the health care team.

Causes

Differential diagnosis is complex and includes bronchopulmonary, cardiovascular, hematologic, and other systemic disorders (Box 3-1). A history of pulmonary or cardiovascular disease; cigarette smoking and tobacco use; trauma; aspiration of a foreign body; repeated and severe lung infections; bleeding disorder; use of anticoagulant agents (warfarin or heparin), aspirin, nonsteroidal anti-inflammatory agents, or chemotherapeutic agents; or inhaling crack cocaine suggests the possible cause of hemoptysis. A history of travel to places where tuberculosis or fungal infections, such as coccidioidomycosis or histoplasmosis, are prevalent, including central Africa (tuberculosis) and the San Joaquin Valley of California (coccidioidomycosis), may also help identify the underlying disorder.

The site of bleeding may be anywhere in the respiratory tract, including the nose or mouth. The amount and mechanisms of bleeding are varied. Tissues engorged by inflammation or backpressure from heart failure or other cardiac problems may bleed easily and cause frothy pink sputum. Trauma bruises tissue or may tear a vessel. Chronic or repeated respiratory infections resulting in bronchiectasis can predispose the patient to bleeding. A tumor or granuloma can erode surrounding tissue or the bronchial

Box 3-1	Notable Causes of Hemoptysis

FREQUENT CAUSES OF HEMOPTYSIS
Acute bronchitis with severe coughing
Bronchogenic carcinoma
Bronchiectasis*
Chronic bronchitis*
Tuberculosis*

LESS FREQUENT CAUSES OF HEMOPTYSIS
PULMONARY
Aspiration of a foreign body
Bronchoarterial fistula*
Broncholithiasis
Deep mycotic infection*
Metastatic carcinoma
Pulmonary abscess*
Pulmonary embolism, infarction
Trauma, pulmonary contusion

CARDIOPULMONARY
Arteriovenous malformation
Mitral stenosis
Cardiac pulmonary edema
Pulmonary hypertension

SYSTEMIC
Coagulation disorders*
Goodpasture syndrome
Sarcoidosis, Wegener granulomatosis

OTHER PSEUDOHEMOPTYSES
Emesis
Oropharyngeal or nosebleed

---

*Potential causes of massive hemoptysis.

TABLE 3-4

Distinguishing Characteristics of Hemoptysis and Hematemesis

Characteristic	Hemoptysis	Hematemesis
History	Cardiopulmonary disease	Gastrointestinal disease
As stated by the patient	Coughed up from lungs/chest	Vomited from stomach
Associated symptoms	Dyspnea, pain or tickling sensation in chest	Nausea, pain referred to stomach
Blood: pH	Alkaline	Acid
Mixed with	Sputum	Food
Froth	May be present	Absent
Color	Bright red	Dark, clotted, "coffee grounds"

Careful evaluation and description of hemoptysis is crucial because it can include clots of blood as well as blood-tinged sputum. Coughing up clots of blood is a symptom of extreme importance suggesting serious illness. Massive hemoptysis (400 mL in 3 hours or more than 600 mL in 24 hours) is seen with lung cancers, tuberculosis, bronchiectasis, and trauma. It is an emergency condition associated with possible mortality. Immediate action is required to maintain an adequate airway, and emergency bronchoscopy and surgery may be necessary.

Associated symptoms may also provide a clue to the source of bleeding. Sometimes patients can describe a sensation, often warmth, in the area where the blood originates. Others perceive a bubbling sensation in the tracheobronchial tree followed by expectoration of blood. Hemoptysis associated with sudden onset of chest pain and dyspnea in a patient at risk for venous stasis of the legs must prompt evaluation for pulmonary embolism and possible infarction. Frothy, blood-tinged sputum associated with paroxysmal cough accompanies cardiac-induced pulmonary edema.

Hemoptysis without severe coughing suggests a cavitary lesion in the lung or bronchial tumor.

Hemoptysis versus Hematemesis

"Spitting up blood," as patients frequently call it, may be confused with blood originating in the oropharynx, esophagus, or stomach. The patient with a nosebleed at night could cough up blood in the morning. The presence of symptoms, such as nausea and vomiting, especially with a history of alcoholism or cirrhosis of the liver, may suggest the esophagus or stomach as the source. Conversely, vomiting of blood may sometimes manifest from bronchopulmonary bleeding. When bleeding occurs during the night and the blood reaches the oropharynx, it may be swallowed without the patient waking. The swallowed blood may act as an irritant, and the patient may vomit early in the morning. Careful questioning and often examination of the bloody sputum are required to distinguish hemoptysis from **hematemesis** (vomited blood) (Table 3-4). It is

---

wall. An acute infective process can create an abscess in the bronchial tree or lung parenchyma, which can erode into another structure (e.g., bronchopleural fistula) or completely through a vessel wall. If the vessel is an artery, hemorrhage can be sudden and massive and may lead to death due to excessive blood loss.

Historically, tuberculosis and bronchiectasis were the most common causes of hemoptysis. Erosive bronchitis in smokers with chronic bronchitis and bronchogenic carcinoma are now also recognized as frequent causes of hemoptysis. In fact, blood-streaked sputum may be the only hint that bronchogenic cancer has developed in the smoker.

Descriptions

Obtaining a description of the amount, odor, color, and appearance of blood produced, as well as the acuteness or chronicity of the bleeding, may provide a clue to the source of bleeding. The most common causes of streaky hemoptysis are pulmonary infection (chronic bronchitis, bronchiectasis, or bacterial pneumonias), lung cancer, and thromboemboli. Small stones or gravel mixed with the sputum and blood suggests broncholithiasis.

important to obtain a detailed sequence of events to determine whether the blood originated in the respiratory tract and was swallowed and then vomited, or the blood was vomited, aspirated, and later expectorated.

QUESTIONS TO ASK

Hemoptysis

Ask the patient the following questions to help obtain an accurate and impartial history:

- Do you smoke? If so, how much and what do you smoke?
- Do you use smokeless tobacco? If so, how much and what do you use?
- Did you start coughing up blood suddenly?
- How long have you noticed the blood?
- Do you have a fever? Do you have a cough?
- Do you cough up anything else with the blood? Can you describe what it looks like?
- Is the sputum blood-tinged or are there actual clots of blood?
- Have there been recurrent episodes of coughing up blood?
- Do you have chest pain?
- What seems to bring on the coughing up of blood? Is it brought on by vomiting, coughing, or nausea?
- Have you felt any unusual sensations in your chest after you cough up the blood? Before you cough up the blood? If yes, where? Can you tell me how it feels?
- Have you had a recent nosebleed?
- Have you been involved in a recent accident or had an injury to your chest, side, or back?
- Have you traveled lately?
- Have you ever had tuberculosis? Have you been exposed to anyone who has had tuberculosis?
- Are you HIV positive? Do you have a history of cancer?
- Have you had recent surgery?
- Have you had night sweats? Shortness of breath? Irregular heartbeats? Hoarseness? Weight loss? Swelling or pain in your legs?
- Is there a family history of coughing up blood? Are you aware of any bleeding tendency in you or your family?
- Have you been exposed to anything at work or hobbies?
- Do you take any blood thinners or aspirin? If yes, how much and how often? Do you take oral contraceptives? Do you use injection drugs?

Shortness of Breath (Dyspnea)

Shortness of breath (SOB), as it is commonly abbreviated in the medical record) or difficult breathing as perceived by the patient is the most distressing symptom of respiratory disease and is also a cardinal symptom of cardiac disease. Dyspnea may also be associated with metabolic diseases, hematologic disorders, toxic ingestion, or psychiatric conditions. Difficult breathing impairs the ability to work or exercise and may interfere with the simplest activities of daily living such as walking, eating, bathing, speaking, and sleeping. In patients with pulmonary disease, it is the single most important factor limiting their ability to function on a day-to-day basis and is frequently the reason the patient seeks medical care.

Dyspnea (*dys*, difficult; *pnea*, breathing) is defined as a subjective experience of breathing discomfort that consists of qualitatively distinct sensations that vary in intensity. The sensations associated with dyspnea range from a slight awareness of breathing to severe respiratory distress and may be mixed with anxiety in severe cases. The sensations experienced by the patient are a product of various factors such as the severity of the physiologic impairment and the psychological makeup of the patient.

Subjectiveness of Dyspnea

Dyspnea may be difficult to evaluate because it is so subjective. The sensation of dyspnea is made up of the following components:

1. *Sensory input to the cerebral cortex.* Multiple sources of sensory information from mechanoreceptors in the upper airway, thorax, and muscles are integrated in the central nervous system and sent to the sensorimotor cortex in the brain. In general, the sensation of dyspnea is related to the intensity of the input from the thoracic structures and from chemoreceptors. It varies directly with ventilatory demand such as exercise and inversely with ventilatory capacity (ability to move gas in and out of the lung). The more stimulation of the drive to breathe when ventilatory abnormalities exist, the greater the dyspnea.

2. *Perception of the sensation.* Perception relies on interpretation of the information arriving at the sensorimotor cortex, and interpretation is highly dependent on the psychological makeup of the person. The emotional state, distraction, and belief of significance can influence the perception of dyspnea.

A patient's perception of dyspnea may have no relation to the patient's breathing appearance. Remember, dyspnea is subjective—a symptom—and what the patient feels. A patient may have labored and rapid breathing and deny feeling short of breath. Conversely, a patient may appear to be breathing comfortably and slowly but may feel breathless. You can never assume that a patient with a rapid respiratory rate is dyspneic. In addition, a patient's complaint of dyspnea must be considered a symptom of a medical problem and must be taken seriously until proved otherwise. In fact, the onset of dyspnea may be the first clue to identifying serious problems.

Patients' perceptions of dyspnea vary greatly. A healthy person notices the increased ventilatory demand required to climb stairs or to exercise but expects it and does not interpret it as unpleasant. In fact, the athlete may consider the breathlessness occurring after a sprint to be exhilarating and even a necessary aspect of physical conditioning.

<table>
<tr><td colspan="2">TABLE 3-5</td></tr>
</table>

TABLE 3-5

Modified Borg Scale for Estimation of Subjective Symptoms

Rating	Intensity of Sensation
0	Nothing at all
0.5	Very, very mild/weak
1	Very mild/weak
2	Mild/weak
3	Moderate
4	Somewhat severe/strong
5	
6	
7	Very severe/strong
8	
9	Very, very severe/strong
10	MAXIMAL

TABLE 3-6

American Thoracic Society Shortness of Breath Scale

Degree	Description	Grade
None	No breathlessness except with exercise	0
Slight	Troubled by shortness of breath when hurrying on the level or walking up a slight hill	1
Moderate	Walks more slowly than people of the same age on the level because of breathlessness or has to stop for breath when walking at own pace on the level	2
Severe	Stops for breath after walking about 100 yards or after a few minutes on the level	3
Very severe	Too breathless to leave the house; breathless when dressing or undressing	4

(From Muza SR, Silverman MY, Gilmore GC et al: Comparison of scales used to quantitate the sense of effort to breath in patients with chronic obstructive pulmonary disease, Am Rev Respir Dis 141:909, 1990.)

Patients, on the other hand, may describe the feeling as "breathless," "short winded," "feeling of suffocation," or a sensation of "air hunger" at rest or during minimal exercise.

Dyspnea Scoring Systems

A variety of methods have been devised to help quantify dyspnea at a single point in time or to help track changes in dyspnea over time or with treatment. In the clinical setting, patients are frequently asked to rate the severity of a symptom, such as dyspnea or pain, using a severity scale of 0 to 10. The patient is asked a question such as "On a scale of 0 to 10, how would you rate your shortness of breath when you are resting? Using this scale, 0 means no shortness of breath, and 10 means the worst or maximum shortness of breath." The patient's response may be recorded simply as "SOB at rest 7/10."

Visual analog scales are straight lines, usually 10 cm long, with the words "Not Breathless" at one end and "Extremely Breathless" at the other end. The patient marks the line to indicate his or her level of respiratory discomfort. The score is measured as the length of the line between "Not Breathless" and the mark made by the patient. The score may be recorded as 5.5/10 or simply as 5.5 (the 10 is implied).

A Modified Borg Scale, such as shown in Table 3-5, also uses a 0 to 10 scoring system with descriptive terms to depict the perceived intensity of a symptom such as dyspnea after a specified task. Tools like the frequently used American Thoracic Society Shortness of Breath Scale (Table 3-6) specify the degree of dyspnea (slight, moderate, severe, or very severe) using descriptive terms as well as a numerical grading system. In addition, there are also questionnaires that attempt to quantify the severity of dyspnea by asking patients to rate their shortness of breath while performing a variety of activities of daily living.

More recently, other scales have emerged for rating dyspnea in cardiopulmonary disease. One such scale is the Dyspnea-12 Survey, or "D-12," which quantifies a patient's level of breathlessness using 12 physical and psychosocial descriptors. This rating scale is showing particular promise in determining the severity of dyspnea in patients who have asthma.

Causes, Types, and Clinical Presentation of Dyspnea

Dyspnea is most often related to pulmonary or cardiac disease, but it is also seen with hematologic, metabolic, chemical, neurologic, psychogenic, and mechanical disorders. Dyspnea may be described by clinical type as shown in Table 3-7, or the causes of dyspnea may be grouped by body system as listed in Table 3-8.

Attempts to understand the physiologic bases of dyspnea have evolved around several separate concepts, including mechanics of breathing, ventilatory performance, work and efficiency of breathing, oxygen cost, length-tension inappropriateness, chemoreception, and exercise testing. The discussion of each concept and its related disorders is beyond the scope of this text. However, it is helpful to remember that patients with respiratory disorders will complain of dyspnea when any of the following are present alone or in combination:

1. The work of breathing is abnormally high for the given level of exertion. This is common with narrowed airways as in asthma and when the lung is stiff as in pneumonia.
2. The ventilatory capacity is reduced. This is common when the vital capacity is abnormally low as seen in patients with neuromuscular disease.
3. The drive to breathe is elevated beyond normal (e.g., hypoxemia, acidosis, or exercise).

Clinical Types of Dyspnea

The physiologic cause of a patient's dyspnea often results in the patient using unique terms to describe his or her discomfort. The patient with asthma frequently describes

TABLE 3-7

Clinical Types of Dyspnea

Dyspnea	Associated with	Associated Signs and Symptoms
Physiologic	Exercise, acute hypoxia (e.g., high altitude)	Awareness of increased ventilation
	Breathing high concentration of CO_2 in a closed space	If space is also devoid of O_2, confusion and unconsciousness may occur before dyspnea warns of danger
Pulmonary		
Restrictive	Pulmonary fibrosis	Comfortable at rest
	Chest deformities	Intensely dyspneic when exertion nears patient's limited breathing capacity
	Pleural effusion	
	Pneumothorax	
Obstructive	Asthma	Increased ventilator effort
	Obstructive emphysema	Dyspnea at rest
		Breathing labored and retarded, especially during expiration
Cardiac	Heart failure	Orthopnea, paroxysmal nocturnal dyspnea, "cardiac asthma," periodic respiration
Circulatory	Chronic anemia	Dyspnea only with exertion unless anemia is extreme
	Exsanguinating hemorrhage	"Air hunger" a grave sign
Chemical	Uremia (kidney failure)	Dyspnea with severe panting caused by acidosis, heart failure, pulmonary edema, and anemia
Central	Head injury	Hyperventilation
	Cerebral lesion	Intense hyperventilation
		Sometimes noisy and stertorous
		Biot respiration
Psychogenic	Pain-related dyspnea	Continuous hyperventilation or deep sighing respirations at maximal depth
	Hysterical overbreathing	
	Sighing dyspnea	

TABLE 3-8

Causes of Dyspnea by Body System

System	Common Causes of Dyspnea
Respiratory	Airway obstruction, asthma, COPD, pneumonia, pulmonary embolus, pneumothorax, pulmonary fibrosis, pleural effusion
Cardiac	Congestive heart failure, pericardial effusion, cardiac shunts, valvular lesions
Hematologic	Severe anemia, carbon monoxide poisoning, hemoglobinopathies
Neurologic	Brain tumor, CNS inflammation, increased intracranial pressure, hypertensive encephalopathy, CVA
Metabolic and endocrine	Toxins, uremia, hepatic coma, thyrotoxicosis, myxedema
Psychiatric	Pain-related dyspnea, severe anxiety, hyperventilation syndrome
Mechanical factors	Chest wall deformities, diaphragmatic paralysis, hepatosplenomegaly, massive ascites, tumors, pregnancy, obesity

CNS, central nervous system; COPD, chronic obstructive pulmonary disease; CVA, cerebrovascular accident.

dyspnea as "tightness in the chest." Patients with congestive heart failure (CHF) often describe a sensation of "suffocation" or "air hunger." Patients with COPD and interstitial lung disease often complain of "increased effort to breathe," probably because of the increased work of breathing associated with these disorders. These results suggest that dyspnea may vary from patient to patient according to the underlying pathophysiology.

Cardiac- and circulatory-related dyspnea occurs primarily when there is an inadequate supply of oxygen to the tissues. In early heart failure, dyspnea is seen primarily during exercise when the decreased pumping power of the heart cannot keep up with the demands created by exercise. The shortness of breath may be accompanied by hyperventilation and be associated with fatigue or a feeling of smothering or sternal compression. In later stages, the lungs become congested with blood and edema, causing an increase in the work of breathing and dyspnea at rest and when lying down. Dyspnea is also associated with anemia and occurs primarily with exertion unless the anemia is extreme. "Air hunger" is a grave sign indicating the need for immediate transfusion in the anemic patient.

Psychogenic dyspnea, or *panic disorder* as it is sometimes called, is a hysterical type of overbreathing that usually presents as breathlessness. A precipitating event other than a stress can rarely be identified. The event is not related to exertion; testing and physical examination are negative. Hyperventilation is common in patients with panic disorder.

Hyperventilating is breathing at a rate and depth in excess of the body's metabolic need, which causes a decrease in arterial carbon dioxide ($Paco_2$) and results in a decrease in cerebral blood flow. Patients with psychogenic dyspnea are usually very anxious and may describe feeling faint or lightheaded, with numbness and tingling around

---

Box 3-2   Common Causes of Acute and Chronic Dyspnea

ACUTE DYSPNEA

Asthma*
Chest trauma
Physical exertion
Pleural effusion
Pneumonia
Pulmonary edema
Pulmonary embolism
Pulmonary hemorrhage
Spontaneous pneumothorax
Cardiac pulmonary edema
Acute interstitial lung disease (e.g., hemorrhage, ARDS)
Upper airway obstruction (e.g., aspirated foreign body, laryngospasm)

CHRONIC DYSPNEA

(usually progressive)

Asthma*
CHF, left ventricular failure*
Cystic fibrosis
Pleural effusion
Interstitial lung diseases
Pulmonary vascular disease
Pulmonary thromboembolic disease
COPD
Severe anemia
Psychogenic dyspnea
Hypersensitivity disorders
Chest wall abnormalities (e.g., neuromuscular disease, kyphoscoliosis, diaphragm paralysis)

---

*Asthma and left ventricular failure represent chronic causes of dyspnea with paroxysmal exacerbations.
ARDS, acute respiratory distress syndrome; CHF, congestive heart failure; COPD, chronic obstructive pulmonary disease.

---

their mouth and in their extremities. They may report having visual disturbances. If they continue to hyperventilate, they may lose consciousness.

Acute and Chronic Dyspnea

Dyspnea may be acute or chronic, progressive, recurrent, paroxysmal, or episodic. Acute dyspnea in children is most frequently associated with asthma, bronchiolitis, croup, and epiglottitis. In adults, the causes are more varied (Box 3-2). Pulmonary embolism should be suspected if a patient is in the postoperative period or has a history of prolonged bed rest, phlebitis, or cardiac arrhythmia. Women who are pregnant or taking birth control pills are also at higher risk for pulmonary embolism. Asthma, upper airway obstruction, foreign body aspiration, pneumonia, pneumothorax, pulmonary edema, hyperventilation, and panic disorder may also cause acute dyspnea.

Chronic dyspnea is almost always progressive. It begins with dyspnea on exertion and over time progresses to dyspnea at rest. Most patients with chronic dyspnea do not seek medical help until their lung disease is advanced, and treatment options are limited. Instead, as their lung disease progresses, they adopt a sedentary lifestyle that requires very little exertion to avoid feeling short of breath.

COPD and chronic CHF are the most common causes of chronic dyspnea in adults. Determining whether the dyspnea is related to the lungs versus the heart can be difficult, especially in older patients. Pulmonary function testing, electrocardiogram, and chest radiographs often prove helpful.

Descriptions

Patients may complain of dyspnea occurring at certain times of the day, in association with a position, or during a specific phase of the respiratory cycle. Inspiratory dyspnea is usually associated with upper airway obstruction, whereas expiratory dyspnea occurs with obstruction of smaller bronchi and bronchioles.

Paroxysmal nocturnal dyspnea (PND) is the sudden onset of difficult breathing that occurs when a sleeping patient is in the recumbent position. It is often associated with coughing and is relieved when the patient assumes an upright position. In patients with CHF, PND usually occurs 1 to 2 hours after lying down and is caused by the gradual transfer of fluid in the lower extremities to the lungs.

Orthopnea is the inability to breathe when lying down. It is often described as two- or three-pillow orthopnea, depending on the number of pillows the patient must use to elevate the upper portion of the body and obtain relief. PND and orthopnea are most commonly associated with left-sided heart failure and occur when reclining causes fluid to collect in the lungs.

Trepopnea is dyspnea caused by lying on one side that does not occur when the patient turns to the other side. Trepopnea is most often associated with disorders of the chest that occur on only one side such as unilateral lung disease, unilateral pleural effusion, or unilateral airway obstruction.

Platypnea, the opposite of orthopnea, is dyspnea caused by upright posture and relieved by a recumbent position. **Orthodeoxia** (*ortho*, positional; *deoxia*, decrease of oxygen) is arterial oxygen desaturation (hypoxemia) that is produced by assuming an upright position and relieved by returning to a recumbent position. Orthodeoxia and platypnea are seen in patients with right-to-left intracardiac shunts from congenital heart disease and in patients with venous-to-arterial shunts in the lung related to severe lung disease or chronic liver diseases such as cirrhosis. Simply stated, when these patients are upright, there is an increased amount of blood being shunted from the right side of the heart to the left without being adequately oxygenated. When orthodeoxia is severe, patients experience increasing dyspnea (platypnea) while standing. Orthodeoxia also may occur after a pneumonectomy (removal of a lung). Terms commonly used to describe dyspnea are listed in Table 3-9.

Occurrences of dyspnea should be chronologically recorded, including related symptoms such as coughing, wheezing, pain, position, and exertion. Coughing in conjunction with dyspnea occurs with acute or chronic infection, asthma, aspiration, CHF, COPD, and many of the diffuse lung diseases. Dyspnea with minimal exertion is frequently associated with poor conditioning, inactivity, obesity, and heavy smoking. Shortness of breath during exercise or excitement is also a common complaint associated with chronic severe anemia (e.g., hemoglobin concentration <6 to 7g/dL). Table 3-10 lists associated symptoms, precipitating and relieving factors, and characteristics of the dyspnea-related disorders.

The effects of dyspnea on activities of daily living (dressing, eating, sleeping, or walking) must be reviewed. Patients with COPD tend to decrease their exercise progressively to prevent being short of breath until their activities of daily living are compromised out of proportion to their actual cardiorespiratory potential. It is essential to gain a picture of the patient's daily habits and routines as well as the physical, emotional, familial, and occupational environment. The potential for relief of the factors contributing to dyspnea should be assessed and recorded.

TABLE 3-9

Terms Commonly Used to Describe Breathing

Medical Term	Definition
Apnea	Absence of spontaneous ventilation
Dyspnea	Unpleasant awareness of difficulty breathing, shortness of breath, or breathlessness
Eupnea	Normal rate and depth of breathing
Bradypnea	Less than normal rate of breathing
Tachypnea	Rapid rate of breathing
Hypopnea	Decreased depth of breathing
Hypernea	Increased depth of breathing with or without an increased rate
Orthopnea	Dyspnea in the recumbent position but not in the upright or semivertical position
Trepopnea	Dyspnea in one lateral position but not in the other lateral position
Platypnea	Dyspnea caused by upright posture and relieved by a recumbent position
Orthodeoxia	Arterial oxygen desaturation (hypoxemia) that is produced by assuming an upright position and relieved by returning to a recumbent position
Hyperventilation	Increased alveolar ventilation caused by an increased rate or increased depth of breathing or both
Hypoventilation	Decreased alveolar ventilation caused by a decreased rate or decreased depth of breathing or both
Air hunger	A grave sign associated with extreme shortness of breath, indicating the need for immediate treatment

QUESTIONS TO ASK
Shortness of Breath

Ask the patient to describe the shortness of breath in his or her own words; if unable to give a description, then give suggestions of descriptive words (e.g., smothering? hard to catch your breath? suffocating? chest tightness? hard to take a deep breath?).

- What do you do when you experience breathlessness? Can you continue to do what you were doing or do you have to sit down or lie down? Can you continue to speak?
- Does the difficult breathing alter your normal activities during the day? Does it make it hard for you to sleep at night? What makes it better? What makes it worse?
- Are you always short of breath or do you have attacks of breathlessness? (The onset of dyspnea may be gradual or sudden or intermittent.)
- What relieves the attacks? Relaxing? Changing location? Changing position? Taking medication?
- Does a body position, time of day, or certain activity affect your breathing?
- Do the attacks cause your lips or nail beds to turn blue?
- How many stairs can you climb or how many blocks can you walk before you begin to feel short of breath? Do activities like taking a shower, getting dressed, or shopping make you feel short of breath?
- When you feel breathless, do you feel any other symptoms like sweating, cough, or chest discomfort?
- Do you make any sounds like wheezing, whistling, or snoring?
- Does the shortness of breath seem to be getting better or worse or staying the same?
- Have you ever had exposure to asbestos? Sandblasting? Pigeon breeding?
- Have you ever been exposed to anyone with tuberculosis?
- Have you started taking any new medications or has the dose or frequency changed for current medications?
- Do you have any known allergies to food, insects, or latex? (Anaphylaxis)
- Do you have any weakness in your arms or legs, difficulty speaking, or swallowing? (Neuromuscular diseases)
- Do you have any numbness or tingling in your fingertips? Do you feel a sense of fear or doom? Do you have panic attacks or anxiety disorder?
- Have you ever lived near the San Joaquin Valley in California (coccidioidomycosis) or in the Midwest or southeastern United States (histoplasmosis)?

Chest Pain

The causes of chest pain vary greatly and can range from a self-limited orthopedic injury such as a pulled chest muscle to much more serious conditions including cardiac ischemia (low blood supply to the myocardium) or inflammatory disorders affecting thoracic or abdominal structures or organs. As a result, it is important to promptly and correctly determine the cause of a patient's chest pain. However,

TABLE 3-10

Causes and Characteristics of Shortness of Breath

Cause	Type of Dyspnea	Associated Symptoms	Precipitating and Aggravating Factors	Patient Characteristics	Usual Physical Findings
Acute or Recurrent Dyspnea					
Asthma	Acute dyspnea Episodic	Cough indicates asthmatic bronchitis	Allergies, noxious fumes, exercise, recumbency, respiratory tract infection	Most common cause of recurrent dyspnea in children	Bilateral wheezing, prolonged expiration
		Dyspnea may be exertional and/or worse at night	Exposure to cold or use of certain types of β-blockers		
Pneumothorax	Acute onset	Sudden, sharp pleuritic pain	Spontaneous, COPD, trauma, cystic fibrosis	Often a prior history of similar episode, may be familial	Decreased or absent breath sounds Tracheal shift if tension pneumothorax
Foreign-body aspiration	Acute dyspnea			Most common in children and intoxicated or semiconscious people during eating	Tachypnea, inspiratory stridor, localized or unilateral wheeze, suprasternal retraction with respiration
Pulmonary emboli	Acute onset	Chest pain, faintness, loss of consciousness	Prolonged recumbency; women using birth control pills, especially those who smoke	Postoperative, phlebitis, postpartum, arrhythmia (atrial fibrillation and flutter)	Tachypnea, crackles, low blood pressure, wheezing → pleural friction rub
Pulmonary edema	Acute onset Episodic	Dyspnea on exertion Orthopnea, PND			Gallop rhythm crackles at bases
Hyperventilation and anxiety	Acute dyspnea, "sighing" respiration	Lightheaded, palpitations, paresthesias (especially around mouth and extremities)	Stress panic	Usually anxious	Signs of anxiety but no signs of dyspnea
Poor physical conditioning	Dyspnea on minimal exertion			Obese, physically inactive	After exercise, pulse slows very gradually
Chronic Dyspnea					
Congestive heart failure	Chronic dyspnea with gradual onset, PND	Edema, dyspnea remains long after exercise is stopped	Exercise, recumbency, trauma, anesthesia, shock, hemorrhage, calcium channel blockers or β-blockers	Older patients, nocturnal dyspnea relieved by sitting	Shallow respirations but not necessarily rapid, basilar crackles, jugular venous distention, edema, third heart sound, hepatomegaly
Chronic bronchitis	Dyspnea not necessarily presenting symptom	Persistent, productive cough	Infection, exertion	Overweight	Coarse crackles, cyanosis
Emphysema	Progressive, usually no dyspnea at rest	Weak cough	Exertion	Malnourished	Hyperinflated lungs, decreased breath sounds, increased resonance, increased AP chest diameter, use of accessory muscles at rest

AP, anteroposterior; COPD, chronic obstructive pulmonary disease; PND, paroxysmal nocturnal dyspnea.

uncovering the root cause can be challenging for many reasons, including the complexity of the nerve structure of the chest, which can result in pain from other locations being referred to the chest and pain from the chest being referred to other sites. For example, pain from indigestion is often referred to the chest. Pain from a dissecting aneurysm of the thoracic aorta may start just below the sternum (anterior substernal location) but then migrates or tears toward the back. Despite such challenges, by investigating the characteristics of a patient's chest pain, the RT can assist in making a correct diagnosis and optimizing patient care.

Chest pain can also occur from musculoskeletal disorders, trauma, drug therapy, indigestion, and anxiety. It can range in character from sharp or stabbing to a vague feeling of heaviness or discomfort. It may be steady or intermittent, mild or acute. It may be caused or aggravated by stress, exertion, deep breathing, coughing, moving, or eating certain foods. The precise cause of chest pain cannot always be determined by taking a history, but it is usually possible to determine whether the origin is from the chest wall, the pleurae, or viscera and whether emergency care is needed. *History taking and the patient interview are key to evaluating chest pain.*

For example, chest pain is the cardinal symptom of heart disease. In its classic presentation, a patient may report "viselike" chest pain radiating down the arms, most often the left, which may spread to the shoulders, neck, jaw, or back. This type of chest pain is known as **angina** and signals a medical emergency. Intervention to open a clogged coronary artery and reestablish blood flow to the heart muscle should occur within about 90 minutes from the onset of pain, or else irreversible damage to the heart muscle is likely. Unfortunately, not all heart pain presents with this classic picture. In fact, in some people, there is only a weak relationship between the severity of the chest pain and the importance of the underlying cause. Therefore, *all chest pain must be taken seriously.*

> **SIMPLY STATED**
>
> Cardiac chest pain in men is most often located in the center of the chest and may radiate to the arm, jaw, or back; in women, it is located across the center of the chest, may radiate to the back and down the legs, and may be accompanied by nausea and dizziness.

The characteristics of the more common causes of chest pain are summarized in Table 3-11.

Pulmonary Causes of Chest Pain

Chest pain caused by pulmonary disease is usually the result of involvement of the chest wall or parietal pleura (the serous membrane that lines the inner chest wall), both of which are well supplied with pain fibers. The lung parenchyma has no pain receptors. However, acute pulmonary diseases such as pneumonia, lung abscess, and pulmonary infarction often involve the overlying pleura and may induce pleuritic pain. Mediastinitis (inflammation of mediastinal structures) causes aching, oppressive retrosternal sensations that may be severe. Chronic disorders of the large airway, such as tracheal or bronchial tumors or ulcers, usually do not cause pain. But the inflammation of tracheobronchitis may induce substernal discomfort that changes to a tearing, rasping, and sharp substernal pain with coughing.

Pleuritic pain, often described as inspiratory pain, is the most common symptom of disease causing inflammation of the pleura (pleurisy). It is sharp, often abrupt in onset, and severe enough to cause the patient to seek medical help (often within hours of onset). It increases with inspiration, a cough, a sneeze, a hiccup, or laughing. Pleuritic pain is usually localized to one side of the chest, frequently the lower, lateral aspect. It may be only partially relieved by splinting and pain medication. Pleuritic pain increases with pressure and movement but not to the same degree as pain originating from the outer chest wall. In contrast, the lung parenchyma and the visceral pleura that cover the lungs are relatively insensitive to pain; therefore, pain with breathing usually indicates involvement of the parietal pleura.

Chest wall pain may originate from the intercostal and pectoral muscles, ribs, and cartilages or from stimulation of a neural pathway (neuralgia) anywhere along a dermatome (skin area innervated by a particular spinal cord segment). It is usually described as a well-localized, constant aching soreness that increases with direct pressure on the area of tenderness and with any arm movement that stretches the thoracic muscles.

Descriptions

The patient's body language, as well as his or her descriptive terms, gives clues about the cause of chest pain. Patients with pleuritic pain may be bent to the side, taking shallow breaths, and holding their chest to decrease the amount of movement. They describe their pain as "sharp," "stabbing," "raw," or "burning," progressing to "excruciating" when they breathe or laugh. A patient with chest wall pain may complain of aching pain or soreness at a specific site and will pull away from being touched. Esophageal pain may be described as "knotlike," "like a big bubble trapped inside," or "burning." Patients with spontaneous pneumothorax or dissecting aortic aneurysm may describe the pain as excruciating "tearing" or "knifelike."

Patients with heart pain (angina) will frequently hold a clenched fist over their sternum as they describe the pain as "aching," "squeezing," "pressing," or "viselike." Their pain is worse with exercise and may prevent them from performing physical activity. The pain may diminish with rest. Patients with this type of chest pain must be evaluated by a physician.

Pain is a purely subjective symptom. The perception of pain varies not only with the source of pain but also with previous experience, culture, personality traits, amount of rest, and emotional implications of the pain. Since chest pain varies from relatively benign neuromuscular skeletal pain (the most common) to life-threatening angina (caused by a decreased blood supply to the heart muscle),

TABLE 3-11

Causes and Characteristics of Chest Pain

Condition	Location and Characteristics	Etiology/Precipitating Factors	Associated Findings
Chest Wall Pain			
Myalgia	Intercostal and pectoralis muscles	Trauma, seizure, nonisometric and isometric exercise, COPD, steroid therapy	Usually no visible erythema or ecchymosis with occult trauma
	Localized dull aching Increases with movement Usually long-lasting	Persistent severe cough	
Chondro-ostealgia	Ribs and cartilages, precisely located (chondral pain in sternal area) Increases with pressure to area, movement, respiration, coughing Can be severe and disabling	Trauma (e.g., steering wheel, cardiopulmonary resuscitation), severe coughing, osteoporosis, tumor, myelocytic leukemia, systemic autoimmune disease, Tietze syndrome, COPD	Rib fractures, chondral dislocations, periostitis, fever with some systemic causes
Neuralgia	Dermatome distribution Superficial tingling to deep burning pain	Thoracic spine disease, metastatic tumor, blunt trauma, herpes zoster (shingles)	Specific changes on x-ray films, fever with infection
Pleuritic and Pulmonary Pain			
Pleuritis (pleurisy)	Pleura, usually well localized Sharp, stabbing, raw, burning Often rapid onset, increased by inspiration, coughing, laughing, hiccupping	Infection/inflammation of pleura, trauma, autoimmune and connective tissue disease	Fever, productive cough, tachypnea, splinting of affected side
Pulmonary embolus, pulmonary infarction	Usually at base of lung, may radiate to abdomen or costal margins Stabbing, sudden onset, increased by inspiration	Immobilization, obesity, pelvic surgery	Symptoms vary with size of embolus Anxiety to panic Dyspnea, tachypnea, tachycardia, coughing with blood-tinged to hemoptoic sputum
Pneumothorax	Lateral thorax, well localized	Interstitial lung disease, bullous emphysema, asthma, idiopathic	Dyspnea, tachypnea, decreased breath sounds on affected side
	Sharp, tearing Sudden onset Increased by inspiration	May follow deep inspiration, Valsalva maneuver, or exercise, or occur at rest	Mediastinal shift and jugular venous distention if tension pneumothorax develops
Tumors	May be localized or diffuse	Invasion of primary or metastatic tumor through parenchyma to parietal pleura, mesothelioma	Symptoms vary with type and location
	Constant, sharp, boring, or dull		Evidence from x-ray films History of asbestos exposure
Pulmonary hypertension (primary)	Substernal, dull, aching, similar to angina Related to stress and exertion	Unknown Seen most commonly in young women	Dyspnea, tachypnea, anxiety, syncope, jugular venous distention
Cardiac Pain			
Angina pectoris	Substernal, may radiate to arms, shoulders, neck, and jaw, and back	Coronary artery blockage or spasm	Anxiety, feeling of impending doom, dyspnea, sweating, nausea
	Tightness or dull, heavy pressure-like pain not related to respiration	Hot, humid weather, large meals, intense emotion, exercise	Relieved by nitroglycerin and rest
Myocardial infarction	Substernal, radiating like angina Sudden crushing, viselike pain lasting minutes to hours		As above, diaphoresis, vomiting Not relieved by nitroglycerin or rest
Pericardial pain	Substernal or parasternal radiating to neck, shoulder, and epigastrium (rarely to arms) Sharp, stabbing, intermittent Intensified by respiration and lying on left side	Inflammation of pericardium, infection, metastatic tumor, trauma, irradiation, autoimmune diseases	Pericardial friction rub Tachycardia, distended neck veins, paradoxical pulse with tamponade, dyspnea

Continued

TABLE 3-11

Causes and Characteristics of Chest Pain—cont'd

Condition	Location and Characteristics	Etiology/Precipitating Factors	Associated Findings
Mediastinal Pain			
Esophageal	Substernal, retrosternal, epigastric	Esophagitis aggravated by bending over, lying down, smoking, ingestion of coffee, fats, large meals	Regurgitation of sour-tasting acid secretions relieved by antacids or may be relieved by nitroglycerin
	Radiates toward shoulders	Esophageal spasm	Hematemesis, shock
	Deep burning pain	Esophageal tear	
	Sudden tearing pain		
Dissecting aortic aneurysm	Tearing midline chest or posterior thoracic pain	Blunt trauma, hypertension, inflammatory or degenerative diseases	May have lower blood pressure in legs or one arm, paralysis, murmur of aortic insufficiency, paradoxical pulse, hypertension, shock, death
	Sudden onset, may last hours		
Tracheobronchitis	Substernal burning discomfort	Acute viral infections, prolonged cigarette smoking	Cough may or may not be productive
	May have fever with infection		May be referred to anterior chest
Other causes	Substernal, retrosternal, epigastric pain or burning	Referred abdominal pain: hiatal hernia, peptic ulcer, gallbladder, acute pancreatitis	Symptoms vary with disease
	Vague tightness to severe crushing		Respiratory distress, tachypnea, diaphoresis, numbness of fingers and around mouth
		Hyperventilation syndrome	Respiratory alkalosis

the interviewer must be careful to obtain an accurate and impartial history. The following characteristics must be reviewed in detail: onset, location, radiation, frequency, duration, severity (a 0 to 10 scale is often used, with 10 being the worst), precipitating and relieving factors, and specific descriptions (e.g., tearing, stabbing, dull, sharp, crushing, or burning). Clues to locating the source of chest pain include a history of trauma, surgery, or muscle strain; local tenderness; swelling; and relationship to inhaling, coughing, position, and activity.

QUESTIONS TO ASK

Chest Pain

Ask the patient the following questions to help obtain an accurate and impartial history:

- Where is the pain?
- Did the pain start suddenly or gradually? Is it more severe now than when it started?
- Have you ever had a pain like this before? What did you do to relieve the pain? Did you take medication to relieve the pain? What medicine did you take?
- How would you describe the pain? (Let the patient describe the character of the pain in his or her own words; if unable to give a description, then use suggestions of descriptive words.) Would you describe the pain as aching? Throbbing? Knifelike? Sharp? Constricting? Sticking? Burning? Dull? Shooting? Tearing?
- Can you rate your pain on a scale of 0 to 10, with 10 being the worst pain you have ever felt?
- How long have you had the pain?
- Do you have recurrent episodes of pain? How often do you get the pain? How long does the pain last?
- What makes the pain worse? Breathing? Lying flat? Moving your arms or neck?
- Is the pain associated with coughing? Shortness of breath? Palpitations? Coughing up blood? Nausea or vomiting? Leg pain? Dizziness? Weakness? Headache? Muscle fatigue?
- Does the pain occur at rest? Exercise? While sleeping? With stress? After eating?
- What do you do to make it better?
- Have you ever had a heart attack? Has anyone in your family had heart disease? At what age?
- Have you had a recent respiratory infection? Do you have pulmonary disease?
- Have you had trauma to your chest? A hip or leg fracture? Been involved in an accident?
- What medications are you taking? Have you recently changed the dose or how you take them?
- Do you take any other type of legal or illegal drugs? If so, what are the drugs, how much and and how often do you take such drugs?

Dizziness and Fainting (Syncope)

Definition

Syncope is a temporary loss of consciousness caused by reduced blood flow and therefore a reduced supply of oxygen and nutrients to the brain. Reduced cerebral blood flow may be localized (as in cerebral thrombosis, embolism, or atherosclerotic obstruction) or generalized, as occurs with obstruction to blood flow from the heart, cardiac arrhythmias, and hypovolemia (decreased available blood volume).

Causes

Pulmonary causes of syncope include pulmonary embolism (obstruction of blood flow from the right heart into the left heart), prolonged bouts of coughing (tussive syncope), and hypoxia (low levels of blood oxygen) or hypocapnia (low levels of carbon dioxide). Holding one's breath after a deep inspiration (Valsalva maneuver) results in high intrathoracic pressure and decreased venous return to the heart. Causes of syncope are listed in Box 3-3. Although some of these causes of syncope are not associated with poor long-term outcomes, others can be serious problems.

The activity that preceded syncope and the position of the patient give clues to the causes of syncope. Primary pulmonary hypertension and some cardiac causes are associated with syncope during exercise. An irregular heart rhythm or palpitations before syncope suggest cardiac arrhythmia as the cause.

Vasovagal syncope, or "common dizziness and fainting," is the most common type of syncope and results from a loss of peripheral venous tone. It can occur with all forms of physical and emotional stress, including (but not limited to) pain; venipuncture; prolonged standing, especially in hot weather; and anxiety. Special attention must be given to careful review of all parts of the history and to the physical examination to rule out the organic causes of syncope.

Orthostatic hypotension is an excessive drop in blood pressure when a person stands up. In normal individuals, standing suddenly causes pooling of blood in the venous capacitance vessels of the legs and trunk, but compensatory mechanisms in the autonomic system maintain blood pressure and the blood supply to the brain. When portions of the reflex arc are impaired by disease processes, drugs, or an inadequate blood volume, these homeostatic mechanisms may be inadequate for restoring the lowered blood pressure. If the patient stands suddenly, the adaptive reflexes do not compensate fast enough, and there is a sudden drop in blood pressure. The patient will experience dizziness, blurring vision, profound weakness, and syncope. Orthostatic hypotension is suggested when a patient reports fainting after suddenly getting up from a chair or after rising suddenly from bed in the middle of the night to run to answer the telephone. Medications that affect vascular tone or vascular volume can lead to orthostatic

---

| Box 3-3 | Causes of Syncope |

CIRCULATORY CONTROL ABNORMALITIES
Drugs (very common)
Vasovagal syncope
Orthostatic hypotension
Hypovolemia
Carotid sinus hypersensitivity
Autonomic failure

CARDIOPULMONARY ABNORMALITIES
VALVULAR AND MYOCARDIAL DISEASE
Prosthetic valve dysfunction
Aortic stenosis
Mitral valve prolapse
Pulmonary stenosis
Pulmonary embolism
Hypertrophic obstructive cardiomyopathy
Acute myocardial ischemia/infarction

INADEQUATE CARDIAC FILLING
Coughing, Valsalva maneuver
Atrial myxoma

CARDIAC ARRHYTHMIAS
Sick sinus syndrome
Atrioventricular block
Supraventricular tachycardia
Ventricular tachycardia
Wolff-Parkinson-White syndrome
Long Q-T syndrome

METABOLIC CONDITIONS
Hypoxia
Hypocapnia
Hypoglycemia
Intoxication

NEUROLOGIC CONDITIONS
Neurovascular disease
Convulsive disorders
Generalized seizures
Transient ischemic attack

PSYCHOLOGICAL CONDITIONS
Hysterical fainting
Panic attacks

---

hypotension. Elderly patients are more prone to orthostatic hypotension because of dehydration.

Carotid sinus syncope is associated with a hypersensitive carotid sinus and is seen more commonly in elderly people. Whenever a patient with carotid sinus syncope wears a tight shirt collar or turns the neck in a certain way, there is an increased stimulation of the carotid sinus. This slows the pulse rate and causes a sudden fall in systemic pressure, resulting in syncope.

Cough (tussive) syncope is the transient loss of consciousness after severe coughing. It occurs most commonly in middle-aged men with underlying COPD who are outgoing and moderately obese and have a great appetite for food, alcohol, and smoking. It rarely occurs in women. The cough may be chronic and is usually dry and unproductive. Typically, there is a "tickle" in the patient's throat precipitating a coughing paroxysm; then the patient's face becomes red, vision dims, the eyes become fixed, and the patient suddenly loses consciousness. The attacks usually last only a few seconds, but the patient may fall or slump in a chair as the muscles relax completely. Some patients have reported more than 20 episodes a day. Cough syncope is usually a benign symptom, and patients return to their previous activity with little recall of the episode. However, deaths and serious injury have been reported when the syncope occurred while driving.

Descriptions

A precise description of the syncopal event should include a description of the preceding events as well as coexisting symptoms, including dyspnea, nausea, neurologic events, angina (chest pain), and palpitations or irregular heartbeat. A careful interview of witnesses (if available) and ambulance personnel can be extremely helpful. In addition, a detailed review of medications and medical history, including known neurologic or heart disease, arrhythmia, pacemaker placement, or known sudden death of a family member, will provide clues to the cause of the syncope.

QUESTIONS TO ASK
Dizziness and Fainting

Ask the patient the following questions to help obtain an accurate and impartial history:

- What do you mean when you say you were dizzy? Felt faint? Did you lose consciousness?
- What were you doing just before you fainted? Did you have any warning that you were going to faint?
- Have you had recurrent fainting spells? If so, how often do you have these attacks?
- What position were you in when you fainted?
- Was the fainting preceded by any other symptom? Nausea? Chest pain? Palpitations? Confusion? Numbness? Hunger? Cough?

Swelling of the Ankles (Dependent Edema)

Definition

Edema is soft tissue swelling resulting from an abnormal accumulation of fluid. It may be generalized (anasarca), may appear only in dependent body areas (feet and ankles in ambulatory patients or the sacral area in patients on bed rest), or may be limited to a single extremity or organ (such as pulmonary edema). Edema is associated with kidney disease, liver disease, cardiac and pulmonary disease, and obstruction of venous or lymphatic drainage of an extremity.

Causes

Peripheral (dependent) edema caused by pulmonary diseases occurs when the disease process causes narrowing of the capillaries in the lung, requiring the right ventricle to generate higher and higher pressures to move blood through the lungs. Gradually, the overworked right ventricle becomes enlarged and unable to pump all of its blood through the lungs. This results in a damming effect that causes the venous system to become engorged with blood. Because of the high pressure in the veins, fluid is pushed out into the tissues. At first, the edema is seen only in the dependent (lower) areas of the body. When the patient has been standing or sitting, the edema is seen in the feet and ankles and is relieved by rest and elevation of the legs. Because patients on bed rest have their legs elevated near the heart level, dependent edema accumulates in the sacral area (back hip area) or at the side of the hip in patients who prefer to lie on their side.

As right heart failure worsens, dependent edema is no longer relieved by rest or changing position, and the edema occurs in the abdominal organs as well as the extremities and dependent areas of the body. As the liver becomes enlarged (hepatomegaly) because of the edema, the patient may also complain of pain just below the ribs on the right side (right upper quadrant pain). Edema of the bowel and ascites (collection of fluid in the abdomen) cause complaints of anorexia, nausea, and sometimes vomiting. Patients may also complain of slowed healing and even skin breakdown in the edematous areas.

Bilateral peripheral, or dependent, edema suggests pulmonary hypertension, heart failure, or venous insufficiency. Unilateral peripheral edema (edema in only one extremity) is most frequently caused by some type of venous obstruction in that extremity, which can occur because of constrictive clothing, jewelry, or wound dressings that surround the extremity and compress venous return. It may also be a danger sign suggesting a deep vein thrombosis (blood clot).

Descriptions

Patients may report that when they press on their swollen ankles or when they remove their shoes and socks, they notice a depression that remains in place for at least several minutes. When compression of an edematous area produces a depression that does not fill immediately, pitting edema is present. In the medical history, pitting edema is usually described in general terms such as "the patient denies pitting edema" or "the patient reports pitting edema in both ankles that remains for at least 5 minutes after leg elevation." When the history and physical examination are reported together, pitting edema may be recorded using the scale shown in Table 3-12.

Peripheral edema is a sign and a symptom. The examiner may find edematous ankles that the patient had not noticed. The presence of edema is such an important factor that the history of the edema should be traced.

TABLE 3-12

Pitting Edema Scale

Scale	Degree	Refill
1+ Trace	Slight	Rapid
2+ Mild	0-0.6 cm (0-¼ in)	10-15 sec
3+ Moderate	0.6-1.3 cm (¼-½ in)	1-2 min
4+ Severe	>1.3 cm (>½ in)	>2 min

Precipitating and alleviating factors and associated symptoms should be documented with the history of present illness.

QUESTIONS TO ASK
Swelling of the Ankles

Ask the patient the following questions to help obtain an accurate and impartial history:

- When did you first notice the swelling? Where else does it occur?
- Does it occur only when you have been standing or sitting for a long time? Or is it present when you first get up in the morning? How does it change throughout the day?
- If you press on the swelling, does it leave a fingerprint in the tissue? How long does the indentation remain?
- What happens to the swelling when you sit with your legs elevated?
- What makes it worse? What makes it better?
- Is the swelling associated with any other activities such as exercise or when you eat food that has a lot of salt?
- Do you have any other symptoms when you have the swelling? [use the following suggestive cues when the patient is unable to answer] Like cough? Difficulty breathing? Pain?

Fever, Chills, and Night Sweats

Normal body temperature (euthermia) varies between 97.0° and 99.5° F (36° and 37.5° C) orally and is 1° to 2° F (0.5° to 1° C) higher in the late afternoon than in the early morning. This normal change of temperature during the day is known as the *diurnal variation.* Body temperature is also affected by age (higher in infants and lower in elderly people), exercise (increases to as high as 100° F during exertion and returns to normal within 30 minutes), excitement, sudden changes in environmental temperature, digestion, technique, and route of measurement (about 1° F higher rectally and about 1° F lower axillary), and use of medications containing antipyretics (drugs that decrease temperature).

Definitions

Fever (hyperthermia or pyrexia) is an elevation of body temperature above the normal range resulting from disease. Fever may be described as sustained (continuously

TABLE 3-13

Terms Used to Describe Fever

Fever, pyrexia	Abnormally high body temperature
High-grade fever	>101° F (38.2° C) orally
Low-grade fever	99.5°-101° F (37.5°-38.2° C) orally
Intermittent fever	Daily elevation with a return to normal or subnormal between spikes
Remittent fever	Continuously elevated with wide, usually diurnal variations
Relapsing fever	Recurring in bouts of several days interspersed with periods of normal temperature
Hyperthermia	Elevation of core body temperature above normal
Mild hyperthermia	99°-102° F (37.2°-38.9° C)
Moderate hyperthermia	102°-105° F (38.9°-40.6° C)
Critical hyperthermia	>105° F (>40.6° C); medical emergency
Malignant hyperthermia	Core body temperature increases 2° F (1° C) every 15 min; occurs in people with an inherited predisposition to the condition
Fever of unknown origin (FUO)	Fever >101° F that has occurred several times in the past 3-4 weeks with no known cause
Hypothermia	Temperature that is below the normal range

elevated, varying little more than 1° F during a 24-hour period), remittent (continuously elevated with wide, usually diurnal, variations), intermittent (daily elevation with a return to normal or subnormal between spikes), or relapsing (recurring in bouts of several days interspersed with periods of normal temperature). Terms used to describe fever are listed in Table 3-13.

Normally, humans increase sweat production about threefold with their diurnal drop in temperature at night. However, when the temperature falls abruptly, as occurs with intermittent fever, sweat production may increase fivefold to eightfold, resulting in **diaphoresis**. When this profuse sweating occurs at night, soaking the bedclothes, it is clinically significant and is termed **night sweats**. Night sweats are common in patients with lymphoma, tuberculosis, and some types of pneumonia.

Causes

Fever is a nonspecific symptom and may be caused by multiple factors, most commonly infection; exposure to a hot environment; dehydration (inadequate fluid volume in the body); reactions to chemical substances, drugs, or protein breakdown; damage to the heat-regulating center in the hypothalamus; malignant neoplasms; connective tissue disease; and a variety of other diseases (Table 3-14). In some patients, a cause is never found, thus the term *fever of unknown origin* (FUO) is used.

TABLE 3-14

Common Causes and Characteristics of Fever

Type	Nature of Fever/Patient	Associated Symptoms	Clinical Findings
Acute			
Upper Respiratory Infection (URI)			
Viral	Usually <101.5°F orally	Cough, signs of URI, may be	Oropharynx infected
	Any age	systemic symptoms	Exposure to URI
Bacterial	Often high temperature, >101° F	Marked signs of URI, few	Pharyngotonsillar exudates
	More common in children	systemic symptoms	Pulmonary findings
			Children are restless
Other Bacterial and Viral Syndromes			
Influenza	Usually mild fever	Muscle aches	Minimal
	Any age		
Acute otitis media (middle ear infection)	More common in children, usually >100° F, often follows URI	Ear and face pain, hearing loss	Ear is sensitive to touch, tympanic membrane appears red and bulging
Gastroenteritis	Any age	Nausea, vomiting, cramps, diarrhea	Dehydration
Urinary tract infection	Often high temperature with chills Adults more common	Backache Usually frequency and urgency	Costovertebral angle tenderness Positive urinalysis
Bacterial sepsis	Often high temperature	Chills	
Factitious fever	Usually >105° F, can be low grade	No weight loss	Disparity between rectal or oral and urine temperature
	Associated with health care	Pulse rate not proportional to fever	May be emotionally disturbed
Drug reaction	Often high temperature, acute or chronic	Occasional rash	Taking prescription or OTC medications Fever abates when drug discontinued
Chronic			
Infectious mononucleosis	Usually low grade Teenagers, young adults	Fatigue	Enanthema, fever, pharyngitis, splenomegaly, adenopathy (especially postcervical)
Tuberculosis	Usually low grade More common in diabetic patients	Cough, fatigue	Chest findings Positive TB test and chest radiograph
Hepatitis	Usually low grade More common in intravenous drug users	Fatigue, jaundice, anorexia	Hepatomegaly, jaundice, liver tender to palpation

OTC, over-the-counter; TB, tuberculosis.

Fever is a concern for two important reasons. First, it often signifies that disease is present. The patient with fever should be evaluated for evidence of infection or other causes. Second, fever causes an increase in the metabolic rate of the patient that is proportional to the degree of temperature elevation. This is of little consequence to the patient with a healthy cardiopulmonary system but may represent a major problem to the patient with chronic lung or heart disease. As the body temperature elevates, the demand for oxygen utilization and carbon dioxide removal both increase. As a result, the patient with chronic cardiopulmonary disease is at higher risk for respiratory failure when significant fever is present.

Fever is usually accompanied by many other constitutional symptoms, such as vague aching, malaise (vague discomfort, or uneasiness), irritability, increased heart rate (9 to 10 beats per minute for each 1° F of elevation), and if high enough, confusion, delirium, or convulsions. A rapidly increasing body temperature may be accompanied by chills and shivering or even rigors (bone-shaking,

teeth-rattling chills) as peripheral vasoconstriction occurs to conserve heat.

Fever with Pulmonary Disorders

Because fever is the most common manifestation of infection, it is usually assumed to be caused by an infectious process until proved otherwise. Pulmonary infections, including lung abscess, empyema (infection within the pleural space), tuberculosis, and pneumonia, are accompanied by fever in most patients. Acute bacterial infections are usually accompanied by shaking chills, although the occurrence of a single rigor followed by sustained fever suggests pneumococcal pneumonia. Remittent fever is seen with mycoplasma, pneumonia, legionnaires disease, and acute viral respiratory infections.

It cannot be assumed that the patient does not have an infection because there is no fever. Patients vary greatly in the degree of fever accompanying a disease process. Patients taking high doses of steroids and other drugs that can be used as immunosuppressants may have no fever in the presence of a massive infection. In addition, patients with a compromised immune system (e.g., leukemia, acquired immunodeficiency syndrome (AIDS)) may have minimal fever despite the presence of severe infection.

Fever, like swelling and wheezing, can be a sign or a symptom. Once the temperature is taken during the physical examination, it is clearly evident that fever is present. However, many patients report fever or chills but have never taken their temperature. It is important to clarify why patients think they have a fever and whether the temperature was taken, to document the route and the patient's technique. The patient should be asked to present any temperature charts that have been made and to describe the pattern of the fever and the accompanying symptoms.

When a cause for fever is not readily apparent, careful attention should also be given to the history of travel, recreation, occupation, and exposure to toxins or carriers of infectious diseases. All drugs used, including over-the-counter (OTC) medications, vitamins, and illicit drugs, should be listed because many drugs, including antibiotics and blood products, can cause drug-related fever.

QUESTIONS TO ASK

Fever, Chills, and Night Sweats

Ask the patient the following questions to help obtain an accurate and impartial history:

- How long have you had fever? How did you measure your temperature? What readings did you get?
- Has there been any pattern to the fever? Did it start gradually or suddenly? Did it rise, then disappear, then reappear?
- Have you had other symptoms with the fever such as chills, headache, fatigue, cough, diarrhea, or pain?
- Has your neck felt swollen? Have you had a sore throat or earache?
- Do you have pain when you take a deep breath or cough? Where is the pain?
- Have you had an infection recently? Can you recall a recent exposure to someone who may have had an infection?
- Have you had a recent wound? How did it heal? Is the area still painful?
- Have you traveled to an area where you may have been bitten by a tick? Insect? Spider? Animal?
- Have you been exposed to high temperatures for a prolonged period of time such as playing sports or working out in the heat? How long were you out in the heat? How much water did you drink while you were working or playing?
- Have you had any unusual physical or emotional stress lately? Injury? Anesthetic? Surgery? Blood transfusion?
- Have you taken any new medications in the last few weeks?
- Are you taking thyroid medication? Antidepressants? Amphetamines or diet pills? Medications that keep you from sweating, such as anticholinergics, phenothiazines, monamine oxidase (MAO) inhibitors?
- Have you ever been told that you have pneumonia? HIV? Cancer?

SIMPLY STATED

In the patient with lung disease, fever usually, but not invariably, signifies infection. However, it cannot be assumed that the patient does not have an infection because there is no fever. Patients taking high doses of steroids and immunosuppressants may have no fever in the presence of massive infection.

Headache, Altered Mental Status, and Personality Changes

There are many causes of headaches and psychosocial changes; some are related to pulmonary problems, whereas other causes may be secondary to medications, neurologic dysfunction, or injury. The patient interview and history outlined in Chapter 2 and the physical examination and laboratory studies can provides important clues to the RT or other member of the patient care team about the cause of such symptoms.

It is important to know that many patients with moderate to severe pulmonary disease experience headaches or some form of mood change. In many instances, such problems are related to insufficient oxygen or excessive carbon dioxide in the arterial blood. When patients cannot get adequate oxygen into their blood, as happens with lung disorders, or when the amount of oxygen in the inspired air is low (as at high altitude), the amount of oxygen available to the brain is decreased (cerebral hypoxia), and headache can occur. Likewise, as the carbon dioxide level in the blood increases, the cerebral arterial vessels dilate, causing vascular headaches with throbbing pain over the entire head. Because hypercapnia worsens during sleep in patients with pulmonary disorders, early-morning headaches may be the first indication that the patient is retaining abnormally high amounts of carbon dioxide. If the hypercapnia persists, headaches may be present throughout the day.

As cerebral hypoxia and hypercapnia worsen, progressive changes occur in the patient's mental status. Thought processes and memory deteriorate, the mind wanders, and the patient is easily distracted. Headaches, tremors, uncontrolled movements, hallucinations, and nightmares may occur. If the hypercapnia continues, alertness is affected, progressing to drowsiness, disorientation, stupor, and then coma.

SIMPLY STATED

Early-morning headache may be the first indication that the patient is retaining abnormally high amounts of carbon dioxide.

Personality changes are not uncommon with advanced pulmonary disorders. The patient may complain of forgetfulness or inability to concentrate. On the other hand, the family may report the patient is depressed, anxious, irritable, demanding, or denying the disease process and refusing to follow the treatment regimen. When chronic lung disease develops from occupational hazards, the patient may be hostile and embittered. Such personality changes may be due to chronic hypoxia or stress or may result from the chronic use of certain medications.

As chronic pulmonary disease progresses, lifestyle options are decreased for the patient and family. Choices of work, play, and even places to live become more limited, and dependency on others increases. Patients must use more of their limited energy to breathe and perform the basic tasks of everyday living. Fears of acute respiratory failure, coughing up blood, another hospitalization, and the possibility of death are always present. As a result, it is not uncommon for patients to deny their illness and refuse to cooperate with treatment, use the illness to demand attention, or channel all of their concerns to the illness and use it as a threat to control others.

However, sudden personality changes or alterations in mental status are indicative of an acute problem. Although such changes are nonspecific and may be seen with neurologic or cardiac disease or intoxication, they also result from hypoxia and hypercapnia. A patient with chronic pulmonary disease who experiences an additional insult, such as trauma, surgery, unusual stress or exertion, pneumothorax, or inhalation of pollutants, may be stressed beyond the ability to adequately oxygenate and remove carbon dioxide from the blood. The patient may have a total change of personality and then deteriorate in a matter of hours. A patient who has been resting quietly and becomes restless deserves the same thorough investigation that would be carried out for the patient who becomes less responsive.

SIMPLY STATED

Sudden personality changes or alteration in mental status are indicative of an acute problem. The patient who suddenly becomes restless deserves the same thorough investigation as the patient who becomes less responsive.

Snoring and Daytime Somnolence (Sleepiness)

Snoring is often a benign symptom that is reported by the patient's spouse or bed partner. However, it can be a symptom of serious concern when it is accompanied with periods of apnea during sleep, sometimes called **sleep disordered breathing**. Patients with this combination and accompanying symptoms such as **daytime somnolence (sleepiness)** must be evaluated for **obstructive sleep apnea (OSA)** by a polysomnograph (sleep study), as discussed in Chapter 19.

Incidence and Causes of Snoring

Snoring occurs in about 10% to 12% of children and 10% to 30% of adults. In children, snoring occurs equally in boys and girls, but in adults, it occurs about twice as often in men. The peak incidence of snoring and OSA occur at ages 50 to 59 years in men and at ages 60 to 64 years in women.

Snoring is caused by excessive narrowing of the upper airway with breathing during sleep. Some narrowing of the hypopharynx is normal with sleep and is the result of muscle relaxation. Excessive narrowing is common when obesity causes a buildup of redundant tissue in the airway. For this reason, obesity is one of the most common causes of snoring and OSA. Enlarged tonsils, a large tongue, a short and thick neck, nasal obstruction, a large soft palate, abuse of alcohol or sleeping pills, and anatomic defects of the upper airway are possible precipitating factors in selected patients. In addition, snoring is influenced by sleeping position because gravity influences the position of the tongue and lower jaw. In the supine position, the lower jaw and tongue tend to flop back into the hypopharynx. Thus, snoring increases in the supine position and is reduced in the lateral or prone position.

Patients who snore most often have inspiratory snoring. Inspiratory snoring is common because the upper airway tends to narrow naturally during each inspiratory effort as air rushes through. Factors that result in narrowing of the upper airway, therefore, become more of an issue on inspiration. The addition of sleep to the picture further complicates the problem when the upper airway support muscles relax. In addition, the greater the inspiratory effort, the greater the drop in pressure within the upper airway, and the more narrow the airway becomes.

The patient with habitual snoring snores each night and often snores loudly. The occasional snorer most often snores only when he or she is excessively tired, has used alcohol or a sleeping medication, or is sleeping in the supine position.

Clinical Presentation

Patients who snore and who have OSA or sleep disordered breathing will complain of excessive daytime somnolence (sleepiness) (EDS). If EDS is not present in the patient who snores, the snoring may be relevant only to the spouse or significant other. The EDS associated with OSA is related to the poor quality of sleep that occurs. Upper airway narrowing increases with the effort to breathe and eventually results in total obstruction and apnea. The apnea continues until the patient arouses somewhat (fragmenting the sleep), and the upper airway muscle tone increases in response to the arousal. The patient then is able to breathe until the deeper stage of sleep returns and the pattern cycles again. These cycles may occur hundreds of times each night of sleep. The result is a night of poor-quality sleep in which the deeper stages are not sustained. The patient awakens feeling fatigued and experiences EDS.

EDS often results in serious consequences, such as occupational accidents, motor vehicle crashes, loss of employment, and social dysfunction. In many cases, there is no association made between daytime sleepiness and snoring by the patient, the family, or the patient's family physician.

Poor daytime concentration, bedwetting, impotence, high blood pressure, and other complicating factors are seen, especially in more severe cases.

SIMPLY STATED

Patients with loud snoring and excessive daytime sleepiness should be evaluated for obstructive sleep apnea (OSA).

Gastroesophageal Reflux

Gastroesophageal reflux disease (GERD) is defined as symptoms produced by the abnormal reflux of gastric contents into the esophagus. This reflux occurs when the lower esophageal sphincter opens inappropriately. Usually, patients experience heartburn and regurgitation when reflux is present. These symptoms are considered "troublesome" when they adversely affect the patient's quality of life. In addition to heartburn, patients with reflux may experience a number of extraesophageal symptoms such as laryngitis or hoarseness, asthma, chronic and nocturnal, dry cough, chest pain, and dental erosion. Persistent reflux that occurs more than twice a week is often referred to as GERD. People of all ages can have GERD. Obesity, cigarette smoking, and pregnancy are common associated factors. GERD may contribute to the worsening of symptoms in patients with asthma.

KEY POINTS

- Cough is one of the most common symptoms in patients with pulmonary disease. It is the powerful protective reflex arising from stimulation of receptors located in the pharynx, larynx, trachea, large bronchi, and even the lung and the visceral pleura.
- An acute self-limited cough is usually due to a viral infection involving the upper airway. It usually resolves in a few days. Chronic persistent cough is most commonly caused by postnasal drip syndrome, asthma, COPD, allergic rhinitis, or GERD.
- Sputum is the substance expelled from the tracheobronchial tree, pharynx, mouth, sinuses, and nose by coughing or clearing the throat. The term *phlegm* refers strictly to secretions from the lungs and tracheobronchial tree.
- Excessive sputum production is most often caused by inflammation of the mucous glands that line the tracheobronchial tree.
- Hemoptysis, expectoration of sputum containing blood, varies in severity from slight streaking to frank bleeding.
- Erosive bronchitis in smokers with chronic bronchitis now accounts for nearly half of the cases of hemoptysis. Bronchogenic carcinoma is the second most frequent cause.
- Dyspnea (*dys*, difficult; *pnea*, breathing) is defined as a subjective experience of breathing discomfort that consists of qualitatively distinct sensations that vary in intensity.
- Dyspnea occurs when the work of breathing is abnormally high for the given level of exertion. This is common with narrowed airways as in asthma and when the lung is stiff as in pneumonia.

KEY POINTS—cont'd

- Orthopnea is present when the patient complains of shortness of breath when lying down.
- Chest pain is the cardinal symptom of heart disease. In its classic presentation, the "viselike" pain of a heart attack is referred down the arms, most often the left, and may radiate into the shoulder, neck, jaw, or back. This type of chest pain is known as *angina* and signals a medical emergency.
- Syncope is a temporary loss of consciousness caused by reduced blood flow and therefore a reduced supply of oxygen and nutrients to the brain.
- Cough (tussive) syncope is the transient loss of consciousness following severe coughing.
- Bilateral peripheral or dependent edema suggests pulmonary hypertension, heart failure, or venous insufficiency.
- Fever (hyperthermia, pyrexia) is an elevation of body temperature above the normal range resulting from disease.
- Patients with snoring and sleep disordered breathing will complain of EDS.

CASE STUDY

A 66-year-old woman is brought to the emergency department (ED) complaining of rapid onset of SOB, stating, "I cannot catch my breath." She also admits to coughing up a tablespoon of yellowish sputum every 30 minutes to 1 hour, sweating, and feeling warm, although she has not taken her temperature.

Questions
1. What other key questions should be asked by the interviewer?
2. What pulmonary problems are suggested by the symptoms at this point?
3. Is the fact that the patient complains of sweat significant? If so, why?

Answers
1. The interviewer should ask the patient if she has chest pain, nausea, dizziness, or blood in her sputum, or a history of lung disease or cigarette smoking.
2. The pulmonary problems suggested at this point include pneumonia, acute bronchitis, asthma, and acute exacerbation of COPD.
3. The sweating is significant because it is consistent with a fever that may be caused by an infection. If a fever is present, it may be contributing to the patient's SOB because of an increase in oxygen consumption and an increase in the drive to breathe.

CASE STUDY

A 60-year-old man is brought to the ER complaining of acute chest pain. He was mowing his lawn when he suddenly felt ill. He went indoors to tell his wife, and she called 911. The patient is breathing rapidly while breathing supplemental oxygen through a nasal cannula.

Questions
1. What questions should the interviewer ask the patient about his chest pain?
2. What other symptoms should the interviewer ask the patient about?
3. What clinical problems may explain the chest pain?

Answers
1. The interviewer should ask the patient to point to the position of the chest pain on his chest. The patient should also be asked to describe the characteristics of the chest pain; if it radiates to the jaw, shoulder, or back; and if it increases with a deep breath.
2. The patient should be asked about nausea, fever, pedal edema, shortness of breath, cough, and dizziness. The patient's smoking history is important to obtain at some point.
3. If the patient has pain in the center of his chest that radiates to his shoulder or jaw and is accompanied by nausea and/or dizziness, it would be consistent with myocardial ischemia, and the patient may be having a heart attack. If the pain is sharp and located peripherally on the chest, the pain may be related to pleural disease or lung infection.

CASE STUDY

A 48-year-old morbidly obese construction worker is brought to the ED after crashing his truck into a parked car in the early afternoon. He has sustained a minor head laceration and a bruised forearm. His partner drove him to the ED and says he believes the patient fell asleep while driving. He added that the patient has frequently has been making stupid mistakes on the job, cannot do estimates anymore, and has been found snoring loudly during breaks. The patient now seems to be breathing normally while receiving low-flow supplemental oxygen through a nasal cannula.

Questions
1. What questions should the interviewer ask of the patient about his condition?
2. What clinical problems may explain the daytime sleepiness?
3. What further studies would you recommend?

Answers
1. The interviewer should ask if the patient believes he fell asleep while driving. Beyond this and more importantly, the patient should be asked about alternations in sleeping habits or medications, day-time sleepiness, and other changes, such as difficulty concentrating.

2. Given the predisposing factors of morbid obesity and male gender, as well as the complaints of daytime sleepiness, snoring, and work difficulties, obstructive sleep apnea (OSA) should be strongly suspected.
3. Given the clinical suspicion, the patient should be referred for a polysomnogram (sleep study), as discussed in Chapter 19.

ASSESSMENT QUESTIONS

See Appendix for answers.

1. Which of the following factors may lead to a weak cough?
   a. Reduced lung recoil
   b. Bronchospasm
   c. Weak inspiratory muscles
   d. All of the above
2. A cough described as being persistent for more than 3 weeks would be called which of the following?
   a. Acute
   b. Paroxysmal
   c. Chronic
   d. Nocturnal
3. Which of the following problems is associated with hemoptysis?
   a. Tuberculosis
   b. Lung carcinoma
   c. Pneumonia
   d. All of the above
4. A patient's complaint of breathlessness or air hunger would be defined as which of the following?
   a. Hemoptysis
   b. Wheezing
   c. Dyspnea
   d. Cyanosis
5. What term is used to describe shortness of breath in the upright position?
   a. Orthopnea
   b. Platypnea
   c. Eupnea
   d. Apnea
6. Which of the following is least associated with causing dyspnea?
   a. An increase in the work of breathing
   b. A decrease in the ventilatory capacity
   c. An increase in the drive to breathe
   d. An increase in lung compliance
7. What term is used to describe difficult breathing in the reclining position?
   a. Apnea
   b. Platypnea
   c. Orthopnea
   d. Eupnea

8. Which of the following characteristics is least associated with pleuritic chest pain?
   a. Sharp
   b. Inspiratory
   c. Radiates to the neck
   d. Located laterally

9. Which of the following may cause syncope?
   a. Severe coughing
   b. Pulmonary embolism
   c. Hypovolemia
   d. All of the above

10. Which of the following is (are) true regarding dependent edema caused by lung disease?
    a. It is caused by pulmonary vasodilation
    b. Accompanying hepatomegaly may be present
    c. It is caused by acute systemic hypertension
    d. All of the above

11. Chronic pulmonary hypertension may lead to which of the following clinical findings?
    a. Pedal edema
    b. Inspiratory crackles
    c. Hepatomegaly
    d. a and c

12. Which of the following is associated with night sweats?
    a. Tuberculosis
    b. Congestive heart failure
    c. Asthma
    d. Interstitial pulmonary fibrosis

13. In what decade of life is snoring and obstructive sleep apnea (OSA) most likely to be present in adult males?
    a. 20 to 29 years
    b. 30 to 39 years
    c. 40 to 49 years
    d. 50 to 59 years

14. Which of the following symptoms is least likely to be associated with GERD?
    a. Pedal edema
    b. Hoarseness
    c. Coughing
    d. Wheezing

Bibliography

Bafadhel M, McCormick M, Sahra S, et al. Profiling of sputum inflammatory mediators in asthma and chronic obstructive pulmonary disease. *Respiration* 2011;**22**:88.

Benich JJ, Carek PJ. Evaluation of the patient with chronic cough. *Am Fam Physician* 2011;**84**:887.

Dicprinigaitis PV. Angiotensin-converting enzyme inhibitor-induced cough: AACP evidence-based clinical practice guidelines. *Chest* 2006;**129**:1695.

Dudha M, Lehman S, Aronow WS, Rosa J. Hemoptysis: diagnosis and treatment. *Compr Ther* 2009;**35**:139.

Eakin EG, Resnikoff PM, Prewitt LM, et al. Validation of a new dyspnea measure: the UCSD Shortness of Breath Questionnaire. *Chest* 1998;**113**:619.

Heuer AJ, Geisler SL, Kamienski M, et al. Introducing medical students to the interdisciplinary health care team: piloting a case-based approach. *J Allied Health* 2010;**39**:76.

Janssen DJ, Spruit MA, Leue C, et al. Symptoms of anxiety and depression in COPD patients entering pulmonary rehabilitation. *Chron Respir Dis* 2010;**7**:147.

Jarvis C. *Physical exam and health assessment.* 6th ed. St Louis: Mosby-Elsevier; 2012.

Kacmarek RM, Stoller JK, Heuer AJ. *Egan's fundamentals of respiratory care.* 10th ed. St. Louis: Mosby-Elsevier; 2013.

Seidel HM, Ball J, Dains J, Flynn JA, et al. *Mosby's guide to physical examination.* 7th ed. St. Louis: Mosby-Elsevier; 2011.

Shumway NM, Wilson RL, Howard RS, et al. Presence and treatment of air hunger in severely ill patients. *Respir Med* 2008;**102**:27.

Sinz E, Navarro K, Soderberg ES. *Advanced cardiovascular life support provider manual.* Dallas: American Heart Association; 2011.

Yorke J, Russell AM, Swigris J, Shuldham C, et al. Assessment of dyspnea in asthma: validation of The Dyspnea-12. *J Asthma* 2011;**48**:602.

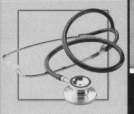

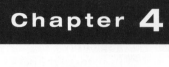

Chapter 4

Vital Signs

ALBERT J. HEUER*

CHAPTER OUTLINE

LEARNING OBJECTIVES

After reading this chapter, you will be able to:

1. Identify the four classic vital signs and the value of monitoring their trends.
2. Recognize the clinical significance of other bedside clinical findings including abnormal sensorium and level of pain.
3. Describe the normal values of the following vital signs and common causes of deviation from normal in the adult:
   a. Pulse rate
   b. Respiratory rate
   c. Blood pressure
   d. Body temperature
4. Describe the following issues related to body temperature measurement:
   a. Types of devices commonly used
   b. Factors affecting the accuracy of devices
   c. Common sites and temperature ranges of those sites for measurement
5. Describe how fever affects the following:
   a. Oxygen consumption and carbon dioxide production
   b. Respiratory rate
   c. Pulse
6. Define the following terms:
   a. Fever
   b. Tachycardia
   c. Bradycardia
   d. Bradypnea
   e. Pulsus paradoxus
   f. Pulsus alternans
   g. Tachypnea
   h. Systolic blood pressure
   i. Diastolic blood pressure
   j. Hypertension

*Dr. Robert Wilkins, PhD, RRT, contributed much of the content for this chapter as the coeditor of the prior edition of this text.

KEY TERMS

bradycardia	hypertension	sensorium
bradypnea	hypotension	systolic blood pressure
diastolic blood pressure	postural hypotension	tachycardia
fever	pulse pressure	tachypnea
Holter monitor	paradoxical pulse	telemetry

The previous two chapters focused on subjective data—those that are perceived by the patient. We now turn our attention to more objective data—those that can be measured. Although subjective data are important, objective data are factual information that is generally not influenced by patient opinion or feelings. Therefore, they are most often relied on to make important clinical decisions. This chapter focuses mainly on vital signs, the most frequently measured objective data for monitoring vital body functions and often the first and most important indicator that the patient's condition is changing. Given that obtaining vital signs generally requires direct patient interaction, the respiratory therapist (RT) or other member of the patient care team should give proper consideration to the principles relating to preparing for the patient encounter, as outlined in Chapter 1.

Vital signs are used for the following purposes:

- Help determine the relative status of vital organs, including the heart, blood vessels, and lungs, which may be helpful in making many clinical decisions such as when to admit the patient to the hospital
- Establish a baseline (a record of initial measurements against which future recordings are compared)
- Monitor response to therapy, such as surgery and medication administration, as well as selected diagnostic tests.
- Observe for trends in the health status of the patient
- Determine the need for further evaluation, diagnostic testing, or intervention

Obtaining Vital Signs and Clinical Impression

The four classic vital sign measurements are temperature, pulse, respirations, and blood pressure. Although they are not always listed as vital signs, the patient's height and weight, level of consciousness and responsiveness (sensorium), level and type of pain, and the RT or other patient care team member's general clinical impression are also important observations often included with the vital sign assessment.

Patients who have intravenous or arterial lines and traumatic or surgical wounds have catheter insertion sites, wounds, and extremity checks performed as part of "routine vitals." In addition, pulse oximetry with continuous heart rate and electrocardiogram (ECG) is often monitored along with vital signs of patients in acute care settings.

It should be noted that the vital signs, like other clinical findings, are only as accurate as the clinician or caregiver obtaining them and interpreting the results. Thus, it is important to properly obtain and monitor vital signs to help optimize patient care and avoid costly medical errors. In addition, significant inconsistencies among vital signs, clinical impression, and other clinical data can signal an error in measurement or the presence of a potentially serious medical condition despite certain normal findings. For example, a patient who has relatively normal vital signs but whose facial expression and general appearance suggest severe distress may still have an acute medical problem. As a result, it is recommended that RTs "don't treat numbers." Instead, they should rely on the critical analysis of several clinical findings, including but not limited to vital signs, in assessing the patient and making related recommendations.

SIMPLY STATED

Vital signs are only as accurate as the way in which they are obtained and may be subject to error. Vital signs may also be only minimally affected by serious medical conditions. Therefore, they should be considered along with other clinical data to help ensure an accurate diagnosis.

Frequency of Vital Signs Measurement

The frequency of vital signs measurement depends on the condition of the patient; the nature and severity of the disorder; and the procedures, surgery, or treatments being performed. A baseline measurement should be taken on admission and at least at the beginning of each shift.

For acutely ill patients in an intensive care setting, vital signs may be monitored continuously with remote electronic monitoring and alarm interface. For patients with conditions affecting only selected organ systems such as the heart, monitoring can be focused on specific vital signs including heart rate and rhythm and can be done continuously through electronic transmitting devices known as **telemetry**. Similarly, patient's heart rate and rhythm can be continuously monitored and digitally recorded for review by a physician, outside of the hospital or clinic using a **Holter monitor**. However, for more stable patients such as those on medical-surgical floors, "routine vitals" are generally measured and recorded every 4 to 6 hours (at beginning of shift and midshift), unless changes in conditions dictate otherwise.

In addition to acuity, certain procedures may determine the frequency with which vital signs are monitored. For example, patients undergoing a bronchoscopy (see Chapter 17) generally have baseline measurements taken before the procedure, at a maximum of 5-minute intervals during the procedure, and at similar intervals until they recover from moderate sedation and any lingering effects of the procedure. After surgery, vital signs are generally measured frequently to ensure the patient's safety—often every 15 minutes for 2 hours, then every 30 minutes for 1 to 2 hours, then hourly until the patient is stable. The physician's order in the chart is often written as "Vitals q15m × 2-4h, q30m × 4h, Q1H until stable, then per protocol." Likewise, certain vital signs such as heart rate and respiratory rate should be monitored at a minimum before and after certain standard respiratory treatments like bronchodilator administration, to evaluate effectiveness of the treatment and for possible side effects.

Of course, vital signs should always be monitored and recorded as often as necessary for the safety of the patient. If the patient's condition worsens unexpectedly, the patient appears to have an adverse reaction to a medical intervention, or the patient suddenly comments about "not feeling well," vital signs should be measured immediately and strong consideration given to activating the Rapid Response Team (also known as the Medical Emergency Teams) in the hospital setting or calling 911 in an alternate care setting.

SIMPLY STATED

Vital signs should be monitored and recorded as often as necessary for the safety of the patient. In general, the frequency with which patients' vital signs are assessed is dictated by the acuity or degree of illness, with those of the more acutely ill patient being assessed more frequently.

Trends in the Vital Signs

A single vital sign measurement gives information about the patient at that moment in time. Each measurement may be evaluated to see whether it is high or low compared with the normal value for the patient's age; however, an isolated measurement does not provide much information about what is normal for the individual patient or how the patient is changing or responding to therapy over time. To evaluate whether an individual patient has "normal" vital signs, you must understand what is normal for them, given factors such as age, disease, and treatment protocols. Sometimes, chronic disease or treatment modalities cause expected alterations in heart rate, respiratory rate, blood pressure, or body temperature, which changes what is normal for an individual patient. If you doubt a finding, repeat the measurement and be sure the patient's position and your technique are correct for the parameter you are measuring. If you still doubt the measurement or if you think the patient may be getting into trouble, get help.

The initial reading is generally referred to as the baseline measurement. A series of vital sign measurements over time establishes a trend and is far more important clinically than any single measurement. Each time vital signs are measured, they should be compared with the baseline values and the most recent measurements. Sometimes, the patient's condition may be changing slowly, and comparison with one or two previous measurements does not indicate the trend, whereas comparison over an entire shift or 24 hours of vital signs may indicate clearly that the patient is slowly deteriorating. Because the trend of vital signs is so important, many physicians insist that vital signs on hospitalized patients be recorded on a multiple-day graph.

Additionally, the patient's vital signs should be viewed in relation to their normal level or the values that can typically be obtained for them, even when they are not necessarily ill. For instance, a heart rate of 96 beats/minute is within normal limits for an adult but may be relatively high and have clinical significance for a patient whose heart rate is generally in the low 60s.

SIMPLY STATED

To evaluate whether a patient has "normal" vital signs, you must understand what is normal for the patient's age, disease, and environment. A vital sign measurement is only as accurate as the technique used to obtain it.

Comparing Vital Signs Information

Clues to whether a patient's condition may be stable or changing may be obtained by comparing changes in vital signs and other signs and symptoms. For example, patients who are not maintaining adequate blood oxygen levels develop specific changes in general appearance, level

TABLE 4-1

Signs of Hypoxemia Assessed During Vital Signs Measurement

Vital Signs Measurement	Sign
General clinical presentation	Impaired coordination or cooperation
	Cool extremities* (can be felt while taking the heart rate and blood pressure)
	Diaphoresis (profuse sweating)
Sensorium (level of consciousness)	Decreased mental function
	Impaired judgment, confusion
	Loss of consciousness
	Decreased pain perception
Respiration	Increased rate and depth of breathing
	Difficulty breathing, use of accessory muscles
Heart rate	Tachycardia
	Arrhythmia (irregular heart rate), especially during sleep
Blood pressure	Increased blood pressure initially

*Temperature of the extremities, as well as diaphoresis, can be felt at the time the heart rate and blood pressure readings are obtained.

of consciousness, heart and respiratory rates, and blood pressure. Table 4-1 lists these common signs of developing acute hypoxemia (partial pressure of arterial oxygen [PaO_2] < 75 to 80 mm Hg).

In the field of medicine, this comparison of multiple signs and symptoms to arrive at the patient's diagnosis is called the *differential diagnosis*. Of course, it takes time for the beginning student to learn all these relationships, but remember, the difference between the novice and expert clinician is not just knowledge. The distinction is also the ability to assess and compare multiple types of subjective and objective data over time and to identify patterns and relationships in an individual patient. The key to expert assessment of vital signs at the bedside is to be constantly aware and to look for change, as follows:

- Look at the patient: watch facial expressions, body movements, coordination, position, color, skin, anatomic landmarks, and effort to breathe or move.
- Listen to the patient: hear words, tones, sounds, rhythms, patterns, silence, feelings, and fears.
- Touch: feel moisture, temperature, air movement, change in temperature, muscle and skin tone, resistance, and quality of pulses.
- Analyze: collect information in a timely manner; compare it with normal values and the patient's baseline and the disease procession. Mentally update this information whenever you are around the patient. Validate its accuracy. Does the information make sense? Is something wrong with the picture?
- Trend, trend, trend: what has changed about the patient? How has the patient changed and why? What has not changed? Why? What does it mean? Does the change indicate a need for immediate action?

Height and Weight

Height and weight are routinely measured as part of the physical examination and usually as part of every outpatient appointment. A patient's height is normally taken without shoes or boots, and their weight is obtained while wearing only a hospital gown or indoor clothing. For hospitalized patients, the admitting height and weight are obtained and recorded either when the patient goes to a preadmitting testing service or by the admitting nurse; thereafter, weight is usually measured every day or two. If there is concern about either dehydration or fluid overload, fluid intake and output and weight may be recorded each shift until the patient's fluid balance is stable. Because weight is often used to calculate medication doses and ventilator settings related to ventilator volumes, the weight may be recorded in kilograms (1 kg = 2.2 lb) on the patient's medication record and, if appropriate, the ventilator-patient flow sheet, in addition to the vital signs record. Scales and measurement standards should be selected in sizes and styles appropriate for the age of the patient and should be calibrated regularly to ensure accuracy.

General Clinical Presentation

General observation begins the moment you first see the patient and continues throughout the examination and care. The patient's general appearance gives clues to the level of distress and severity of illness as well as information about the patient's personality, hygiene, culture, and reaction to illness. This first step may dictate the order of care or physical examination. If the patient is in distress, the priority is to evaluate the problem in the most efficient and rapid way possible and to intervene or locate someone who can assist the patient. A more complete examination can be performed when the patient is more stable. Some visual signs of distress include the following:

- Cardiopulmonary distress is suggested by labored, rapid, irregular, or shallow breathing that may be accompanied by coughing, choking, wheezing, dyspnea, chest pain, or a bluish color (cyanosis) of the oral mucosa, lips, and fingers. The patient with cardiopulmonary distress often speaks in short, choppy sentences because of severe dyspnea.
- Anxiety is recognized by restlessness, fidgeting, tense looks, and difficulty communicating normally and may be accompanied by cool hands and sweaty palms.
- Pain is suggested by drawn features, moaning, shallow breathing, guarding (protecting the painful area), and refusal to deep-breathe or cough.

- Bleeding and loss of consciousness are signs of extreme distress that require immediate intervention.

When a patient is not in acute distress, this initial observation provides an opportunity to see the patient as a whole person. Using all your senses—hearing, smelling, seeing, touching, and perception—during this head-to-toe inspection gives information about the patient's apparent age, state of health, body structure, nutritional status, posture, motor activity, physical and sensory limitations, and mental acuity. It helps assess the reliability of the patient as a historian. It also helps identify what type of assistance and teaching the patient may need.

QUESTIONS TO ASK

The Clinical Presentation

Questions to ask yourself while doing this portion of the examination include the following:

- What are the general appearance and attitude of the patient?
- Are there inconsistencies between (or among) objective and subjective clinical findings?
- Is the patient in distress and in immediate need of additional care?
- How is the patient responding to the assessment or treatment?
- Are there abnormalities in the patient's face or movements?
- Does the patient have any motor or sensory limitations?
- Will this patient require assistance, safety precautions, or teaching?

A written description of these initial observations helps others involved in the patient's care know how to plan care and relate to the patient's needs. Usually, these descriptive statements are written in language everyone can understand (e.g., "J.C. is a cooperative, alert, well-nourished, 43-year-old man who appears younger than his stated age and exhibits no indication of distress. He shows no signs of acute or chronic illness and is admitted for …"). You may occasionally find that more specific terms for body types have been used in the written physical examination report. Box 4-1 lists and defines some of those terms.

A statement is usually made in the documentation of the patient's general appearance regarding the apparent age of the patient relative to his or her stated age. Patients who appear much older than their stated age often suffer from chronic illness such as heart disease, diabetes, or chronic pulmonary disease. For example, the patient with chronic obstructive pulmonary disease often appears older than his or her stated age.

Pain Level and Type

Pain is referred to by some clinicians as the "fifth vital sign." In the past, the assessment of pain was considered to be mainly a subjective measure. More recently, pain intensity scales have been developed and validated to help accurately quantify a patient's level of pain. One commonly used pain measurement instrument uses a 10-point scale, with 10 being "hurts worst," and corresponding facial expressions and verbal description to assess pain level. In assessing pain, it is important to be mindful of certain cultural differences that may affect the patient's accurate reporting of pain, or lack thereof. For example, some cultures may deny or understate massive pain because of cultural beliefs and stigmas. With this in mind, when a patient's accurate pain rating score is coupled with additional information regarding its location and actions that worsen or alleviate it, this information can be quite useful in clinical assessment. For example, chest pain originating from the cardiac versus the pulmonary system (e.g., myocardial infarction versus pleuritis) can vary in features such as intensity, location, and duration. As a result, rapid assessment and characterization of pain may assist in making a differential diagnosis and implementing the appropriate treatment.

The use of analgesic (pain-relieving medication) before assessing a patient is somewhat controversial in that the immediate administration of such medications can cause the patient to understate the pain severity, altering the assessment. However, in extreme cases, the pain may be so severe that it interferes with the

Box 4-1	Terms Used to Describe Body Types
Ectomorphic	Slight development, body linear and delicate with sparse muscular development
Endomorphic	Soft, roundness throughout the body; large trunk and thighs with tapering extremities
Mesomorphic	Preponderance of muscle, bone, and connective tissue, with heavy hard physique of rectangular outline (between endomorphic and ectomorphic)
Sthenic	Average height; well-developed musculature, wide shoulders, flat abdomen; oval face
Hypersthenic	Short, stocky, may be obese; shorter, broader chest; thicker abdominal wall; rectangular-shaped face
Hyposthenic	Tall, willowy, musculature poorly developed; long, flat chest; abdomen may sag; long neck; triangular face
Asthenic	Exaggeration of hyposthenic body type
Cachectic	Profound and marked malnutrition; wasting; ill health
Debilitated	Weak, feeble, lack of strength (with weakness and loss of energy)
Failure to thrive	Physical and developmental delay or retardation in infants and children; seen in children with illness but more often in children with psychosocial or maternal deprivation

assessment of the patient. In such cases, it may be necessary to administer a modest initial dose of analgesic to assess the patient.

QUESTIONS TO ASK

Pain

To ensure a thorough patient examination, the presence and features of pain should be assessed by asking yourself the following questions:

- Does the patient appear to be in pain?
- Is the patient's subjective response consistent with the presence of pain?
- If the patient is in pain, what are the intensity and location?
- What makes the pain better or worse?
- Was the onset of pain gradual or sudden?
- Is the pain affecting the patient's breathing pattern?
- Did you notify the nurse and the doctor that the patient is in pain?

SIMPLY STATED

Pain is often an important clinical feature and should be quickly evaluated in regard to location, intensity, onset, and what makes it worse or better.

Level of Consciousness (Sensorium)

Evaluation of the patient's level of consciousness is a simple but important task. Adequate cerebral oxygenation must be present for the patient to be conscious, alert, and oriented. The conscious patient also should be evaluated for orientation to time, place, and person. This is referred to as evaluating the patient's **sensorium** or mental status. The alert patient whose orientation to time, place, and person is accurate is said to be "oriented × 3," and the sensorium is considered normal.

An abnormal sensorium and loss of consciousness may occur when cerebral perfusion is inadequate or when poorly oxygenated blood is delivered to the brain. As cerebral oxygenation deteriorates, the patient initially is restless, confused, and disoriented. If tissue hypoxia continues to deteriorate, the patient eventually becomes comatose. An abnormal sensorium also may occur as a side effect of certain medications and in drug overdose cases. Deterioration of the patient's sensorium often indicates the need for mechanical ventilation in the presence of acute respiratory dysfunction.

Evaluation of the patient's sensorium helps determine not only the status of tissue oxygenation but also the ability of the patient to cooperate and participate in treatment. Patients who are alert and oriented can take an active role in their care, whereas those who are disoriented or comatose cannot. The treatment plan is often adjusted according to the evaluation of sensorium.

QUESTIONS TO ASK

Level of Consciousness

Asking yourself questions, such as the following, while obtaining vital signs will help you assess the patient's sensorium:

- Is the patient conscious? If the patient is medicated, can he or she be aroused easily?
- Is the patient responding and is the response appropriate for the stimulus?
- Is the patient alert?
- Is the patient oriented to person, place, and time?
- Can the patient see, hear, and sense touch?
- Is the patient restless, fidgety, or easily distracted?
- Has the patient's responsiveness or behavior changed?

Glasgow Coma Scale

Many systems for evaluating the patient's level of consciousness have been developed. One such assessment tool is the Glasgow Coma Scale, which allows for objective evaluation based on behavioral response in three areas: motor function, verbal function, and eye-opening response. This scale can be quite useful in assessing trends in the neurologic function of patients who have been sedated, have received anesthesia, have suffered head trauma, or are near coma. The Glasgow Coma Scale is described in more detail in Chapter 6.

SIMPLY STATED

An abnormal sensorium may be caused by inadequate oxygenation of the brain resulting from respiratory or cardiac failure.

Temperature

Normal body temperature for most people is approximately 98.6° F (37° C), with a normal range from 97.0° to 99.5° F and daily variations of 1° to 2° F (Table 4-2). The body temperature usually is lowest in the early morning and highest in the late afternoon. Most metabolic functions occur optimally when body temperature is within the

---

TABLE 4-2

Normal Temperature Values by Site and Time Requirements for Accuracy when Using a Glass Thermometer

Site	NORMAL TEMPERATURE RANGES		Time Required
	Fahrenheit	Celsius	
Oral	97.0°-99.5°	36.5°-37.5°	3-5 min*
Axillary	96.7°-98.5°	35.9°-36.9°	9-11 min
Rectal	98.7°-100.5°	37.1°-38.1°	2-4 min
Ear	Expected to be very close to rectal if measured correctly		2-3 sec

*Wait 15 minutes after eating or drinking.

normal range. Temperature elevation to between 99° and 100° F occurs normally during exercise and takes about 15 minutes to return to normal after exercise. In women, normal temperature increases approximately 1° F during ovulation and during the first 4 months of pregnancy.

Body temperature is maintained in the normal range by balancing heat production with heat loss. If the body had no ability to rid itself of the heat generated by metabolism, the body temperature would rise rapidly. The hypothalamus plays an important role in regulating heat loss and can initiate peripheral vasodilation and sweating in an effort to dissipate body heat.

The respiratory system also helps in the removal of excess heat through ventilation. When the inhaled gas is cooler than the body temperature, the airways warm the gas to body temperature. This warming and subsequent exhalation with each breath aids in removing excess body heat. When the inhaled gas is heated to near body temperature before inhalation, this heat loss mechanism is not functional. This most often occurs when the patient is intubated and receiving mechanical ventilation with a heated humidifier in place.

Fever

An elevation of body temperature above normal (hyperthermia) can result from disease or from normal activities such as exercise. When the temperature is elevated from disease, this elevation is called **fever**, and the patient is said to be febrile. Terms used to describe fever and its patterns are given in Chapter 3.

Fever most often results from infection somewhere in the body. Infection in the respiratory system can occur in the sinuses, airways, or lungs. However, fever can occur when infection is not present as a side effect of certain medications, with aspiration pneumonia or atelectasis, and after a blood transfusion. Infection is most likely to be the cause of the fever when the body temperature exceeds 102° F.

It is important to remember that not all patients with an infection develop a fever. Some patients are unable to generate a significant fever despite the presence of major infection. Patients with an inadequate immune system are most prone to this finding. In addition, patients who would otherwise have an elevated body temperature but are taking fever-reducing medication, such as acetaminophen or aspirin, may not be febrile. As a result, a complete assessment of body temperature should address the presence of such medications.

A fever results in an increase in the metabolic rate of the body functions and produces an increase in oxygen consumption and carbon dioxide production by the body tissues. For every 1° C elevation of body temperature, oxygen consumption and carbon dioxide production increase approximately 10%. The demand for an increase in the oxygen supply to the tissues and removal of carbon dioxide must be met by an increase in circulation and ventilation. Examination of the febrile patient often reveals increased heart rate and breathing rate. For the patient with significant cardiac or pulmonary disease, the increased demand on these systems may represent an intolerable stress.

Hypothermia

When the body temperature is below normal, hypothermia exists. Hypothermia is not common but can occur in persons with severe head injuries that damage the hypothalamus and in persons exposed to cold environmental temperatures. When the body temperature is below normal, the hypothalamus initiates shivering in an effort to generate energy and vasoconstriction to conserve body heat.

Because hypothermia reduces oxygen consumption and carbon dioxide production by the body tissues, the patient with hypothermia usually has slow and shallow breathing and a reduced pulse rate. Mechanical ventilator settings may need significant adjustments in the depth and rate of delivered tidal volumes as the body temperature of the patient varies above and below normal. Likewise, special respiratory interventions, such as heated aerosol, may be helpful in raising the body temperature in hypothermic patients.

Measurement of Body Temperature

Body temperature is most often measured at one of four sites: the mouth, ear, axilla, or rectum. Rectal temperatures accurately reflect actual body core temperature but are difficult to obtain in most patients. Feeling the skin temperature to determine elevation of temperature is not reliable because skin temperature varies, depending on the body's need to store or release heat, the ambient temperature, and the adequacy of blood circulation to the area.

Temperature is recorded in degrees Fahrenheit (°F) or degrees Celsius (°C), depending on the policies and equipment in each practice setting. Formulas for converting temperature between Fahrenheit and Celsius and an abbreviated conversion table are shown as follows:

$$°F = (°C \times 9/5) + 32$$
$$°C = (°F - 32) \times 5/9$$

Temperature normals vary with the site and method of temperature measurement. When glass thermometers are used, accuracy depends on the length of time the thermometer is allowed to register (see Table 4-2). Electronic thermometers can accurately measure the temperature in approximately 30 seconds or less, provided the probe is positioned correctly and the device is correctly calibrated. To trend temperature over time, the same site and same device must be used for each temperature measurement.

Accurate body temperature measurement is important as variations can be an important clue in properly diagnosing and treating patients. For example, a patient with an elevated body temperature is said to be "febrile", which is often associated with bacterial and viral infections. In addition, variations in body temperature can impact lab results, most notably arterial blood gases (see Chapter 8).

Therefore, it is often recommended that the patient's body temperature be obtained and recorded just prior to drawing blood for such purposes.

Rectal Measurement

Rectal temperatures may be used for patients who are comatose, in intensive care, or confused. The average normal rectal temperature is 99.5°F (37.5°C). A minimum of 2 minutes is required for the glass thermometer to register an accurate rectal temperature. Rectal temperatures are often a few tenths of a degree higher than core temperature. However, despite the relative accuracy of rectal temperatures, the following methods have become increasingly popular alternatives.

Axillary Measurement

The axillary method is safe for infants and small children who do not tolerate rectal temperatures. It is the method of choice for neonates because it approximates their core temperature and avoids injury to the rectal tissues. In adults, axillary temperature measurement assesses peripheral or skin temperature rather than core temperature and has poor correlation to other forms of temperature measurement in febrile adults. Average normal axillary temperature in adults is 97.7°F (36.5°C), approximately 1°F lower than oral temperature and 2°F lower than rectal temperature. It can take up to 11 minutes to obtain an axillary temperature in an adult and approximately 5 minutes in a child. For these reasons, axillary temperature is rarely assessed in the adult.

Oral Measurement

Oral temperature measurement remains a common, convenient, and acceptable method for awake adult patients. This method should not be used with infants, comatose patients, or orally intubated patients. Average normal oral temperature in adults is 98.6°F (37°C). Proper placement of the thermometer tip into the posterior sublingual pocket on either side of the mouth is essential, because the temperature in other parts of the mouth may vary as much as 1.7°C. A 10- to 15-minute waiting period is required if a patient has ingested hot or cold liquid or has been smoking. A glass mercury thermometer requires 3 to 5 minutes to register but may take as long as 7 minutes.

The oral temperature is not affected significantly by oxygen administration via nasal cannula, simple mask, or air-entrainment mask. Therefore, it is not necessary to remove the oxygen or take rectal temperatures in patients receiving oxygen via cannula or mask to obtain accurate oral temperature readings. Heated aerosol or cool mist by face mask may alter oral temperature slightly but probably not enough to alter clinical decisions.

Tympanic (Ear) Measurement

Tympanic infrared thermometry uses a hand-held probe placed in the ear canal to detect infrared emissions from the surfaces of the tympanic membrane and ear canal. No direct contact is made with the tympanic membrane. The temperature is digitized by a computer processor and displayed on a liquid crystal screen in less than 3 seconds. The first ear thermometer was introduced to the US market in 1986 after 2 decades of use in the aerospace industry. This method has the advantage of being fast, clean, and noninvasive and avoids the embarrassment and time delays associated with the classic forms of temperature measurement. It is commonly used in pediatric outpatient offices and emergency departments around the country. However, there are concerns about its accuracy and use in the hospital setting.

One end of the ear canal is immersed in the body near the tympanic membrane and the other end is exposed to the outside, with a temperature gradient of 0.5° to 1.0° C or more down the canal. Temperature is warmest at the tympanic membrane where it is within several tenths of a degree of core body temperature. The ear canal of an adult is an elliptical S-shaped tube approximately 3 cm long with varied size and shape. Because the otoscope-like probe is placed in the outer part of the ear canal and has a relatively wide-view angle through a curved ear canal, the probe detects both the tympanic membrane temperature and ear canal temperature. The computer processor then uses a mathematical formula to adjust for these temperature differences. Different companies use different mathematical equations, so ear temperature measurement also varies slightly by manufacturer.

Multiple studies have been performed in different populations and age groups to evaluate correlations with other types of temperature measurement. The effects of examiner technique, ambient temperature changes, middle ear infection, and the influence of wax and exudate in the ear have also been evaluated; results have been mixed. It is clear that there is not 100% equivalence between the temperatures in the ear canal and those in other body sites; however, there is a significant correlation between ear and rectal, oral, and core temperatures. In most cases, ear temperature measurements run a few tenths of a degree below core temperature.

QUESTIONS TO ASK

Temperature

To ensure the accuracy of the temperature measurement, ask yourself the following questions:

- What type of thermometer was used?
- What site was used: oral, axillary, rectal, or tympanic?
- Was an appropriate amount of time used to obtain the temperature for the method of measurement?
- Had the patient just had a treatment, food, liquid, medication (antipyretic), or other event that could alter the accuracy of the measurement?
- Was the patient observed during temperature measurement? Is there any reason to believe that an elevated temperature was "factitious fever," or one artificially created by the patient?
- What is the time of day? Is the temperature highest in the late afternoon and lowest in the early morning, as expected?

TABLE 4-3

Pulse and Respiratory Rates Referred to Age

Age	Resting Pulse (beats/min)	Respiratory Rate (breaths/min)
Newborn	90-170	35 to 45-70 with excitement
1 year	80-160	25-35
Preschool	80-120	20-25
10 years	70-110	15-20
Adult	60-100	12-20
Athlete	40-60	12-20

SIMPLY STATED

A body temperature higher than 102° F usually indicates infection.

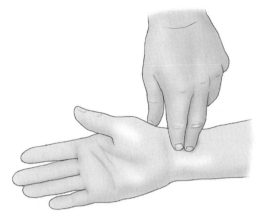

FIGURE 4-1 Technique for assessment of radial pulse.

Pulse

The pulse rate should be evaluated for rate, rhythm, and strength. Normal pulse rate varies with the age and status of the patient. As shown in Table 4-3, the younger the patient, the faster the pulse rate. The normal pulse rate for adults is 60 to 100 beats/min and is regular in rhythm.

A pulse rate exceeding 100 beats/min in an adult is termed **tachycardia**. Common causes of tachycardia include anxiety, fear, exercise, fever, high ambient temperature, low blood pressure, anemia, reduced arterial blood oxygen levels, and certain medications such as bronchodilators.

A pulse rate lower than 60 beats/min is termed **bradycardia**. This is less common but can occur when the heart is diseased, as a side effect of certain medications, or in well-conditioned athletes who typically have resting pulse rates in the 50s. Irregularity of the pulse suggests arrhythmias, which are discussed in Chapter 11.

The amount of oxygen delivered to the tissues depends on the ability of the heart to pump oxygenated blood. The amount of blood pumped through the circulatory system (cardiac output) is a function of pulse rate and stroke volume (volume of blood ejected with each contraction of the left ventricle). When the oxygen content of the arterial blood falls below normal, usually from lung disease, the heart tries to compensate by increasing cardiac output to maintain adequate oxygen delivery to the tissues. An increase in cardiac output is accomplished by an increase in pulse rate in most persons. For this reason, the heart rate is important to monitor in patients with lung disease.

Measurement of Pulse Rate

The radial artery is the most common site for evaluation of the pulse. The patient's arm and wrist should be relaxed, with the hand at or below heart level. If the patient's wrist is held above the level of the heart, the pulse may be difficult to obtain. The pads of the RT's or other clinician's index and middle fingers are placed lightly over the patient's pulse point and then compressed until the maximal pulsation is felt (Fig. 4-1). The thumb is not used because

pulsations from the artery in the examiner's thumb can be confused with the patient's pulse. The rhythm and strength of pulse are evaluated, the pulse rate is evaluated, and then the pulse rate is counted.

Other common sites available for assessment of the pulse include the brachial, femoral, and the carotid arteries. When the blood pressure is abnormally low, the more centrally located pulses, such as the carotid pulse in the neck and femoral pulses in the groin, can be identified more easily than the peripheral pulse.

Ideally, the pulse rate is counted for a full minute to evaluate rate, rhythm, and strength accurately. When the pulse is regular and rhythm and strength are normal, the pulse rate may be counted for 15 seconds and multiplied by 4 or counted for 30 seconds and multiplied by 2. However, if any irregularity is felt, the pulse is counted for a full minute. The pulse rate, or heart rate as it is called on some vital signs records, is always recorded as beats per minute.

Pulse Rhythm and Pattern

The rhythm of the pulse is the relative equality of the intervals between beats. The rhythm can be described as regular, regularly irregular, or irregularly irregular. A regularly irregular rhythm is a pulse with an irregularity that occurs in a continuous pattern (e.g., beat, beat, pause, beat, beat, pause). Bigeminy is a rhythm coupled in pairs. Trigeminy is a rhythm grouped as three beats and a pause. An irregularly irregular pulse has no pattern and is generally an unfavorable clinical finding.

When the rhythm is very irregular, it may be necessary to count the heart rate using a stethoscope placed over the heart (auscultation). During very irregular heart rhythms, some heartbeats cannot generate a strong enough pulse wave to be felt in the peripheral pulse. The difference between the number of auscultated beats and peripheral pulse beats is termed the pulse deficit. Irregular pulse rhythms are best evaluated by an ECG and may indicate the need for continuous ECG monitoring (see Chapter 11).

The strength of the pulse is assessed by how the artery feels as the blood flows through it with each beat. The strength of the pulse can be described as bounding, full, normal, weak, thready, or absent. A normal pulse is easy to feel, does not fade in and out, and is not easily obliterated by finger pressure. A bounding pulse is a full pulse that is difficult to depress with the fingertips. A weak, thready, or feeble pulse is not strong and can be compressed easily. An absent pulse cannot be felt.

There are slight variations in numeric systems used to describe pulses; some scales are 0 to 3, others are 0 to 4, and some rating systems add plus signs (+). Because of this variation, it is important to clarify which scale is used in each health care facility. Two commonly accepted grading systems for pulse strength are shown later. If the preferred grading system is not indicated on the charting forms, it is better to use the descriptive terms for pulse strength.

The fullness of the pulse can be reduced for many reasons, including an arterial blood clot, atherosclerosis, diabetes mellitus, dehydration, or any other condition that would cause the blood flow through the artery to decrease.

Spontaneous ventilation may influence the strength of the pulse. When the patient's pulse strength notably decreases with spontaneous inhalation, it is referred to as pulsus paradoxus. Pulsus alternans is an alternating succession of strong and weak pulses and usually is not related to respiratory disease. These concepts are described in more detail in the discussion of blood pressure later in this chapter.

QUESTIONS TO ASK

Pulse

To ensure the accuracy of the pulse rate, ask yourself the following questions:

- What is the pulse rate? Rhythm? Quality?
- Has the patient been doing something that might raise the pulse temporarily? Is the patient usually anxious at this time?
- Should I take the pulse again later when the patient is resting?
- If the pulse is irregular, did I count it for a full minute?
- Does the pulse vary with respirations?
- How does the current measurement compare with previous measurements?

SIMPLY STATED

An irregular pulse should be counted for a full minute to determine heart rate accurately.

Respiratory Rate and Pattern

Respiratory rates vary by age and condition of the patient. Table 4-3 gives reference ranges for patients of various ages. A respiratory rate of 40 breaths/min is unusual for an adult, and greater than 60 breaths/min is abnormal at any age. If carefully measured, respiratory rate is a sensitive and

TABLE 4-4

Terms Commonly Used to Describe Breathing Patterns

Medical Term	Definition
Apnea	Absence of spontaneous ventilation
Eupnea	Normal rate and depth of breathing
Bradypnea	Less than normal rate of breathing
Tachypnea	Rapid rate of breathing
Hypopnea	Decreased depth of breathing
Hyperpnea	Increased depth of breathing with or without an increased rate
Sighing respiration	Normal rate and depth of breathing with periodic deep and audible breaths
Intermittent breathing	Irregular breathing with periods of apnea

reasonably specific marker of acute respiratory distress. Likewise, the respiratory pattern relates to the regularity and depth of the breaths, which can vary in the presence of certain diseases.

Tachypnea is the term used to describe respiratory rates above normal. Rapid respiratory rates may occur as the result of certain respiratory disorders such as atelectasis, reduced arterial blood oxygen content, and increased arterial carbon dioxide. Tachypnea in the postoperative patient is common when significant fever develops or when the lungs partially collapse (atelectasis) as a side effect of the surgery. Atelectasis causes the lung volumes to decrease below normal, and the patient adopts a breathing pattern that is made up of rapid and shallow breaths as a compensatory mechanism. The degree of atelectasis determines the degree of tachypnea in such cases.

Alternatively, tachypnea can stem from nonrespiratory conditions such as anxiety, pain, and exertion. In addition, various forms of metabolic acidosis place extra stress on the respiratory system as a compensatory response and can cause an increase in rate and depth of breathing. In the case of ketoacidosis resulting from uncontrolled diabetes, a fast and deep breathing pattern known as Kussmaul's breathing is often evident. Evaluation of abnormal respiratory patterns is described in Chapter 5. In any event, a thorough history and interview, as well as an appropriate bedside patient assessment, will often help distinguish the root cause of tachypnea and thus facilitating appropriate treatment.

A slow respiratory rate, referred to as **bradypnea**, is uncommon but may occur in patients with head injuries or hypothermia, as a side effect of certain medications such as narcotics, and in patients with drug overdose.

Other medical terms used to describe respiratory rate and depth are listed in Table 4-4. Intermittent breathing, flaring nostrils, external sounds (e.g., wheezing, or stridor), intercostal and sternal retractions, and use of accessory muscles when breathing are all indications that the patient is in acute distress and requires immediate intervention (see Chapter 5).

Measurement of Respiratory Rate and Pattern

The respiratory rate is counted by watching the abdomen or chest wall move in and out with breathing. With practice, even the subtle breathing movements of the healthy person at rest can be identified easily. In some patients, the RT or other clinician may need to place his/her hand on the patient's abdomen to identify the breathing rate.

Never ask the patient to "breathe normally" while you are assessing the rate of respiration. When individuals think about their breathing, they often voluntarily change their breathing rate and pattern. A better technique is to observe the patient's chest as you finish counting the radial pulse and evaluate the respirations while still holding the wrist. The patient will not be aware that you stopped counting the pulse, so voluntary changes in breathing usually do not occur. When the respiratory rate is regular, counting the number of respirations in 30 seconds and multiplying the number by 2 provides an accurate respiratory rate. The depth and pattern of breathing should also be assessed and recorded with the respiratory rate. Assessment of breathing pattern is discussed in Chapter 5.

QUESTIONS TO ASK

Respiratory Rate

To ensure the accuracy of the respiratory rate, ask yourself the following questions:

- What is the respiratory rate? Regularity? Pattern?
- What is the depth of respiration?
- Are accessory muscles used for respiration?
- Did the patient's awareness that respirations were being counted alter the rate or pattern of respiration?
- Did I count the rate for a full minute if the rate was unusually fast, slow, or irregular?
- How does this current respiratory rate compare with previous measurements?
- Does the change in respiratory rate originate from nonrespiratory causes such as pain, anxiety, or a metabolic problem?

SIMPLY STATED

The respiratory rate should be assessed without the patient being aware of the assessment.

SIMPLY STATED

An abnormal respiratory rate and pattern may indicate respiratory distress but can also be caused by other problems such as pain, anxiety, or metabolic problems.

Blood Pressure

Arterial blood pressure is the force exerted against the walls of the arteries as the blood moves through the arterial vessels. Arterial **systolic blood pressure** is the peak force exerted during contraction of the left ventricle. **Diastolic blood pressure** is the force occurring when the heart is relaxed. Blood pressure is recorded with the systolic pressure listed over diastolic pressure: 120/80 mm Hg.

Pulse pressure is the difference between systolic and diastolic pressures. Normal pulse pressure is 35 to 40 mm Hg. When pulse pressure is less than 30 mm Hg, the peripheral pulse is difficult to detect. Patients with heart failure and inadequate stroke volume usually have a reduced pulse pressure.

Arterial blood pressure is determined by the force of left ventricular contraction, the peripheral vascular resistance, and the blood volume. The normal values for blood pressure change with age, as shown in Table 4-5. Blood pressure lower than 120/80 mm Hg is considered normal for an adult and is associated with a favorable cardiovascular risk.

A blood pressure persistently higher than 140/90 mm Hg is termed **hypertension**. Persistent pressures above this level are associated with an escalating risk for development of heart, vascular, and renal diseases. Risk increases progressively: the higher the blood pressure and number of concurrent risk factors, the more advanced the degree of target organ damage.

Although hypertension is one of the major modifiable risk factors for stroke, coronary heart disease, congestive heart failure, and peripheral vascular disease, it is estimated that approximately half of those affected are not aware of their hypertension. Table 4-6 lists adult blood pressure and hypertension classifications.

Although hypertension is a common problem in the United States and around the world, the exact cause in most cases is not known. Hypertension most often occurs when either the contractility of the heart or the peripheral vascular resistance is abnormally increased. In most cases of hypertension, the cause is complex and involves many factors, including genetics, environment, diet, smoking history, and stress level. In addition, the presence of select disorders, such as obstructive sleep apnea, may cause chronic hypertension.

TABLE 4-5

Median Blood Pressure by Age and Sex

Age	MEDIAN BLOOD PRESSURE (mm Hg)*	
	Male	Female
1 year	85/37	86/40
5 years	95/53	93/54
10 years	102/61	102/60
13 years	108/62	107/63
17 years	118/67	111/66
20+ years	120/80	120/80

*For 50% percentile for height.
Data from The Fourth Report on the Diagnosis, Evaluation, and Treatment of High Blood Pressure in Children and Adolescents. *American Family Physician* 2005;**71**:1014.

Hypotension is defined as blood pressure that is significantly less than 120/80 mm Hg in adults. Low blood pressure is relative and may be clinically significant if it drops suddenly, is unusually low, or is associated with symptoms such as dizziness or fainting. Hypotension may occur as the result of peripheral vasodilation, left ventricular failure, or low blood volume. Perfusion of vital body organs may be significantly reduced with hypotension. Without adequate circulation, oxygen delivery to the tissues is impaired, and tissue hypoxia occurs. Adequate pressure and perfusion must be reestablished to prevent organ failure. In cases of hypotension caused by dehydration, this can often be accomplished by the administration of intravenous fluids. However, in other cases, severe hypotension may need to be managed with medication.

Changes in posture may produce abrupt changes in the arterial blood pressure, especially in the hypovolemic patient. Normally, when the patient moves from the supine to the sitting position, blood pressure changes very little, but when hypovolemia or vasodilation is present, blood pressure may fall significantly when the patient sits up; this is referred to as **postural** (or orthostatic) **hypotension**.

Measurement of Blood Pressure

The most common technique for measuring arterial blood pressure uses a sphygmomanometer (an occluding cuff, stethoscope, and manometer). This technique measures blood pressure indirectly by determining the pressure required to collapse the artery in an arm or leg (Fig. 4-2).

TABLE 4-6

Classification of Blood Pressure and Hypertension for Adults (18+ Years)

Category	Systolic Blood Pressure (mm Hg)	Diastolic Blood Pressure (mm Hg)	Potential Management and Treatment Recommendations
Normal	<120	<80	
Prehypertensive Hypertension	120-139	80-89	Lifestyle modification with possible drug therapy
Stage 1 (mild)	140-159	90-99	Lifestyle modification, drug therapy, frequent monitoring
Stage 2 (moderate)	>159	>99	Lifestyle modification, drug therapy, possibly with multiple drugs, frequent monitoring

Data from the Seventh Report of the Joint National Committee on Prevention, Detection, Evaluation and Treatment of High Blood Pressure. *JAMA* 289:2560-2571, 2003.

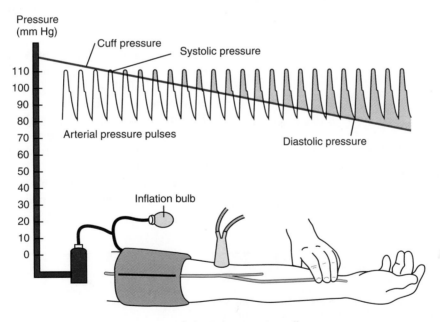

FIGURE 4-2 When the pressure within the sphygmomanometer cuff is increased above arterial blood pressure, the arteries under the cuff are occluded, and no pulse can be palpated at the wrist. As the cuff pressure is gradually released, the systolic peaks of pressure finally exceed cuff pressure, and blood spurts into the arteries below the cuff, producing palpable pulses at the wrist. The sudden acceleration of blood below the cuff produces vibrations that are audible through a stethoscope. The pressure in the mercury manometer at the time the pulse is heard or felt indicates systolic pressure. As cuff pressure is diminished, the sounds increase in intensity and then rather suddenly become muffled at the level of diastolic pressure where the arteries remain open throughout the entire pulse wave. At still lower pressures, the sounds disappear completely when laminar flow is reestablished. (Modified from Rushmer RF: *Cardiovascular dynamics,* ed 3, Philadelphia, 1970, WB Saunders.)

The cuff is applied to the extremity, usually the upper arm, and inflated. When the pressure in the cuff exceeds the systolic blood pressure, blood flow through the artery is occluded and the pulse can no longer be felt. When the cuff is gradually deflated, blood flow in the artery resumes and the pulsations can be felt, heard with a stethoscope, or sensed by a flow probe or sensor. The cuff pressure at the time the blood flow resumes is used as the systolic arterial pressure.

The blood pressure cuff consists of an inflatable rubber bladder encased in a nondistensible cuff. Blood pressure cuffs are made in many different sizes to accommodate various sizes and ages of patients. Some of the most commonly used sizes are listed in Table 4-7. The bladder inside the cuff can be removed for cleaning or repair, so it is important to ensure that the correct size bladder is inside the cuff. Selection of the proper size cuff and bladder is essential to obtain an accurate pressure reading. The length of the bladder should be long enough to cover 80% of the distance around the arm in an adult and 100% of the arm circumference of a child. Overlapping the end of the

bladder in children does not produce an error in the measurement. Using too wide a bladder produces a pressure that is lower than actual pressure. Using a bladder that is too narrow or too short results in overestimation of the blood pressure. The error of overestimation is greater, so if the correct size cuff is not available, a larger cuff should be selected.

Auscultatory Blood Pressure Measurement

The auscultatory method of pressure measurement uses the stethoscope to listen for the sounds produced by the arterial pulse waves (Korotkoff sounds) when blood flow in the artery resumes. As the pressure is reduced during deflation of the occluding cuff, the Korotkoff sounds change in quality and intensity. The five phases of this change are characterized in Table 4-8.

The pressure at which the first sound is heard corresponds to the systolic pressure. There has been debate over whether to use the muffling or disappearance of the sounds as the diastolic pressure. There is now general consensus that Phase V, disappearance of sounds, should be used as the diastolic pressure for most children, adolescents, and adults. In situations where sounds can be heard at levels far below those at which muffling occurs, such as that which may occur in pregnant women and patients with aortic insufficiency, Phase IV may be used as the diastolic pressure. When there is a large discrepancy between muffling and disappearance of sounds, both pressures should be recorded (e.g., 110/60/30 mm Hg).

Occasionally, the Korotkoff sounds disappear during Phases II or III and reappear as the cuff pressure decreases. The period of silence is called the auscultatory gap and is most common in older patients with high blood pressure. The auscultatory gap can generally be eliminated by elevating the arm overhead for 30 seconds before inflating the cuff then bringing the arm to the usual position to continue measurement.

The technique for obtaining an auscultatory blood pressure as specified by the American Heart Association is

---

TABLE 4-7

Acceptable Bladder Dimensions for Arms of Different Sizes

Cuff	Bladder Width (cm)	Bladder Length (cm)	(Maximum) Arm Circumference* (cm)
Newborn	4	8	10
Infant	6	12	15
Child	9	18	22
Small adult	10	24	26
Adult	13	30	34
Large adult	16	38	44
Adult thigh	20	42	52

*Calculated so that the largest arm would still allow the bladder to encircle the arm by at least 80%.
Data from the National High Blood Pressure Education Program Working on High Blood Pressure in Children and Adolescents: the Fourth Report on the Diagnosis, Evaluation, and Treatment of High Blood Pressure in Children and Adolescents. *American Family Physician* 2005;71:1014.

TABLE 4-8

Korotkoff Sounds and Characteristics

Korotkoff Sounds	Characteristic	Pressure Measured
Phase I	First appearance of clear, repetitive tapping sounds; coincides approximately with the reappearance of a palpable pulse	Systolic pressure
Phase II	Sounds are softer and longer, with the quality of an intermittent murmur	Auscultatory gap may occur
Phase III	Sounds become crisper and louder	Auscultatory gap may occur
Phase IV	Sounds are muffled, less distinct, and softer	Diastolic pressure in pregnant women, patients with high cardiac outputs or peripheral vasodilation, and some small children
Phase V	Sounds disappear completely	Diastolic pressure in adults and children

included in Box 4-2. The student is encouraged to obtain a copy of the recommendations and to check periodically for updates.

Errors in Blood Pressure Measurement

Causes of arterial blood congestion above the cuff that result in erroneously high cuff pressure measurements include the following (Fig. 4-3):

- Too narrow a cuff
- Cuff applied too tightly
- Cuff applied too loosely (when the loose bladder is inflated, the edges rise, so the portion pressing on the artery has a tourniquet effect)
- Excessive pressure placed in the cuff during measurement

- Inflation pressure held in the cuff
- Incomplete deflation of cuff between measurements

A low pressure reading is obtained if the cuff is too wide; however, this produces errors in the range of 3 to 5 mm Hg rather than the 40-mm Hg error often obtained when using too narrow a cuff.

Erroneous diastolic pressures occur when pressure is maintained on the artery so that laminar flow is not reestablished. Because turbulent flow can be heard, muffling or disappearance of sound may not occur. Causes include applying the cuff too tightly and pressing the stethoscope too tightly over the artery. Static electricity, ventilators, extraneous room sounds, and the presence of an auscultatory gap may also cause erroneous cuff measurements.

Box 4-2   Technique for Measurement of Blood Pressure by Sphygmomanometry and Auscultation

The intent and purpose of the measurement should be explained to the patient in a reassuring manner, and every effort should be made to put the patient at ease and properly prepare for the patient encounter as described in Chapter 1.

The sequential steps for measuring the blood pressure in the upper extremity should include the following:

1. Prepare for the actual patient encounter (Chapter 1), including scanning the medical record, gathering all necessary equipment, and ensuring there is a means to record the blood pressure readings immediately after being obtained.
2. Identify the patient and explain the procedure to the patient.
3. Have the patient sit up, if possible, and minimize noise and other potential distractions , which can artificially alter measurements or interfere with the measurement process.
4. Position the patients with their bare arm resting so that the middle portion of the upper arm is approximately at the level of the heart.
5. Estimate the circumference of the bare upper arm at the midpoint between the shoulder and elbow and select an appropriately sized cuff. The bladder inside the cuff should encircle about 80% of the arm in adults and about 100% of the arm in children younger than 13 years. If in doubt, use a larger cuff.
6. Palpate the brachial artery and apply the cuff so that the midline of the bladder is over the arterial pulsation, then wrap and secure the cuff snugly around the patient's bare upper arm. Avoid rolling up the sleeve too tightly to prevent constricting blood flow. Loose application of the cuff results in overestimation of the pressure. The lower edge of the cuff should be 1 inch or about 2 cm above the inside bend (antecubital fossa).
7. Place the manometer so that the center of the pressure reading dial or mercury column is easily visible at about eye level and the tubing from the cuff is unobstructed.
8. First inflate the cuff rapidly to 70 mm Hg, and then increase it in 10–mm Hg increments while palpating the radial pulse. Note the level of pressure at which the pulse disappears. Then gradually deflate the cuff and note the pressure at which the pulse subsequently reappears during deflation. This procedure, called the *palpatory method*, provides a necessary preliminary approximation of the systolic blood pressure to ensure an adequate level of inflation when the actual auscultatory measurement is made. It may be useful to avoid underinflation of the cuff in patients with an auscultatory gap and overinflation in those with very low blood pressure.

9. Place the stethoscope ready to auscultate, and ensure that the stethoscope head is in the low-frequency position (bell).
10. Place the head of the stethoscope over the brachial artery pulsation, just above and medial to the inside of the elbow (antecubital fossa) but below the lower edge of the cuff, and hold it firmly in place, making sure that the head makes contact with the skin around its entire circumference.
11. Inflate the bladder rapidly to a pressure 20 to 30 mm Hg above the level previously determined by palpation, then partially unscrew (open) the valve and gradually deflate the bladder at 2 mm/sec while listening for the appearance of the Korotkoff sounds.
12. As the cuff pressure declines, note the level of the pressure on the manometer at the first appearance of repetitive sounds (phase I), at the muffling of these sounds (phase IV), and when they disappear (phase V). While the Korotkoff sounds are audible, the rate of deflation should be no more than 2 mm per pulse beat, thereby compensating for both rapid and slow heart rates.
13. After the last Korotkoff sound is heard, deflate the cuff slowly for at least another 10 mm Hg, to ensure that no further sounds are audible, and then rapidly deflate it.
14. Both systolic (phase I) and diastolic (phase V) pressures should be promptly recorded, rounded off (upward) to the nearest 2 mm Hg. All values should be recorded in the medical record with the date and time of the measurement, the arm on which the measurement was made, the patient's position, and the cuff size (when a nonstandard size is used).
15. The procedure should be repeated after at least about 1 minute, and the two readings averaged.

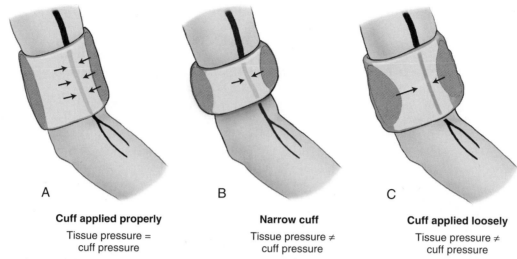

A — **Cuff applied properly**
Tissue pressure =
cuff pressure

B — **Narrow cuff**
Tissue pressure ≠
cuff pressure

C — **Cuff applied loosely**
Tissue pressure ≠
cuff pressure

FIGURE 4-3 A, When a sphygmomanometer cuff of sufficient width in relation to the diameter of the arm is properly applied, the tissue pressure around deep arteries under the cuff equals cuff pressure. However, pressure under the edge of the cuff does not penetrate as deeply as that under the center of the cuff. **B,** A cuff that is too narrow in relation to the diameter of the limb does not transmit its pressure to the center of the limb. Under these conditions, the cuff pressure must greatly exceed arterial pressure to produce complete occlusion of the artery, and erroneously high systolic and diastolic pressures are read from the mercury manometer. **C,** If a cuff of sufficient width is applied too loosely, it becomes rounded before exerting pressure on the tissues and produces the same sort of error as a narrow cuff produces.

Effects of the Respiratory Cycle on Blood Pressure and Pulse Intensity

Systolic blood pressure usually decreases slightly (by 2 to 4 mm Hg) with normal inhalation. This decrease in systolic blood pressure is more significant during a forced maximal inhalation. When the systolic pressure drops more than 10 mm Hg during inhalation at rest, a definite abnormality exists; this is termed paradoxical pulse. **Paradoxical pulse,** also called pulsus paradoxus, occurs in various circulatory and respiratory conditions such as asthma and cardiac tamponade. The most probable mechanism responsible for this fluctuation in blood pressure centers around the negative intrathoracic pressure created by the respiratory muscles during inhalation. The negative intrathoracic pressure encourages venous blood to return to the right ventricle and discourages arterial blood flow out of the left ventricle. The increased venous return to the right ventricle during inspiration increases the right ventricular filling pressures, which causes the interventricular septum to distend toward the left ventricle. This results in reduced left ventricular filling, reduced stroke volume, and decreased systolic blood pressure simultaneous with inhalation. It should be noted that the pulsus paradoxus should not be confused with abdominal paradox (see Chapter 5), which is the inward movement of the abdomen on inhalation and is associated with diaphragmatic fatigue.

The fluctuation in systolic blood pressure with breathing can be identified most accurately with a sphygmomanometer; however, if the pulse can be felt to wane with inspiration in several accessible arteries, paradoxical pulse is probably present. To confirm and quantify the presence of paradoxical pulse, a blood pressure cuff is used. The cuff is inflated until no sounds are heard with the stethoscope bell over the brachial artery, and then it is gradually deflated until sounds are

heard on exhalation only. The cuff pressure then is reduced slowly until sounds are heard throughout the respiratory cycle. The difference between the systolic pressure heard only during expiration and systolic pressure heard throughout the respiratory cycle indicates the degree of paradoxical pulse. A reading in excess of 10 mm Hg is significant.

Pulsus paradoxus is commonly seen in patients with restrictions around their heart such as cardiac tamponade, constrictive pericarditis, or restrictive cardiomyopathy. It may also occur in patients with severe pulmonary disease such as acute asthma.

QUESTIONS TO ASK

Blood Pressure

To ensure the accuracy of the blood pressure reading, ask yourself the following questions:

- Is the correct cuff size being used? Is the cuff applied correctly?
- Is the arm in the standard position when the blood pressure is measured?
- Is the same arm used as was used in previous measurements? Which arm has higher blood pressure?
- If using a mercury column or gauge, is it at eye level?
- Has the patient been in the same position long enough to obtain a stable reading?
- Does the blood pressure change when the patient changes position from supine or sitting to standing?
- Does the patient complain of symptoms such as dizziness when changing position?
- Are things occurring in the environment that would artificially alter the patient's blood pressure?
- If the blood pressure is high, does it decrease if measured again in a few minutes?

SIMPLY STATED

Hypotension occurs when the left ventricle is weak, the blood volume is reduced, or vasodilation is excessive. These problems can occur as a side effect of certain medications (e.g., β-blockers, diuretics).

KEY POINTS

▶ The respiratory therapist (RT) who accurately measures vital signs, properly trends these data, and views such information collectively with other clinical findings can be a valuable asset in diagnosing and treating patients with respiratory dysfunction.

▶ Vital signs are only as accurate as the way in which they are obtained. Therefore, vital signs should be analyzed along with other clinical data to help ensure an accurate diagnosis.

▶ The four classic vital signs are temperature, pulse, respirations, and blood pressure.

▶ Other clinical indicators available to RTs include general clinical impression, height and weight, sensorium, and pain.

▶ The frequency for obtaining vital signs depends on the patient's condition and the procedures being performed, but vital signs should be obtained at least every 4 to 6 hours and as often as every 15 minutes or even continuously for acutely ill patients.

▶ The RT should trend vital signs to monitor a patient's status over time.

▶ The normal body temperature is 98.6° F (37.0° C) with daily variations of 1° to 2° F. A patient with a temperature above that is febrile and below that range is hypothermic.

▶ For every 1° C elevation of body temperature, oxygen consumption and carbon dioxide production increase approximately 10%.

▶ For an adult, the normal pulse rate is 60 to 100 per minute. A pulse rate above that is termed tachycardia and below that is bradycardia.

▶ The normal respiratory rate for an adult is 12 to 20 per minute. Tachypnea is a respiratory rate higher than 20, and bradypnea is when the respiratory rate is below 12.

▶ In addition to assessing pulse and respiratory rate, the RT should also assess the pattern and intensity of a patient's pulse and respirations.

▶ Pulsus paradoxus (or paradoxical pulse) is a decrease in systolic blood pressure and pulse intensity during inhalation should not be confused with abdominal paradox, which is the inward movement of the abdomen on inhalation and is associated with diaphragmatic fatigue.

▶ A blood pressure slightly below 120/80 mm Hg is considered normal for an adult. Hypertension is a blood pressure above 140/90 mm Hg, and hypotension is significantly below 120/80 mm Hg.

▶ There are several errors that can occur when measuring blood pressure. For example, using a cuff that is too narrow or tight can result in falsely high readings.

▶ A paradoxical pulse occurs when systolic pressure drops more than 10 mm Hg during inhalation and may occur during a severe asthma attack or during cardiac tamponade.

ASSESSMENT QUESTIONS

See Appendix for answers.

1. All of the following are included in the measurement of vital signs, except which one?
   a. Pulse
   b. Respiratory rate
   c. Urinary output
   d. Blood pressure

2. Which of the following changes is consistent with a fever?
   a. Decreased respiratory rate
   b. Increased pulse rate
   c. Decreased oxygen consumption
   d. Decreased blood pressure

3. Which of the following methods of temperature measurement is recommended for neonates?
   a. Oral
   b. Axillary
   c. Rectal
   d. Ear

4. What is the normal value of the resting pulse rate in the adult?
   a. 30-60 beats/min
   b. 60-100 beats/min
   c. 80-120 beats/min
   d. 100-150 beats/min

5. What is the normal range of the respiratory rate for adults?
   a. 6-10 breaths/min
   b. 8-12 breaths/min
   c. 12-20 breaths/min
   d. 15-25 breaths/min

6. Which of the following causes tachycardia in the adult?
   a. Hypothermia
   b. Hypoxemia
   c. Hypertension
   d. Polycythemia

7. Which of the following arterial sites is the most common for evaluating the pulse in the adult patient?
   a. Pedal
   b. Temporal
   c. Radial
   d. Femoral

8. Which of the following causes tachypnea in the adult?
   a. Hypothermia
   b. Narcotic overdose
   c. Metabolic acidosis
   d. Hyperoxia

9. Which of the following causes an erroneously low blood pressure measurement?
   a. Inflation pressure held in the cuff between measurements
   b. Use of blood pressure cuff that is too narrow

   c. Not enough pressure used in the cuff during measurement

   d. Tachycardia

10. Hypotension may often be associated with all of the following, except which one?

   a. Reduced perfusion

   b. Less oxygen delivery to the tissues

   c. Excessive salt intake

   d. Dehydration

11. The peak pressure in the arteries is known as which of the following?

   a. Pulse pressure

   b. Diastolic pressure

   c. Systolic pressure

   d. Pulse pressure

12. A decrease in the intensity of the palpated pulse during inhalation is a definition of which of the following?

   a. Abdominal paradox

   b. Pulse pressure

   c. Pulsus paradoxus

   d. Pulsus alternans

13. What is the normal range for pulse pressure?

   a. 10-20 mm Hg

   b. 20-25 mm Hg

   c. 30-50 mm Hg

   d. 35-40 mm Hg

14. If a patient experiences syncope when moving from the supine to the upright position, what is the likely cause?

   a. Left ventricular failure

   b. Postural hypotension

   c. Excessive vasoconstriction

   d. Pulsus paradoxus

Bibliography

DesJardins T, Burton GG. *Clinical manifestations and assessment of respiratory disease.* 6th ed. Maryland Heights, MO: Mosby-Elsevier; 2011.

Hellekson K. The fourth report on the diagnosis, evaluation, and treatment of high blood pressure in children and adolescents. *Am Fam Physician* 2005;**71**:1014.

Jarvis C. *Physical examination and health assessment.* 6th ed. St. Louis: Saunders-Elsevier; 2012.

Kacmarek RM, Stoller JK, Heuer AJ. *Egan's fundamentals of respiratory care.* 10th ed. St. Louis: Mosby-Elsevier; 2013.

LeBlond RF, Brown DD, DeGowin RL. *DeGowin's diagnostic examination.* 9th ed. New York: McGraw-Hill; 2009.

Schindler MB. Treatment of atelectasis: where is the evidence? *Crit Care* 2005;**9**:341.

Seidel HM, Ball J, Dains J, Flynn JA, et al. *Mosby's guide to physical examination.* 7th ed. St. Louis: Mosby-Elsevier; 2011.

Chapter 5

Fundamentals of Physical Examination

CARA DENUNZIO AND ALBERT J. HEUER*

CHAPTER OUTLINE

Examination of the Head and Neck
Head and Face
Eyes
Neck
Lung Topography
Imaginary Lines
Thoracic Cage Landmarks
Lung Fissures
Tracheal Bifurcation
Diaphragm
Lung Borders
Examination of the Thorax
Inspection
Palpation
Percussion of the Chest to Assess Resonance
Auscultation of the Lungs

Examination of the Precordium
Review of Heart Topography
Inspection and Palpation
Auscultation of Heart Sounds
Examination of the Abdomen
Examination of the Extremities
Clubbing
Cyanosis
Pedal Edema
Capillary Refill
Peripheral Skin Temperature
Assessment of Hydration: Skin Turgor

LEARNING OBJECTIVES

After reading this chapter, you will be able to:
1. Describe the four components of the physical examination.
2. Explain the importance of reviewing the history of present illness before performing a physical examination.
3. Describe the significance of the following during examination of the head and neck:
   a. Nasal flaring
   b. Cyanosis
   c. Pursed-lip breathing
   d. Diaphoresis
   e. Changes in pupillary size in response to light
   f. Deviated tracheal position
   g. Jugular venous distention
4. Identify the correct method for measuring jugular venous pressure and expected normal findings.
5. Locate the topographic position of the following:
   a. Thoracic cage landmarks (suprasternal notch, sternal angle [angle of Louis], vertebral spinous processes [C7 and T1])
   b. Lung fissures (oblique [major] and horizontal [minor])

---

*Dr. Robert Wilkins, PhD, RRT, contributed much of the content for this chapter as the coeditor of the prior edition of this text.

LEARNING OBJECTIVES—cont'd

    c. Tracheal bifurcation anteriorly and posteriorly
    d. Right and left diaphragm anteriorly and posteriorly
    e. Lung borders

6. Define the following terms used to classify thoracic configuration during inspection of the chest:
    a. Pectus carinatum
    b. Pectus excavatum
    c. Kyphosis
    d. Scoliosis
    e. Kyphoscoliosis
    f. Barrel chest
    g. Flail chest

7. Define the following terms used to describe breathing pattern during inspection of the chest:
    a. Apnea
    b. Biot breathing
    c. Cheyne-Stokes breathing
    d. Kussmaul breathing
    e. Apneustic
    f. Paradoxical breathing

8. Describe the breathing patterns associated with restrictive and obstructive lung disease.
9. Identify the muscles of inspiration.
10. Describe the clinical significance of accessory muscle use and retractions and bulging.
11. Define the following terms and state their significance:
    a. Abdominal paradox
    b. Respiratory alternans
    c. Peripheral cyanosis
    d. Central cyanosis
    e. Hoover sign

12. Describe the clinical significance of peripheral versus central cyanosis.
13. List causes of increased and decreased tactile fremitus.
14. List causes of decreased thoracic expansion as assessed during chest palpation.
15. Describe subcutaneous emphysema and its clinical significance.
16. List causes of increased and decreased resonance during percussion of the lung.
17. Identify the four basic parts of a stethoscope and their uses.
18. Describe the proper technique for auscultation of the lungs.
19. Identify the four characteristics of breath sounds that should be evaluated during auscultation.
20. Define the following terms used to describe lung sounds and the mechanisms responsible for producing the sounds:
    a. Adventitious
    b. Tracheal
    c. Bronchovesicular
    d. Vesicular (normal)
    e. Diminished/absent
    f. Harsh/bronchial

21. Define the following terms used to describe abnormal lung sounds and the mechanisms responsible for producing the sounds:
    a. Crackles
    b. Rhonchi
    c. Wheezes
    d. Stridor
    e. Pleural friction rub

22. Use qualifying adjectives to describe lung sounds and explain the importance of using these qualifying adjectives.
23. Describe the significance of the following auscultatory findings:
    a. Early inspiratory crackles
    b. Late inspiratory crackles
    c. Monophonic wheezes
    d. Polyphonic wheezes
    e. Stridor
    f. Late inspiratory crackles
    g. Inspiratory and expiratory crackles
    h. Pleural friction rub

LEARNING OBJECTIVES—cont'd

24. Define bronchophony and its cause.
25. Identify the topographic location of the apex and base of the heart during examination of the precordium.
26. Identify the point of maximal impulse, its normal location, and the factors that may cause it to shift to the right or left.
27. Describe the best location for auscultating sounds produced by the aortic, pulmonic, mitral, and tricuspid valves.
28. Describe what produces the first (S_1) and second (S_2) heart sounds, which are normal, as well as the third (S_3) and fourth (S_4) heart sounds, which are typically not normal.
29. Describe what is meant by a gallop rhythm and what it signifies.
30. List the factors that increase or decrease the intensity of the heart sounds.
31. Describe the clinical significance of a loud P_2 heard during auscultation of the heart.
32. Describe the factors that cause systolic and diastolic heart murmurs.
33. Define the term *hepatomegaly* and its significance in the cardiopulmonary patient.
34. Define the following terms and their significance during examination of the extremities:
    a. Digital clubbing
    b. Cyanosis
    c. Pedal edema
    d. Capillary refill
    e. Peripheral skin temperature and turgor

KEY TERMS

abdominal paradox	gallop rhythm	peripheral cyanosis
accessory muscles	harsh breath sounds	pleural friction rub
acrocyanosis	heave	pleurisy
adventitious	hepatomegaly	point of maximal impulse (PMI)
angle of Louis	Hoover sign	precordium
ascites	hyperresonant	ptosis
attenuation	intercostal	respiratory alternans
auscultation	kyphosis	retractions
barrel chest	kyphoscoliosis	rhonchi
bronchial breath sounds	late inspiratory crackles	scalene
bronchophony	loud P_2	scoliosis
bulging	lymphadenopathy	sternocleidomastoid
central cyanosis	miosis	stridor
clubbing	mydriasis	subcutaneous emphysema
crackles	nystagmus	tactile fremitus
cyanosis	palpation	tracheal breath sound
diaphoresis	pectus carinatum	vesicular breath sound
diplopia	pectus excavatum	vocal fremitus
early inspiratory crackles	pedal edema	wheeze
flail chest	percussion	

Physical examination is the process of examining the patient for the physical signs of disease. It is an inexpensive way to obtain immediate and pertinent information about the patient's health status. The four basic components of the physical examination are inspection, palpation, percussion, and auscultation.

The patient initially is examined to help the physician and other members of the patient care team determine the correct diagnosis and to establish the patient's baseline clinical status. Once a tentative diagnosis is made, subsequent examinations are valuable in monitoring the patient's hospital course and evaluating the results of treatment. Each examination should be modified according to the patient's history and the purpose of the assessment.

Through experience, the clinician learns which of the techniques described in this chapter should be used in any situation. Each examination should be performed in a quiet, well-lighted private setting, and the respiratory therapist (RT) or other clinician should avoid exposing the patient to unnecessary physical or emotional discomfort.

The skills described in this chapter are not difficult to learn; however, proficiency is attained only with practice. The beginner first should practice the skills on healthy persons to improve technique and, more important, to obtain an appreciation for normal variations. Abnormalities can be detected only by clinicians who have developed an understanding of normal body functions for comparison.

Box 5-1	Typical Format for Recording the Physical Examination

INITIAL IMPRESSION
Age, height, weight, general appearance, and gender

VITAL SIGNS
Pulse rate, respiratory rate, temperature, and blood pressure

HEENT (HEAD, EARS, EYES, NOSE, AND THROAT)
Inspection findings

NECK
Inspection and palpation findings

THORAX
Lungs: inspection, palpation, percussion, and auscultation findings
Heart: inspection, palpation, and auscultation findings

ABDOMEN
Inspection, palpation, percussion, and auscultation findings

EXTREMITIES
Inspection and palpation findings

This chapter emphasizes the techniques of examination used in assessment of the patient with cardiopulmonary disease. Because cardiopulmonary disease may indirectly alter other body systems, examination of the whole patient is important. The techniques used in examination of the thorax and other body systems for the abnormalities often associated with respiratory disease are reviewed. The typical order in which the initial physical examination is performed and recorded is presented in Box 5-1. See Chapter 4 for a complete discussion of the initial impression and assessment of the vital signs.

A review of the patient's history of present illness and past medical history before examination is helpful, especially if the RT or other clinician was not involved in acquiring the patient's medical history. This review gives the patient care team insight into the expected physical examination findings and suggests the techniques to emphasize.

Examination of the Head and Neck

Head and Face

An examination of the head should first identify the patient's facial expression. This may help determine whether the patient is in acute distress or is experiencing physical pain. The facial expression can also help evaluate alertness, mood, general character, and mental capacity. Nasal flaring is identified by observing the external nares flare outward during inhalation. This may occur in patients of any age but is most often seen in neonates and young children with respiratory distress. It suggests that an increase in the work of breathing is present. It may be seen in a large variety of clinical conditions, including

upper airway obstruction (e.g., croup), bronchiolitis, pneumonia, and respiratory distress syndrome.

Cyanosis may be detected, especially around the lips and oral mucosa, when respiratory disease results in reduced oxygenation of the arterial blood. Cyanosis is a bluish cast to the skin that clinically may be difficult to detect, especially in a poorly lighted room, in patients with dark-pigmented skin, and in those with moderate to severe anemia. The presence of cyanosis is strong evidence that tissue oxygenation may be less than optimum; further investigation (e.g., arterial blood gas analysis) is indicated. The absence of cyanosis does not indicate that tissue oxygenation is adequate because a sufficient hemoglobin concentration must exist before cyanosis can be identified (see Inspection for Central Cyanosis).

Patients with chronic obstructive pulmonary disease (COPD) may use pursed-lip breathing during exhalation. This technique often is taught to patients and may even be used by patients who have not had instruction on its benefits. Some patients naturally begin to pucker their lips during exhalation to provide a slight resistance to the exhaled breath. This resistance provides a modest backpressure in the airways during exhalation and prevents their premature collapse. This exhalation technique alters the inspiratory-to-expiratory (I:E) ratio, extending expiratory time and thus allowing a more complete exhalation.

Excessive sweating by the patient is known as **diaphoresis**. It usually occurs at many sites in the body at the same time but is often first appreciated during inspection of the patient's face. It is a common finding in patients in acute respiratory distress and in those having severe pain. It also may be seen with exercise, eating spicy foods, fever, menopause, and other scenarios. Diaphoresis is also common in patients experiencing a myocardial infarction. For this reason, diaphoresis should always be taken seriously especially in the patient at risk for heart disease.

Eyes

The pupillary reflexes are evaluated as part of the neurologic examination. Cranial nerves II and III must be intact for normal pupillary reflexes to be present. If the pupils are equal in size, round, and reactive to light and accommodation, the physician may simply write PERRLA (*pupils equal, round, reactive to light and accommodation*) in the patient's chart. Head trauma, tumors, central nervous system disease, and certain medications can cause abnormal findings. Brain death, catecholamines, and atropine can cause the pupils to become dilated and fixed (**mydriasis**). Atropine is a common medication used during cardiopulmonary resuscitation, and its administration minimizes the use of assessing pupillary reflexes as a measure of the patient's neurologic status. Parasympathetic stimulants and opiates can cause pinpoint pupils (**miosis**). Examination of the pupillary reflexes is also discussed in Chapter 6.

Examination of the eyelids is useful when the RT or other clinician suspects disease of the cranial nerves. Drooping of the upper lid (**ptosis**) may be an early sign of disease involving the third cranial nerve. Congenital defects, cranial tumors, and neuromuscular diseases, such as myasthenia gravis, may cause ptosis. Ptosis may be an early warning sign of respiratory failure when a descending neuromuscular disease, such as myasthenia gravis, is occurring. Neuromuscular diseases affecting the cranial nerves also may result in blurred or double vision (**diplopia**) and involuntary, cyclic movement of the eyeballs known as **nystagmus**.

Neck

Inspection and palpation of the neck are of value in determining the tracheal position, estimating the jugular venous pressure (JVP), and identifying whether the patient's accessory muscles are in use. Normally, the trachea is located centrally in the neck when the patient is facing forward. The midline of the neck can be identified by palpation of the suprasternal notch at the base of the anterior neck. The midline of the trachea should be directly below the center of the suprasternal notch.

The trachea may be shifted from midline with atelectasis, pneumothorax, pleural effusion, or lung tumors. In instances of atelectasis or lung resection (removal of one part of a lung), the trachea shifts toward the affected side as it moves toward the side with reduced lung volumes. Conversely, the trachea often shifts (deviates) away from a tension pneumothorax, pleural effusion, or lung tumor because of the effect that excessive air, fluid, or tissue outside of the lung has on pushing the trachea away from the affected side toward the unaffected side. It should also be noted that abnormalities in the lower lung fields may not shift the trachea unless the defect is severe.

The JVP is estimated by examining the level of the column of blood in the jugular veins. JVP reflects the volume and pressure of the venous blood in the right side of the heart. Both the internal and external jugular veins can be assessed, although the internal jugular is most reliable. Persons with an obese or muscular neck may not have visible neck veins, even with distention.

In the supine position, the neck veins of a healthy person are full. When the head of the bed is elevated gradually to a 45-degree angle from horizontal, the level of the column of blood descends to a point no more than a few centimeters above the clavicle with normal venous pressure. With elevated venous pressure, the neck veins may be distended as high as the angle of the jaw, even when the patient is sitting upright (Fig. 5-1). The degree of venous distention can be estimated by measuring the distance the veins are distended above the sternal angle. The sternal angle has been chosen universally because its distance above the right atrium remains nearly constant (approximately 5 cm) in all positions. With the head of the bed elevated to a 45-degree angle, venous distention greater than 3 to 4 cm above the sternal angle is abnormal (Fig. 5-2).

Exact quantification of the jugular pressure in terms of centimeters above the sternal angle is difficult and

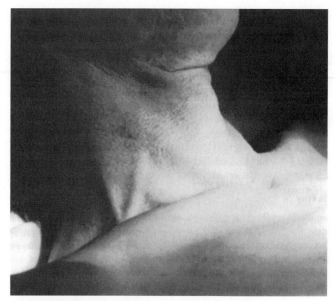

FIGURE 5-1 Photograph of jugular venous distention. (From Daily EK, Schroeder JP: *Techniques in bedside hemodynamic monitoring*, 5th ed. St. Louis: Mosby; 2000.)

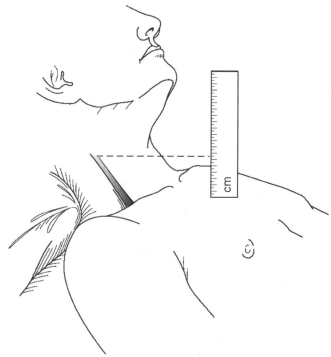

FIGURE 5-2 Estimation of jugular venous pressure. (Modified from Malasanos L, Barkauskas V, Stoltenberg-Allen K: *Health assessment*, 4th ed. St. Louis: Mosby; 1990.)

probably exceeds the accuracy needed for most observers. A simple grading scale of normal, increased, and markedly increased is acceptable.

The level of jugular venous distention may vary with breathing. During inhalation, the level of the column of blood may descend toward the thorax and return to the previous position with exhalation. For this reason, JVP should always be estimated at the end of exhalation.

The most common cause of jugular venous distention is right-sided heart failure. Right-sided heart failure may occur secondary to left-sided heart failure or chronic hypoxemia. Hypoxemia initiates pulmonary vasoconstriction and increases the resistance to blood flow through the pulmonary vasculature, increasing the workload of the right ventricle. Persistent lung disease with hypoxemia may result in right-sided heart failure and jugular venous distention. Jugular venous distention also may occur with hypervolemia and when the venous return to the right atrium is obstructed by tumors in the mediastinum.

SIMPLY STATED

Jugular venous distention most often is the result of right-sided heart failure. Right-sided heart failure occurs with chronic left-sided heart failure or when chronic hypoxemic lung disease is present.

Contraction of the sternocleidomastoid muscle in the neck is an indication that the patient's work of breathing is increased. It is a common finding in patients with airway obstruction and is discussed in the section on chest inspection.

The attending physician often examines the patient's neck for enlarged lymph nodes (**lymphadenopathy**) during the initial examination. Lymphadenopathy is a common finding in patients with respiratory infections, and the lymph nodes usually are tender to palpation in this situation. Nontender lymphadenopathy may be caused by malignancy or HIV.

The carotid pulse in the neck is palpated to evaluate the strength of the left ventricular contraction and the condition of the aortic valve. Heart disease that results in poor left ventricular contraction causes the carotid pulse to become weak. Stenosis of the aortic valve also causes a weak carotid pulse along with a systolic murmur (see Examination of the Precordium). An incompetent aortic valve that causes regurgitation of blood back into the left ventricle results in a pulse that rises and descends sharply. This is called a water-hammer pulse. The left and right carotid pulses must not be palpated simultaneously because this may significantly reduce blood flow to the brain.

The strength of the pulse at any location is described on a scale of 0 to 4, as follows:

0 = Absent, not palpable
1 = Diminished, barely palpable
2 = Expected normal amplitude
3 = Full and stronger than expected
4 = Bounding

Lung Topography

Understanding how the lungs are situated within the chest is vital when preparing to perform an accurate physical

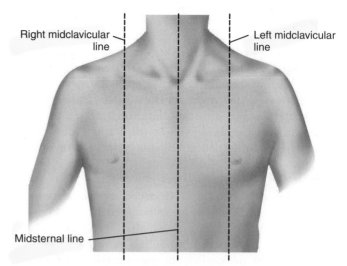

FIGURE 5-3 Imaginary lines on anterior chest wall. (From Kacmarek RM, Stoller JK, Heuer AJ: *Egan's fundamentals of respiratory care,* ed 10, St. Louis, 2013, Mosby-Elsevier.)

assessment of the respiratory system. Topographic (surface) landmarks of the chest are helpful in identifying the location of underlying structures and describing the location of abnormalities.

Imaginary Lines

On the anterior chest, the midsternal line divides the chest into two equal halves. The left and right midclavicular lines parallel the midsternal line and are drawn through the midpoints of the left and right clavicles, respectively (Fig. 5-3).

The midaxillary line divides the lateral chest into two equal halves. The anterior axillary line parallels the midaxillary line and is situated along the anterolateral chest. The posterior axillary line is also parallel to the midaxillary line and is located in the posterolateral chest (Fig. 5-4).

Three imaginary vertical lines are drawn on the posterior chest. The midspinal line divides the posterior chest into two equal halves. The left and right midscapular lines parallel the midspinal line and pass through the inferior angles of the scapulae in the relaxed upright patient (Fig. 5-5).

Thoracic Cage Landmarks

On the anterior chest, the suprasternal notch is located at the top of the manubrium and can be located by palpation of the depression at the base of the neck. Directly below this notch is the sternal angle, which is also called the **angle of Louis**. The sternal angle can be identified by palpating down from the suprasternal notch until the ridge between the gladiolus and the manubrium is identified. This important landmark is visible in most persons. The second rib articulates with the top of the gladiolus at this point (Fig. 5-6). Rib identification on the anterior chest can now be accomplished with this as a reference point. It is recommended that ribs be counted to the side of the

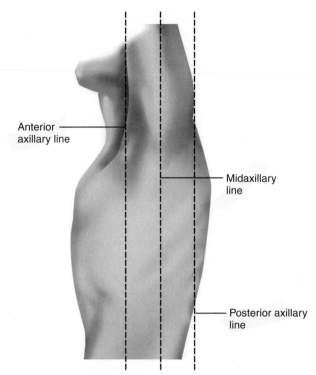

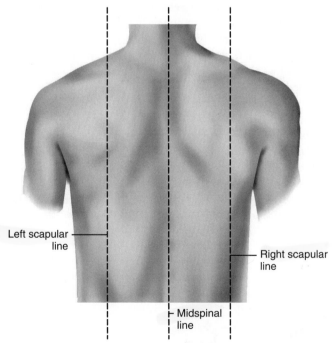

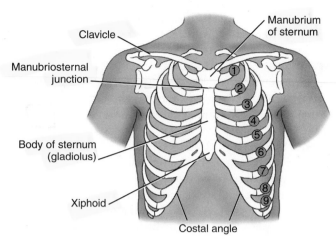

FIGURE 5-6 Thoracic cage landmarks on anterior chest.

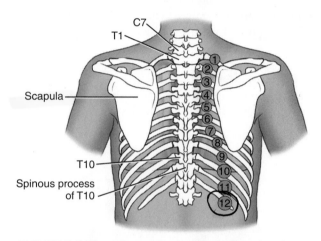

FIGURE 5-7 Thoracic cage landmarks on posterior chest.

FIGURE 5-4 Imaginary lines on lateral chest wall. (From Kacmarek RM, Stoller JK, Heuer AJ: *Egan's fundamentals of respiratory care,* ed 10, St. Louis, 2013, Mosby-Elsevier.)

FIGURE 5-5 Imaginary lines on posterior chest wall. (From Kacmarek RM, Stoller JK, Heuer AJ: *Egan's fundamentals of respiratory care,* ed 10, St. Louis, 2013, Mosby-Elsevier.)

sternum because individual costal cartilages that attach the ribs to the sternum are not identified as easily near the sternum.

On the posterior chest, the spinous processes of the vertebrae are useful landmarks (Fig. 5-7). The spinous process of the seventh cervical vertebra (C7) usually can be identified by having the patient extend the head and neck forward and slightly down. At the base of the neck, the most prominent spinous process that can be visualized and palpated is C7. The spinous process just below C7 belongs to the first thoracic vertebra (T1). The scapular borders also can be useful landmarks on the posterior chest. With the patient's arms raised above the head, the inferior border of the scapula lies almost directly over the oblique fissure that separates the upper from the lower lobes on the posterior chest.

Lung Fissures

Between the lobes of the lungs are the interlobar fissures. Both lungs have an oblique fissure that begins on the anterior chest at approximately the sixth rib at the midclavicular line. This fissure extends laterally and upward until it crosses the fifth rib on the lateral chest in the midaxillary line and continues on the posterior chest to approximately T3 (Figs. 5-8 and 5-9).

The right lung also has a horizontal fissure that separates the right upper lobe from the right middle lobe. The horizontal fissure extends from the fourth rib at the sternal border around to the fifth rib at the midaxillary line. The left lung rarely has a horizontal fissure.

Tracheal Bifurcation

On the anterior chest, the carina (tracheal bifurcation) is located approximately beneath the sternal angle (angle of Louis) and on the posterior chest at approximately T4.

Diaphragm

The diaphragm is a dome-shaped muscle that lies between the thoracic and abdominal cavities and moves up and down during normal ventilation. At the end of a tidal expiration, the right dome of the diaphragm is located at the level of T9 posteriorly and the fifth rib anteriorly. On the left, the diaphragm comes to rest at the end of expiration at T10 posteriorly and the sixth rib anteriorly. The right hemidiaphragm is usually a little higher anatomically than the left hemidiaphragm because of the placement of the liver.

Lung Borders

Superiorly on the anterior chest, the lungs extend 2 to 4 cm above the medial third of the clavicles. The inferior borders on the anterior chest extend to approximately the sixth rib at the midclavicular line and to the eighth rib on the lateral chest wall. On the posterior chest, the superior border extends to T1, and the inferior border varies with ventilation between approximately T9 and T12 (see Fig. 5-9).

Examination of the Thorax

Inspection

Visual examination of the chest is of value in assessing the thoracic configuration and the pattern and effort of breathing. For inspection to be adequate, the room must be well lighted, and the patient should be sitting upright. If the patient is too ill to sit up, the clinician must roll the patient carefully onto one side to examine the posterior chest. Male patients should be stripped to the waist. Female patients should be given some type of drape to prevent possible embarrassment from exposure of their breasts.

Thoracic Configuration

The normal adult thorax has an anteroposterior diameter less than the transverse (side-to-side) diameter. The anteroposterior diameter normally increases gradually with age and prematurely increases in patients with COPD. This abnormal increase in anteroposterior diameter is called a **barrel chest** and is commonly seen in patients with emphysema due to hypertrophy of the accessory muscles of breathing and chronic hyperinflation of the lungs. When the anteroposterior diameter increases, the ribs lose their normal 45-degree angle of slope in relation to the spine and become horizontal (Fig. 5-10). Other abnormalities of the thoracic configuration include the following:

Pectus carinatum: outward sternal protrusion anteriorly
Pectus excavatum: depression of part or all of the sternum
Kyphosis: spinal deformity in which the spine has an abnormal anteroposterior curvature (Fig. 5-11)
Scoliosis: spinal deformity in which the spine has a lateral curvature (see Fig. 5-11)

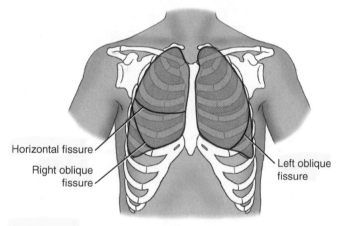

Horizontal fissure
Right oblique fissure
Left oblique fissure

FIGURE 5-8 Topographic position of lung fissures on anterior chest.

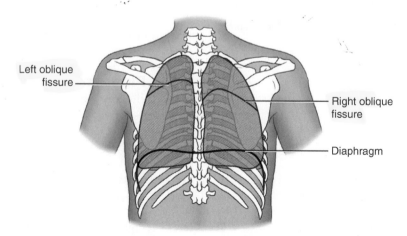

Left oblique fissure
Right oblique fissure
Diaphragm

FIGURE 5-9 Topographic position of lung fissures on posterior chest.

Kyphoscoliosis: combination of kyphosis and scoliosis (see Fig. 5-11)

It should be noted that several of the above abnormalities, depending on their severity, can result in a restrictive lung defect. In particular, the abnormalities of pectus excavatum and kyphoscoliosis may produce such a restriction. Severe trauma to the chest cage can result in fractures of the ribs and sternum. Abnormal configuration of the thoracic cage may result, especially if multiple ribs are broken. A section of the rib cage may move paradoxically with breathing when multiple ribs are fractured at more than one site. The paradoxical motion is seen as a sinking inward of the affected region with each spontaneous inspiratory effort and an outward movement with subsequent exhalation. This paradoxical motion of the affected rib cage is called **flail chest**.

Breathing Pattern and Effort

The healthy adult at rest has a consistent rate and rhythm of ventilation. The diaphragm and the intercostal muscles are the primary muscles of ventilation, actively working to increase the thoracic cavity dimension during normal inspiratory effort. During normal breathing at rest, the diaphragm performs the majority of the work of breathing. The effort of breathing is minimum on inhalation and passive on exhalation. Men typically breathe with the diaphragm, causing the stomach to move slightly outward during inhalation. Women tend to use a combination of intercostal muscles and the diaphragm, producing more chest wall movement than men. Table 5-1 describes the abnormal patterns of breathing. See Chapter 4, Table 4-4 for further descriptions of terms commonly used to describe breathing rates associated with patterns of breathing.

Additional muscles of ventilation, called **accessory muscles**, are also slightly active during normal, resting breathing. When ventilatory demands increase, these accessory muscles become more active in assisting the primary muscles of ventilation in the work of breathing. The predominant accessory muscles include the intercostal, scalene, sternocleidomastoid, pectoral, trapezius, and abdominal wall muscles. The accessory muscles of inspiration specifically include the external intercostals, scalene, sternocleidomastoids, trapezius, pectoralis minor, and pectoralis major. Changes in the patient's breathing pattern can provide important clues to the type of respiratory problem present. Patients with restrictive lung disease (reduced lung volumes) typically breathe with a rapid (tachypnea) and

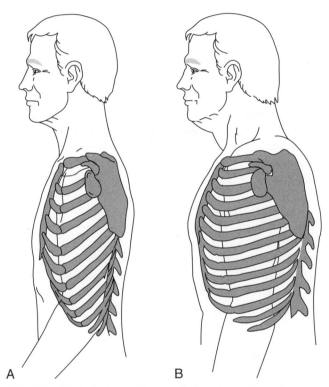

FIGURE 5-10 A, Patient with normal thoracic configuration. **B,** Patient with increased anteroposterior diameter. Note contrasts in angle or slope of ribs and development of accessory muscles.

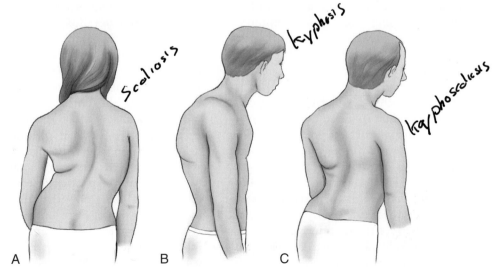

FIGURE 5-11 Examples of chest cage abnormalities. **A,** Scoliosis. **B,** Kyphosis. **C,** Kyphoscoliosis.

TABLE 5-1

Abnormal Breathing Patterns

Pattern	Characteristics	Causes
Tachypnea	Rapid rate of breathing	Loss of lung volume, arterial hypoxemia, metabolic acidosis
Apnea	No breathing	Cardiac arrest
Biot	Irregular breathing with long periods of apnea	Increased intracranial pressure
Cheyne-Stokes	Irregular type of breathing; breaths increase and decrease in depth and rate with periods of apnea	Diseases of central nervous system, congestive heart failure
Kussmaul	Deep and fast	Metabolic acidosis
Apneustic	Prolonged inhalation	Brain damage
Paradoxical	Injured portion of chest wall area moves in the opposite direction to the rest of the chest	Chest trauma
Abdominal paradox	Contraction of accessory muscles to aid inspiratory effort; diaphragm is pulled upward and abdomen sinks inward during inspiration	Fatigue of diaphragm, paralysis

shallow (hypopnea) pattern (see Chapter 4, Table 4-4 for further discussion of breathing rate and pattern terminology). The more lung volume lost, the greater increase in the respiratory rate. Acute obstruction of intrathoracic airways, as occurs with asthma, results in a prolonged exhalation time. The approximate I:E ratio can be determined by timing the two phases of breathing. Normal I:E ratio is approximately 1:2. With more severe cases of airway obstruction, the I:E ratio may be 1:3, 1:4, or even longer at 1:5 or greater. Acute upper airway obstruction, as occurs with croup or epiglottitis, often results in a prolonged inspiratory time.

> ### SIMPLY STATED
>
> The patient's breathing pattern often provides strong clues to the underlying pathologic condition. Rapid and shallow breathing suggests a loss of lung volume, a prolonged expiratory time indicates intrathoracic airway obstruction, and a prolonged inspiratory time indicates upper airway obstruction.

Any respiratory abnormalities that increase the work of breathing may cause the accessory muscles of breathing (most visibly the **scalenes** and **sternocleidomastoids**) to become active during breathing at rest. This is common in acute and chronic diffuse airway obstruction, acute upper airway obstruction, and disorders that reduce lung compliance such as pneumonia or acute respiratory distress syndrome.

Significant increases in the effort of breathing cause large swings in pleural pressure. As a result, the skin overlying the chest cage may sink inward between the ribs during inspiration and bulge outward during exhalation, when the work of breathing is increased. Inward depression of the skin during inspiration is known as **retractions**. Retractions may be seen between ribs (**intercostal**), below the ribs (subcostal), or above the clavicles (supraclavicular).

The opposite movement of the skin during exhalation is known as **bulging**. Obesity and muscular chest walls prevent retractions and bulging from occurring unless the abnormality is severe.

The diaphragm may be nonfunctional in patients with spinal injuries or neuromuscular disease and severely limited in patients with COPD. When this occurs, the accessory muscles of breathing become active, even at rest. The respiratory accessory muscles may also become active during acute airway obstruction. However, its absence does not rule out the possibility that severe airway obstruction is present.

In patients with emphysema, the lungs lose their elastic recoil and become hyperinflated. This results in the diaphragm assuming a lower, less functional position. The accessory muscles must assist ventilation by raising the anterior chest in an effort to increase thoracic volume. Significant use of the accessory muscles of breathing at rest is a sign of more severe chronic obstructive lung disease.

Normally, the abdomen moves gently outward with inspiration and inward with exhalation. When the diaphragm becomes fatigued, the accessory muscles of breathing attempt to maintain ventilation by becoming more active. As the accessory muscles contract in an effort to cause gas to flow into the lung, negative intrathoracic pressure causes the diaphragm to be pulled upward and the abdomen to sink inward during inspiration. This is known as **abdominal paradox**, which is an important finding that occurs with paralysis or fatigue of the diaphragm. Diaphragm fatigue is common in patients with COPD, especially during weaning from mechanical ventilation. It should be noted that abdominal paradox should not be confused with the term paradoxical pulse (also known as pulsus paradoxus), which is when the systolic blood pressure drops by more than 10 mm Hg during inspiration, described in more detail in Chapter 4.

Abdominal paradox may be accompanied by respiratory alternans. **Respiratory alternans** consists of periods of breathing using only the chest wall muscles alternating with periods of breathing entirely by the diaphragm. It is not as common as abdominal paradox but also is an indication that the diaphragm is fatigued. Not all patients with diaphragm dysfunction develop abdominal paradox or respiratory alternans, but when these clinical signs are present, they indicate significant inspiratory muscle fatigue.

COPD patients with severe hyperinflation have a low, flat diaphragm with limited mobility. Contraction of the flattened diaphragm pulls the lateral margins of the chest wall inward during each inspiratory effort. This abnormal movement of the lateral chest wall during breathing in COPD patients with severe hyperinflation is known as **Hoover sign**.

Patients with brain injury may have an abnormal pattern of breathing. The pattern of breathing often proves useful in determining the degree of brainstem function, which is discussed in Chapter 6.

Inspection for Central Cyanosis

Central cyanosis is present when the patient's trunk or oral mucosa is cyanotic. This occurs when the lungs are not oxygenating the blood adequately or when congenital heart disease causes venous blood to be shunted into the arterial system without passing through the lungs. Central cyanosis is an indication that tissue oxygenation may not be adequate and that further investigation is needed (e.g., arterial blood gas analysis). Cyanosis is apparent only when a significant amount of reduced (deoxygenated) hemoglobin is present. In patients with severe anemia (hemoglobin of 4 to 5 grams or less per deciliter of blood), cyanosis is generally not detected until advanced oxygenation problems are present.

> ### SIMPLY STATED
> Central cyanosis generally indicates hypoxemia or cyanotic heart disease. Further investigation is needed.

Palpation

Palpation is the act of touching the chest wall in an effort to evaluate underlying lung structure and function. Palpation is performed to evaluate vocal fremitus, estimate thoracic expansion, and assess the skin and subcutaneous tissues of the chest. Palpation is used in selected patients to confirm or rule out suspected problems suggested by the history and initial physical examination.

Vocal Fremitus

The term **vocal fremitus** refers to the vibrations created by the vocal cords during phonation. These vibrations are transmitted down the tracheobronchial tree and through the alveoli to the chest wall. When these vibrations are felt on the chest wall, they are called **tactile fremitus**.

During the assessment of tactile fremitus, the patient is directed to repeat the word "ninety-nine" while the clinician systematically palpates the thorax. The clinician can use the palmar aspect of the fingers or the ulnar aspect of the hand as illustrated in Figure 5-12. If one hand is used, it should be moved from one side of the chest to the corresponding area on the other side. The anterior, lateral, and posterior chest wall should be evaluated.

The vibrations of tactile fremitus may be increased, decreased, or absent. Increased fremitus results from the transmission of the vibration through a more solid medium. The normal lung structure is a combination of solid and air-filled tissue. Any condition that tends to increase the density of the lung, such as the consolidation of pneumonia, atelectasis, lung tumors or masses, results in an increased intensity of fremitus. If the area of consolidation or atelectasis is not in connection with a patent bronchus, for instance, due to mucous obstruction of a bronchus, fremitus will be absent or decreased.

A reduced tactile fremitus is often present in patients who are obese or overly muscular. In addition, when there is a bronchial obstruction such as a mucous plug or foreign object, or when the pleural space lining the lung becomes filled with air (pneumothorax) or fluid (pleural effusion), the vocal fremitus is reduced significantly or is absent.

The lungs become hyperinflated, with a significant reduction in the density of lung tissue, in patients with emphysema. In this situation, the vocal vibrations from the larynx transmit poorly through the lung tissue, resulting in a bilateral reduction in tactile fremitus. The bilateral reduction in tactile fremitus is more difficult to detect than the unilateral increase in fremitus associated with lobar consolidation. The causes of abnormal tactile fremitus are summarized as follows:

Increased
- Pneumonia
- Lung tumor or mass
- Atelectasis (with patent bronchiole)

Decreased
- Unilateral
  - Bronchial obstruction with mucous plug or foreign object
  - Pneumothorax
  - Pleural effusion
- Diffuse
  - COPD with hyperinflation
  - Muscular or obese chest wall

The passage of air through airways contaminated with thick secretions may produce palpable vibrations called rhonchial fremitus. Rhonchial fremitus often is identified during inhalation and exhalation and may clear if the patient produces an effective cough. It often is associated with a coarse, low-pitched sound that is audible without a stethoscope.

Thoracic Expansion

The normal chest wall expands symmetrically during deep inhalation. This expansion can be evaluated on the anterior and posterior chest. Anteriorly, the RT or other clinician's hands are placed over the anterolateral chest with the thumbs extended along the costal margin toward the xiphoid process. On the posterior chest, the hands are positioned over the posterolateral chest with the thumbs meeting at approximately T8 (Fig. 5-13). The patient is instructed to exhale slowly and completely while the clinician's hands

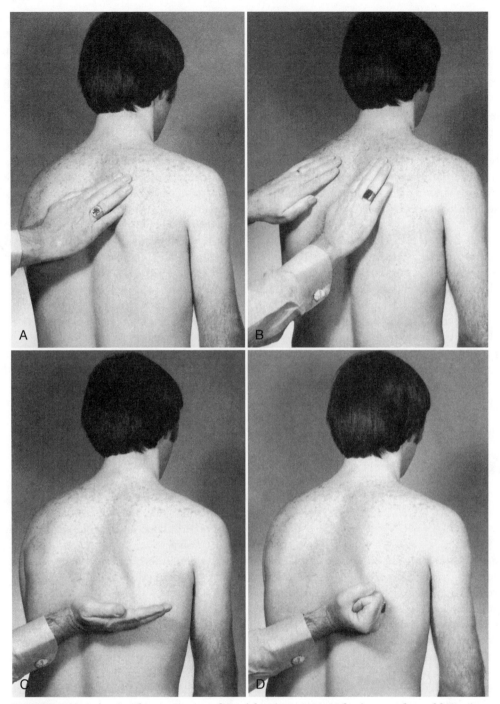

FIGURE 5-12 Palpation for assessment of vocal fremitus. **A,** Use of palmar surface of fingertips. **B,** Simultaneous application of fingertips of both hands. **C,** Use of ulnar aspect of hand. **D,** Use of ulnar aspect of closed fist. (From Prior JA, Silberstein JS: *Physical diagnosis: the history and examination of the patient,* ed 6, St. Louis, 1982, Mosby.)

are positioned as described. When the patient has exhaled maximally, the clinician gently secures the tips of his or her fingers against the sides of the chest and extends the thumbs toward the midline until the tip of each thumb meets at the midline. The patient is then instructed to take a full, deep breath. The clinician should make note of the distance each thumb moves from the midline. Normally, each thumb moves an equal distance of approximately 3 to 5 cm.

Diseases that affect expansion of both lungs cause a bilateral reduction in chest expansion. This is seen commonly with neuromuscular diseases and COPD. A unilateral (one-sided) reduction in chest expansion occurs with respiratory diseases that reduce the expansion of one lung or a major part of one lung. This may occur with lobar consolidation, atelectasis, pleural effusion, and pneumothorax.

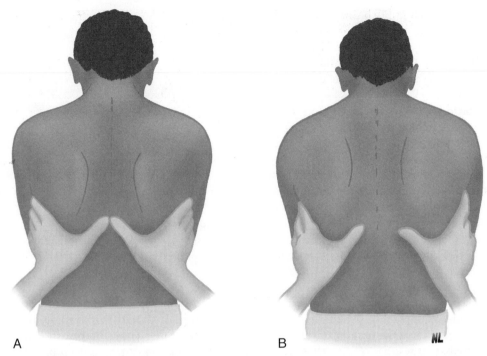

FIGURE 5-13 Estimation of thoracic expansion. **A,** Exhalation. **B,** Maximal inhalation. (From Kacmarek RM, Stoller JK, Heuer AJ: *Egan's fundamentals of respiratory care,* ed 10, St. Louis, 2013, Mosby-Elsevier.)

Skin and Subcutaneous Tissues

The chest wall can be palpated to determine the general temperature and condition of the skin. When air leaks from the lung into subcutaneous tissues, fine beads of air produce a crackling sound and sensation when the chest wall is palpated. This is called **subcutaneous emphysema**.

Percussion of the Chest to Assess Resonance

Percussion is the act of tapping on a surface in an effort to evaluate the underlying structure. Percussion of the chest wall produces a sound and a vibration useful in the evaluation of the underlying lung tissue. The vibration created by percussion penetrates and thus evaluates the lung to a depth of 5 to 7 cm below the chest wall.

The technique most often used in percussion of the chest wall is called mediate or indirect percussion. The RT or other clinician places the middle finger of the left hand (if the clinician is right-handed) firmly against the chest wall parallel to the ribs with the palm and other fingers held off the chest. The tip of the middle finger on the right hand or the lateral aspect of the right thumb strikes the finger against the chest near the base of the terminal phalanx with a quick, sharp blow. Movement of the hand striking the chest should be generated at the wrist and not the elbow or shoulder (Fig. 5-14).

The percussion note is clearest if the clinician remembers to keep the finger on the chest firmly against the chest wall and to strike this finger and immediately withdraw. The two fingers should be in contact for only an instant.

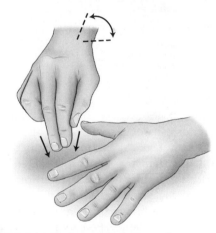

FIGURE 5-14 Technique for indirect chest percussion.

Percussion over Lung Fields

Percussion of the lung fields should be performed systematically, testing comparable areas on both sides of the chest consecutively. Percussion over the bony structures and breasts of the female patient is not of value and should be avoided. The RT or other clinician can ask the patient to raise his or her arms above the shoulders, which helps move the scapulae laterally and minimizes interference with percussion on the posterior chest wall.

The sounds generated during percussion of the chest are evaluated for intensity (loudness) and pitch. Percussion over normal lung fields produces a moderately low-pitched sound that can be heard easily. This sound is best described as normal resonance. When the percussion note is louder and lower in pitch than normal, the resonance is said to be increased. A hollow-sounding pitch during percussion is said to be **hyperresonant**. Percussion may produce a sound with characteristics just the opposite of resonance, referred to as dull or flat. This sound is high pitched, short in duration, and not loud. It is simply described as decreased resonance.

Clinical Implications. By itself, percussion of the chest is of little value in making a diagnosis. When the percussion note is considered along with the history and other physical findings, it may contribute significantly. Any abnormality that tends to increase the density of the lung tissue, such as the consolidation of pneumonia, lung tumors, or alveolar collapse (atelectasis), results in a loss of resonance and a dull percussion note over the affected area. Percussion over pleural spaces filled with fluid, such as blood or water, also results in decreased resonance.

An increase in resonance is detected in patients with hyperinflated lungs. Hyperinflation can occur as a result of acute bronchial obstruction (asthma) and chronic bronchial obstruction (emphysema). When the pleural space contains large amounts of air (pneumothorax), the percussion note increases in resonance over the affected side.

SIMPLY STATED

Increased resonance to percussion indicates excessive air trapped in the pleural space or lung; decreased resonance to percussion indicates fluid in the pleural space or consolidation of the lung.

Unilateral abnormalities are easier to detect than are bilateral abnormalities because the normal side provides an immediate comparison. The decreased resonance heard from percussion over consolidation is a distinct sound that is easier to detect than the subtle increase in resonance associated with hyperinflation or pneumothorax.

Percussion of the chest has limitations that are often clinically important. Abnormalities of the lungs are difficult to detect if the patient's chest wall is obese or overly muscular. Abnormalities that are small or more than 5 cm below the surface are not likely to be detected during percussion of the chest. Percussion to assess lung resonance is not performed routinely on most patients. However, it is useful in selected situations such as in the acutely ill patient suspected of having tension pneumothorax.

Diaphragmatic Excursion

The range of diaphragm movement may be estimated by percussion and is assessed best on the posterior chest wall (Fig. 5-15). For the clinician to estimate diaphragm movement, the patient first is instructed to take a deep, full inspiration and to hold it. The clinician then determines the lowest margin of resonance by percussing over the lower lung field and moving downward in small increments until a definite change in the percussion note is detected. The patient then is instructed to exhale maximally, holding

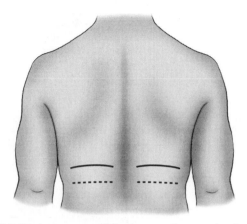

FIGURE 5-15 Assessment of diaphragmatic excursion by percussion. Horizontal lines indicate position of diaphragm at maximal inhalation (*dashed line*) and exhalation (*solid line*).

this position while the percussion procedure is repeated. The clinician should work rapidly to prevent the patient from becoming short of breath. The normal diaphragmatic excursion during a deep breath is approximately 5 to 7 cm. The range of diaphragm movement is less than normal in certain neuromuscular diseases and in patients with severe pulmonary hyperinflation (e.g., emphysema).

The exact range of movement and position of the diaphragm is difficult to determine by percussion. This probably is because the diaphragm is a dome-shaped muscle, with the center of the dome 15 cm beneath the surface of the posterior chest. Percussion can only approximate the position and degree of movement of the diaphragm.

Auscultation of the Lungs

Auscultation is the process of listening for sounds produced in the body. Auscultation over the thorax is performed to identify normal or abnormal lung sounds. Careful assessment of the patient's lung sounds is useful in making the initial diagnosis and evaluating the effects of treatment. A stethoscope is used during auscultation for better transmission of sounds to the clinician. The room must be as quiet as possible whenever auscultation is performed.

Stethoscope

The stethoscope includes four basic parts: a bell, a diaphragm, tubing, and earpieces (Fig. 5-16). The bell detects a broad spectrum of sounds and is of particular value in listening to low-pitched heart sounds. It is also valuable in auscultation of the lungs in certain situations such as in the emaciated patient whose rib protrusion restricts placement of the diaphragm flat against the chest. The bell piece should be pressed lightly against the chest when the clinician is attempting to auscultate low-frequency sounds. If the bell is pressed too firmly against the chest wall, the skin will be stretched under the bell and may act as a diaphragm, filtering out certain low-frequency sounds.

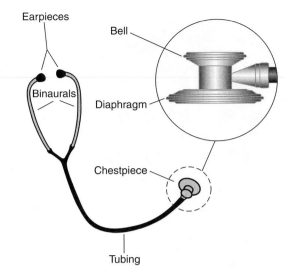

Earpieces

Bell

Binaurals

Diaphragm

Chestpiece

Tubing

FIGURE 5-16 Acoustic stethoscope. (From Kacmarek RM, Stoller JK, Heuer AJ: *Egan's fundamentals of respiratory care*, ed 10, St. Louis, 2013, Mosby-Elsevier.)

The diaphragm piece is used most often in auscultation of the lungs because most lung sounds are high frequency. It is also useful in listening to high-frequency heart sounds. The diaphragm piece should be pressed firmly against the chest so that external sounds are not heard.

The ideal tubing should be thick enough to exclude external noises and should be approximately 19 inches in length, with the total length of the stethoscope from the binaurals to the diaphragm being a standard 27 inches. Longer tubing may compromise transmission of lung sounds, and shorter tubing often is inconvenient in reaching the patient's chest.

The stethoscope should be examined regularly for cracks in the diaphragm, wax or dirt in the earpieces, and other defects that may interfere with the transmission of sound. It should be wiped with isopropyl alcohol regularly to prevent a buildup of microorganisms.

Technique

The patient should be sitting upright in a relaxed position when possible. The patient is instructed to breathe a little deeper than normal with the mouth open. Inhalation should be an active process and exhalation passive. The bell or diaphragm is placed directly against the chest wall to eliminate clothing as a factor in most cases. However, a thin gown or shirt/blouse probably offers little interference and may make the female patient more comfortable during the procedure. The tubing should not be allowed to rub against any objects because this may produce extraneous sounds. Auscultation of the lungs should be systematic, including all lobes on the anterior, lateral, and posterior chest. It is recommended that clinicians begin at the bases, compare side with side, and work toward the lung apices. The examination begins at the lung bases because certain abnormal lung sounds (described later) that occur

primarily in the dependent lung zones may be altered by several deep breaths (Fig. 5-17). The clinician should listen to at least one full ventilatory cycle at each position on the chest wall. Auscultation over the neck is useful whenever upper airway narrowing may be present.

Four characteristics of breath sounds are to be identified. First, the pitch, either high or low pitch (vibration frequency), is identified. Second, the amplitude or intensity (loudness) is noted. Third, the clinician listens for the distinctive characteristics. Fourth, the duration of inspiratory sound is compared with that of expiration. The acoustic characteristics of breath sounds can be illustrated in breath sound diagrams (Fig. 5-18). RTs and other members of the patient care team must have a clear understanding of the characteristics of the normal breath sounds described in Table 5-2 to identify subtle changes that may signify respiratory disease.

Terminology

In healthy persons, the sound heard over the trachea has a loud, tubular quality called a **tracheal breath sound**. Tracheal breath sounds are high-pitched sounds with an expiratory component equal to or slightly longer than the inspiratory component.

A slight variation to the tracheal breath sound is heard around the upper half of the sternum on the anterior chest and between the scapulae on the posterior chest (Fig. 5-19). This is not as loud as the tracheal breath sound, is slightly lower in pitch, and has equal inspiratory and expiratory components. It is called a bronchovesicular breath sound. It is not evaluated in most clinical situations.

Auscultating over the lung parenchyma of a healthy person yields a soft, muffled sound. This is called a **vesicular breath sound**, or normal breath sound, and is lower in pitch and intensity (loudness) than the tracheal breath sound. The vesicular sound is somewhat difficult to hear and is heard primarily during inhalation with only a minimal exhalation component (see Table 5-2).

Respiratory disease may alter the intensity of normal breath sounds heard over the lung fields. A slight variation in intensity is difficult to detect even for experienced clinicians. Breath sounds are described as diminished when the intensity decreases and absent in extreme cases. Breath sounds are described as harsh when the intensity increases. **Harsh breath sounds** may have an expiratory component equal to the inspiratory component and are described as **bronchial breath sounds** in such cases.

Abnormal lung sounds produced by the movement of air in the lungs are called adventitious sounds. The term **adventitious** refers to sounds that are added sounds or extra sounds produced within a normal sound, or heard in a place within the lung where that particular sound is not normally heard, such as tracheal or bronchial breath sounds heard over lung parenchyma. Health care workers also may often use the term adventitious as a synonym to mean abnormal lung sounds. Most adventitious lung

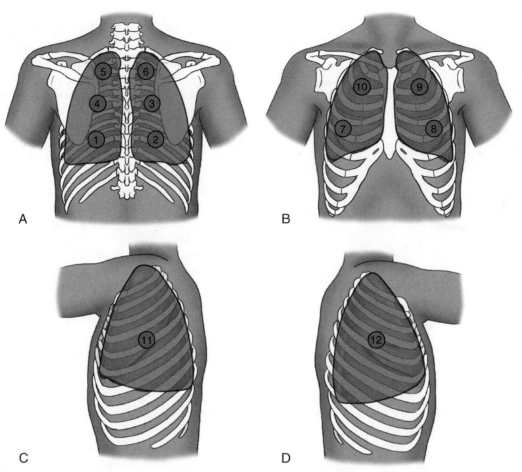

FIGURE 5-17 The normal sequencing for auscultation of the posterior (**A**); anterior (**B**); left lateral (**C**); and right lateral chest wall (**D**). Note that the clinician compares the breath sounds from side to side using the corresponding location on each side of the chest.

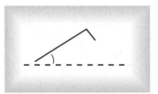

FIGURE 5-18 Diagrammatic representation of normal breath sound. Upstroke represents inhalation, downstroke represents exhalation, length of upstroke represents duration, thickness of stroke represents intensity, and angle between upstroke and horizontal line represents pitch. The example in this figure illustrates a normal vesicular breath sound. (Modified from Kacmarek RM, Stoller JK, Heuer AJ: *Egan's fundamentals of respiratory care,* ed 10, St. Louis, 2013, Mosby-Elsevier.)

SIMPLY STATED

Lung sounds are classified in two basic categories: normal breath sounds and adventitious lung sounds. The normal breath sounds are the expected sounds of breathing heard when auscultating each area of the lung, and the adventitious lung sounds are the abnormal sounds superimposed on the normal breath sounds or sounds not normally heard in the particular area of auscultation.

sounds can be classified as either continuous or discontinuous sounds. Continuous lung sounds are defined as those having a duration longer than 25 msec. (This definition is derived from recording and spectral analysis of lung sounds. Clinicians are not expected to time the lung sounds.) Discontinuous lung sounds are characteristically intermittent, crackling, or bubbling sounds of short duration (Fig. 5-20).

Experts have debated for many years about the terms to use in the description of abnormal lung sounds. Rales is an outdated term that had a long, evolving history and in the past was used to describe discontinuous abnormal lung sounds. Like the term rales, the term rhonchi has a confusing history and has been applied to more than one type of abnormal lung sound by various health care professionals. However, the American Thoracic Society (ATS) and the American College of Chest Physicians (ACCP) Joint Committee on Pulmonary Nomenclature has suggested that the term **crackles** be used to describe discontinuous, abnormal lung sounds, and the term **rhonchi** be used to describe low-pitched, continuous, abnormal lung sounds. Crackles may be heard

TABLE 5-2

Characteristics of Normal Breath Sounds

Breath Sound	Pitch	Intensity	Location	Diagram of Sound
Vesicular or normal	Low	Soft	Peripheral lung areas	
Bronchovesicular	Moderate	Moderate	Around upper part of sternum, between scapulae	
Tracheal	High	Loud	Over trachea	

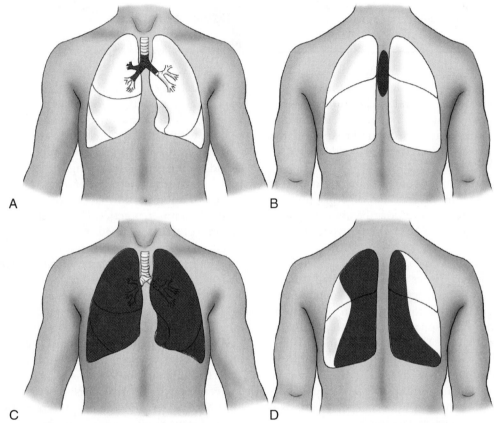

FIGURE 5-19 Location on chest wall where normal bronchovesicular and vesicular breath sounds are heard. **A,** Anterior bronchovesicular. **B,** Posterior bronchovesicular. **C,** Anterior vesicular. **D,** Posterior vesicular.

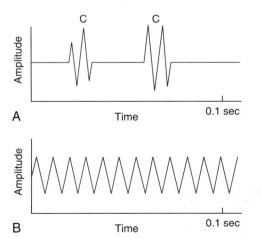

FIGURE 5-20 Time-expanded waveforms demonstrating inspiratory crackles (**A**) and expiratory polyphonic wheezes (**B**). (Modified from Wilkins RL, et al: Lung sound terminology used by respiratory care practitioners. *Respir Care* 34:36, 1989.)

when air moves through excessive fluid or secretions in the airways, when collapsed airways pop open during inspiration

Low-pitched "coarse" crackles (a crackling sound) that are continuous are often referred to as rhonchi.

The term **wheeze** is used to describe the musical sounds heard from the chest of the patient with intrathoracic airway obstruction (e.g., asthma). Wheezes are classified as continuous sounds and are easily recognized in most cases.

SIMPLY STATED

The term *crackles* should be used for discontinuous abnormal lung sounds. Both the terms *wheeze* and *rhonchi* are classified as continuous adventitious lung sounds. Wheeze is an abnormal musical sound, and rhonchi describes low-pitched, continuous, abnormal lung sounds.

TABLE 5-3

Recommended Terminology for Lung Sounds and Other Terms Used

Recommended Term	Classification	Other Terms Used
Crackles	Discontinuous	Rales
		Crepitations
Rhonchi	Low-pitched, continuous	Coarse crackles
Wheezes	High-pitched, continuous	Sibilant rales
		Musical rales
		Sibilant rhonchus

Another continuous type of adventitious lung sound, heard primarily over the larynx and trachea during inhalation when upper airway obstruction is present, is known as **stridor**. This is a loud, high-pitched sound that often may be heard without the aid of a stethoscope. Stridor is readily recognized by most clinicians.

Because there is a lack of standardization of lung sound terminology among clinicians, authors of other publications may use different terms to describe abnormal lung sounds. Table 5-3 provides a list of alternative terms that may be used by others.

When abnormal lung sounds are identified, their location and specific characteristics should be noted. Abnormal lung sounds may be high or low pitched, loud or faint, scanty or profuse, and inspiratory or expiratory (or both). The timing during the respiratory cycle should also be noted (e.g., late inspiratory). The RT or other clinician must pay close attention to these characteristics of abnormal lung sounds because they help determine the functional status of the lungs. The importance of using appropriate qualifying adjectives to describe abnormal lung sounds is further emphasized in the next paragraphs.

Mechanisms and Significance of Lung Sounds

The exact mechanisms responsible for the production of normal and abnormal lung sounds are not understood in detail. However, there is enough agreement among investigators to allow a general description. This knowledge should provide a better understanding of the lung sounds often heard through a stethoscope.

Normal Breath Sounds. Lung sounds heard over the chest of the healthy person are generated primarily by turbulent flow in the larger airways. Turbulent flow creates audible vibrations in the airways, producing sounds that are transmitted through the lung and the chest wall. As the sound travels to the lung periphery and the chest wall, it is altered by the normal lung. Normal lung tissue acts as a low-pass filter, which means it preferentially passes low-frequency sounds. This filtering effect can be demonstrated easily by listening over the periphery of the lung while a subject speaks. The muffled voice sounds are difficult to understand because of the filtering properties of the normal lung. The alteration of sounds that travel through the lung is known as **attenuation**. Attenuation accounts for the characteristic differences between tracheal and bronchovesicular breath sounds heard directly over larger airways and vesicular sounds heard over the periphery of the lung.

Normal vesicular lung sounds are at least partly produced locally in the underlying lobe being auscultated.

SIMPLY STATED

All normal breath sounds are produced primarily by turbulent flow in the airways.

The stability of normal breath sounds over time has been studied. Results indicate that normal vesicular breath sounds remain very stable from one day to the next in healthy persons with regard to pitch and amplitude. This suggests that significant changes in the pitch or loudness of breath sounds in the patient breathing with a similar pattern over time is not normal, and further investigation is indicated.

Auscultation for normal breath sounds following intubation is common practice. This is performed in an attempt to confirm that the tube is placed properly in the trachea and not in the esophagus or one of the mainstem bronchi. The finding of bilateral vesicular breath sounds is strong evidence that the tube is in the trachea. Confirmation by a chest film is recommended because the breath sounds may be difficult to hear in some patients, and air entering the esophagus may be misinterpreted as breath sounds.

Abnormal Bronchial Breath Sounds. Bronchial breath sounds may replace the normal vesicular sound when the lung increases in density, as occurs in pneumonia and certain types of atelectasis. When the normal air-filled lung becomes consolidated, the attenuation of sound is reduced, and similar sounds are heard over large upper airways and the consolidated lung (Fig. 5-21).

Diminished Breath Sounds. Diminished breath sounds occur when the sound intensity at the site of generation (larger airways) is reduced or when the sound transmission properties of the lung or chest wall are reduced. The intensity of sound created by turbulent flow through the bronchi is reduced with shallow or slow breathing patterns (e.g., major sedation). Obstructed airways (e.g., mucous plugs) and hyperinflated lung tissue (e.g., emphysema) increase attenuation of breath sounds through the lungs. Air (pneumothorax) or fluid (e.g., pleural effusion) in the pleural space and obesity reduce the transmission of breath sounds through the chest wall.

SIMPLY STATED

Diminished breath sounds are produced by shallow breathing or when the turbulent flow sounds of the larger airways are not transmitted through the lung or chest wall. This attenuation of breath sounds is increased with mucous plugging or pleural effusion that absorbs or reflects sound.

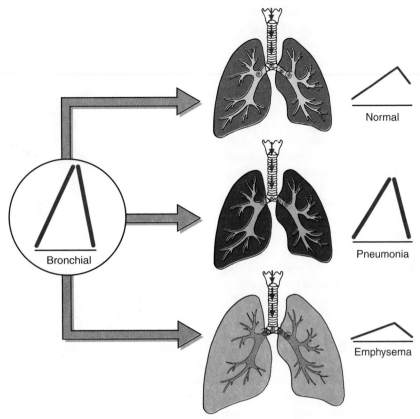

FIGURE 5-21 Examples of how the normal bronchial breath sound is altered as it passes through normal (*top*), consolidated (*middle*), and emphysematous (*bottom*) lung tissue.

Wheezes. Wheezes are generated by the vibration of the wall of a narrowed or compressed airway as air passes through at high velocity (Fig. 5-22). The diameter of an airway may be reduced by bronchospasm, mucosal edema, increased mucus production, or foreign object obstruction. The pitch of the wheeze is independent of the length of the airway but is related directly to the degree of airway compression—the tighter the compression, the higher the pitch. Low-pitched continuous sounds often are associated with the presence of excessive sputum in the airways. A sputum flap vibrating in the airstream may produce low-pitched wheezes that clear after the patient coughs.

When wheezes are identified, certain characteristics should be noted. RTs and other clinicians should identify the pitch and intensity and the portion of the respiratory cycle occupied by the wheezing. Improvement in the patient's airway caliber with bronchodilator therapy often results in a decrease in pitch and intensity of the wheezing and in a reduction in the portion of the respiratory cycle occupied by wheezing. For example, before treatment, the patient may have loud, high-pitched wheezing that is heard during inspiration and expiration. After bronchodilator therapy, the wheezing may decrease in pitch and intensity and be heard only during the latter part of exhalation. Because the intensity of wheezing is related to the flow, loud wheezing indicates that air movement is occurring, whereas soft wheezing may occur with fatigue and the

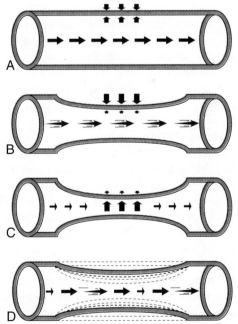

FIGURE 5-22 Proposed mechanism for wheezing. **A,** Normal airway, where internal and external airway wall pressures are equal. **B,** Slight narrowing of the airway, which causes an increase in the velocity of airflow and a decrease in the lateral wall pressure inside the airway relative to the outside. **C,** Greater narrowing of the airway to the point that forward flow is inhibited and lateral wall pressure increases relative to outside pressure. **D,** Fluttering of the airway walls between position of **B** and **C.**

onset of respiratory failure. The clinician must never rely solely on changes in the intensity (loudness) of wheezing in assessing the patient's response to therapy.

Wheezing may be polyphonic (having several different musical notes) or monophonic (having a single note). Polyphonic wheezing is limited to exhalation, and its many different musical notes begin and end simultaneously, indicating that multiple airways are obstructed, as in asthma. Monophonic wheezes may occur in one or more than one bronchus, with each one indicating obstruction of a bronchus. When multiple monophonic wheezes are present, the multiple notes often begin and end at different times; therefore, these single-note wheeze sounds may overlap. The illusion of widespread airway obstruction results from a few loud notes transmitting to most areas of the chest wall. A single monophonic wheeze indicates obstruction of a single airway. This may be present in the patient with an airway tumor that is partially obstructing a major airway or with aspiration of a foreign object. The clinician who hears a monophonic wheeze over the patient's chest should also auscultate over the patient's neck. If the wheeze is heard loudest over the neck, the upper airway is the source of the sound.

Stridor. Stridor is produced by mechanisms similar to those of wheezing. Rapid airflow through a narrow site of the upper airway causes the lateral walls to vibrate and produce a high-pitched sound often heard without a stethoscope. The diameter of the upper airway is most often narrowed because of infection, as in croup or epiglottitis, or with inflammation after extubation. Stridor is most often heard during inhalation because the upper airway tends to narrow with significant inspiratory efforts. It may also be heard during inhalation and exhalation when the upper airway obstruction is severe and fixed (airway opening does not vary with breathing). This is seen in patients with laryngeal tumor.

Stridor can be a life-threatening sign that indicates ventilation may be compromised. The patient with stridor should be monitored closely, and equipment and personnel needed to perform emergency intubation, cricothyroidotomy, or tracheostomy should be nearby. The simultaneous presentation of stridor and cyanosis is a particularly ominous sign because the cyanosis probably is the result of hypoxemia caused by hypoventilation. Like wheezing, stridor can occur only when significant airflow is present through the site of obstruction. As a result, the lack of stridor should never be interpreted as a sign of a healthy upper airway in the patient with a history or other clinical findings consistent with upper airway abnormalities.

Crackles. Crackles often are produced by the movement of excessive secretions or fluid in the airways as air passes through. In this situation, crackles usually are coarse and heard during inspiration and expiration. They often clear if the patient coughs, and they may be associated with rhonchial fremitus.

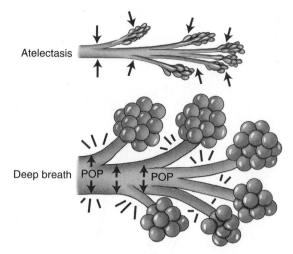

FIGURE 5-23 Proposed mechanism for late inspiratory crackles. Peripheral airways pop open when inspiratory effort is sufficient to overcome the forces causing the atelectasis.

Airway closure may occur in peripheral bronchioles or in more proximal bronchi. Crackles also occur in patients without excess secretions when collapsed airways pop open during inspiration. The crackling sound in this situation is caused by the explosive equalization of pressure between the collapsed airways and the patent airways above. The source of the crackles in this situation may be suggested by certain characteristics described in the next paragraphs.

Larger, more proximal bronchi may close during expiration when there is an abnormal increase in bronchial compliance, such as in the case of severe emphysema. In this situation, crackles usually occur early in the inspiratory phase and are called **early inspiratory crackles**. Early inspiratory crackles are usually few in number but may be loud or faint. They often are transmitted to the mouth and are not silenced by a cough or change in position. They occur most often in patients with COPD, as in chronic bronchitis, and emphysema, and may indicate that a more severe airway obstruction is present.

Peripheral alveoli and airways may close during exhalation when the surrounding intrathoracic pressure increases. Crackles produced by the sudden opening of peripheral airways usually occur late in the inspiratory phase and are called **late inspiratory crackles** (Fig. 5-23). They are more common in the dependent regions of the lungs, where the gravitational stress predisposes the peripheral airways to collapse during exhalation. They are often identified in several consecutive respiratory cycles, producing a recurrent rhythm. They may clear with changes in posture or if the patient performs several deep inspiratory maneuvers. Coughing or maximal exhalation by the patient may produce the reappearance of late inspiratory crackles. Patients with respiratory disorders, such as atelectasis, pneumonia, pulmonary edema, and fibrosis, that reduce lung volume (restrictive disorders) are most likely to have the late inspiratory type of crackles (Table 5-4).

TABLE 5-4			
Application of Adventitious Lung Sounds			
Lung Sounds	Possible Mechanism	Characteristics	Causes
Rhonchi	Airflow through mucus	Discontinuous, coarse	Pneumonia, bronchitis, bronchiectasis, cystic fibrosis, other lung infections
Wheezes	Rapid airflow through obstructed airways caused by bronchospasm, mucosal edema	High-pitched; most often occur during exhalation	Asthma, congestive heart failure (CHF), bronchitis
Stridor	Rapid airflow through obstructed upper airway caused by inflammation or fixed obstruction	High-pitched; often occurs during inhalation	Croup, epiglottitis, post-extubation airway edema, laryngeal tumor
Crackles			
Inspiratory and expiratory	Excess airway secretions moving with airflow	Coarse and often clears with cough	Bronchitis, respiratory infections
Early inspiratory	Sudden opening of proximal bronchi	Scanty, transmitted to mouth; not affected by cough	Bronchitis, emphysema, congestive heart failure
Late inspiratory	Sudden opening of peripheral airways	Diffuse, fine; occur initially in the dependent regions	Atelectasis, pneumonia, pulmonary edema, fibrosis

SIMPLY STATED

Wheezing indicates intrathoracic airway obstruction, whereas late inspiratory crackles suggest atelectasis or other conditions of the lung that cause a loss of lung volume. Fine crackles indicate the sudden opening of airways. Rhonchi or coarse crackles indicate excess airway mucus moving with airflow into and out of the lung.

Pleural Friction Rub. A **pleural friction rub** is a creaking or grating type of sound that occurs when the inflamed pleural membranes (**pleurisy**) rub together. It may be heard only during inhalation but often is identified during both phases of breathing, with the intensity of sound increasing during deep breaths. Pleural rubs are rarely encountered in the clinical setting and for this reason often are not identified correctly when present. Pleural rubs may be heard in patients with pneumonia, pulmonary fibrosis, or pulmonary embolism, or after thoracic surgery.

Voice Sounds

If inspection, palpation, percussion, or auscultation of the patient's chest suggests any respiratory abnormality, vocal resonance may be useful. Vocal resonance is produced by the same mechanism as vocal fremitus, described earlier. The vibrations created by the vocal cords during phonation travel down the tracheobronchial tree and through the peripheral lung units to the chest wall. The patient is instructed to repeat the words "one, two, three" or "ninety-nine" while the clinician listens over the chest wall with the aid of a stethoscope, comparing side with side. The normal, air-filled lung tissue filters the voice sounds, resulting in a significant reduction in intensity and clarity. Pathologic abnormalities in lung tissue alter the transmission of voice sounds, resulting in either increased or decreased vocal resonance.

An increase in intensity and clarity of vocal resonance is called **bronchophony**. Bronchophony occurs as a result of an increase in lung tissue density, as in the consolidation of pneumonia, and is the result of the better transmission of vocal vibrations through consolidation. Bronchophony is easier to detect when it is unilateral and is often associated with bronchial breath sounds, dull percussion note, and increased vocal fremitus.

Egophony is when the spoken voice sounds increase in intensity through the chest wall and the quality sounds nasal or bleating. This is assessed by the clinician when the patient is asked to say "e-e-e" but the sound is heard as "a-a-a" through the stethoscope. The area where it is heard may indicate a compressed lung above a pleural effusion. Whispering pectoriloquy is a technique to assess a patient for lung consolidation. Whispering of the words "one, two, three" by the patient creates high-frequency vibrations that are selectively filtered by normal lung tissue. Normally, whispers are heard as muffled, low-pitched sounds through the stethoscope. If the clinician hears high-pitched sounds, this is evidence that consolidation is present in the lung.

Vocal resonance is reduced in similar lung abnormalities that result in reduced breath sounds and decreased tactile fremitus. Hyperinflation of lung parenchyma, pneumothorax, bronchial obstruction, and pleural effusion reduce the transmission of vocal vibrations through the lung or chest wall, producing decreased vocal resonance.

Examination of the Precordium

As mentioned previously, chronic diseases of the lungs may and often do cause abnormalities in other body systems. Recognition of these abnormalities is helpful in identifying respiratory disease and in quantifying its severity. Because of the close working relationship between the heart and lungs, the heart is especially at risk for developing problems secondary to lung disease. The techniques for physical examination of the chest wall overlying the heart (**precordium**) include inspection, palpation, and auscultation. Percussion is of little or no value in the examination and is omitted. For the sake of convenience, most clinicians perform the examination of the precordium simultaneously with the examination of the lungs.

Review of Heart Topography

The heart lies between the lungs within the mediastinum and is situated so that the right ventricle is more anterior than the left ventricle. The upper portion of the heart consists of both atria and commonly is called the *base of the heart*. The base lies directly beneath the upper-middle portion of the gladiolus (sternum). The lower portion of the heart, which consists of the ventricles, is called the *apex*. The apex points downward and to the left, extending to a point near the midclavicular line, and usually lies directly beneath the lower left portion of the gladiolus and near the costal cartilage of the fifth rib (Fig. 5-24).

Inspection and Palpation

The purpose of inspecting and palpating the precordium is to identify any normal or abnormal pulsations. Pulsations on the precordium are affected by the thickness of the chest wall and the quality of the tissue through which the vibrations must travel. The normal apical impulse is produced by the thrust of the contracting left ventricle and usually is identified near the midclavicular line in the fifth intercostal space. This systolic thrust may be felt and visualized in many healthy persons; it may be called the **point of maximal impulse (PMI)**.

Right ventricular hypertrophy, a common manifestation of chronic lung disease, often produces a systolic thrust (**heave**) that is felt and may be visualized near the lower left sternal border. The palmar aspect of the clinician's right hand is placed over the lower left sternal border for identification. Right ventricular hypertrophy may be the result of chronic hypoxemia, pulmonary valve disease, or pulmonary hypertension.

In patients with chronic pulmonary hyperinflation (emphysema), identification of the apical impulse is more difficult. The increase in anteroposterior diameter and the alteration in lung tissue contribute to poor transmission of the vibrations of systole to the surface of the chest. Therefore, in patients with pulmonary emphysema, the intensity of the PMI often is reduced or not identifiable.

The PMI may shift to the left or right with shifts in the mediastinum. Pneumothorax or lobar collapse often shifts the mediastinum, resulting in a shift of the PMI toward the lobar collapse but usually away from the pneumothorax. Patients with emphysema and low, flat diaphragms may have the PMI located in the epigastric area.

The second left intercostal space near the sternal border is called the *pulmonic area* and is palpated in an effort to identify accentuated pulmonary valve closure. Strong vibrations may be felt in this area with pulmonary hypertension (Fig. 5-25).

Auscultation of Heart Sounds

Normal heart sounds are created primarily by the closure of the heart valves. The first normal heart sound is S_1, produced by the sudden closure of the mitral and tricuspid valves (often called the *atrioventricular [AV] valves*), which happens virtually simultaneously during contraction of the ventricles (systole). The second normal heart sound is S_2. When systole ends, the ventricles relax and the pulmonic and aortic (semilunar) valves close, which signals the onset of diastole and creates the second heart sound (S_2). Because the left side of the heart has a significantly higher pressure created during systole, closure of the mitral valve is louder and contributes more to the S_1 sound than the closure of the tricuspid valve in the healthy person. For the same reason, closure of the aortic valve usually contributes more to the production of S_2. Both S_1 and S_2 heart sounds are normally heard in all populations. The S_3 and S_4 heart sounds are only normal in small children and may indicate a murmur in adults.

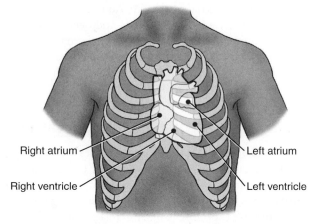

FIGURE 5-24 Topographic position of the heart.

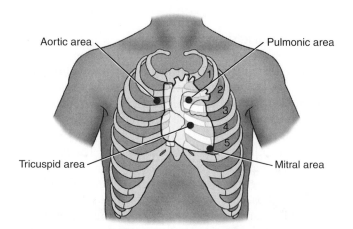

FIGURE 5-25 Position on the chest where each heart valve is best auscultated. Note that the stethoscope chest piece is placed between the ribs to better hear the underlying heart sounds and to avoid interference by bony structures.

A split in the S_1 sound is heard when the tricuspid valve closure is delayed, and the sounds of the mitral and tricuspid valve are heard separately. This significant splitting of S_1 usually indicates heart disease. Defects in the electrical conduction system of the heart, such as bundle branch block, cause the two ventricles to lack synchrony during systole, causing a splitting of S_1.

Splitting of S_2 occurs when the semilunar valves (pulmonic and aortic) do not close simultaneously. A physiologically normal, narrow splitting of S_2 is due to the effects of spontaneous breathing on blood flow into the heart. During inhalation, there is a decrease in intrathoracic pressure, increasing venous return to the right side of the heart, which further delays pulmonic valve closure. The splitting of S_2 decreases or disappears on exhalation. Wide splitting of the second heart sound (significantly delayed closure of the pulmonic valve after the aortic valve) is usually a sign of disease and is seen with pulmonary hypertension, right bundle branch block, pulmonary embolism, and right-sided heart failure.

A third heart sound (S_3) may be identified early in diastole. S_3 is thought to be produced by rapid ventricular filling immediately after systole. The rapid distention of the ventricles causes the walls of the ventricles to vibrate briefly and produce a sound of low intensity and pitch. It is best heard over the apex with the bell of the stethoscope. It is normal in young healthy children and is called physiologic S_3 in this situation. However, in patients older than 40 years of age and especially in those with a history of heart disease, an S_3 is usually a sign of disease. S_3 usually indicates a ventricular abnormality (e.g., myocardial infarction) or some condition in which ventricular filling in volume or pressure is increased, such as an enlarged, failing ventricle. A fourth heart sound (S_4) also may be identified during diastole. S_4 occurs late in diastole just before S_1. S_4 is produced by active filling of the ventricles from atrial contraction just before systole. It may occur in healthy persons but most often is considered a sign of heart disease. The presence of an S_4 heart sound suggests decreased ventricular compliance with increased resistance to filling (increased end-diastolic pressure) as occurs with systemic hypertension, ventricular hypertrophy with outflow obstruction, ischemic heart disease, aortic stenosis, and acute mitral valve regurgitation. Most patients with an acute myocardial infarction have an S_4 if a sinus rhythm is present as seen on the electrocardiogram (see Chapter 11). The patient with an S_4 is often incorrectly thought to have a split S_1 because the timing of S_4 is normally very close to the first heart sound (Fig. 5-26).

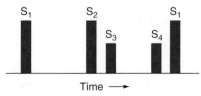

FIGURE 5-26 Timing of the first, second, third, and fourth heart sounds.

A **gallop rhythm** is an abnormal condition in which a third (S_3) or fourth (S_4) heart sound is present. The spacing of the heart sounds results in a unique sequence of sounds that resembles the gallop of a horse. A gallop rhythm suggests that the left or right ventricle is being overdistended during diastole. When an S_3 or S_4 is present and originates in the right ventricle, it is best heard at the left sternal border near the apex. When the S_3 or S_4 originates in the left ventricle, it is best heard at the midclavicular line over the apex of the heart.

Auscultation of the heart sounds may identify alterations in the loudness of S_1 or S_2. A reduction in the intensity of the heart sounds may be the result of cardiac or extracardiac abnormalities. Extracardiac factors include alteration in the tissue between the heart and the surface of the chest. Pulmonary hyperinflation, pneumothorax, and obesity make identification of both S_1 and S_2 difficult. S_1 and S_2 intensity may also be reduced when the force of ventricular contraction is poor, as in heart failure, or when valvular abnormalities exist.

Pulmonary hypertension increases intensity of S_2 as a result of more forceful closure of the pulmonic valve; this is called an increased or **loud P$_2$**. A loud P_2 is a common finding in patients with pulmonary hypertension, cor pulmonale, and pulmonary embolism because high pulmonary artery pressures cause the pulmonic valve to close with more force. An increased P_2 is identified best over the pulmonic area of the chest (see Fig. 5-25). A loud aortic valve component (loud A_2) is commonly heard in patients with systemic hypertension. The best location to auscultate each heart valve is presented in Figure 5-25.

> **SIMPLY STATED**
>
> A gallop rhythm is an abnormal condition in which a third (S_3) or fourth (S_4) heart sound is present in the adult. A loud pulmonic valve component to the second heart sound is called a *loud P_2* and suggests pulmonary hypertension, cor pulmonale, and/or pulmonary embolism. A loud aortic valve component (*loud A_2*) is commonly heard in patients with systemic hypertension.

Cardiac murmurs are identified whenever the heart valves are incompetent (incomplete closure) or stenotic (narrowed). Murmurs usually are classified as either systolic or diastolic. Systolic murmurs occur during systole and are heard following S_1. These murmurs are produced by an incompetent AV valve as in mitral valve regurgitation or a stenotic semilunar valve as in aortic valve stenosis. An incompetent mitral valve allows a backflow of blood into the left atrium, usually producing a high-pitched whooshing noise simultaneously with S_1. A stenotic aortic valve produces a similar sound because a narrowed valve creates an obstruction of blood flow out of the ventricle during systole.

Diastolic murmurs occur during diastole and are heard following S_2. These murmurs are created by either an incompetent semilunar valve, as in aortic regurgitation, or a stenotic AV valve, as in mitral stenosis. In aortic regurgitation, an incompetent aortic valve allows a backflow (reflux) of blood from the aorta into the left ventricle simultaneously with or immediately after S_2. A stenotic mitral valve obstructs blood flow from the left atrium into the left ventricle creating a turbulent murmur sound.

A murmur may also be created by rapid blood flow across normal valves. In summary, murmurs are created by a backflow of blood through an incompetent valve, forward flow through a stenotic valve, and rapid flow through a normal valve.

When indicated, auscultation of heart sounds is usually performed at the same time as auscultation of lung sounds. The diaphragm of the stethoscope is most useful for higher-frequency sounds such as S_1, S_2, and systolic murmurs. The bell side of the stethoscope is best used for low-frequency sounds such as gallops (S_3 and S_4) and diastolic murmurs. The heart sounds may be easier to identify if the patient leans forward or lies on the left side because anatomically this moves the heart closer to the chest wall. When the peripheral pulses are difficult to identify, auscultation over the precordium may be an easier method of assessing the heart rate.

Examination of the Abdomen

An in-depth discussion of the abdominal examination is beyond the scope of this text; however, the abnormalities associated with respiratory disease are reviewed here.

The abdomen should be inspected and palpated for evidence of distention and tenderness. Abdominal distention may cause impairment of excursion of the diaphragm and contribute to respiratory failure. Distention may also inhibit the patient from coughing and deep breathing, both of which are extremely important in preventing respiratory complications in the postoperative patient.

Palpation and percussion are used on the right upper quadrant (Fig. 5-27) of the abdomen in an effort to estimate the size of the liver. An enlarged liver may be found when chronic right-sided heart failure has occurred as a consequence of chronic respiratory disease. Any respiratory disease that results in a reduction of the oxygen level in the blood causes pulmonary vasoconstriction. If this occurs over a period of months or years, the right ventricle becomes enlarged and fails to pump blood effectively. The venous blood flow returning to the right ventricle is reduced, and engorgement of major veins and organs may occur. The hepatic vein that empties into the inferior vena cava may become engorged in this situation, and the liver may increase in size. This is called **hepatomegaly**.

To identify hepatomegaly, the clinician locates the superior and inferior borders of the liver by percussion. Normally, the liver spans approximately 10 cm at the right midclavicular line. If the liver extends more than 10 cm, it is considered enlarged.

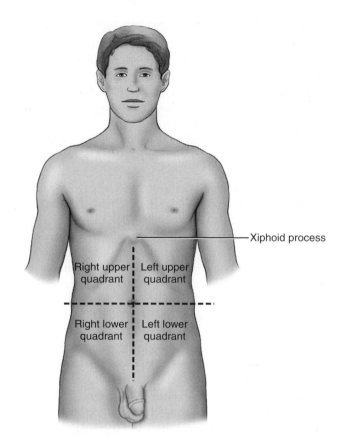

FIGURE 5-27 Division of the abdomen into quadrants.

Hepatomegaly may be accompanied by the collection of serous fluid in the peritoneal cavity known as **ascites**. Ascites most often results from interference with venous return to the right side of the heart, as occurs in heart failure. Cirrhosis of the liver, depletion of plasma proteins, and sodium retention are common contributing factors. Severe ascites may restrict diaphragm movement, as mentioned earlier, and contribute to the onset of respiratory failure.

Obesity causes the abdomen to enlarge as a result of the collection of fatty tissue in the abdominal wall. This will restrict movement of the diaphragm especially during exertion when larger tidal volumes are needed. For this reason, obese patients often complain of shortness of breath during minimal exercise.

Examination of the Extremities

Respiratory disease may result in numerous abnormalities, identified during inspection of the extremities. These abnormalities include digital clubbing, cyanosis, and pedal edema, and each is discussed briefly.

Clubbing
Clubbing of the digits is a significant manifestation of cardiopulmonary disease. The mechanism responsible for clubbing is not known, but it is often associated with a chronic cardiopulmonary disease. It is identified most

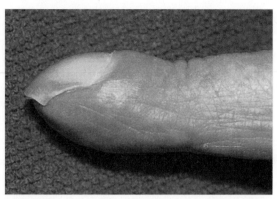

FIGURE 5-28 Lateral view of digital clubbing of the index finger. (Courtesy of Lawrence Cox. From Seidel HM, Ball J, Dains J, Flynn JA, Solomon BS, et al: *Mosby's guide to physical examination,* ed 7, St. Louis, 2011, Mosby-Elsevier.)

commonly in patients with cyanotic congenital heart disease, bronchogenic carcinoma, COPD, cystic fibrosis, and bronchiectasis.

Clubbing is characterized by a painless bulbous enlargement of the terminal phalanges of the fingers and toes, developing over many years. The angle of the fingernail to the nail base advances past 180 degrees, and the base of the nail feels spongy. The profile view of the digits allows easier recognition of clubbing (Fig. 5-28).

SIMPLY STATED

Clubbing of the digits is most commonly seen in patients with cyanotic congenital heart disease, bronchogenic carcinoma, COPD, cystic fibrosis, and bronchiectasis.

Cyanosis

Examination of the fingertips and toes indicates the presence or absence of **cyanosis**, a blue, gray, or purplish appearance of the skin, common in patients with severe cardiopulmonary disease. The ability to observe cyanosis depends on the patient's skin pigmentation and lighting in the room and may be masked by severe anemia. The presence of cyanosis in the digits (**peripheral cyanosis** or **acrocyanosis**) indicates that the blood flow contains a reduction in oxygen-saturated hemoglobin. The patient with peripheral cyanosis resulting from poor perfusion also has extremities that are cool to the touch because vasoconstriction may occur due to cold ambient temperature. Tissue oxygenation may be compromised in such situations.

SIMPLY STATED

The ability to see peripheral or acrocyanosis depends on the lighting in the room, the patient's skin pigmentation, and the patient's hemoglobin level. This is different from the condition of central cyanosis. If a patient is anemic, central and peripheral cyanosis will be masked and unapparent on visual examination.

Pedal Edema

Pedal edema may be a manifestation of chronic lung disease. Because hypoxemia produces pulmonary vasoconstriction, the right ventricle must work harder than normal whenever significant hypoxemia exists. This chronic workload on the right ventricle may result in right ventricular hypertrophy and poor venous blood flow return to the heart. When the venous return to the right side of the heart is reduced, the peripheral blood vessels engorge, resulting in an accumulation of fluid in the subcutaneous tissues of the ankles, called **pedal edema**. The ankles most often are affected because they naturally are maintained in a gravity-dependent position throughout the day. The edematous tissues pit (indent) when pressed firmly with the fingertips. The severity of edema usually is characterized by the examining physician using a scale of 1+ to 4+, with 1+ indicating slight edema and 4+ indicating severe edema. Pitting edema, or that which leaves an indentation on the patient's leg after the clinician's gloved finger releases moderate pressure, should be evaluated for the level of occurrence above the ankle in an effort to quantify the degree of right-sided heart failure. For example, pitting edema occurring at a level well above the knee is much more significant than pitting edema around the ankles only.

SIMPLY STATED

Pedal edema may occur in patients with chronic lung disease that has resulted in cor pulmonale or chronic right-sided heart failure.

Capillary Refill

Capillary refill is assessed by pressing firmly for a brief period on the fingernail and identifying the speed at which the blood flow returns. When cardiac output is reduced and digital perfusion is poor, capillary refill is slow, taking several seconds to appear. In normal persons with good cardiac output and digital perfusion, capillary refill should take less than 3 seconds.

Peripheral Skin Temperature

When the heart does not circulate the blood at a sufficient rate, compensatory vasoconstriction occurs in the extremities to shunt blood toward the vital organs. The reduction in peripheral perfusion results in a loss of warmth in the extremities. Palpation of the patient's feet and hands may provide general information about perfusion. Cool extremities usually indicate inadequate perfusion.

Actual extremity temperature can be compared with room temperature. The extremity should be at least 2° C warmer than room temperature (unless room temperature is equal to or greater than body temperature). When there is less than 2° C difference, perfusion is reduced; a 0.5° C difference indicates that the patient has serious perfusion problems.

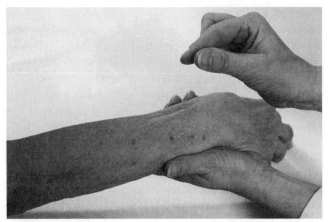

FIGURE 5-29 Skin turgor is assessed by first grasping a fold of skin on the back of the patient's hand, sternum, forearm, or abdomen. Note the ease and speed with which the skin returns to place. (From Christensen B, Kockrow E: *Foundations and adult health nursing,* ed 6, St. Louis, 2010, Mosby-Elsevier.)

Assessment of Hydration: Skin Turgor

Physical assessment also includes assessing the skin for clues as to the hydration status of the patient. Skin turgor is the normal tension or resiliency of the skin attributable to the outward pressure of cells and interstitial fluid. It is assessed by pulling up on the skin on the back of the patient's hand or wrist in a gentle pinching motion with the thumb and pointer finger. The skin of the patient will tent upward as the clinician pinches it. When the skin is released, it should immediately return to its original state of tension on the hand or wrist, indicating adequate hydration of the patient. When the skin does not immediately snap back and return to its original state, but remains in a pinched or tented position with a slower return to its original state, this is an indication of possible dehydration (Fig. 5-29).

KEY POINTS

▶ Physical examination of the patient with cardiopulmonary disease is performed to determine the cause and severity of the patient's problem and the effects of treatment. A review of the patient's history of present illness and past medical history before examination gives the clinician insight into the expected physical examination findings and suggests the techniques to emphasize.

▶ Diaphoresis is a sign of severe stress in the patient with cardiopulmonary disease. In patients prone to heart disease, it is consistent with myocardial infarction.

▶ Distention of the neck veins is consistent with right heart failure and cor pulmonale.

▶ Lymphadenopathy in the neck is often palpated when respiratory infection is present.

▶ The degree of venous distention can be estimated by measuring the distance the veins are distended above the sternal angle. With the head of the bed elevated to a 45-degree angle, venous distention greater than 3 to 4 cm above the sternal angle is abnormal.

KEY POINTS—cont'd

▶ In unilateral lung disease, the trachea tends to shift toward large-scale atelectasis and away from the side with a pneumothorax, pleural effusion, or lung mass.

▶ On the anterior chest, directly below the suprasternal notch is the sternal angle (the angle of Louis). The carina (tracheal bifurcation) is located approximately beneath the angle of Louis.

▶ A barrel chest is seen as an abnormal enlargement in the anteroposterior diameter of the chest due to accessory muscle hypertrophy and lung hyperinflation. It is a common finding in patients with COPD.

▶ The diaphragm and the intercostal muscles are the primary muscles of ventilation, actively working to increase the thoracic cavity dimension during normal inspiratory effort.

▶ When ventilatory demands increase, these accessory breathing muscles become more active in assisting the primary muscles of ventilation in the work of breathing.

▶ Abdominal paradox is a sign of diaphragm fatigue and impending respiratory failure and should not be confused with a paradoxical pulse, which is characterized by a drop in systolic blood pressure during inspiration.

▶ Patients with restrictive lung disease breathe with a rapid and shallow breathing pattern.

▶ Patients with obstructive lung disease breathe with a prolonged expiratory time.

▶ Retractions are a sign of significant respiratory distress.

▶ Any respiratory abnormalities that increase the work of breathing may cause the accessory muscles of breathing to become active during breathing at rest.

▶ Increased tactile fremitus results from the transmission of the vibration through a more solid medium such as the consolidation of pneumonia, atelectasis, lung tumors, or masses.

▶ A reduced tactile fremitus is often found in patients with obesity, overly muscular body type, hyperinflation (COPD), a bronchial obstruction such as a mucous plug or foreign object, or pleural space lining the lung that becomes filled with air (pneumothorax) or fluid (pleural effusion).

▶ A unilateral decrease in chest expansion is always abnormal and is consistent with pneumonia, pneumothorax, or atelectasis.

▶ Subcutaneous emphysema is when air leaks from the lung into subcutaneous tissues and fine beads of air produce a crackling sound and sensation when the chest wall is palpated. It may be caused by barotrauma to the alveoli due to positive-pressure ventilation.

▶ An increase in resonance during percussion of the chest indicates hyperinflation of the lungs as in emphysema or an accumulation of air in the pleura as in pneumothorax.

▶ A decrease in resonance during percussion of the chest is consistent with an abnormality that causes consolidation of the lungs such as pneumonia, atelectasis, or pleural effusion.

▶ The four characteristics of breath sounds to be identified during auscultation include the pitch (vibration frequency), the amplitude or intensity (loudness), distinctive characteristics, and the duration of inspiratory sound compared with expiratory sound.

KEY POINTS—cont'd

▶ All normal breath sounds are created by turbulent flow in the airways. Listening directly over the trachea allows direct auscultation of this sound. Listening over the lung provides an attenuated, softer version of the turbulent flow sounds in the larger airways.

▶ Diminished breath sounds occur with shallow breathing or when attenuation of the breath sounds is increased due to hyperinflation of the lung (e.g., emphysema).

▶ Adventitious bronchial breath sounds are heard when the lung attenuation ability is reduced due to consolidation of the lung (e.g., pneumonia).

▶ Wheezes are consistent with diseases of airway obstruction such as asthma and bronchitis.

▶ Coarse crackles are heard when air moves through excessive airways secretions, whereas fine crackles are most commonly heard with the sudden opening of collapsed peripheral airways during deep breathing in the patient with restrictive lung disease or with fluid filled alveoli.

▶ Stridor is a high-pitched sound and an ominous sign that indicates the patency of the upper airway is compromised.

▶ The normal point of maximal impulse (PMI) is created by contraction of the ventricles. Normal location is near the fifth intercostal space at the left midclavicular line. A shift to the left or right of the mediastinum, as occurs in lower lobe atelectasis, will cause the PMI to shift to one side.

▶ The normal heart sounds are created by closure of the atrioventricular valves during systole (S_1) and closure of the semilunar valves during diastole (S_2).

▶ S_3 is thought to be produced by rapid ventricular filling immediately after systole. S_4 is produced by active filling of the ventricles from atrial contraction just before systole.

▶ A gallop rhythm is present when S_3 and S_4 are present. A gallop rhythm is consistent with cardiac disease, including a recent myocardial infarction.

▶ Pulmonary hypertension increases intensity of S_2 as a result of more forceful closure of the pulmonic valve. A loud P_2 is also consistent with cor pulmonale and pulmonary embolism.

▶ A loud aortic valve component (loud A_2) is considered an increase in the intensity of a heart sound and is commonly heard in patients with systemic hypertension.

▶ Cardiac murmurs are identified whenever the heart valves are incompetent (incomplete closure) or stenotic (narrowed).

▶ An enlarged liver (hepatomegaly) is frequently seen in patients with right heart failure caused by chronic lung disease (cor pulmonale).

▶ Cyanosis of the oral mucosa provides evidence that the lungs are not oxygenating the blood at normal levels.

▶ Pedal edema is a sign of heart failure. Edema that extends above the ankles suggests a more severe case of heart failure.

▶ Skin turgor is the normal tension or resiliency of the skin attributable to the outward pressure of cells and interstitial fluid and can indicate hydration status of patient.

ASSESSMENT QUESTIONS

See Appendix for answers.

1. Which of the following is not a typical component to physical examination?
   a. Inspection
   b. Palpation
   c. Auscultation
   d. Interviewing

2. Pursed-lip breathing is most often seen in patients with which of the following diseases?
   a. Pulmonary fibrosis
   b. COPD
   c. Pneumonia
   d. Congestive heart failure

3. Which of the following is an unlikely cause of diaphoresis?
   a. Myocardial infarction
   b. Fever
   c. Pulmonary fibrosis
   d. Exercise

4. In which of the following conditions is lymphadenopathy of the neck seen?
   a. Infection of the upper airway
   b. Asthma
   c. Cystic fibrosis
   d. Atelectasis

5. Which of the following may cause an increased jugular venous distention?
   1. Chronic hypoxemia
   2. Right-sided heart failure secondary to left-sided heart failure
   3. Right-sided heart failure alone
   a. 1 and 2 only
   b. 2 and 3 only
   c. 1, 2, and 3

6. What spinous process is most prominent with the patient sitting and with the head bent forward?
   a. T1
   b. C1
   c. C7
   d. S3

7. At which of the following topographic locations is the bifurcation of the trachea located on the anterior chest?
   a. Over the upper part of the manubrium
   b. Beneath the sternal angle
   c. The fourth rib at the sternum
   d. Under the xiphoid process

8. The minor (horizontal) fissure begins at which of the following locations on the anterior chest?
   a. Second rib at the sternal border
   b. Fourth rib at the sternal border
   c. Sixth rib at the sternal border
   d. Seventh rib at the sternal border

9. "An inward depression of the sternum" describes which of the following thoracic configurations?
   a. Kyphosis
   b. Pectus excavatum
   c. Flail chest
   d. Barrel chest

10. What type of lung problem is associated with severe kyphoscoliosis?
    a. COPD
    b. Restrictive lung disease
    c. Pneumothorax
    d. Pulmonary fibrosis

11. Which of the following best describes an apneustic breathing pattern?
    a. Prolonged exhalation
    b. Prolonged inhalation
    c. Deep and fast
    d. Absence of breathing

12. What is indicated by the presence of retractions?
    a. Heart failure
    b. An increase in the work of breathing
    c. Pneumothorax
    d. Restrictive lung disease

13. Which of the following I:E ratios is consistent with a severe asthma attack?
    a. 3:1
    b. 2:1
    c. 1:1
    d. 1:3

14. Which of the following breathing patterns is associated with narrowing of intrathoracic airways?
    a. Prolonged inspiratory time
    b. Prolonged expiratory time
    c. Rapid and shallow
    d. Rapid and deep

15. Which of the following indicate diaphragmatic fatigue?
    1. Paradoxical pulse
    2. Abdominal paradox
    3. Respiratory alternans
    4. Biot breathing pattern
       a. 1 and 2 only
       b. 2 and 3 only
       c. 3 and 4 only
       d. 1 and 4 only

16. Which of the following causes an increased tactile fremitus?
    a. Atelectasis with a patent bronchiole
    b. Pleural effusion
    c. Emphysema
    d. Obesity

17. Which of the following causes a bilateral decrease in chest expansion?
    a. Lung tumor
    b. Pneumothorax
    c. COPD
    d. Pleural effusion

18. Which of the following causes an increased resonance to percussion of the chest?
    a. Lobar consolidation
    b. Pneumothorax
    c. Pleural effusion
    d. Atelectasis

19. What clinical condition would cause the range of diaphragm movement to be reduced bilaterally?
    a. Severe emphysema
    b. Left lower lobe atelectasis
    c. Congestive heart failure
    d. Pneumonia

20. Normal tracheal breath sounds are produced by which of the following mechanisms?
    a. Turbulent airflow through large airways
    b. Filtered sounds through lung tissue
    c. Passage of air through secretions
    d. Passage of air through narrowed airways

21. Which of the following terms is used to describe discontinuous adventitious lung sounds?
    a. Wheeze
    b. Crackles
    c. Rhonchi
    d. Stridor

22. The finding of late inspiratory crackles on auscultation of a patient might indicate which of the following?
    1. Atelectasis
    2. Pulmonary fibrosis
    3. Bronchospasm
    4. Pneumonia
       a. 1 only
       b. 1 and 3 only
       c. 1, 2, and 3 only
       d. 1, 2, and 4 only

23. What clinical condition is most closely associated with polyphonic wheezing?
    a. Pneumonia
    b. Pneumothorax
    c. Asthma
    d. Pulmonary fibrosis

24. Which of the following lung sounds is commonly heard in the patient with upper airway obstruction?
    a. Polyphonic wheeze
    b. Fine inspiratory crackles
    c. Coarse inspiratory and expiratory crackles
    d. Inspiratory stridor

25. Which of the following is the normal topographic location of the PMI?
    a. Third intercostal space at the anterior axillary line
    b. Fourth intercostal space at the anterior axillary line
    c. Fifth intercostal space at the midclavicular line
    d. Sixth intercostal space at the midsternal line

26. Which of the following locations is best for auscultating the mitral valve?
    a. Third intercostal space at the anterior axillary line
    b. Fourth intercostal space at the anterior axillary line
    c. Fifth intercostal space at the midclavicular line
    d. Sixth intercostal space at the midsternal line
27. What produces the sounds associated with the first heart sound?
    a. Closure of the atrioventricular (AV) valves
    b. Closure of the semilunar valves
    c. Left ventricular muscle movement
    d. Blood flow through normal valves
28. What clinical condition is most closely associated with a gallop heart rhythm?
    a. Pneumonia
    b. Pericarditis
    c. Congestive heart failure
    d. Aortic stenosis
29. Which of the following may cause an increased P_2 component of the second heart sound?
    1. Pulmonary hypertension
    2. Pulmonary embolism
    3. Cor pulmonale
    4. Systemic hypertension
       a. 1 and 3 only
       b. 2 and 3 only
       c. 1, 2, and 3 only
       d. 1, 2, 3, and 4

30. Which of the following is/are associated with right heart failure?
    1. Jugular venous distention
    2. Hepatomegaly
    3. Pedal edema
    4. Systemic hypertension
       a. 1 only
       b. 1 and 2 only
       c. 1 and 3 only
       d. 1, 2, and 3

Bibliography

DesJardins T, Burton GG. *Clinical manifestations and assessment of respiratory disease.* ed 6 Maryland Heights, MO: Mosby-Elsevier; 2011.

Jarvis C. *Physical examination and health assessment.* 6th ed. St. Louis: Saunders-Elsevier; 2012.

Kacmarek RM, Stoller JK, Heuer AJ. *Egan's fundamentals of respiratory care.* 10th ed. St. Louis: Mosby-Elsevier; 2013.

LeBlond RF, Brown DD, DeGowin RL. *DeGowin's diagnostic examination.* 9th ed. New York: McGraw-Hill; 2009.

Seidel HM, Ball J, Dains J, Flynn JA, Solomon BS, et al. *Mosby's guide to physical examination.* 7th ed. St. Louis: Mosby-Elsevier; 2011.

Shumway NM, Wilson RL, Howard RS, Parker JM, Eliasson AH. Presence and treatment of air hunger in severely ill patients. *Respir Med* 2008;**102**:27.

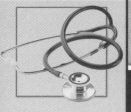

Chapter 6

Neurologic Assessment

RUBEN D. RESTREPO AND ZAZA COHEN

CHAPTER OUTLINE

LEARNING OBJECTIVES

After reading this chapter, you will be able to:
1. Define key terms related to neurologic assessment.
2. Describe the functional anatomy of the nervous system.
3. Explain the cortical function of the different lobes of the brain.
4. Describe the functions of the brainstem, the cerebellum, and the12 pairs of cranial nerves.
5. Describe common techniques used to assess the mental status.
6. Obtain and interpret Glasgow Coma Scale assessment.
7. Describe the importance of assessing level and content of consciousness in intensive care unit patients.
8. Describe common techniques used to assess the cranial nerves, the sensory system, the motor system, coordination, and gait.
9. Describe common techniques used to assess deep, superficial, and brainstem reflexes.
10. Explain the control of the breathing and circulation by the central nervous system.
11. Briefly describe ancillary tests used in neurologic assessment.
12. Identify the importance of intracranial pressure monitoring and the value of assessing cerebral perfusion pressure.
13. Give an overview of brain death declaration.

KEY TERMS

afferent
anisocoria
ataxia
ataxic breathing
Babinski sign
Biot breathing
brain death
central nervous system (CNS)

cerebral perfusion pressure
  (CPP)
Cheyne-Stokes respiration
content of consciousness
corneal reflex
Cushing triad
decerebrate posture
decorticate posture

deep tendon reflexes
delirium
doll's eyes reflex
efferent
electroencephalogram (EEG)
encephalopathy
gag reflex
gait

KEY TERMS—cont'd

Glasgow Coma Scale (GCS)	mydriasis	phrenic nerves
intracranial pressure (ICP)	nystagmus	plantar reflex
level of consciousness	oculocephalic reflex	proprioception
lower motor neuron (LMN)	oculovestibular reflex	pupillary reflex
lumbar puncture (LP)	patellar reflex	sensory dissociation
Mini-Mental State Examination (MMSE)	PERRLA	upper motor neuron (UMN)
miosis	peripheral nervous system	
	persistent vegetative state	

Neurologic assessment is a method of obtaining specific data in relation to the function of a patient's nervous system. It is a comprehensive evaluation that covers several areas: mental status, cranial nerve function, motor system, coordination, sensory system, and various reflexes. Although different aspects of neurologic examination are often done by the respiratory therapist (RT), nurse (RN), or other member of the health care team, a detailed and in-depth assessment is usually the ultimate responsibility of the attending physician or the neurologist. Injuries that involve the nervous system often affect the patient's respiratory system and the ability of the patient to cooperate with respiratory care procedures; therefore, the RT should become familiar with the key components of the neurologic assessment. The challenges of examining an intubated, restrained, and often sedated patient in the intensive care unit (ICU) make neurologic assessment difficult in many patients. This chapter covers in detail the clinical neurologic assessment and the terminology usually used to describe it. Ancillary tests, neurologic control of vital organ function, and determination of brain death are discussed briefly at the end of the chapter. The reader is reminded that the terminology used in the description of neurologic assessment is often misused and misinterpreted in clinical practice, even by highly qualified professionals. For documentation and communication purposes, it is generally preferred to give a descriptive assessment of the neurologic status, such as stimuli applied to the patient and the responses they elicited.

SIMPLY STATED

Injuries that involve the nervous system often affect a patient's respiratory system and the ability to cooperate with respiratory care procedures; thus, the RT should become familiar with the key components of the neurologic assessment, especially when managing critically ill patients.

Proper clinical assessment of the nervous system emphasizes the neurologic history and examination. Obtaining a thorough history from the patient or family members can help the clinician characterize the dysfunction, whereas the neurologic examination will assist in localizing and quantifying its severity. The neurologic examination is often brief if initial interactions with the patient are normal (e.g., the patient responds appropriately to verbal stimuli) and the patient has no symptoms suggesting neurologic disease. This initial interaction with the patient could provide insights about the patient that might affect the patient's adherence to respiratory care and performance of complex tasks that require coordination of multiple sensorimotor systems (e.g., the use of a pressurized metered-dose inhaler). A more extensive examination is performed when abnormalities are suspected and may involve the expertise of a neurologist. The initial examination establishes baseline data with which to compare subsequent assessment findings. Neurologic observation allows monitoring and evaluation of changes in the nervous system that aid in the diagnosis and treatment that later affect patient prognosis and rehabilitation. It also gauges the patient's response to the clinician's interventions. After a thorough evaluation is done on admission or at the beginning of each shift, subsequent assessments should be tailored to the patient's condition. The frequency of these assessments will depend on the patient's diagnosis, acuity of the condition, and how rapidly changes are occurring or expected to occur.

SIMPLY STATED

The frequency and depth of neurologic assessments depend on the patient's diagnosis, acuity of the condition, and how rapidly changes are occurring or expected to occur.

Functional Neuroanatomy

To perform or understand a neurologic assessment, the examiner needs a basic understanding of anatomy and function of the nervous system. The neurologic system is made up of two major parts: the central and peripheral nervous systems. The **central nervous system (CNS)** contains the brain and spinal cord (Fig. 6-1), whereas the **peripheral nervous system** is composed of the 12 cranial nerves and the 31 spinal nerves. The brain consists of three parts: the cerebrum, which contains two hemispheres; the brainstem (midbrain, pons, and medulla); and cerebellum.

The peripheral nervous system is organized according to its function into sensory (**afferent**, from the Latin word *afferens*, to bring to) and motor (**efferent**, from Latin

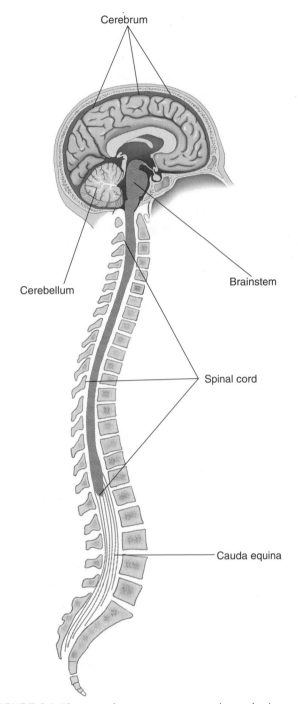

Cerebrum

Brainstem

Cerebellum

Spinal cord

Cauda equina

FIGURE 6-1 The central nervous system: cerebrum, brainstem, cerebellum, and spinal cord.

efferens, to bring out) divisions. This functional organization allows the clinician to understand how signals are transmitted to and from the CNS (Fig. 6-2).

The cerebrum is the largest part of the brain and is made up of two hemispheres and areas that control specific intellectual or motor functions (Fig. 6-3). Lesions in the cerebrum can lead to abnormalities in functions such as movement, level of consciousness, ability to speak and write, emotions, and memory.

The brainstem is the lower part of the brain where it connects to the spinal cord. It consists of the midbrain, pons, and the medulla oblongata (Fig. 6-4). Most of the cranial nerves originate in the brainstem. Many neurologic functions of particular importance to the RT, such as regulation of heart rate, blood pressure, and breathing, are located in the brainstem. In addition, the brainstem contains reflex centers for certain cranial nerve functions such as the pupillary reflex, which is discussed later in this chapter. Lesions in the brainstem can cause a wide range of breathing problems from hyperventilation to apnea.

In addition to the centers that control the function of various organs and organ systems, the brainstem also contains multiple afferent and efferent pathways that connect the brain to the spinal cord. An important feature of these pathways is that they cross over to the other side in the medulla, an area called the *pyramidal tract.* Therefore, if a disease affects these pathways above the pyramidal tracts, the neurologic deficit will be on the contralateral (opposite) side, but if the pathways are affected below the pyramidal tract, the neurologic deficit will be on the ipsilateral (same) side.

SIMPLY STATED

Many neurologic functions of particular importance to the RT, such as regulation of heart rate, blood pressure, and breathing, are located in the brainstem.

The cerebellum is located in the posterior part of the brain and is responsible for controlling equilibrium, muscle tone, and coordination of muscle movements. Lesions in the cerebellum cause characteristic symptoms such as loss of muscle coordination (**ataxia**), tremors, and disturbances in gait and balance.

The spinal cord lies within the center of the vertebral bodies and extends from the base of the brain down to the level of the first lumbar (L1) vertebra (see Fig. 6-1). The rest of the space between the vertebral bodies is taken up by the loose collection of the nerve roots that originate in the lower portion of the spinal cord and the cerebrospinal fluid (see Lumbar Puncture). This collection of nerve roots is called the cauda equina (Latin for horse's tail). The fact that the spinal cord does not extend below L1 will become important when we discuss the anatomy of lumbar puncture. The spinal cord spans a distance of approximately 45 cm in the average adult. It serves the purpose of connecting the brain to the various parts of the body for motor and sensory function. It is an oval cylinder that has two tapering bulges: one in the cervical region and one in the lumbar region. The bulges are formed by the accumulation of extra neurons for the innervations of the upper and lower extremities, respectively.

Two sets of nerve fibers called *spinal nerves* project from both sides of the spinal column at 31 locations along the spine. Sensory and motor nerve roots separate as they exit

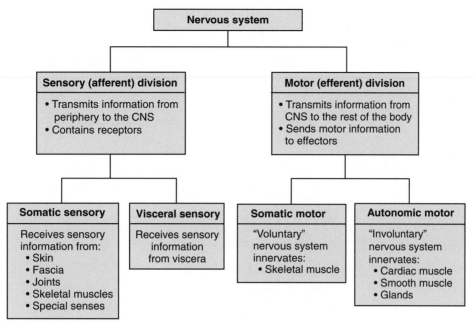

FIGURE 6-2 Functional organization of the central nervous system (CNS).

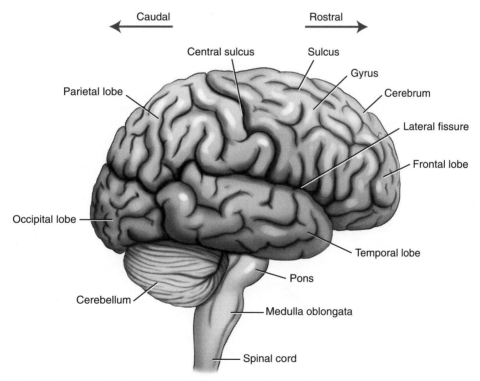

FIGURE 6-3 Left lateral view of the cerebrum showing the four cerebral lobes (frontal, parietal, temporal, and occipital) and its anatomic relationship with the cerebellum and the brainstem.

the spinal cord until their fibers combine at the level of the dorsal root ganglion. The dorsal nerve root consists of posterior nerve fibers that carry sensory information into the spinal cord. The ventral nerve root consists of anterior nerve fibers that conduct motor impulses out of the spinal cord. Because all spinal nerves contain both motor and sensory fibers, they are called *mixed nerves*. Each has the

ability to provide sensory input to the brain (e.g., feel pain) and the ability to cause muscle movement (e.g., extend the arm on command) (Fig. 6-5).

These spinal nerves have no specific name but rather are numbered according to the level of the vertebral column at which they exit the spinal column. There are 8 cervical (C1 to C8), 12 thoracic (T1 to T12), 5 lumbar

(L1 to L5), 5 sacral (S1 to S5), and 1 coccygeal pair of spinal nerves. It must be noted that the number of spinal nerves does not always equal the number of the corresponding vertebrae (8 cervical nerves vs. 7 vertebrae), which might lead to some confusion.

A herniated vertebral disk is the most common nerve root pathology that results in compression on the nerve roots. This usually results in pain with radiation into the affected area of skin (dermatome) supplied with afferent nerve fibers by a single posterior spinal root (Fig. 6-6).

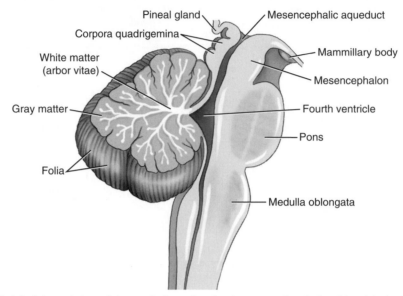

FIGURE 6-4 Left lateral view of the cerebellum showing its anatomic relationship with the brainstem.

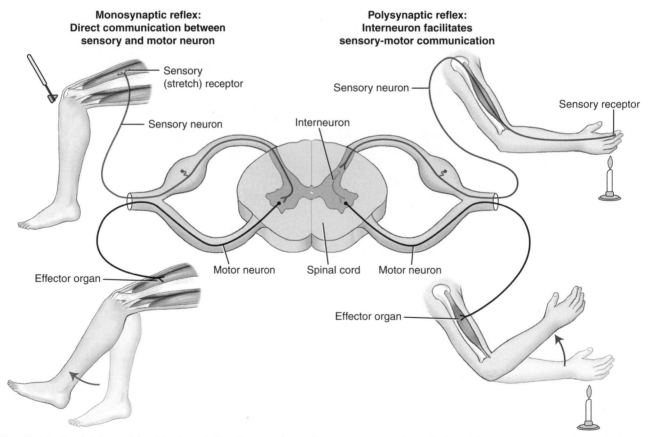

FIGURE 6-5 Caudal view of the spinal cord. The diagram shows the motor neuron (anterior) and the sensory neuron (posterior) before they come together as a spinal nerve. The sensory neuron provides sensory input to the brain to elicit a motor response.

Two spinal nerves important for respiratory function are the right and left **phrenic nerves** that innervate the diaphragm to control breathing. The phrenic nerves arise from the cervical spine roots of C3 to C5. Damage to this portion of the spinal cord (or above) can result in complete paralysis of the diaphragm as well as the intercostal muscles and make the patient dependent on a ventilator for life.

The additional muscles of respiration, such as intercostal muscles, are innervated by the spinal nerves that originate in the thoracic portion of the spinal cord. These nerves, although normal, will be cut off from the efferent impulses originating above the injury (C3 to C5 level, or above) and will be rendered ineffective. Figures 6-6 and 6-7 illustrate the typical outcome after spinal cord or root injury.

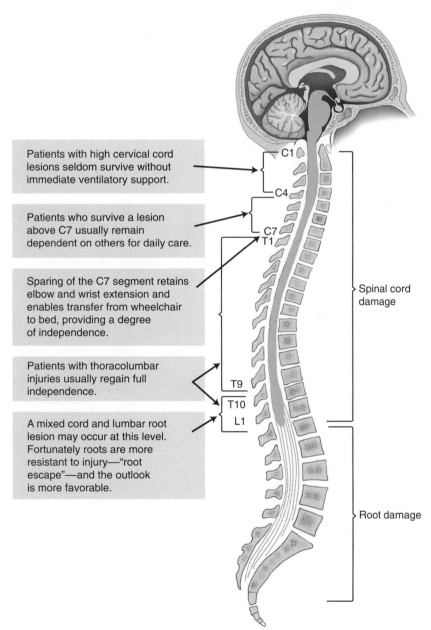

Patients with high cervical cord lesions seldom survive without immediate ventilatory support.

Patients who survive a lesion above C7 usually remain dependent on others for daily care.

Sparing of the C7 segment retains elbow and wrist extension and enables transfer from wheelchair to bed, providing a degree of independence.

Patients with thoracolumbar injuries usually regain full independence.

A mixed cord and lumbar root lesion may occur at this level. Fortunately roots are more resistant to injury—"root escape"—and the outlook is more favorable.

FIGURE 6-6 Outcome after spinal cord or root injury.

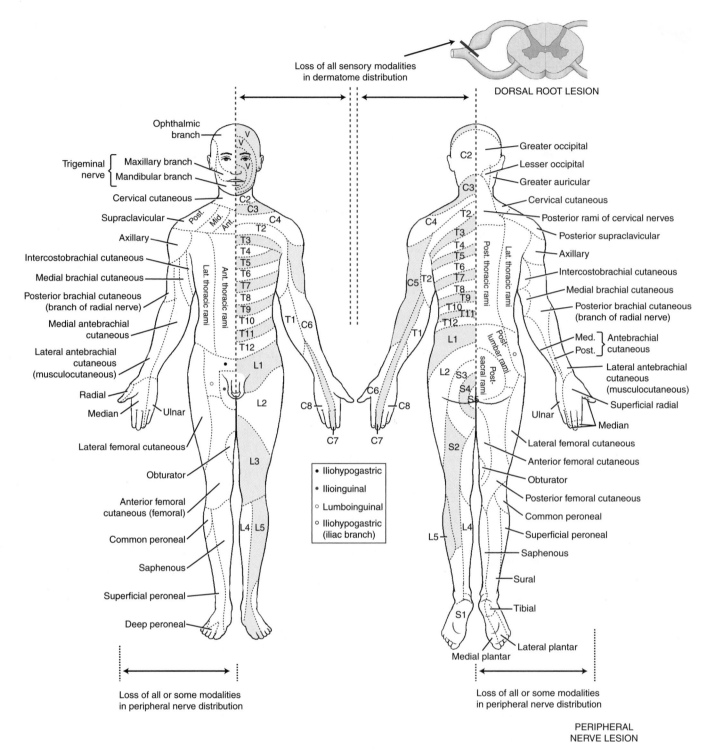

FIGURE 6-7 Schematic representation of dermatomes.

Assessment of Consciousness

The cerebral hemispheres (or lobes) represent the highest and most complex level of neurologic function. Although a great deal of the mental status reflects integration of cortical function, it can still be divided into functional areas that correspond to anatomic regions of the cerebral hemispheres (Fig. 6-8). Table 6-1 gives a brief overview of areas

of cortical function that can be assessed by components of the mental status examination.

Assessing Consciousness

Whenever evaluating consciousness, it is important to assess the **level of consciousness** (wakefulness and alertness) as well as the **content of consciousness** (awareness and thinking). A change in either is usually the first clue to

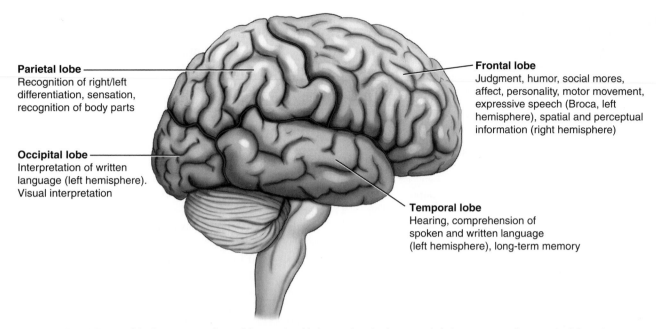

Parietal lobe
Recognition of right/left differentiation, sensation, recognition of body parts

Occipital lobe
Interpretation of written language (left hemisphere). Visual interpretation

Frontal lobe
Judgment, humor, social mores, affect, personality, motor movement, expressive speech (Broca, left hemisphere), spatial and perceptual information (right hemisphere)

Temporal lobe
Hearing, comprehension of spoken and written language (left hemisphere), long-term memory

FIGURE 6-8 Graphical representation of the cerebral lobes or hemispheres and their corresponding cortical function.

TABLE 6-1

Assessment of Cerebral Cortical Function

Cerebral Lobe	Cortical Function	Assessment
Frontal	Attention: working memory	Digit span, spelling backward, and naming months of the year backward
	Judgment: abstract reasoning	Problem solving, verbal similarities, and proverbs
	Set generation	Verbal fluency and the ability to generate a set of items
Temporal	Orientation, memory	Questions about month, date, day of week, and place
		Three-word recall (recent memory)
		Naming U.S. presidents (remote memory)
Frontal-temporal	Receptive language	Following commands (spoken and written language)
	Expressive language	Fluency and correctness of content and grammar
		Reading comprehension
Parietal (dominant)	Gnosis	Identifying objects placed in the hand and numbers written on the hand with eyes closed
	Constructional	Attending to the contralateral side of the body
		Drawing a face, clock, or geometric figures
		Right-left orientation, naming fingers, and calculations
Parietal (nondominant)	Praxis	Performing skilled motor tasks without any nonverbal prompting
Occipitotemporal	Visual recognition	Recognition of colors and faces

CNS dysfunction. The initial goals of the examination of a patient with altered mental status are to determine whether the patient is conscious and then to determine awareness.

Assessment of consciousness begins when you first encounter the patient. A neurologically healthy patient will be awake and interacting with those around. If asleep, the patient can be easily aroused to an awake, alert state. Different levels of consciousness from full alertness to coma have been defined (Box 6-1). These and other terms used to categorize consciousness are frequently used imprecisely, so it is often recommended to avoid using them. Instead, a brief description of the applied stimulus and arousal pattern is preferred.

The assessment of the content of consciousness starts with orientation. The patient will often be asked to state his or her name, the current date, and the present location. A fully conscious patient will be expected to answer those questions in detail—for example, first and last name, month, day and year, and the ward and name of the hospital. Such patients can be described as *alert and oriented times three* (one score for each name, date, and location). However, a patient who just woke up from coma or heavy sedation may not be able to answer these questions in such detail. A partial response (e.g., first name only, month and year, but not the exact date) may substitute for a correct answer in such situations. The content of consciousness

Box 6-1	Levels of Consciousness

Full consciousness: The patient is alert and attentive, follows commands, responds promptly to external stimulation if asleep, and once awake, remains attentive.

Lethargy: The patient is drowsy but partially awakens to stimulation; the patient will answer questions and follow commands but will do so slowly and inattentively.

Obtundation: The patient is difficult to arouse and needs constant stimulation to follow a simple command. Although there may be verbal response with one or two words, the patient will drift back to sleep between stimuli.

Stupor: The patient arouses to vigorous and continuous stimulation; typically, a painful stimulus is required. The only response may be an attempt to withdraw from or remove the painful stimulus.

Coma: The patient does not respond to continuous or painful stimulation. There are no verbal sounds and no movement, except possibly by reflex.

has multiple additional components, many of which are outside of the scope of this chapter.

The two common conditions often present in hospitalized patients are coma and delirium. Although coma is characterized by the absence of arousal and awareness, a patient with **delirium** has a fluctuating course with alternating levels of consciousness as well as marked deficits in attention and organized thinking (confusion). Several studies have shown that delirium occurs in 60% to 80% of mechanically ventilated patients and that it is independently associated with longer stay in the hospital, higher mortality, and poor long-term cognitive function. Once again, when referring to a patient with delirium, it is better to give a descriptive evaluation of the patient's behavior and thinking, rather than a simple statement of "confusion" or "delirium," which can often be misleading. The causes of delirium are frequently multifactorial, including some combination of hypoxia, electrolyte or acid-base imbalance, concomitant medical illness, sleep deprivation, use (previous or current) of sedation, unfamiliarity with surroundings, and side effects of medications. A patient with preexisting dementia may present similarly to a patient with delirium, and it may be difficult to tell them apart without knowledge of the patient's medical history.

SIMPLY STATED

Coma and delirium are two common dysfunctions of the level and content of consciousness, respectively, that are often present in hospitalized patients, especially in the ICU. Delirium occurs in 60% to 80% of mechanically ventilated patients and is associated with longer stay in the hospital, higher mortality, and poor long-term cognitive function.

Some patients who recover from their initial severe neurologic injury will remain in a **persistent vegetative state**. The patient's eyes may be open, but the patient cannot be engaged. Patients with this condition may appear to be, but actually are not, aware of their surroundings, do not respond to verbal stimuli or commands in a meaningful way, do not track object or individuals, and do not respond to environmental changes. Overall prognosis is usually poor, even though breathing may not be impaired if the brainstem is unaffected by the injury. The term *persistent vegetative state* is frequently misused by medical and non-medical professionals and should be avoided in favor of more descriptive statements.

Another commonly misused term is encephalopathy. When translated from Latin, it simply means suffering of the brain. Naturally, any condition affecting the brain can be classified as **encephalopathy**, but the term is usually reserved for patients with a combination of alteration in both level and content of consciousness (e.g., lethargy and confusion in patients with advanced liver disease, a condition often called *hepatic encephalopathy*).

Glasgow Coma Scale

The **Glasgow Coma Scale (GCS)** was published in 1974 by Graham Teasdale and Bryan J. Jennett at the University of Glasgow as the neurologic assessment tool in patients with head injury. It has multiple limitations outside of its initial scope in acute traumatic brain injury patients, especially in ICU patients, but the simplicity of the scale makes it widely useful for nearly every member of the health care team from emergency medical services personnel for initial evaluation to ICU staff in daily neurologic assessment. The GCS is commonly incorporated in other, more complex and comprehensive acute illness scoring systems in the ICU. It is the most widely used instrument for quantifying neurologic impairment. The GCS is used to test best motor response, best verbal response, and eye opening. Although it is easy to perform and readily reproducible, it is poorly suited to patients who have impaired verbal responses caused by aphasia, hearing loss, or tracheal intubation or more subtle alterations of consciousness, such as delirium. A scale that goes from 3 (deep coma or death) to 15 (fully awake) is useful for rapid triage (Table 6-2). Endotracheal intubation makes it impossible to test the patient's verbal response, so the letter "T" is often attached to the GCS score to indicate the presence of the tube (e.g., GCS 5T).

Patients with GCS scores of 12 to 15 often do not require ICU admission. Scores of 9 to 12 on the GCS indicate a significant insult with a moderate coma. Patients with GCS scores lower than 9 have a severe coma and typically require endotracheal intubation for airway protection and ventilatory assistance (other textbooks may use the mnemonic "less than eight, intubate" to easily remember this concept). Such absolute dependence on the neurologic status and the GCS score in decision making for endotracheal intubation may be warranted only in certain situations. For example, patients with head trauma and low GCS score may need to be intubated because they will have a prolonged recovery period, but patients with more transient neurologic deficit

TABLE 6-2		
Glasgow Coma Scale		
Action	Response	Score
Eyes open	Spontaneously	4
	To speech	3
	To pain	2
	None	1
Best verbal response	Oriented	5
	Confused	4
	Inappropriate words	3
	Incomprehensive sounds	2
Best motor response	Obeys commands	6
	Localized pain	5
	Flexion withdrawal	4
	Abnormal flexion	3
	Abnormal extension	2
	Flaccid	1
	Total	15

TABLE 6-3	
Richmond Agitation Sedation Scale (RASS)	
Target RASS	RASS Description
+4	Combative, violent, danger to staff
+3	Pulls or removes tube(s) or catheter(s); aggressive
+2	Frequent nonpurposeful movement, fights ventilator
+1	Anxious, apprehensive, but not aggressive
0	Alert and calm
−1	Awakens to voice (eye opening/contact) >10 sec
−2	Light sedation, briefly awakens to voice (eye opening/contact) <10 sec
−3	Moderate sedation, movement, or eye opening; no eye contact
−4	Deep sedation, no response to voice, but movement or eye opening to physical stimulation
−5	Unarousable, no response to voice or physical stimulation

(such as drug or alcohol overdose) may not benefit from intubation based solely on their GCS score.

SIMPLY STATED

The GCS is the most widely used instrument for quantifying neurologic impairment. Patients with GCS scores lower than 9 have a severe coma and typically require endotracheal intubation.

Mini-Mental State Examination

The **Mini-Mental State Examination (MMSE)**, or Folstein test, is a brief, 30-point quantitative questionnaire used to assess cognition. It can be used to screen for cognitive impairment, to estimate the severity of cognitive impairment at a given point in time, to follow the course of cognitive changes in an individual over time, and to document an individual's response to treatment. It samples various functions, including arithmetic, memory, and orientation. It was introduced by Folstein and colleagues in 1975 and is widely used with small modifications. Any score higher than 27 (out of 30) is normal; scores between 20 and 26 indicate mild dementia; scores of 10 to 19 indicate moderate dementia, and scores below 10 indicate severe dementia. The normal value is also corrected for degree of schooling and age.

Assessment of Consciousness in the Intensive Care Unit

The Richmond Agitation Sedation Scale (RASS) helps to measure the sedation and agitation of patients in an ICU and is often considered when titrating sedation medications (Table 6-3). Delirium is frequently evaluated with the Confusion Assessment Method for the ICU (CAM-ICU). Delirium is an acute change or fluctuation in mental status plus inattention and either disorganized thinking or an altered state of consciousness at the time of assessment. Delirium occurs in many mechanically ventilated patients and has been associated with longer hospital stays and poor clinical outcomes. Because many aspects of delirium in the ICU may be preventable or treatable (see earlier discussion of causes of delirium), it is recommended that RTs become familiar with these assessment tools (see Bibliography).

Cranial Nerve Examination

There are 12 cranial nerves (CNs) connected to the undersurface of the brain, with most coming from the brainstem (Fig. 6-9). Assessment of the CNs allows the clinician to examine the brainstem all the way from its rostral to its caudal extent. The brainstem can be divided into three levels: the midbrain, the pons, and the medulla. There are 2 CNs for the midbrain (III and IV), 4 CNs for the pons (V to VIII), and 4 CNs for the medulla (IX to XII). Because CNs never cross, except for CN IV, clinical findings are always on the same side as the CN involved (Table 6-4).

Each nerve is named according to its distribution or function. Some of the CNs are sensory only, some are motor only, and others have both functions. Therefore, they are evaluated by using a combination of sensory and motor function tests. Those that have both functions allow sensory input to the brain for interpretation and control of muscles for function. Some functions are controlled by several CNs. For example, an acoustic problem will be assessed by testing the acoustic nerve (CN VIII) and the nearby facial nerve (CN VII). Extraocular movements (EOMs) are controlled by CNs III, IV, and VI, which are tested together. Other functions, such as the pupillary response (CNs II and III), the corneal reflex (CNs V and VII), and the gag reflex

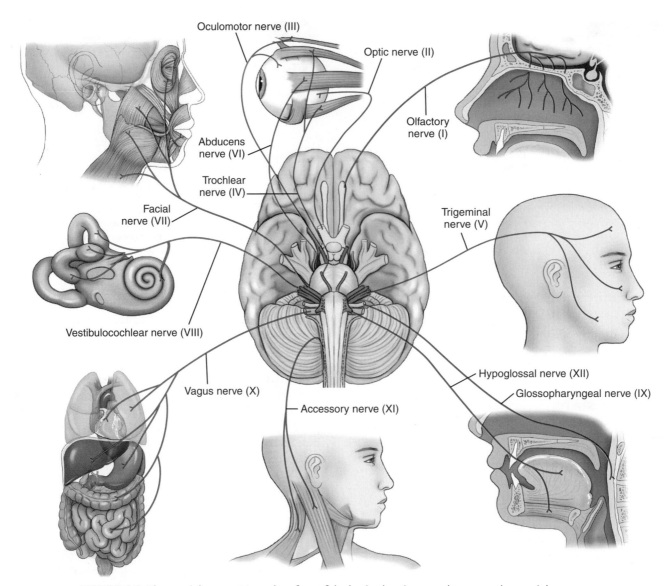

FIGURE 6-9 The cranial nerves. Ventral surface of the brain showing attachment to the cranial nerves.

(CNs IX and X), depend on more than one CN. Although a stroke is the most common cause of CN dysfunction, other abnormalities should be considered (Table 6-5). Many of the nerves cannot be tested without the patient's cooperation, so the cranial nerve assessment of a comatose patient may not be viewed as complete.

SIMPLY STATED

The gag reflex (CNs IX and X), the pupillary reflex (CNs II and III), and the corneal reflex (CNs V and VII) depend on more than one CN.

Sensory Examination

Clinically, there are two major somatosensory pathways that are examined. The first is the spinothalamic (ST) part of the anterolateral system, and the second is the dorsal column–medial lemniscus (DCML) system. The principal sensory modalities for the ST system are pain and temperature. The principal sensory modalities for the DCML system are vibratory, position sense, and discriminatory or integrative sensation. Spinal cord and lower brainstem lesions can result in **sensory dissociation**, which means one sensory system is affected, but the other is not.

Sensory evaluation is performed by having the patient respond to stimuli at a specific location. It evaluates the ability to perceive and identify specific sensations with the patient's eyes closed. The patient must be able to cooperate with the examination by communicating whether the sensation is felt and whether both sides of the body feel it equally. The assessment of light touch, pinprick, and temperature sensation can be achieved by applying a cotton swab, clean pin, and a cold or warm object, respectively, to various parts of the body. The clinician should begin with the patient's feet and move upward. Comparing

TABLE 6-4

Assessment of the Cranial Nerves

Cranial Nerve	Classification	Major Functions	Assessment
I: Olfactory	Sensory	Smell	Have patient identify a familiar scent with eyes closed (usually deferred).
II: Optic	Sensory	Vision (acuity and field of vision) Pupil reactivity to light and accommodation (afferent impulse)	Have patient read from a card, one eye at a time. Test visual fields by having patient cover one eye, focus on your nose, and identify the number of fingers you are holding up in each of four visual quadrants.
III: Oculomotor	Motor	Eyelid elevation Pupil size and reactivity (efferent impulse) Most EOM	Check pupillary responses by shining a bright light on one pupil; both pupils should constrict (consensual reflex). Do the same for the other eye. To check for accommodation, move your finger toward the patient's nose; the pupils should constrict and converge. Check EOMs by having patient look up, down, laterally, and diagonally.
IV: Trochlear	Motor	EOM (turns eye downward and laterally)	Have patient look down and in.
V: Trigeminal	Both	Chewing	Ask patient to hold the mouth open while you try to close it and to move the jaw laterally against your hand. With patient's eyes closed, touch her face with cotton and have her identify the area touched. In comatose patients, brush the cornea with a wisp of cotton; the patient should blink.
		Facial and mouth sensation Corneal reflex (sensory)	Facial and mouth sensation Corneal reflex (sensory)
VI: Abducens	Motor	EOM (turns eye laterally)	Have patient move the eyes from side to side.
VII: Facial	Both	Facial expression	Ask patient to smile, raise eyebrows, and keep eyes and lips closed while you try to open them.
		Taste Corneal reflex (motor) Eyelid and lip closure	Have patient identify salt or sugar placed on the tongue.
VIII: Acoustic	Sensory	Hearing Equilibrium	To test hearing, use tuning fork, rub your fingers, or whisper near each ear.
IX: Glossopharyngeal	Both	Gagging and swallowing (sensory) Taste	Touch back of throat with sterile tongue depressor or cotton-tipped applicator. Have patient swallow.
X: Vagus	Both	Gagging and swallowing (motor) Speech (phonation)	Assess gag and swallowing with CN IX. Assess vocal quality.
XI: Spinal accessory	Motor	Shoulder movement Head rotation	Have patient shrug shoulders and turn head from side to side.
XII: Hypoglossal	Motor	Tongue movement	Have patient stick out tongue and move it internally from cheek to cheek.
		Speech (articulation)	Assess articulation.

CN, cranial nerve; EOM, extraocular movements.

one side with the other is valuable in localizing the specific site of abnormality. To test vibratory sensation, use a low-frequency tuning fork.

To test **proprioception**, or position sense, have the patient with the eyes closed distinguish whether the finger or toe is moved up or down. Patients should be able to discriminate between two different points 2 to 10 mm apart on their fingers and hands and up to 75 mm apart on their thigh and back.

Motor Examination

A bedside neurologic assessment almost always includes an evaluation of motor function. The clinician assesses the patient's ability to move on command; therefore, the patient must be awake, willing to cooperate, and able to understand what the examiner is asking.

Motor strength is assessed bilaterally by having the patient flex and extend the arm against the clinician's hand, squeezing the clinician's fingers, lifting the leg while the clinician presses down on the thigh, holding the leg straight and lifting it against gravity, and flexing and extending the foot against the clinician's hand. Each extremity is graded using a motor scale from 0 (no movement) to +5 (full range of motion with full strength). In an unconscious patient, the assessment of motor response is performed by applying a noxious stimulus and observing the patient's response to it. Central stimulation, such

TABLE 6-5

Etiology of Cranial Nerve Malfunction

Cranial Nerve	Cause of Impairment
I	Trauma to the cribriform plate, frontal lobe mass or stroke, and nasal problems (e.g., allergic or viral)
II	Eye disease or injury, diabetic retinopathy and glaucoma major causes, occipital lobe mass or stroke
III, IV, and VI	Brainstem injury or compression (e.g., tumor, stroke, intracranial bleeding, diabetic neuropathy [can cause temporary palsies])
V	Stroke in the contralateral sensory cortex
VII	Stroke induced (central palsy)
VIII	Sensorineural hearing loss as a result of age or noise exposure, tumors at cerebellopontine angle, acoustic neuroma, earwax, or middle ear disease can cause temporary hearing loss
IX and X	Stroke
XI	Neck injury
XII	Stroke

as sternal pressure, produces an overall body response and is more reliable than peripheral stimulation. In an unconscious patient, peripheral stimulation, such as nail bed pressure, can elicit a reflex response, which is not a true indicator of motor activity. If central stimulation is necessary, it should be performed judiciously because deep sternal pressure can easily bruise the soft tissue above the sternum. A less traumatic alternative to sternal pressure is to squeeze the trapezius muscle. Supraorbital pressure should not be used for central stimulation in patients with facial fractures or vagal nerve sensitivity. The response to pain varies depending on the level of neurologic function. Normally, pain causes the patient to attempt to remove the source of the pain or to withdraw from the painful stimulation. If the cerebral cortex is functioning, there is withdrawal from painful stimuli in a predictable and reflexive manner. The symmetry and pattern of the motor response to noxious stimuli, as well as associated neurologic symptoms, should be documented for all patients suspected of having a neurologic disease.

The motor system is usually divided into the direct corticospinal tract or **upper motor neuron (UMN)** and **lower motor neuron (LMN)**. The corticospinal tract has its main influence on the motor neurons that innervate the muscles of the distal extremities such as the hand and the foot.

The clinical findings from a UMN lesion include loss of distal extremity strength, dexterity, and a Babinski sign (see the next section) plus increased tone, hyperreflexia, and the clasp-knife phenomenon (from loss of control of the indirect brainstem centers). A UMN lesion above the level of the red nucleus (a collection of neurons in the anterior part of the midbrain) will result in **decorticate posture** (thumb tucked under flexed fingers in fisted

position, pronation of forearm, and flexion at elbow with the lower extremity in extension with foot inversion), whereas a lesion below the level of the red nucleus will result in **decerebrate posture**, in which the upper extremity is in pronation and extension and the lower extremity is in extension (Fig. 6-10). The reason for this is that the red nucleus output reinforces antigravity flexion of the upper extremity. When its output is eliminated, the unregulated tracts reinforce extension tone of both upper and lower extremities. If there is a lesion in the medulla, all of the brainstem motor nuclei, as well as the direct corticospinal tract, would be out, and the patient would be acutely flaccid.

SIMPLY STATED

A UMN lesion above the level of the red nucleus will result in decorticate posture (thumb tucked under flexed fingers in fisted position, pronation of forearm, and flexion at elbow with the lower extremity in extension and foot inversion), whereas a lesion below the level of the red nucleus will result in decerebrate posture (upper extremity in pronation and extension and the lower extremity in extension).

Lesions of the LMN result in loss of strength, tone, and reflexes, with muscle showing wasting and fasciculations. Table 6-6 summarizes some of the clinical findings of UMN and LMN lesions.

Deep Tendon, Superficial, and Brainstem Reflexes

Reflex assessment encompasses deep tendon, superficial, and brainstem reflexes.

Deep Tendon Reflexes

Deep tendon reflexes evaluate spinal nerves and include the triceps, biceps, brachioradialis, patellar, and Achilles tendon. They should be tested in any patient with a spinal cord injury or symptoms consistent with a neurologic problem. The **patellar reflex** or *knee jerk* is tested by tapping on the patellar tendon with a reflex hammer while the patient's leg hangs loosely at a right angle with the thigh. Normally, the lower leg jerks forward when this reflex is intact (Fig. 6-11).

The reflexes are graded on a scale from 0 to 5, with 0 being no reflex, 2 being normal, and 5 being hyperreflexia with clonus (repeated rhythmic contractions). Abnormal or absent deep tendon reflexes indicate abnormalities in anatomic components required for the reflex arc to occur. These structures include the muscle, the nerve fibers going from the tendon to the spinal cord, and the nerve fibers returning from the spinal cord to the muscle. Table 6-7 illustrates the spinal nerve level assessed with each reflex. Absent deep tendon reflexes may be a sign that the patient is at risk for respiratory failure.

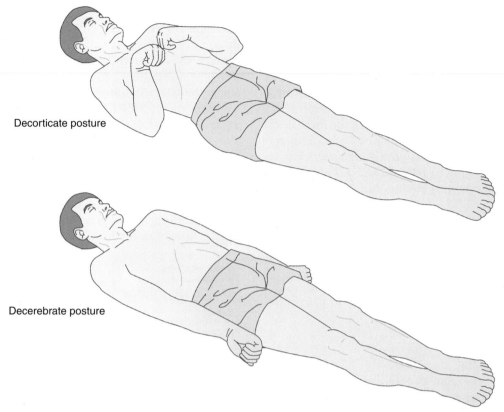

Decorticate posture

Decerebrate posture

FIGURE 6-10 Decorticate posture is indicated by flexed wrist and arm and extended legs and feet. Decerebrate posture is indicated by arm and leg extension. (From McCance K, Heuther S. *Pathophysiology,* 6th ed. St. Louis: Mosby-Elsevier; 2009.)

TABLE 6-6		
Clinical Signs of Upper Motor Neuron (UMN) and Lower Motor Neuron (LMN) Lesions		
Clinical Sign	UMN Lesion	LMN Lesion
Weakness	+	+
Atrophy	−	+
Fasciculation	−	+
Reflexes	↑	↓
Tone	↑	↓
Babinski	+	−

Superficial Reflexes

The plantar reflex is the only superficial reflex that is commonly assessed and should be tested in comatose patients and in those with suspected injury to the L4 to L5 or S1 to S2 areas of the spinal cord. To assess the **plantar reflex**, the examiner strokes the lateral plantar aspect of the foot with the handle of a reflex hammer or thumbnail. The stroke should begin at the heel and move up the foot, in a continuous motion, along the outer aspect of the sole and then across the ball to the base of the big toe. The normal response is plantar flexion (curling under) of the toes. Dorsiflexion of the great toe with fanning of remaining toes (**Babinski sign**) is abnormal, except in children up to 12 to 18 months of age (Fig. 6-12). The presence of Babinski sign

could indicate a lesion of the UMN or brain disease caused by damage to the corticospinal tract.

Brainstem Reflexes

Brainstem reflexes are evaluated in stuporous or comatose patients to determine whether the brainstem is intact. Protective reflexes, such as coughing, gagging, and the corneal response, are usually evaluated as part of the assessment of the CNS.

Gag Reflex

CNs IX and X are especially important to the RT because they control a variety of functions. CN IX controls the muscles of swallowing that are needed to prevent aspiration. This function of CN IX is evaluated by testing the patient's **gag reflex**. This test is performed by gently inserting a tongue depressor into the back of the throat. Although some healthy individuals have a minimal or absent gag reflex, its absence may increase the risk for aspiration, and endotracheal intubation may be necessary to protect the lungs. CN IX also has a branch that extends to the carotid sinus and plays a major role in the control of blood pressure. The ability to cough with suctioning can be tested in an intubated patient and implies an intact CN X. This test should not be attempted in nonintubated patients in the ICU because of the risk for aspiration. Stimulation of CN X while suctioning the airway may result in bradycardia caused by vagal stimulation. Excessively aggressive suctioning may also cause airway injury from the mechanical trauma. To decrease the vagal stimulation, as well as airway injury, it is recommended that suctioning time (catheter in the airway) be limited to 10 to 15 seconds and that an appropriate pressure setting be used during suctioning.

SIMPLY STATED

Although some healthy individuals have a minimal or absent gag reflex (CNs IX and X), its absence may increase the risk for aspiration, and endotracheal intubation may be necessary to protect the airway and lungs. The ability to cough with suctioning can be tested in an intubated patient and implies an intact CN X.

Pupillary Reflex

Pupillary light reflexes provide information regarding the status of the brain and the sympathetic and parasympathetic nervous systems. Pupillary function is controlled by the midbrain and evaluates CNs II and III. **Pupillary reflex** is determined by briefly passing a bright light in front of both open eyes while carefully watching the iris in both eyes for movement. Pupil size, congruency, and response to light and accommodation should be described.

The acronym **PERRLA** is commonly used to refer to normal *p*upils that are *e*qual, *r*ound, and *r*eactive to *l*ight and *a*ccommodation (movement) (see Chapter 5). Any visible change in the pupils' size is noted. **Anisocoria** is a neurologic term indicating that one pupil is larger than the other. **Mydriasis**, or pupillary dilation, may be caused by serious brain injury or inadvertent exposure of the eyes to inhaled anticholinergics. **Miosis**, or small "pinpoint" pupils, usually result from pontine hemorrhage or from

TABLE 6-7

Deep Tendon Reflex

Reflex	Spinal Nerve
Biceps	C5-C6
Triceps	C7-C8
Patellar	L2-L4
Achilles	L5-S1

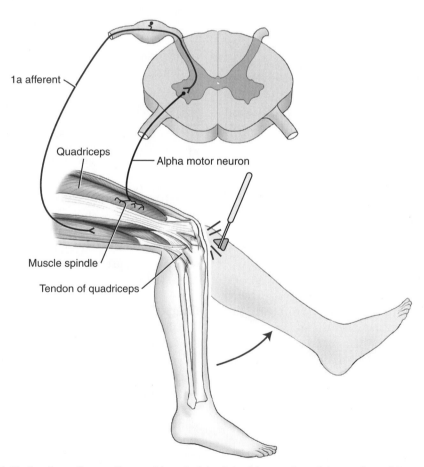

FIGURE 6-11 • Patellar reflex arc. Forward knee jerk is elicited by tapping of the tendon of the quadriceps.

ingestion of narcotics or organophosphates. Pupillary responses almost always remain intact in metabolic causes of coma. Midposition and fixed pupils often indicate severe cerebral damage (Fig. 6-13).

SIMPLY STATED

The acronym PERRLA refers to normal *p*upils that are *e*qual, *r*ound, and *r*eactive to *l*ight and *a*ccommodation. Pupillary function is controlled by the midbrain and evaluates CNs II and III.

Corneal Reflex

The **corneal reflex** is used to test the afferent CN V and the efferent CN VII. The test is performed by lightly touching the cornea with a cotton swab. The normal response is that the patient blinks both eyes. The presence of this response implies an intact ipsilateral fifth cranial nerve, intact central pons, and intact bilateral seventh cranial nerves. Testing must be performed bilaterally to evaluate both afferent components of the fifth cranial nerve. Most clinicians omit

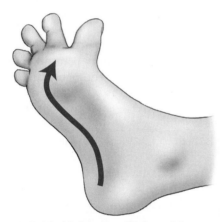

FIGURE 6-12 Babinski sign. Dorsiflexion of the great toe with fanning of remaining toes after stroking the outer aspect of the sole in the direction of the *arrow.*

the corneal reflex test unless there is sensory loss on the face as per history or examination or cranial nerve palsies are present at the pontine level (Fig. 6-14).

Oculocephalic and Oculovestibular Reflexes

Abnormalities of extraocular movement (CNs II, III, IV, and VI) have prognostic importance in the ICU. Normal movement of the eyes requires an intact midbrain connection. The resting position of the gaze, the presence of **nystagmus**, and the response to head movements and cold tympanic membrane stimulation should be identified. To test the **oculocephalic reflex**, or **doll's eyes reflex**, turn the patient's head briskly from side to side; the eyes should turn to the left while the head is turned to the right, and vice versa. If this reflex is absent, there will be no eye movement when the patient's head is moved side to side. Cervical spine stability must be ensured before oculocephalic maneuvers are performed. To test the **oculovestibular reflex**, also known as the *ice caloric* or *cold caloric reflex*, a physician instills at least 20 mL of ice water into the ear of a comatose patient. In patients with an intact brainstem, the eyes will move laterally toward the affected ear. In patients with severe brainstem injury, the gaze will remain at midline.

Coordination, Balance, and Gait Examination

The principal area of the brain that is examined by the coordination, balance, and gait examination is the cerebellum. Although the cortex initiates the volitional movements, the cerebellum ensures its coordination, precision, and timing. Therefore, cerebellar dysfunction results in disintegration of movements and undershooting and overshooting of goal-directed movements (dysmetria). Disintegration of movement and dysmetria are the main elements of ataxia.

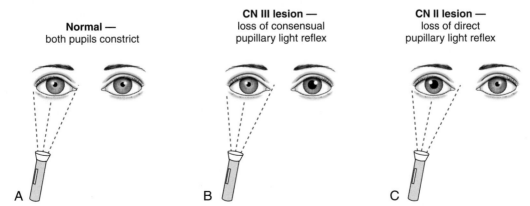

FIGURE 6-13 Pupillary reflex. **A,** Shining of a light source on the right may cause a constriction of both pupils in normal individuals. **B,** Constriction of the pupil only on the right eye in patients with lesions of CN III and loss of consensual reflex. **C,** Pupillary constriction of the opposite eye in lesions of CN II and loss of direct pupillary reflex.

CORNEAL REFLEX

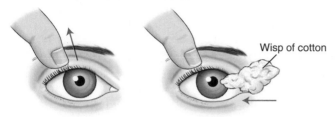

Wisp of cotton

No orbicularis oculi contraction in
response to corneal stimulation

FIGURE 6-14 Corneal reflex. Lightly touching the cornea with a cotton swab should be followed by blinking of both eyes.

SIMPLY STATED

Cerebellar dysfunction results in breakdown of coordinated movements and leads to undershooting and overshooting of goal-directed movements (dysmetria).

Dysfunction of different systems of the cerebellum may result in a myriad of signs and symptoms that include nystagmus, truncal instability, truncal ataxia, ataxia of speech (scanning dysarthria), and ataxia of the extremities (appendicular ataxia). Ataxia caused by disease of the cerebellar hemispheres will be ipsilateral (same side) to the dysfunctional hemisphere.

Cerebellar assessment may not be necessary in a problem-focused examination, and it cannot be done if the patient cannot or does not follow commands. Coordination may be simply assessed by holding up your finger and having the patient quickly and repeatedly move his or her finger back and forth from your finger to his or her nose. Ask the patient to alternately touch his or her nose with the right and left index fingers. Finally, have the patient repeat these tasks with the eyes closed. The movements should be rapid, smooth, and accurate.

Balance can be assessed using the Romberg test if the patient is able to stand and is not restricted to bed. Have the patient stand with the feet together, arms at the sides, and eyes open; the patient should be able to stand upright with no swaying. If the patient can do that, have the patient close the eyes and stand the same way. If the patient falls or breaks the stance after closing the eyes, the Romberg test is positive, indicating proprioceptive or vestibular dysfunction.

All levels of the neural axis contribute to **gait**, although most gait abnormalities are motor in nature. In assessing gait, it is important to watch not only the lower extremities but also the upper extremities for normal associated movements. To assess gait, ask the patient to walk without shoes around the examining room or down the hallway, first with the eyes open, then with the eyes closed. A smooth, regular gait rhythm and symmetrical stride length are expected.

Vital Organ Function and the Neurologic System

Control of Breathing

The nervous system is intricately connected to the mechanics of respiration. From the cerebral cortex to the LMNs, the nervous system regulates respiratory effort. Automatic breathing is regulated primarily by lower brainstem nuclei (Fig. 6-15). A healthy awake individual has rhythmic and regular respiratory cycles, occasionally interrupted by the cortical commands (e.g., hyperventilation during anxiety or irregular breathing during speaking). The breathing is even more regular during sleep, when the responses to the exogenous stimuli are minimal. It is debated whether a true "pacemaker" exists that works at a subconscious level and results in rhythmic contraction and relaxation of the respiratory muscles. Alternatively, it is argued that the respiratory centers in the brainstem receive impulses from multiple receptors and the rhythmic breathing is the result of integration of these various excitatory or inhibitory stimuli. The major receptors that influence the breathing are central and peripheral chemoreceptors. Central chemoreceptors are located in the brainstem and respond to changes in Pa_{CO_2} (Fig. 6-16). It is important to note that the central chemoreceptors respond to the changes in Pa_{CO_2} indirectly. The cellular membrane of these receptor cells is impermeable to the hydrogen ions (H^+), but freely permeable to CO_2 (see Fig. 6-16). As CO_2 travels across the membrane, it combines with water and forms H^+ and HCO_3^-. It is the hydrogen ion that forms from this reaction, not the CO_2 itself, that the central chemoreceptors respond to. Peripheral chemoreceptors are located in the aortic and carotid bodies and are further subdivided into receptors that sense pH and Pa_{O_2}. Unlike the central receptors, peripheral chemoreceptors directly respond to the hydrogen ion concentration. The response to the fluctuation in any one of these individual variables (pH, Pa_{CO_2}, and Pa_{O_2}) depends on the status of the other variables. For example, the response to Pa_{CO_2} elevation is exaggerated during relative hypoxia or acidosis and blunted during relative hyperoxia and alkalosis (Figs. 6-17 and 6-18). A good example of hyperventilation caused by severe acidosis is Kussmaul breathing (Fig. 6-19B).

In a normal awake individual, the brain is very sensitive to even miniscule fluctuations in Pa_{CO_2}. Small changes in Pa_{CO_2} cause great increase in minute ventilation (see Fig. 6-17). This type of response keeps Pa_{O_2} in the 90- to 100-mm Hg range, which does not change the activity of the oxygen-sensing chemoreceptors (Fig. 6-20). For this reason, it is stated that normal individuals have *hypercapnic drive* to breathe. In patients with chronic respiratory acidosis (advanced chronic obstructive pulmonary disease [COPD] or other alveolar hypoventilation syndromes), Pa_{CO_2} is constantly elevated, and the respiratory system's response to Pa_{CO_2} fluctuations is blunted. In such situations, the patient becomes more dependent on the peripheral chemoreceptors (especially the ones that sense Pa_{O_2}).

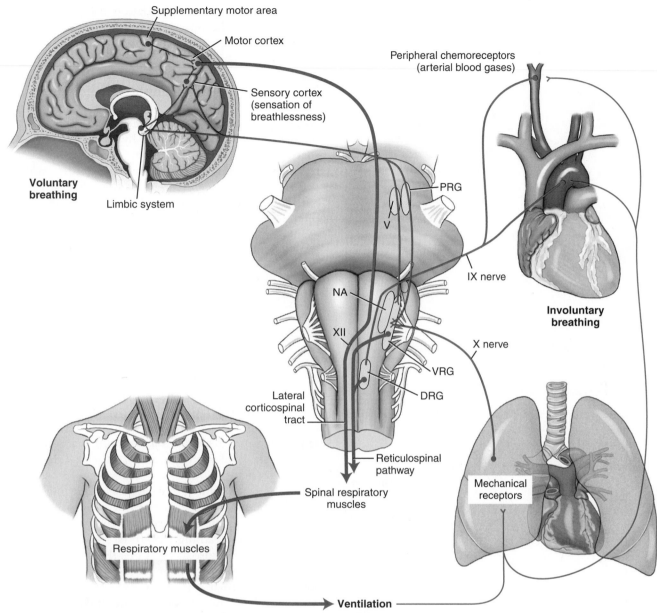

FIGURE 6-15 Schematic representation of the neural control of breathing. Central chemoreceptors; DRG, dorsal respiratory group; NA, nucleus ambiguus; PRG, pontine respiratory group; V, sensory nucleus of V; VRG, ventral respiratory group.

Such patients are said to have *hypoxic drive* to breathe. This mechanism becomes very important when patients with chronic hypercarbia are given supplemental oxygen. Many myths and misconceptions exist regarding the situation when a patient with chronic compensated respiratory acidosis and hypoxia is given oxygen. Some of these patients develop worsening hypercarbia, probably due to various factors, the important ones being ventilation/perfusion ($\dot{V}/\dot{Q}$) ratio mismatch and the abolition of hypoxic drive. Although conceptually easy to understand, the abolition of hypoxic drive has been difficult to prove during experimental research, leading many clinicians to explain the worsening hypercarbia on the basis of $\dot{V}/\dot{Q}$ mismatch: during the periods of hypoxia, there is vasoconstriction of the

pulmonary vessels, which is reversed once supplemental oxygen is given. This reversal leads to perfusion of the lung areas that are not well ventilated—creation of additional lung units with poor ventilation, but good perfusion, an equivalent of alveolar dead space—causing worsening hypercarbia and often requiring intubation. This leads to a dilemma: either leave the patient hypoxic, or give supplemental oxygen at the risk for intubation, with neither option being optimal. In reality, many of these patients will likely benefit from early intubation. However, a small minority of patients may be well managed with low levels of supplemental oxygen (keeping Sp_{O_2} in the 90% to 92% range) and careful monitoring of their clinical status and gas exchange abnormalities.

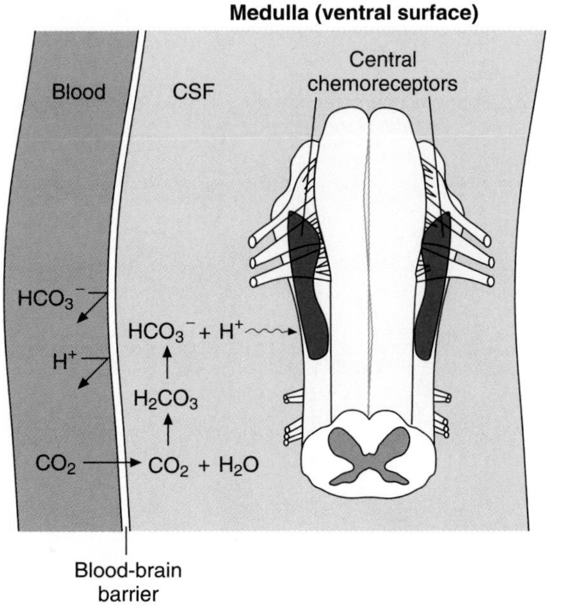

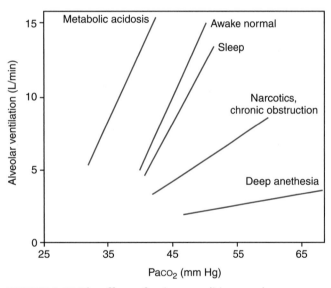

Medulla (ventral surface)

FIGURE 6-16 How carbon dioxide affects respiratory drive. CSF, cerebrospinal fluid. (From Beachey W. *Respiratory care anatomy and physiology.* 2nd ed. St. Louis: Mosby-Elsevier; 2007.)

FIGURE 6-17 The effects of various conditions on the ventilatory response to carbon dioxide. (Redrawn from Raff H, Levitzky M: *Medical physiology: a systems approach,* New York, 2011, Lange Medical Books.- A McGraw Hill Company)

Other peripheral receptors are less important in minute-to-minute control of breathing but still have significant effects on the system. They include receptors that are located in the bronchial tree that sense temperature (bronchospasm and coughing when breathing cold air); stretch receptors located in the lung (after a period of inactivity and relatively low minute ventilation, we all sigh to take a deep breath and "stretch" the lungs—an event mostly dictated by the stretch receptors); and musculoskeletal receptors that sense the movement of the muscles and joints

and increase the minute ventilation even when no extra work is done by the muscles.

Higher brain centers that are located in the amygdala and the cortex have some, but not complete, control of the lower centers located in midbrain. For example, we can all hyperventilate or hold our breath on command. However, at some point, the influence of these higher centers seizes, and the midbrain takes over. Breath holding is usually terminated by the combination of hypoxia and hypercarbia that results from it. Similarly, hyperventilation will lead to syncope, leading to relative hypoventilation until PaO_2 and $PaCO_2$ levels are corrected. Another illustrative example of integrated responses to breathing is high-altitude physiology. When a person dwelling at sea level arrives at high altitude (usually altitudes higher than 3000 m or 10,000 feet), he or she will start to hyperventilate because of relative hypoxia from low inspired PO_2. Although this hyperventilation will only modestly increase the PaO_2, it will cause significant changes in $PaCO_2$ and pH, causing severe respiratory alkalosis and limiting further increases in minute ventilation. Within the next 24 to 48 hours, other compensatory mechanisms (usually bicarbonate wasting by the kidneys) will correct the alkalosis and allow further increases in minute ventilation and PaO_2. For this reason, it is imperative that individuals climbing high altitudes regularly stay at base camps to acclimate before climbing. Use of alcohol and other CNS depressants while at high altitudes is also incrementally dangerous because it adds undue stress to the already strained respiratory drive.

As described earlier, the normal breathing pattern is rhythmic and regular. Lesions at various levels from the cerebrum to the upper cervical cord cause abnormal changes of the breathing pattern (see Fig. 6-19). Despite the nonspecific nature of most breathing patterns, it can still provide valuable clues to the cause of coma. The most common abnormal respiratory pattern seen in patients with neurologic disorders is **Cheyne-Stokes respiration**, which consists of phases of hyperpnea that regularly alternate with episodes of apnea. Figure 6-20 was obtained from a patient with a stroke and shows tidal volume waxing in a smooth crescendo and, once a peak is reached, waning in an equally smooth decrescendo. Cheyne-Stokes respiration usually has an intracranial cause, although it can be caused by hypoxemia and cardiac failure. **Ataxic breathing** (also called **Biot breathing**) is a marker of severe brainstem dysfunction seen as an irregular and unpredictable breathing pattern that indicates that all brain function above the medulla is absent.

SIMPLY STATED

The most common abnormal respiratory pattern seen in patients with neurologic disorders is Cheyne-Stokes respiration, which consists of phases of hyperpnea that regularly alternate with episodes of apnea.

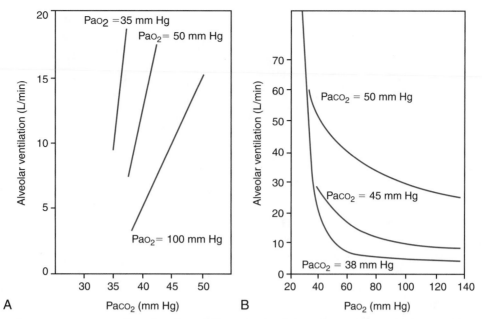

FIGURE 6-18 A, Ventilatory response to carbon dioxide at different levels of Pa_{O_2}. **B,** Ventilatory responses to hypoxia at different levels of Pa_{CO_2}. (Redrawn from Raff H, Levitzky M. *Medical physiology: a systems approach.* New York: Lange Medical Books, A McGraw Hill Company; 2011.)

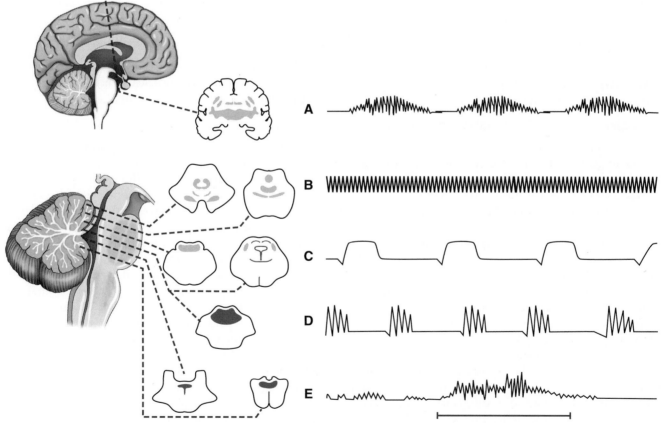

FIGURE 6-19 Correlation of intra-axial brainstem lesions at different levels and the associated type of respiratory dysrhythmia. **A,** Cheyne-Stokes respiration. **B,** Central neurogenic hyperventilation (Kussmaul breathing). **C,** Apneustic breathing. **D,** Cluster breathing. **E,** Ataxic breathing (Biot breathing).

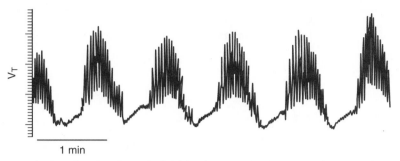

FIGURE 6-20 Cheyne-Stokes respiration showing the typical tidal volume waxing in a smooth crescendo and decrescendo pattern. V$_T$, tidal volume.

Control of Cardiovascular System

Because the brainstem and vagus nerve play an important role in vasomotor tone, conditions affecting these areas can cause vital signs to change. However, a change in vital signs is not a very sensitive indicator of neurologic deterioration because the change often happens too late to prevent irreversible brain damage. Increased **intracranial pressure (ICP)**, such as in herniation syndromes, produces a specific set of changes known as **Cushing triad** (see more details on ICP monitoring in later sections of the chapter). Cushing triad consists of increasing systolic blood pressure with a widening pulse pressure, bradycardia, and bradypnea. Cushing triad is, however, a late sign of increased ICP. Once this pattern of vital signs occurs, brainstem herniation is already in progress, and it may be too late to reverse it.

Ancillary Testing of the Neurologic System

Imaging of the Neurologic System

Computed tomography (CT) scanning and magnetic resonance imaging (MRI) are two commonly used imaging studies to assess structural integrity of the neurologic system (also see Chapter 10). Although CT is quick and easy to perform, MRI provides higher-quality images. Both studies can be enhanced with contrast material, which is often used for the better visualization of the vasculature. When it comes to brain imaging, CT scan is frequently done in the emergency department or in other urgent scenarios for a rapid evaluation, whereas MRI is reserved for more stable patients, in whom detailed information about structural anatomy of the nervous system is necessary. In the evaluation of the spinal cord, MRI is far superior to CT (even with contrast enhancement), so it is often the test of choice. See Chapter 10 for the safety issues and precautions associated with CT and MRI scanning. Special types of imaging (angiography or radionuclide testing) may be performed to confirm brain death (see Declaration of Brain Beath).

Electroencephalography

An **electroencephalogram (EEG)** is a recording of brain's electrical activity, just like an electrocardiogram is a recording of heart's electrical activity. A major role of the EEG is to evaluate a patient with seizures. It is commonly used to distinguish true seizures from false seizures (malingering, conversion disorder, or involuntary movements that resemble seizures). Other common indications include assessment of patients with altered consciousness or as confirmatory test during determination of brain death. Multiple electrodes are placed on the patient's skull to record the electrical activity. The tracings are acquired digitally and interpreted by a physician, typically a neurologist. In most situations, an approximately 1-hour-long recording is enough to make a diagnosis. In complicated or equivocal cases, 24-hour EEG monitoring (to extend the observation period) or video EEG monitoring (to correlate the patient's symptoms and movements with waveform tracings) may be necessary. A simplified version of EEG is also performed during an overnight sleep study (polysomnogram), which is discussed in detail in Chapter 19.

Lumbar Puncture

The brain and the spinal cord are surrounded by the cerebrospinal fluid (CSF) and are often described to be floating in it. CSF is a clear, colorless fluid and serves a number of purposes: to insulate brain from mechanical injury, provide favorable biochemical environment, and decrease the weight of the brain within the skull. **Lumbar puncture (LP)** is done to obtain a sample of CSF. The major utility of CSF analysis is in patients with suspected infection. In other cases, it is done to determine the presence of elevated protein levels (Guillain-Barré syndrome) or to look for inflammatory or malignant conditions. The fluid is typically sent for cell count and differential, smears and culture, and biochemical analysis. Cytology and serologic studies are ordered to diagnose malignancy and other inflammatory conditions. LP is typically done by inserting a long 20-gauge catheter into the space between the lower lumbar vertebrae, at the level of the cauda equina, to avoid injury to the spinal cord. To increase the curvature of the spine and increase the space between the vertebrae, where the needle will be placed, the patient is placed in fetal position with the neck fully flexed forward and the knees brought as close to the chin as possible. In many intubated patients, a number of assistants (nurse as

TABLE 6-8				
Sequence of Loss of Brainstem Function				
Highest Level of Brainstem Function	**Breathing**	**Oculocephalic Reflex**	**Pupils**	**Pain Response**
High midbrain	Normal	Normal	Normal	Withdrawal
Mid-midbrain	Cheyne-Stokes	Present	Small but reactive	Decorticate
Pons	Hyperventilation	Minimal	Mid-fixed	Decerebrate
Medulla	Ataxic	None	Mid-fixed	None

well as RT) are necessary to maintain the patient in this unnatural position for the duration of the procedure and ensure the security of the endotracheal tube and other catheters.

Intracranial Pressure Monitoring

The main purpose of ICP monitoring is to assess cerebral perfusion. As the blood flows across the pressure gradient, the cerebral perfusion will be proportional to the difference between the mean arterial pressure (MAP) and the ICP. This pressure difference is often called **cerebral perfusion pressure (CPP)**. Assuming CPP = MAP − ICP, the cerebral perfusion worsens as ICP increases. Mean ICP of a supine patient is normally 10 to 15 mm Hg. Although small fluctuations are normal during the cardiac cycle, variability greater than 10 mm Hg is suggestive of serious neurologic compromise. Elevations in ICP to 15 to 20 mm Hg compress the capillary bed and compromise microcirculation. At ICP levels of 30 to 35 mm Hg, edema develops, even in normal tissue. Cerebral perfusion cannot be maintained if ICP increases to within 40 to 50 mm Hg of the MAP. When ICP approximates MAP, perfusion stops, and the brain dies.

ICP monitoring is commonly done in patients with increased risk for herniation, such as with stroke or anoxic brain injury. As the brain swells, the pressure rises within the confined space of the skull, and CPP decreases. During incremental elevation of the ICP, brainstem functions are lost in a predictable sequence. The loss of function starts from the top of the midbrain and extends sequentially down through the medulla (Table 6-8). In cases of significant swelling, parts of the brain (commonly the brainstem) are displaced (herniated) from their original location and thus become injured. Hyperventilation (goal $Paco_2 \sim 30$) is sometimes used to decrease the intracranial blood volume and lower ICP, especially because it is one of the fastest ways to decrease the ICP. However, it is extremely important to remember that hypoventilation also affects the overall blood flow to the brain, and its final effect on the CPP (a measure of brain perfusion) may be misjudged by only examining the effects of hyperventilation on ICP. The overall effect of the hyperventilation on CPP is complex and not completely understood. These effects are also short lived, limiting the usefulness of hyperventilation to the initial 24 hours or so. Owing

to the complexity of the situation, the decision about whether to hyperventilate the patient for the purposes of ICP lowering is often made in consultation with various subspecialty physicians.

SIMPLY STATED

Although hyperventilation is associated with lower ICP values, CPP is the most critical element to monitor.

Declaration of Brain Death

Brain death is an irreversible condition that occurs when all perceptible brain activity has seized. It usually follows a devastating brain injury, commonly caused by a prolonged cardiac arrest or a massive stroke. In most situations, the determination of brain death will be the grounds to pronounce the patient dead (even if the heart is still beating) and remove the mechanical ventilator as well as other support devices. Because of the nuances of various protocols and exceptions from this general rule, the reader is encouraged to become familiar with the local laws and regulations regarding brain death. We give only a general overview of the topic here.

Typically, a two-step approach, including a clinical examination by either attending neurologist or critical care specialist and a confirmatory test (EEG or an imaging study), is performed. During the clinical examination, a physician will ascertain that all clinical brain activity has seized, which is usually documented by the absence of pupillary, corneal, gag, and oculovestibular reflexes, as well as the absence of respirations during an apnea test. Other important clinical features that need to be documented by the physician before the declaration of brain death are the absence of reversible conditions, such as the following:

• Hypothermia
• Effects of sedative medications
• Effects of neuromuscular blockade
• Major metabolic disturbances
• Shock

An apnea test is administered by a physician and RT. Many patients with brain injury may have been hyperventilated for various reasons, and respiratory alkalosis will suppress the drive to breathe. For this reason, the arterial blood gases are normalized before the apnea test. After documentation of normal or near-normal Pao_2 and $Paco_2$, the patient is disconnected from the ventilator, and 100% oxygen is administered through an endotracheal tube. Some protocols require administration of oxygen through a transtracheal catheter, but this technique may lead to increased intrathoracic pressures and barotrauma and should be done very carefully. The patient is closely monitored during the apnea test, with the emphasis on spontaneous breathing, oxygenation, and cardiovascular status. Many patients, already terminally ill, will deteriorate during the apnea test, leading to termination of the test by the attending physician. In the absence of spontaneous breathing movement and the evidence of clinical deterioration, the patient is monitored for 8 to 10 minutes, arterial blood gases are redrawn, and the patient is placed back on the ventilator. An increase of $Paco_2$ to 60 mm Hg or 20 mm Hg above the baseline in the absence of spontaneous respirations is indicative of a positive apnea test (i.e., the patient was apneic).

It must be remembered that although designed to measure spontaneous respiratory drive, the apnea test truly measures the respiratory effort. For example, the patient may have a preserved drive but weak effort due to concomitant illness, leading to shallow and ineffective respirations that do not make the chest rise or affect $Paco_2$ levels. Proper and timely administration of brain death protocol is of paramount importance to the patient and the family as well as to ensuring maintenance of other organ functions (e.g., kidney, liver, heart) if organ donation is to ensue.

KEY POINTS

▶ Injuries that involve the nervous system often affect the patient's respiratory system and the ability of the patient to cooperate with respiratory care procedures.
▶ Many neurologic functions of particular importance to the RT, such as regulation of heart rate, blood pressure, and breathing, are located in the brainstem.
▶ Damage to cervical spine roots of C3 to C5 may result in complete paralysis of the diaphragm.
▶ The GCS is the most widely used instrument for quantifying neurologic impairment.
▶ Delirium in ventilated patients is associated with longer stays in the hospital and poor clinical outcomes.
▶ An absent gag reflex (CNs IX and X) may increase the risk for aspiration.
▶ The ability to cough with suctioning implies an intact CN X.
▶ The most common abnormal respiratory pattern seen in patients with neurologic disorders is Cheyne-Stokes respiration.
▶ CPP is the most critical element to monitor in patients with head injury when monitoring ICP.
▶ Brain death is an irreversible condition when all perceptible brain activity has seized. Absence of brainstem reflexes and spontaneous respiratory drive are critical features of brain death.
▶ There several ancillary tests, including ICP and EEG monitoring, as well LP, that can be done to help clinicians assess the patient's neurologic status.

ASSESSMENT QUESTIONS

See Appendix for answers.

1. The knowledge of neurologic function and its assessment is important in the daily practice of the respiratory therapist (RT) because:
   a. The RT is often the first health care professional to encounter a patient with stroke
   b. The RT is an important member of neurology clinic staff
   c. Many respiratory conditions also affect the central nervous system
   d. Many central nervous system conditions also affect the respiratory system

2. Anatomically, the brain is divided into:
   a. Cerebrum, cerebellum, and brainstem
   b. Cerebrum, cerebellum, brainstem, and cranial nerves
   c. Cerebrum, cerebellum, brainstem, and spinal cord
   d. Cerebrum, cerebellum, brainstem, spinal cord, cranial and spinal nerves

3. The centers that regulate autonomous respiratory function are located in:
   a. Brain cortex
   b. Brainstem
   c. Cerebellum
   d. Spinal cord

4. Which of the following is the most common cause of nerve root pathology caused by compression?
   a. Herniated vertebral disk
   b. Spinal tumor
   c. Spinal cord injury
   d. Infection

5. A patient with C3-level spinal cord injury is likely to demonstrate:
   a. Normal respiratory drive
   b. Babinski sign
   c. Normal patellar reflex
   d. Altered content of consciousness

6. Injury to the cervical spine roots C2 to C4 is associated with which of the following abnormalities?
   a. Absence of deep tendon reflexes
   b. Babinski sign
   c. Paralysis of the diaphragm
   d. Doll's eyes reflex

7. A patient in stupor will have a major deficit during this part of the neurologic assessment:
   a. Sensory examination
   b. Motor examination
   c. Level of consciousness
   d. Deep tendon reflexes

8. What is the most widely used instrument to quantify neurologic impairment?
   a. Merck Gait Evaluation
   b. Glasgow Coma Scale
   c. APACHE III score
   d. Apnea test

9. A Glasgow Coma Scale score below this number is typically an indication for endotracheal intubation:
   a. 9
   b. 10
   c. 12
   d. 14

10. Which of the following cranial nerves are evaluated with the gag reflex?
    a. II and III
    b. V and VII
    c. I and II
    d. IX and X

11. Dislodgment of the endotracheal tube is most likely to occur during:
    a. Lumbar puncture
    b. ICP monitoring
    c. CAM-ICU assessment
    d. EEG lead placement

12. The presence of dorsiflexion of the great toe with fanning of remaining toes while testing the plantar reflex is known as which of the following?
    a. Babinski sign
    b. Jerk reflex
    c. Patellar reflex
    d. Quadriceps reflex

13. Which of the following is the most useful test in assessing delirium?
    a. Glasgow Coma Scale
    b. Richmond Agitation Sedation Scale
    c. CAM-ICU assessment
    d. Cranial nerve examination

14. PERRLA is used to describe findings while examining
    a. Pupils
    b. Gag reflex
    c. Deep tendon reflexes
    d. Level of consciousness

15. A patient with Kussmaul breathing is likely to have:
    a. Severe acidosis
    b. Hypoxic drive to breathe
    c. Brain death
    d. Normal minute ventilation

16. Which of the following respiratory patterns consists of phases of hyperpnea that regularly alternate with episodes of apnea?
    a. Biot
    b. Kussmaul
    c. Apnea
    d. Cheyne-Stokes

17. Which of the following is the most critical parameter to keep in mind when managing a patient with intracranial hypertension?
    a. Mean arterial pressure
    b. Cerebral perfusion pressure
    c. Intracranial pressure
    d. Pulse pressure

Bibliography

Bleck TP. Levels of consciousness and attention. In: Goetz CG, editor. *Textbook of clinical neurology.* 3rd ed. Philadelphia: WB Saunders; 2007.

Caruana-Montaldo B, Gleeson K, Zwillich CW. Control of breathing in clinical practice. *Chest* 2000;**117**:205.

DeMyer WE. *Technique of the neurologic examination.* 5th ed. New York: McGraw-Hill; 2004.

Dunn WF, Nelson SB, Hubmayr RD. Oxygen-induced hypercarbia in obstructive pulmonary disease. *Am Rev Respir Dis* 1991;**144**:526.

Ely EW. *Confusion Assessment Method for the ICU (CAM-ICU): complete training manual.* Retrieved July 26, 2012, from October 2010, http://www.mc.vanderbilt.edu/icudelirium/docs/CAM_ICU_training.pdf:Last revised.

Kacmarek RM, Stoller JK, Heuer AJ. *Egan's fundamentals of respiratory care.* 10th ed. St. Louis: Mosby-Elsevier; 2013.

Teasdale G, Jennett BJ. Assessment of coma and impaired consciousness: A practical scale. *The Lancet* 1974; **2**(7872):81–4.

Zuercher M, Ummenhofer W, Baltussen A, Walder B. The use of Glasgow Coma Scale in injury assessment: a critical review. *Brain Inj* 2009;**23**:371.

Chapter 7

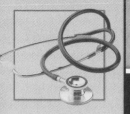

Clinical Laboratory Studies

NADINE A. FYDRYSZEWSKI AND ELAINE M. KEOHANE*

CHAPTER OUTLINE

Clinical Laboratory Overview
Phases of Laboratory Testing
Composition of Blood
Specimen Integrity and Effect on Test Results
Laboratory Test Parameters
Hematology
Complete Blood Count
Erythrocyte Sedimentation Rate
Coagulation Screening Tests
Chemistry
Basic Metabolic Panel
Renal Panel
Hepatic Panel
Lipid Panel
Cardiac Biomarkers

Microbiology
Pre-analytical Phase: Specimen Selection, Collection, and Transport
Microscopic Examination of Specimens
Culture and Sensitivity
Examination of Pulmonary Secretions
Bronchoalveolar Lavage
Pleural Fluid Examination
Histology and Cytology
Skin Testing
Recommended Laboratory Tests

LEARNING OBJECTIVES

After reading this chapter, you will be able to:
1. Explain the three phases of laboratory testing.
2. Describe the composition of blood.
3. Explain the importance of specimen integrity and effects on laboratory test results.
4. Define laboratory test sensitivity, specificity, and positive and negative predictive value.
5. Discuss the meaning of the term *reference range*.
6. Describe the clinical applications and general clinical significance of increases and decreases for each component of the complete blood count and for the reticulocyte count and erythrocyte sedimentation rate.
7. Define leukocytosis, leukopenia, relative and absolute count, neutrophilia, neutropenia, lymphocytosis, lymphopenia, monocytosis, eosinophilia, basophilia, leukemia, anemia, and hemostasis.
8. Describe the body's response to anemia and the potential effects on the body of uncompensated anemia.
9. Differentiate primary, secondary, and relative polycythemia and describe the adverse effects of polycythemia on the body.
10. Describe the clinical applications of the activated partial thromboplastin time, prothrombin time, and platelet count in assessing hemostasis.
11. Explain the clinical application and significance of the quantitative D-dimer assay.
12. Describe the clinical applications and general clinical significance of increases and decreases in electrolyte concentrations, glucose levels, blood urea nitrogen and creatinine.
13. Discuss the importance of renal and hepatic panel tests as related to the management of patients with respiratory disorders.

---

*Dr. Robert Wilkins, PhD, RRT, contributed much of the content for this chapter as the coeditor of the prior edition of this text.

LEARNING OBJECTIVES—cont'd

14. Relate lipid panel measures to the risk for atherosclerosis and heart disease.
15. Identify the current cardiac biomarkers used to help identify acute coronary syndrome and congestive heat failure.
16. Describe the pre-analytical phase of testing in clinical microbiology.
17. Discuss the common methods of examination of microbiology specimens (e.g., Gram stain, acid-fast stains).
18. Explain the purpose of a microbiology culture and antimicrobial sensitivity test.
19. Describe the collection and transport protocols for pulmonary secretions.
20. Discuss the importance of macroscopic and microscopic examination of sputum.
21. List the microscopic criteria used to assess the quality of a sputum sample.
22. Explain the significance of sputum eosinophilia.
23. Describe the indications and method of performing a bronchoalveolar lavage.
24. Describe the macroscopic, microscopic, and chemical significance of pleural fluid examination.
25. Explain the purpose of histologic and cytologic examinations.
26. List the malignant tumors responsible for producing most primary lung cancers.
27. List the types of pulmonary samples that can be examined cytologically.
28. Discuss the general concept of skin testing and two methods to screen for tuberculosis.
29. Given a variety of patient presentations, identify the common laboratory tests helpful in assessing the problem.

KEY TERMS

analyte	hypochromic	normoblasts
anemia	hypoglycemia	normochromic
anergy	hypokalemia	normocytic
basophilia	hyponatremia	polycythemia
blasts	left shift	polycythemia vera
cytology	leukocytosis	pseudoneutropenia
eosinophilia	leukopenia	pseudoneutrophilia
glycosuria	lymphocytopenia	reticulocyte
hemostasis	lymphocytosis	sensitivity
hyperchloremia	macrocytic	serum
hyperglycemia	macrophage	specificity
hyperkalemia	microcytic	spurious
hypernatremia	monocytosis	thrombocytopenia
hypoalbuminemia	neutropenia	thrombocytosis
hypochloremia	neutrophilia	

Clinical Laboratory Overview

The practice of modern medicine would be impossible without the tests performed by medical laboratory scientists in the clinical laboratory. Laboratory scientists analyze body fluids and other medical specimens, providing laboratory data and vital information to other members of the health care team. Clinical laboratory tests are used to diagnose, treat, monitor, and prevent disease.

The clinical laboratory includes several specialized disciplines: microbiology, hematology, immunology, transfusion medicine, clinical chemistry, and molecular diagnostics. Most hospitalized patients with respiratory disease undergo many laboratory tests, and it is important for respiratory therapists (RTs) to have a basic understanding of the commonly ordered tests. This chapter provides key information related to the pre-analytical, analytical, and post-analytical phases of laboratory testing. Although the emphasis is on laboratory tests and data related to patients with respiratory disease, most of the concepts described here are applicable to any patient.

Phases of Laboratory Testing

Laboratory testing involves a pre-analytical, analytical, and post-analytical phase. The pre-analytical phase is related to specimen selection, collection, and transport. The RT may be involved in this phase, particularly in collection of arterial blood samples and pulmonary secretions for laboratory testing. The analytical phase is the actual testing performed by laboratory scientists. The post-analytical phase involves reporting and interpretation of results.

Most laboratory tests are performed using blood collected from peripheral veins, arteries, or capillaries. For most tests, the site of blood collection has no effect on the analysis or the results. Exceptions include blood gases and lactic acid that vary significantly by collection site. Therefore, it is important that appropriate selection, collection, and transport be used. Blood collection tubes, with various stoppers and additives, must be matched to the analytes being tested. Other specimens submitted for laboratory tests include body fluids, secretions such as sputum, pleural fluid, cerebrospinal fluid, urine, feces, biopsy material, and sweat.

Composition of Blood

Blood consists of two major components: the formed elements (45%) and the plasma (55%). The formed elements are composed of three types of cells: white blood cells (leukocytes), red blood cells (erythrocytes), and platelets (thrombocytes). These formed elements are made in the bone marrow from stem cells. The plasma consists of water and soluble substances including electrolytes, clotting factors, immunologic factors, proteins, lipids, and hormones. Almost every substance the cells use must be transported by the plasma. **Serum** is the fluid remaining when the blood is allowed to clot. It closely resembles plasma, but lacks some coagulation factors.

Specimen Integrity and Effect on Test Results

Specimen integrity is critical to quality, accurate laboratory testing. Test results can be affected by hemolysis, storage times and temperature, method of transport, interfering conditions of the blood (icterus, lipemia, turbidity), inadequate blood volume when using tubes with additives, and using the wrong collection tube. For example, a specimen that is hemolyzed can yield falsely elevated results for several **analytes**, including potassium, magnesium, calcium, and iron. Maintenance of specimen integrity for microbiologic samples commonly gathered by RTs is discussed later in this chapter. Specimen integrity for arterial blood gas samples is covered in Chapter 8.

Laboratory Test Parameters

A quality test results is accurate and precise but also must provide information to clinicians useful for making a diagnosis or in monitoring disease. The usefulness of a test is evaluated in terms of its predictive value model, which includes measurements of clinical sensitivity, clinical specificity, positive predictive value, and negative predictive value. If a patient has a disease, the test results can either be positive or negative. If the test is positive, it is considered a true positive (TP). If the test is negative in a patient with disease, it represents a false negative (FN). If a patient is free of disease, the test results also can either be positive or negative. A negative test in a disease-free patient is considered a true negative (TN). On the other hand, if a positive test occurs in a disease-free patient, the result would be considered a false positive (FP). TP, FN, TN, and FP can be grouped into statistical parameters describing the accuracy of the test results in relation to a particular disease.

- **Sensitivity:** frequency of positive test results of patients with disease. *Example:* A sensitivity of 98% means that 98% of the patients with the disease will be detected by the test (TP), and 2% of the patients with the disease will be negative with the test (FN). Another way to express sensitivity is: "if the patient has the disease, the test will be positive." If, on the other hand, the results of a test with high sensitivity are negative, one can confidently rule out the disorder in question.

- **Specificity:** frequency of negative test results of patients without disease. *Example:* A specificity of 98% means that 98% of the patients without the disease will be negative for the test (TN), and 2% of the patients without the disease will be positive for the test (FP). Another way to express specificity is: "if the patient does *not* have the disease, the test will be negative." Conversely, if the results of a test with high specificity are positive, one can confidently rule-in the disorder in question.

Laboratory test results are often interpreted based on comparison to a reference value or range. This comparison is used to aid in the medical diagnosis, assessment of physiologic state, and therapeutic management. Reference values depend on many factors, including patient age, gender, sample population, and test method. The laboratory report will contain specific reference ranges that have been established for that facility or population. Reference values are expressed as ranges constructed to include 95% of the normal population (2 standard deviations). Each laboratory must determine its own reference values based on population and test methodology. Therefore, the reference ranges mentioned in this chapter represent those typical of many laboratories, but not absolute values. Clinicians should abandon using the terms "normal value" and "normals" because they are misleading. A test result falling outside a reference range does not necessarily mean that the patient has the abnormal condition or disease. Trends in results, comparison with other test results, and evaluation in light of other clinical findings must be taken into consideration. Correlation of clinical findings with laboratory test results leads to appropriate diagnosis and treatment.

Hematology

Clinical laboratory tests in hematology can be divided into two main categories: (1) general hematology tests for evaluating normal and abnormal blood cells and (2) coagulation studies for evaluating blood clotting. General hematology tests covered here include the complete blood count (CBC), white blood cell differential count, reticulocyte count, and erythrocyte sedimentation rate. Routine coagulation tests discussed in this section include the prothrombin time (PT)/international normalized ratio (INR) and the activated partial thromboplastin time (APTT). Routine hematology and coagulation tests are important for assessing wellness and health status, detecting and initial investigation of various disease states, and monitoring certain therapies.

Complete Blood Count

The CBC is an overall assessment of the quantity and morphology (appearance) of the white blood cells (WBCs), red blood cells (RBCs), and platelets. The CBC includes a total WBC count, a count of the different types of WBCs (called a *differential count*), the RBC count, hemoglobin (Hb) level, hematocrit (Hct), the RBC indices, a platelet count, and sometimes a reticulocyte count. Table 7-1 contains sample adult reference ranges for the CBC components in both common units and standard international (SI) units.

CBC analyzers examine whole blood using various technologies and software to count cells and assess their volume and internal structures. However, CBC results are reviewed and verified by laboratory scientists before they are reported. The following discussion focuses first on WBCs and the differential count, and then shifts to RBCs and platelets. Coagulation studies are discussed last.

TABLE 7-1

Sample Reference Ranges for the Complete Blood Count (CBC) in Adults

CBC Component Conventional Units (SI units)	Reference Ranges
WBC count × 10^3/μL (× 10^9/L)	4.5-11.5
RBC count × 10^6/μL (× 10^{12}/L)	M: 4.60-6.00
	F: 4.00-5.40
Hemoglobin g/dL (g/L)	M: 14.0-18.0 (140-180)
	F: 12.0-15.0 (120-150)
Hct % (L/L)	M: 40-54 (0.40-0.54)
	F: 35-49 (0.35-0.49)
Erythrocyte Indices	
Mean cell volume (MCV) (fL)	80-100
Mean cell hemoglobin (pg)	26-32
Mean cell Hb concentration (MCHC) (g/dL)	32-36
Platelet count × 10^3/μL (× 10^9/L)	150-450
Reticulocytes %	0.5-1.5
Reticulocytes × 10^3/μL (× 10^9/L)	25-75

M, male; F, female; RBC, Red blood cell; SI, standard international; WBC, white blood cell.

White Blood Cells

WBCs function as part of the immune system in protecting the body from various pathogenic microorganisms and foreign antigens. WBCs originate from hematopoietic stem cells in the bone marrow, develop into specific cell lineages through the influence of growth factors, and are released into the peripheral blood when mature. The WBCs that are normally present in the peripheral blood include segmented neutrophils, bands, eosinophils, basophils, lymphocytes, and monocytes.

White Blood Cell Differential Count. CBC analyzers determine the total number of WBCs per microliter or liter of blood and perform an automated differential count in which the percentage and absolute number of each type of WBC is determined. If the instrument count is abnormal, or a sample is flagged for suspected abnormal or immature cells, a manual slide review and differential count is performed by a laboratory scientist. In addition, the morphology of all the cells is assessed, and the presence of immature and abnormal cells is noted.

The relative count is the percentage of a particular cell among all the WBCs counted. The absolute count for that cell type is determined by multiplying its percentage or relative count by the total WBC count. CBC analyzers automatically calculate the absolute counts for each type of WBC. Table 7-2 provides sample reference ranges for the relative and absolute counts of each type of WBC.

Because the relative count is influenced by increases or decreases of the other WBC types, the absolute count provides a more useful quantitative assessment. In a simplified example, if an adult patient had a total WBC count of 20 ×10^9/L with a relative count of 85% neutrophils and 15% lymphocytes, the absolute counts would be 17 × 10^9/L for neutrophils and 3 × 10^9/L for lymphocytes. Comparing these results to the reference ranges in Table 7-2, there is both a relative and an absolute increase in neutrophils. On the other hand, although the relative count for the lymphocytes is decreased, the absolute count is well within the reference range.

White Blood Cell Functions. Neutrophils, eosinophils, and basophils are included in a general category

TABLE 7-2

Sample Reference Ranges for the Differential White Blood Cell Count in Adults

Cell Type	Relative	Absolute*
Segmented neutrophils	50-70	2.3-8.1
Bands	0-5	0-0.6
Eosinophils	1-3	0-0.4
Basophils	0-1	0-0.1
Lymphocytes	20-45	0.8-4.8
Monocytes	2-11	0.45-1.3

*% × 10^3/μL (× 10^9/L)

of cells called *granulocytes* because of their prominent granules. However, they have different functions.

Segmented neutrophils (previously called polymorpho-nuclear leukocytes) are the most numerous cell type in the peripheral blood, constituting 50% to 70% of circulating WBCs. A band is a slightly less mature neutrophil in which the nucleus has not yet segmented. Bands normally represent only 0% to 5% of the circulating WBCs.

The primary function of neutrophils is to destroy invading microorganisms, foreign material, and dead cells. They accomplish this by phagocytosis, a process in which the neutrophil engulfs and destroys the particles through release of various enzymes and reactive molecules.

SIMPLY STATED

There are five different types of WBCs, the most common of which is the segmented neutrophil. It is the first line of defense against bacterial infections.

Neutrophils are produced and stored in the bone marrow, a process that takes 8 to 12 days. However, if the demand for neutrophils increases—as may occur in an acute bacterial infection— their time in the bone marrow may be shortened to as few as 2 days. In these cases, some immature neutrophils may be released. Once released into the peripheral blood, neutrophils have a very short half-life of 6 to 8 hours.

In the peripheral blood, neutrophils are continuously exchanged between two intravascular pools, with about half the cells in the circulating pool and half in the marginated pool. The circulating neutrophils are those counted in the CBC. Marginated neutrophils adhere to the walls of the blood vessels and are not counted. Neutrophils are able to rapidly shift from one pool to the other based on physiologic conditions (discussed subsequently).

Eosinophils are a type of granulocyte with large granules that stain bright orange or pink, whereas basophils have large granules that stain dark blue or purple. Eosinophils normally constitute 1% to 3% of WBCs, whereas basophils are even more rare at 0% to 1%. Both cell types are involved in immune system regulation, control of parasitic infections, and allergic reactions. Eosinophils also accumulate at the site of allergic reactions.

Lymphocytes constitute 20% to 45% of circulating WBCs in adults; in healthy children, the relative and absolute lymphocyte count is higher. Lymphocytes are particularly important in the body's defense against foreign microorganisms and cells. There are three major types of lymphocytes: T cells, B cells, and NK (natural killer) cells. T and B cells participate in the body's adaptive or specific immune response by recognizing foreign antigens and tagging them for destruction. T cells are involved in cell-mediated immunity, which is particularly important in eliminating viruses and other intracellular organisms. B cells are involved in humoral immunity and develop into antibody-producing cells. NK cells are able to destroy certain virally infected cells and tumor cells.

The different lymphocyte types appear similar on a peripheral blood smear. Enumeration of the different types of lymphocytes is not done routinely but can be accomplished using monoclonal antibodies. Approximately 85% of circulating lymphocytes are T cells, with B cells making up 10% to 15% and NK cells less than 2%. T lymphocytes also can be separated into subcategories. For example, knowledge of the CD4$^+$ T-lymphocyte cell count provides important information about the severity and prognosis of patients with acquired immunodeficiency syndrome (AIDS; see later discussion of lymphocytopenia).

Monocytes are the largest WBCs normally seen in the peripheral blood and constitute 2% to 11% of circulating WBCs. In tissues, the monocyte is known as a **macrophage**. The primary functions of the monocyte are phagocytosis of organisms and other foreign material invading the body and initiation and regulation of the specific immune response with T lymphocytes. In the lung, alveolar macrophages play a key role in clearing inhaled particulate matter.

Nonmalignant White Blood Cell Abnormalities. **Leukocytosis** is an increase in the WBC count above the reference range, whereas **leukopenia** is a decrease in the WBC count below the reference range. Abnormalities in the WBC count can be defined more specifically by referring to the specific cell type that is increased or decreased using similar terminology. For example, an increase in neutrophils is called neutrophilia, and a decrease is called **neutropenia**. Increases in the cell counts may be primary (a result of uncontrolled proliferation of cells in the bone marrow) or secondary (a result of stimulation of the bone marrow secondary to other diseases or disorders). Similarly, decreases in cell counts may be caused by either primary bone marrow failure or increased destruction of the cells peripherally. Bone marrow failure can occur as a side effect of various drugs and disorders (secondary) or as a result of unknown causes (primary or idiopathic).

Neutrophilia is a common response to acute bacterial infections, such as bacterial pneumonia (Box 7-1). Neutrophilia also may occur in response to fungal, parasitic, or early viral infections. In addition, neutrophilia also occurs in inflammation due to autoimmune disorders or tissue damage that occurs after surgery, burns, myocardial infarction, or traumatic injury. Acute hemorrhage or hemolysis, metabolic disorders (such as acidosis or uremia), and certain drugs, toxins, and chemicals also cause neutrophilia. When the bone marrow is stimulated to release neutrophils at a rate faster than it can produce them, it releases them at increasingly more immature stages. This is called a **left shift**. The degree of the left shift and the severity of the neutrophilia usually correlate with the severity of the infection.

SIMPLY STATED

The typical response to an acute bacterial infection is a neutrophilia with a left shift (increase in bands and presence of immature neutrophils in the peripheral blood).

Box 7-1	Common Causes of Nonmalignant or Reactive Neutrophilia

PATHOLOGIC
Acute bacterial infections
Other infections (fungal, parasitic, early stages of viral infections)
Inflammatory responses
Tissue damage (burns, surgery, traumatic injury, myocardial infarction)
Autoimmune disorders
Acute hemorrhage or hemolysis
Metabolic disorders (acidosis, uremia)
Certain drugs, chemicals, or toxins

PHYSIOLOGIC (PSEUDONEUTROPHILIA)
Physical or emotional stress
Strenuous exercise
Exposure to temperature extremes
Epinephrine administration
Anesthesia

Box 7-2	Causes of Neutropenia

DECREASED NEUTROPHIL PRODUCTION
Drugs, chemicals, physical agents (e.g., chemotherapy, benzene, radiation)
Disorders of stem cells, acquired and inherited
Cancers infiltrating the bone marrow
Vitamin B_{12} or folate deficiency (megaloblastic anemia)
INCREASE IN NEUTROPHIL DESTRUCTION
Overwhelming bacterial infection
Immune disorders (antibody production against neutrophils)
PSEUDONEUTROPENIA
Bacterial endotoxins
Hypersensitivity reactions

SIMPLY STATED

Neutropenia is often a sign of a serious health problem and usually occurs as a result of decreased bone marrow production or increased destruction of neutrophils in the peripheral blood or tissues.

Pseudoneutrophilia, also called physiologic neutrophilia, occurs when marginated neutrophils are shifted to the circulating pool and are counted in the CBC. This type of neutrophilia is immediate and typically transient, lasting less than an hour. Because these are mature neutrophils, there is no spike in band-type cells as seen in pathologic neutrophilia.

Neutropenia may occur as a result of decreased bone marrow production or increased destruction of circulating neutrophils (Box 7-2). Many drugs, some chemicals, and radiation therapy can cause neutropenia by destroying the hematopoietic cells in the bone marrow, thus decreasing bone marrow production. One of the most common causes of neutropenia is cancer chemotherapy. Because of their short half-life, the neutrophils are the first blood cell type to decrease with chemotherapy. The absolute neutrophil count is closely monitored during chemotherapy, and adjustments in therapy are made if it drops too low. Other causes of decreased production include acquired and hereditary defects in hematopoietic stem cells, infiltration of cancer cells into the bone marrow, and deficiencies of vitamin B_{12} or folate. Neutrophils can also be quickly depleted by overwhelming infections or be destroyed as a result of the production of antibodies against them. **Pseudoneutropenia** is a transient shift of the neutrophils in the circulating pool to the marginated pool. It may be caused by bacterial endotoxins or hypersensitivity reactions.

Neutrophils are the first-line defense against microorganisms, so patients with neutropenia have a high risk for developing life-threatening bacterial or fungal infections. The lower the absolute neutrophil count and the longer the duration of the neutropenia, the greater the risk for serious infection.

Eosinophilia (increase in eosinophils) is often seen in parasitic infestations and allergic states (such as hay fever, dermatitis, and drug reactions). Patients with extrinsic or atopic asthma often have eosinophilia. **Basophilia** (increase in basophils) is usually associated with myeloproliferative neoplasms (discussed later in the chapter).

Lymphocytosis (increase in lymphocytes) is typically seen in viral infections and certain bacterial (pertussis) and parasitic (toxoplasmosis) infections. In some viral infections, especially infectious mononucleosis, many of the lymphocytes are enlarged and have a characteristic appearance, being labeled as reactive or variant lymphocytes. Interpretation of lymphocytosis should take into account the patient's age because children normally have higher counts than adults. **Lymphocytopenia** (decrease in lymphocytes) is seen in acquired and congenital immune deficiency states and in various conditions such as acute inflammation, malnutrition, and after treatment with chemotherapy, radiation, or corticosteroids. Lymphocytopenia is an important feature of human immunodeficiency virus (HIV) infection, the virus that causes AIDS. The virus infects and destroys the CD4[+] helper T lymphocytes, resulting in their depletion. As the CD4[+] cells decline, the immune system becomes more compromised, leading to increased risk for certain cancers and infections. Peripheral blood CD4[+] counts, along with the HIV viral load, are used to monitor the progression of the disease. **Monocytosis** (increase in monocytes) is characteristic of certain infections, including tuberculosis, syphilis, typhoid fever, and subacute bacterial endocarditis. A monocytosis often signals the recovery stage of an acute infection. Monocytosis also may occur in inflammatory conditions and autoimmune states.

Malignant White Blood Cell Abnormalities. Leukemias, myeloproliferative neoplasms, and myelodysplastic syndromes are the primary hematologic malignancies involving the bone marrow and peripheral blood. Leukemias result from the uncontrolled proliferation (growth) of a specific type of WBC and may be either acute or chronic. Myeloproliferative neoplasms encompass a spectrum of diseases resulting from an abnormality in stem cells (the precursor of all blood cells). Myeloproliferative neoplasms may have a variable blood picture as the disease progresses, and they sometimes terminate as an acute leukemia. Myelodysplastic syndromes are characterized by decreases in WBCs, RBCs, and platelets in the peripheral blood due to a stem cell defect.

In acute leukemia, there is a mutation that causes a maturation arrest in a blood cell precursor at an early stage of development. Typically, **blasts**, which are the most immature stage of a cell type, accumulate in the bone marrow and peripheral blood. These blasts quickly replace all other cells in the bone marrow and, if left untreated, will cause a rapid death of the patient. WBC counts are variable, but the key feature in the WBC differential is the presence of blasts. The normal WBCs, along with RBCs and platelets, are decreased. Acute lymphoblastic leukemia usually occurs in young children, whereas acute myeloid leukemia most often occurs in infants and older adults. Acute leukemias are classified by the World Health Organization according to the presence of recurrent genetic abnormalities in the leukemia cells.

Chronic leukemias result from a slower proliferation and accumulation of more mature cells in the peripheral blood and bone marrow. Chronic lymphocytic leukemia is the most common type of leukemia and occurs predominantly in elderly people. The WBC count is increased, and the differential shows a preponderance of mature lymphocytes. Chronic myelogenous leukemia (CML) is a myeloproliferative neoplasm that occurs predominantly in middle-aged adults. It is caused by a mutation in a stem cell that results in uncontrolled proliferation of granulocytes. The WBC count is increased, and the bone marrow and peripheral blood contain vast numbers of neutrophils, with immature neutrophils in all stages of maturation, as well as eosinophils and basophils. Platelets are also increased, and there is progressive anemia. Without treatment, CML terminates in acute leukemia, known as *blast transformation*.

Other myeloproliferative neoplasms include polycythemia vera, primary myelofibrosis, and essential thrombocythemia. **Polycythemia vera** is characterized by a proliferation of granulocytic, erythrocytic, and platelet precursors in the bone marrow with an increase in WBCs, RBCs, and platelets in the peripheral blood. Myelofibrosis is characterized by defective hematopoiesis caused by the excessive growth of fibrous tissue (fibrosis) in the bone marrow. Essential thrombocythemia primarily involves the excessive proliferation of megakaryocytes, with increased platelets in the peripheral blood. Myelodysplastic syndromes result from stem cell mutations that cause ineffective blood cell production in the bone marrow and a progressive decrease in WBCs, RBCs, and platelets in the peripheral blood. They occur predominantly in the elderly.

Red Blood Cells

RBCs are produced in the bone marrow by maturation of nucleated erythrocytic precursor cells known as **normoblasts**. Under normal circumstances, as the normoblasts mature, the nuclei become smaller and more condensed, and the cytoplasm acquires a pink color as a result of the development of hemoglobin. Before the RBC is released from the bone marrow to circulate in the peripheral blood, the nucleus is removed. RBCs have a life span of approximately 120 days.

Normal RBCs assume the shape of a biconcave disk to facilitate their primary function of carrying oxygen and to provide maximal deformability to bend as they pass through small capillaries. The major component of mature RBCs (erythrocytes) is hemoglobin, which imparts to blood its normal red color when carrying oxygen. The RBC count is reported in number of cells per microliter or liter of blood (see Table 7-1 for reference ranges). An adequate number of RBCs with an adequate concentration of hemoglobin and a functionally normal hemoglobin molecule are needed for transport of sufficient oxygen from the lungs to the tissues.

> **SIMPLY STATED**
>
> RBCs act as carriers of hemoglobin, which is needed to transport oxygen throughout the body.

Hematocrit (Packed Cell Volume). The Hct is the ratio of the packed RBC volume to the volume of whole blood. A manual Hct is performed by centrifuging whole blood to pack the blood cells to the bottom of a small capillary tube and then measuring the percentage or fraction of the total blood volume occupied by the RBCs (Fig. 7-1). CBC analyzers determine the Hct using various automated technologies. Because it measures the volume of the hemoglobin-containing RBCs, one can estimate the Hct by multiplying the hemoglobin content times a factor of three.

Hemoglobin. Hemoglobin is the protein that carries oxygen to the tissues; it is the major component of RBCs. Hemoglobin also is important in maintaining acid-base balance by acting as a buffer and by carrying carbon dioxide (CO_2) from the tissues to the lungs. The hemoglobin molecule consists of four heme groups, each with an iron molecule capable of binding oxygen, and four globin chains.

Hemoglobin is reported in grams per deciliter or liter of blood. The reference ranges for the RBC count, Hct, and hemoglobin vary by gender, with men having higher levels than women because of the positive influence of

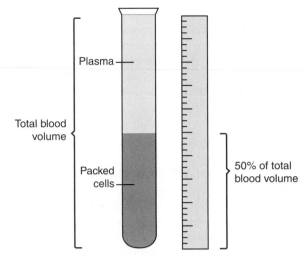

FIGURE 7-1 Determination of hematocrit (Hct) from centrifuging blood sample. Packed cell volume is half the total blood volume; therefore, the Hct is 50% in this example.

testosterone on RBC production (see Table 7-1). Age also affects hemoglobin levels, with higher values in newborns and slightly lower values in elderly people.

Red Blood Cell Indices. Three erythrocyte indices are the mean cell volume (MCV), mean cell hemoglobin (MCH), and mean cell hemoglobin concentration (MCHC). They are calculated from the RBC count, hemoglobin, and Hct. The MCV is the average volume of the patient's RBCs. A decrease in the MCV indicates the RBCs are smaller, or **microcytic**, whereas an increase in the MCV indicates the RBCs are larger, or **macrocytic**. A normal MCV indicates the RBCs are normal in volume, or **normocytic**, although the presence of an equal number of smaller and larger RBCs could produce a normal MCV. The MCH is the average weight of hemoglobin in the patient's RBCs. The interpretation of the MCH correlates with that of the MCV. The MCHC is the concentration of hemoglobin in the patient's RBCs. A decrease in the MCHC indicates the RBCs have less hemoglobin, called **hypochromic**, whereas a normal MCHC indicates the RBCs have a normal complement of hemoglobin, called **normochromic**.

Red Blood Cell Abnormalities. Anemia is a decrease in the oxygen carrying capacity of the blood due to a quantitative deficiency or a functional defect in hemoglobin. Although the RBC count and Hct also decrease, **anemia** is clinically defined by a decrease in the hemoglobin concentration below the reference range for an individual's gender and age.

One of the body's responses to hypoxia is an increase in secretion of erythropoietin by the kidneys, which accelerates the maturation and release of new RBCs into the circulation. The circulatory system also responds to anemia by increasing the heart rate, respiration rate, and cardiac output to deliver oxygen more quickly to the tissues.

General symptoms of anemia include fatigue and dyspnea, but various other symptoms may also occur depending on the cause of the anemia. In severe anemia, tachycardia and hypotension also occur, which if untreated can lead to cardiac failure. The severity of the symptoms depends on the degree of hemoglobin reduction, the state of the patient's cardiovascular system, and the rate of development and duration of the anemia.

Anemias may be classified by pathophysiology into those caused by a decrease in RBC production and those caused by an increase in RBC destruction or loss. However, a more practical approach is to use the MCV to classify anemias into microcytic, macrocytic, or normocytic types.

The most common type of anemia worldwide is the result of iron deficiency. Iron deficiency anemia occurs when there is a dietary deficiency of iron, increased need for iron that is not met (pregnancy, infancy, adolescent growth spurts), malabsorption of iron, or chronic blood loss. In chronic blood loss, the iron contained in the RBCs slowly leaves the body instead of being recycled. Iron is required for hemoglobin synthesis, and with sustained, low iron levels, the bone marrow begins to produce smaller RBCs with a decreased amount of hemoglobin, and the RBC indices become microcytic and hypochromic.

Anemia also can result from chronic inflammation that causes an impairment of iron regulation and RBC production in the bone marrow. The resulting anemia is often normocytic, but it can be microcytic in diseases of long duration. Macrocytic anemia is most often caused by either folate or vitamin B_{12} deficiency. Low folate or vitamin B_{12} levels impair DNA synthesis in the nucleus and result in ineffective blood cell production and macrocytic RBCs.

The hemolytic anemias constitute a large group of disorders in which excessive destruction of RBCs in the circulation exceeds the capacity of the bone marrow to replace the cells that are lost. Hemolytic anemia may be due to intrinsic defects in the RBCs (such as sickle cell anemia) or abnormalities extrinsic to the RBCs (such as hemolysis caused by antibodies, malaria, or drugs).

Hemoglobin may be converted to an inactive form through oxidation, denaturation, or other chemical reaction. The most common forms of inactive hemoglobins are carboxyhemoglobin (COHb) and methemoglobin (metHb). The measurement of these abnormal Hb combinations and their impact on oxygen transport are discussed in detail in Chapter 8.

SIMPLY STATED

Patients with anemia have a decreased oxygen-carrying capacity of the blood. The response to severe and chronic anemia is vasodilation, which increases demands on the heart to maintain blood pressure and can result in high-output cardiac failure.

Polycythemia is an increase in the RBC count, hemoglobin, and Hct and may be primary, secondary, or relative (**spurious**). Primary polycythemia is uncommon and is caused by an uncontrolled proliferation of hematopoietic cells within the bone marrow (polycythemia vera, previously discussed)

Secondary polycythemia is more common and is seen in patients who have chronic stimulation of the bone marrow to produce more RBCs secondary to some other disorder or condition. Examples include patients with chronic hypoxemia due to disease (e.g., chronic obstructive pulmonary disease [COPD]), obstructive sleep apnea, pulmonary fibrosis, chronic heart failure) or as compensation for the low oxygen pressures breathed by those living at high altitude. In these cases, chronic hypoxemia stimulates renal production of erythropoietin, causing the bone marrow to produce and release additional RBCs to compensate for the oxygen deficit.

Heavy smokers also may exhibit secondary polycythemia. The carbon monoxide associated with cigarette smoke binds tightly with the hemoglobin and reduces oxygen transport. This results in a functional anemia to which the bone marrow responds by increasing RBC production.

In the presence of significant hypoxia due to severe anemia, the maturation time of RBCs in the bone marrow is decreased, resulting in the release of immature nucleated RBCs (NRBCs), which are not normally seen in the blood of adults. As a result of the hypoxic conditions in utero, NRBCs are present in fetal blood and newborns but disappear 3 to 4 days after birth. NRBCs also occur in patients with some myeloproliferative neoplasms.

Both primary and secondary polycythemias involve an absolute increase in the total RBC mass. Sometimes, relative polycythemia occurs because of a decrease in the plasma volume. This is seen in patients who are dehydrated. Relative polycythemia does not represent a true increase in the number of circulating RBCs.

Although polycythemia is helpful in increasing the oxygen-carrying capacity of the blood, it can be detrimental to the heart and circulatory system. Polycythemia increases the viscosity of the blood, causing both an increased cardiac workload and a greater risk for clot formation and thrombosis. Treatment focuses on management of the underlying cause and in some patients may include restoring a normal Hct by controlled removal of whole blood through phlebotomy.

SIMPLY STATED

Patients with chronic hypoxemia may develop a secondary polycythemia to compensate for the reduction in blood oxygen levels; polycythemia can increase cardiac workload and the incidence of thrombosis.

Reticulocyte Count. The **reticulocyte** is the final erythrocyte development stage before the RBC is fully mature. These slightly immature RBCs lack a nucleus and differ from mature RBCs in that they are slightly larger and have not yet assumed a biconcave shape. A reticulocyte count is performed by obtaining the percentage of reticulocytes among the RBCs. Normally about 1% of the circulating RBCs are reticulocytes, with slightly higher values in newborns. The reticulocyte count is also reported as an absolute count by multiplying the reticulocyte percentage by the RBC count. Reference ranges are provided in Table 7-1.

The reticulocyte count helps to assess the bone marrow response to an anemia. If the absolute reticulocyte count is high in a patient with anemia, it indicates that the bone marrow is responding to the anemia by increasing production of RBCs. In this case the cause of the anemia is likely due to excessive peripheral blood loss or destruction. However, if the reticulocyte count is low, then the anemia is likely the result of decreased bone marrow production.

Platelet Count

Platelets are the smallest cells in the peripheral blood. After injury to a blood vessel, they participate in clot formation at the site of the injury to stop the bleeding. The platelet count routinely is provided as part of the CBC. Table 7-1 provides the reference range for the platelet count. Like other blood cells, platelets may be decreased as a result of increased destruction in the peripheral blood or decreased production in the bone marrow. A reduction in the platelet count below the reference range is called **thrombocytopenia**.

Thrombocytopenia usually manifests as small skin hemorrhages (petechiae and ecchymoses) and bleeding from mucosal surfaces (such as epistaxis or menorrhagia). When the platelet count is decreased significantly ($<20 \times 10^3/\mu L$), patients are more likely to have bleeding problems, especially with trauma such as surgery or arterial punctures. However, when the platelet count becomes extremely low ($<10 \times 10^3/\mu L$), the patient is at risk for serious spontaneous bleeding, including intracranial hemorrhage. There are many disorders that cause thrombocytopenia, including side effects of drugs such as chemotherapy or heparin, bone marrow diseases, and immune thrombocytopenic purpura, an autoimmune disorder in which autoantibodies are produced against the platelets, marking them for destruction in the spleen.

An increase in platelets (**thrombocytosis**) may be due to a reactive (secondary) process after hemorrhage, surgery, splenectomy, stress, or inflammation, or by a malignant process associated with one of the myeloproliferative neoplasms. A markedly increased platelet count increases the risk for thrombosis.

Erythrocyte Sedimentation Rate

Although not part of the CBC, the erythrocyte sedimentation rate (ESR) is a commonly ordered test to monitor inflammatory diseases. If whole blood is placed in a vertical tube, the RBCs tend to fall to the bottom. The ESR measures the distance (in millimeters) that the RBCs fall in a vertical tube in 1 hour. The ESR is a nonspecific test that is increased in many disorders, especially inflammatory processes. This is largely because of an increase in various plasma proteins (such as globulins and fibrinogen) that reduce the negative charge on the surface of the RBCs, causing them to aggregate or stack on each other and fall at an increased rate. Anemia falsely increases the ESR because the RBCs fall faster in a whole blood specimen with a lower concentration of RBCs per microliter.

Coagulation Screening Tests

Hemostasis (ability to prevent hemorrhage, form a blood clot, keep blood flowing in circulation) involves a complex system of clot-forming and anticoagulant forces that are in balance to promote localized clot formation and to prevent unintended clotting under other circumstances.

Hemostasis testing is complex and is done to evaluate patients who are bleeding as well as those who have excessive clotting. In the clinical laboratory, however, the ability to form a clot is assessed in a plasma-based system (without platelets and vascular cells) and is divided into intrinsic, extrinsic, and common pathways that use different groups of clotting factors. Three basic screening tests are generally used for the initial assessment of bleeding: the platelet count (already discussed), the APTT, and the PT/INR.

The APTT assesses the clotting factors in the intrinsic and common pathways by measuring the length of time required for plasma to form a fibrin clot once the intrinsic pathway is activated. The reference range varies by laboratory but is usually about 25 to 35 seconds. The PT assesses the clotting factors in the extrinsic and common pathways and is performed similarly, using activation of the extrinsic system as an initiation point. The reference range for the PT generally falls between 12 and 15 seconds. An INR is calculated from the PT result using a formula that takes into account the specific reagents and instrument used for the test. Because there are many different reagent-instrument combinations that can affect the PT result, the INR allows for a comparison of results between different laboratories.

Prolongation of the APTT or PT/INR indicates a reduction in blood clotting ability. These tests are abnormal if one or more of the involved clotting factors are decreased significantly. Usually, further studies are required to delineate the specific factors implicated. Factor deficiencies may be either congenital (e.g., hemophilia A, which is a congenital decrease or absence of factor VIII) or acquired (e.g., liver disease with a decrease in multiple clotting factors). The APTT is one of the tests used for monitoring intravenous unfractionated heparin therapy, whereas PT/INR is used for monitoring warfarin (Coumadin) therapy. The INR should be between 2.0 and 3.0 in patients taking warfarin who have atrial fibrillation or a history of pulmonary emboli and generally between 2.5 and 3.5 in patients with a mechanical heart valve. Patients on warfarin with an INR lower than 2 are below the therapeutic range and are at risk for thrombosis. Patients with an INR greater than 4.0 have an increased the risk for hemorrhage, and patients with an elevated INR and anatomic bleeding should be treated as a medical emergency.

> **SIMPLY STATED**
>
> Respiratory therapists should review the patient's platelet count, PT/INR, and APTT before performing an arterial puncture; if results indicate a decrease in blood-clotting ability, extra precautions should be taken to ensure hemostasis.

Tests used for the assessment of excessive thrombosis are complex, but one important assay to consider is D-dimer. D-dimer is produced as a result of the breakdown of fibrin clots that form in the vasculature. The upper reference range for D-dimer in the plasma is about 240 ng/mL, but the value varies depending on each laboratory's methods. An increase in D-dimer is nonspecific and can be observed in many conditions with excessive clotting, as well as in inflammation, renal disease, and even pregnancy. However, because the D-dimer test has high sensitivity, a level below the upper limit of the reference range can help rule out both systemic thrombosis, such as disseminated intravascular coagulation, and local thrombosis, such as pulmonary embolism and deep vein thrombosis.

Chemistry

The clinical chemistry laboratory provides key information to clinicians to assess the health status of the body or disease processes. This is accomplished by measurements of specific biochemical compounds, both those normally present in the body (endogenous chemicals) and external or exogenous substances that are administered or ingested, such as drugs, alcohol, and poisons. It is beyond the scope of this chapter to discuss the hundreds of laboratory tests available. This section will focus on the commonly ordered tests used to assess patient status and those directly related to the needs of the RT for patient management.

It is important to emphasize again that laboratory reference values depend on many factors, including patient age, gender, sample population, and test method. The reference ranges used in this section are based on general averages. However, test interpretation should always be based on the values established within one's institution.

Chemistry tests typically are ordered by clinicians in groupings called *panels*. The common chemistry panels discussed here and the reference ranges for their constituent tests are provided in Table 7-3.

Basic Metabolic Panel

The basic metabolic panel is the most commonly ordered group of chemistry tests. It includes the four major electrolytes, the fasting glucose level and two renal-function tests, blood urea nitrogen (BUN) and creatinine.

TABLE 7-3

Common Chemistry Panels with Sample Test Reference Ranges

Panel and Analytes Measured	Common Reference Ranges
Basic Metabolic Panel	
Sodium (Na⁺)	135-145 mmol/L
Potassium (K⁺)	3.5-5.0 mmol/L
Chloride (Cl⁻)	98-107 mmol/L
Total CO₂	22-30 mmol/L
Glucose (fasting)	70-99 mg/dL
Blood urea nitrogen (BUN)	7-20 mg/dL
Creatinine	0.7-1.3 mg/dL
Renal Panel	
Blood urea nitrogen (BUN)	See basic metabolic panel
Creatinine	See basic metabolic panel
Glomerular filtration rate (GFR)	90-120 mL/min/1.73 m²
Urinalysis	Multiple tests—see discussion
Hepatic Panel	
Albumin	3.5-5.0 g/dL
Total protein	6.3-8.0 g/dL
Alkaline phosphatase (ALP)	38-126 U/L
Alanine aminotransferase (ALT)	10-40 U/L
Aspartate aminotransferase (AST)	5-30 U/L
Bilirubin (total)	0.3-1.9 mg/dL
Lipid Profile	
Total cholesterol	<200 mg/dL
High-density lipoproteins (HDLs)	<40 mg/dL
Low-density lipoproteins (LDLs)	<130 mg/dL
Triglycerides	30-149 mg/dL
Cardiac Biomarkers	
Total creatine kinase (CK)	50-200 U/L
Creatine kinase isoenzyme (CK-MB)	<% total CK
Troponin I (cTnI)	<0.4 µg/L
Myoglobin	19-92 µg/L
B-type natriuretic peptide (BNP)	<20 pg/L

Electrolytes

Normal cell function depends on proper concentrations of electrolytes, and the body must maintain electrolytes in a balanced state. Monitoring electrolyte concentrations is extremely important in patients whose body fluids are being endogenously or exogenously manipulated (e.g., intravenous therapy, renal disease, or diarrhea). Electrolytes are measured in the blood using either a plasma or serum sample. The four primary electrolytes are sodium (Na^+), potassium (K^+), chloride (Cl^-), and total CO_2.

Sodium is the major cation in the extracellular fluid. The kidney, influenced by hormones secreted by the adrenal gland (aldosterone) and hypothalamus (antidiuretic hormone [ADH]), closely regulates the concentration of Na^+ in the blood. Sodium is mainly responsible for the osmotic pressure of the extracellular fluid. Increased serum Na^+ (**hypernatremia**) is seen when the body loses

Box 7-3 Causes of Hypokalemia

DECREASED POTASSIUM INTAKE
Low-potassium diet
Alcoholism

INCREASED LOSS OF POTASSIUM
Gastrointestinal loss
Renal disease
Diuretics

EXTRACELLULAR-TO-INTRACELLULAR SHIFT OF POTASSIUM
Alkalosis
Increased plasma insulin
Diuretic use

water without salt (e.g., profuse sweating, diarrhea, renal diseases, or prolonged hyperpnea), when water intake is insufficient, or when certain hormonal abnormalities are present. Patients with hypernatremia typically complain of excessive thirst and a dry, sticky mouth.

Decreased Na^+ concentration (**hyponatremia**) is caused by either excess water intake/retention or excess sodium loss. Theoretically, healthy people could become hyponatremic by drinking too much water, but water retention is most commonly associated with excessive secretion of ADH. Excessive ADH secretion can occur with many illnesses, most commonly neurologic, pulmonary, or malignant. Patients with these conditions may become severely hyponatremic despite normal total body salt stores. Hyponatremia caused by actual loss of Na^+ is most often seen in patients receiving diuretics but can also be caused by diarrhea, severe sweating, or Addison's disease (impaired production of aldosterone). Patients with severe hyponatremia (<115 mmol/L) may show confusion, abnormal sensorium, muscle twitching, and sometimes, seizures.

Potassium is the major cation within cells. Extracellular concentration normally is low, with serum concentrations typically in the 3.5 to 5.0 mmol/L range. **Hypokalemia** occurs when there is increased loss of potassium or decreased intake, or when K^+ ions shift from the extracellular to intracellular space (Box 7-3). Increased loss of potassium occurs when K^+-containing fluid is lost (e.g., vomiting, nasogastric suctioning), with some kidney diseases, and with the use of some diuretics. Decreased intake of potassium is often a dietary problem. Total body potassium depletion is present in such cases.

Metabolic alkalosis causes a shift of K^+ from the extracellular to the intracellular space, decreasing its serum concentration. This shift occurs in exchange for H^+ and is necessary to maintain electrolytic neutrality between these two spaces (see Chapter 8). This type of hypokalemia is not associated with true depletion of body potassium stores.

Hypokalemia is important to detect because it can be associated with cardiac, skeletal muscle, and gastrointestinal dysfunction. Weaning from mechanical ventilation may

Box 7-4	Causes of Hyperkalemia

INCREASED POTASSIUM INTAKE
High-potassium diet
Oral potassium supplement
Transfusion of old blood

DECREASED POTASSIUM EXCRETION
Renal failure
Hypoaldosteronism

INTRACELLULAR TO EXTRACELLULAR SHIFT OF POTASSIUM
Acidosis
Crush injuries
Tissue hypoxia

PSEUDOHYPERKALEMIA
Hemolysis
Leukocytosis

be difficult if hypokalemia is present. Patients with hypokalemia often have nausea, vomiting, abdominal distention, muscle cramps, lethargy, confusion, muscle weakness, and dysrhythmias. Electrocardiogram (ECG) abnormalities and dysrhythmias include flattened or inverted T waves, ST-segment depression, premature atrial contractions, and atrial or ventricular fibrillation (see Chapter 11).

Hyperkalemia can occur with increased intake, with decreased output, or when K^+ shifts from the intracellular to extracellular space (Box 7-4). Pseudohyperkalemia may occur when K^+ leaks out of RBCs or WBCs. This can be caused by improper collection technique causing hemolysis, delay in processing the specimen, or specimens from patients with abnormally high numbers of platelets, WBCs, or RBCs. As with hypokalemia, hyperkalemia can have major effects on the heart, causing telltale ECG abnormalities such as peaked T waves, shortened QT intervals, increases in the PR interval, and widening of the QRS complex (see Chapter 11). Untreated high serum potassium levels can lead to ventricular fibrillation and asystole.

Hyperkalemia caused by increased intake is often the result of dietary supplementation. Decreased output of K^+ is seen in some kidney disorders and with use of certain diuretics. Metabolic acidosis causes an increased level of H^+ in the extracellular fluid. In an effort to buffer this acidosis, intracellular K^+ ions exchange with extracellular H^+. This helps maintain a more neutral extracellular pH but leads to increased extracellular levels of K^+. Correcting the acidosis usually corrects the hyperkalemia.

Chloride is the chief anion in the extracellular fluid. **Hypochloremia** occurs when there is prolonged vomiting (loss of HCl), chronic respiratory acidosis (which elevates HCO_3^- levels), addisonian crisis, and certain kidney diseases. **Hyperchloremia** is seen with prolonged diarrhea (loss of HCO_3^-), certain kidney diseases, and sometimes hyperparathyroidism.

Total CO_2 is technically not an electrolyte because the measure includes both physically dissolved CO_2 and that dissociated into HCO_3^-. Because about 95% of the total CO_2 consists of HCO_3^-, the two measures are often used interchangeably. As the second most plentiful anion in the serum and the key element in the carbonic acid buffer system, HCO_3^- plays a major role in acid-base balance (see Chapter 8). Increased serum HCO_3^- and CO_2 levels are observed in metabolic alkalosis or as compensation for respiratory acidosis. On the other hand, HCO_3^- and CO_2 levels decrease in metabolic acidosis or as compensation for respiratory alkalosis.

Other electrolyte concentrations that are often measured include calcium (Ca^{2+}), phosphorus (PO_4^-), and magnesium (Mg^{2+}). Ca^{2+} levels are controlled by parathyroid hormone (PTH). Patients with increased PTH have hypercalcemia. Because bone contains a large amount of calcium, certain bone diseases or metastasis of cancer to bone may result in hypercalcemia. Hypocalcemia occurs in vitamin D deficiency (rickets) and in various other hormonal aberrations. PO_4^- metabolism is closely linked to that of Ca^{2+}. Abnormalities of Mg^{2+} concentrations are common in the intensive care unit. Hypomagnesemia and hypocalcemia have been associated with respiratory muscle weakness, which makes ventilator weaning difficult.

SIMPLY STATED

Normal electrolyte concentrations are essential for proper physiologic function of the body. Assessment of a patient's electrolytes can help identify causes of abnormalities such as irregular heart rhythms or respiratory muscle weakness.

Electrolyte values can be used to approximate the anion gap between the measured anions and cations and those that are not measured. Calculating the anion gap helps classify the acid balance status and define the cause of a metabolic acidosis. Chapter 8 provides details on the measurement and interpretation of the anion gap.

Analysis of the electrolyte concentration of sweat can assist in diagnosis of cystic fibrosis. The test is called a *sweat chloride test*, *sweat electrolytes*, or *iontophoretic sweat test*. The sweat glands of patients with cystic fibrosis have a diminished ability to reabsorb Na^+ and Cl^-. As a result, a high concentration of Na^+ and Cl^- (>60 mmol/L) is present in the sweat.

Glucose

Glucose is the major carbohydrate found in the blood. It is produced through digestion of dietary carbohydrates and used as a primary energy source by most body tissues as well as by various blood cells. A common reference range for fasting plasma glucose level (blood drawn after an overnight fast) is 70 to 99 mg/dL. After ingestion of carbohydrates, the glucose level normally rises in the first 60 to 90 minutes and then returns to the normal fasting level within 2 hours.

TABLE 7-4

Interpretation of Tests for Assessing Glucose Imbalances

	Fasting Blood Glucose	Oral Glucose Tolerance Test	Glycosylated Hemoglobin
Normal	<100 mg/dL	<140 mg/dL	<6%
Prediabetes	100-125 mg/dL	140-199 mg/dL	6%-6.5%
Diabetes	>125 mg/dL	>200 mg/dL	>6.5%

Glucose metabolism is regulated primarily by insulin, a hormone produced by the pancreas that decreases blood glucose levels. The most common glucose imbalance is **hyperglycemia**, most frequently caused by type 1 or type 2 diabetes. Patients with type 1 diabetes have decreased blood insulin levels as a result of failure of the pancreas to produce this hormone. Type 1 diabetes accounts for about 10% of cases in the United States. Type 1 diabetic patients require daily doses of insulin for the rest of their life. Type 2 diabetes accounts for 90% of diabetes cases. Type 2 diabetes occurs when insulin made by the body is ineffective because of a problem in structure, function, or release.

Patients with diabetes are at greater risk for stroke, cardiovascular disease, serious infection, and renal failure. For this reason, patients with diabetes must regularly check their blood sugar levels and adjust their medication accordingly. Inadequate insulin dosing can result in impaired glucose metabolism, which forces the body to turn to fats and proteins as an energy source. The result is an abnormal accumulation of ketoacids. This build up of organic acids causes a form of metabolic acidosis called ketoacidosis, which can represent a medical emergency often manifested by Kussmaul respirations (see Chapter 8). On the other hand, administration of too much insulin can cause hypoglycemia, as discussed subsequently.

Medications such as steroids, diuretics, antihypertensive drugs, birth control pills, and some immunosuppressive drugs also can cause hyperglycemia. Other conditions associated with hyperglycemia are acute stress (e.g., trauma, heart attack, stroke), chronic renal failure, excessive food intake, hyperthyroidism, pancreatic cancer, and pancreatitis.

Hypoglycemia is a relatively uncommon problem caused by either pancreatic overproduction or excessive administration of insulin. Excessive production may occur in response to a rapid rise in blood sugar or as a result of insulin-producing pancreatic tumors. Both overproduction and excessive administration have the same effect, that is, a rapid fall in blood glucose. Hypoglycemia causes sweating, shaking, weakness, headaches, lethargy, and in severe cases, coma. Other conditions associated with hypoglycemia are excessive alcohol intake, severe liver disease, hypothyroidism, and starvation.

The American Diabetes Association recommends three tests for differentiating among diabetic-associated glucose imbalances: (1) the traditional fasting blood glucose (FBG), (2) the oral glucose tolerance test (OGTT), and (3) the glycosylated Hb (HbA1c) test. The FBG is performed after an overnight fast. For the OGTT, an initial FBG test is performed. Then patients are required drink a standard amount of glucose solution. Two hours after this "challenge" to their system, a repeat blood glucose test is performed. The HbA1c test measures the percentage of blood sugar attached to hemoglobin. In contrast to the FBG and OGTT tests, which provide "snapshots" of diabetic control, the HbA1c indicates average blood glucose control for the prior 2 to 3 months. However, it does not eliminate the need for patients' daily self-testing of their blood glucose levels. Table 7-4 summarizes the interpretation of these tests for glucose imbalances.

Blood Urea Nitrogen and Creatinine

BUN and creatinine are common screening tests used to assess renal function and as such are included in both the basic metabolic and renal panels (see Table 7-3). Urea is a waste product of protein metabolism and is synthesized in the liver from amino groups and ammonia generated during protein catabolism. Therefore, urea is constantly being formed and is excreted by the kidneys. BUN levels thus depend not only on renal function but also on diet and liver function.

Many kidney diseases result in decreased filtration and thereby increased retention of urea, leading to an elevated BUN level. Other conditions that are associated with elevated BUN include increased metabolism (e.g., fever and stress), malignancy, congestive heart failure, ketoacidosis and dehydration in diabetes, gastrointestinal bleeding, sepsis, high-protein diet, some antibiotics, and burns. Conditions causing a decreased BUN include pregnancy, decreased dietary protein, and some antibiotics.

Creatinine is a waste product of creatine metabolism and produced in muscle. It enters the blood and is filtered out by the kidneys. Diet (e.g., protein intake), water intake, exercise, and urine output do not effect creatinine levels; thus, increased creatinine levels are directly associated with renal function impairment. Creatinine serum levels usually remain nearly constant, reflecting the balance between its production and its filtration by the renal glomerulus. Creatinine can be elevated in shock, hypotension, congestive heart failure, dehydration, muscle atrophy, urinary obstruction caused by kidney stones, prostatic cancer, and anabolic steroid administration. Decreased creatinine levels are seen in muscle wasting conditions. Neither the BUN nor the creatinine level is sensitive to early renal disease.

When the BUN and creatinine are elevated as a result of renal failure, metabolic acidosis may be present (see Chapter 8). To compensate for metabolic acidosis, the respiratory system normally tries to restore the pH by increasing ventilation and reducing $Paco_2$ levels. Therefore, patients with renal failure may have increased respiratory rates and may appear to be short of breath. However, if the patient with metabolic acidosis also has a concurrent respiratory disorder, respiratory compensation may not be possible, and the pH may remain dangerously low.

Renal Panel

The renal panel includes the aforementioned blood tests for BUN and creatinine and two nonblood analyses, the glomerular filtration rate (GFR) and urinalysis.

The ratio of BUN to creatinine can help determine the cause of increases in these analytes. The reference range is usually between 10:1 and 20:1. An increased BUN-to-creatinine ratio can be observed in conditions causing decreased renal blood flow (e.g., congestive heart failure, dehydration). A decreased ratio may be observed with liver disease and malnutrition.

Glomerular Filtration Rate

The GFR is used to screen for early kidney damage. This is not a laboratory test per se, but rather a calculation based on the serum creatinine level and the patient's age, gender, height, weight, and race. All else being equal, as the serum creatinine increases, the GFR decreases. The common reference range is 90 to 120 mL/minute per 1.73 m². Older people will have lower normal GFR levels because GFR decreases with age. Levels below 60 mL/minute per 1.73 m² for three or more months are a sign of chronic kidney disease. A GFR below 15 mL/minute per 1.73 m² indicates renal failure and the need for immediate medical attention.

Urinalysis

Routine urinalysis includes assessment of its appearance, specific gravity, pH, protein, glucose, ketones, blood cells, bilirubin, urobilinogen, and other chemical compounds. A microscopic examination of the urine sediment also may be performed if abnormalities are detected in the chemical analysis.

The appearance simply denotes the color and whether the urine appears clear or cloudy. The specific gravity indicates the concentration of the urine. More concentrated urine (specific gravity > 1.03) is seen in dehydration, whereas more dilute urine (specific gravity < 1.002) occurs with high fluid intake and when the kidneys are unable to concentrate urine normally. The pH of the urine reflects the acid-base status of the patient, typically ranging between 5 and 7. Lower urine pH levels indicate increased acid production.

Normally little to no protein appears in the urine. The presence of protein (proteinuria) usually indicates renal disease. Glucose in the urine (**glycosuria**) appears most commonly in diabetes but sometimes is caused by renal disease. Ketones occur with starvation and in diabetes mellitus. Hematuria, or RBCs in the urine, is a nonspecific finding caused by a variety of problems and some drugs. Bilirubin occurs in the urine in the conjugated form and is seen in liver disease and bile duct obstruction. Urobilinogen is normally present in the urine in small amounts but increases in some liver diseases and hemolytic states. A high urine WBC count suggests inflammation, most commonly associated with a urinary tract infection.

In addition to its analysis in the blood, urine creatinine also may be measured. By comparing creatinine concentrations in the blood and urine, the creatinine clearance test can help clinicians evaluate the efficiency of renal filtration. The average creatinine clearance is 90 to 125 mL/minute for males and 80 to 115 mL/minute for females. Clearance decreases approximately 1 mL/minute per year after the age of 50 years. Levels below the reference values indicate impaired kidney function or decreased renal blood flow.

Hepatic Panel

The hepatic panel includes tests for blood proteins, liver-associated enzymes, and bilirubin. These tests are used primarily to help assess liver function.

Proteins

There are two primary classes of proteins found in the blood, albumin and globulin. Albumin is produced by liver cells and makes up a large percentage of the total serum protein. There are more than 500 proteins classified as globulins, including enzymes and antibodies.

Albumin functions as a transport and storage vehicle for many hormones, drugs, and electrolytes. Albumin is also important in maintaining the oncotic pressure of blood, which helps keep water within the vascular space. In addition, albumin plays a primary role in lipid metabolism. Decreased albumin levels (**hypoalbuminemia**) are seen in various forms of protein malnutrition and in severe liver disease. Significant hypoalbuminemia leads to loss of fluid from the vascular space and can cause edema throughout the body, including in the lungs (pulmonary edema).

Total protein represents the sum of the albumin and globulins in the blood. Total protein analysis provides information on nutritional status and possible disease conditions. A decrease in total protein occurs in severe liver disease (many proteins are produced by the liver), in nephrotic syndrome (albumin lost through kidneys), and in severe malnutrition. Increased total protein is seen in inflammatory disorders and infections such as hepatitis and HIV, or in certain bone marrow disorders such as multiple myeloma.

The total protein level has many limitations, in part because it does not reveal which of the many serum proteins may be abnormal. That information requires serum protein electrophoresis. For example, in multiple myeloma, a characteristic narrow band or spike pattern appears on electrophoresis, indicating a high concentration of a specific immunoglobulin.

Liver-Associated Enzymes

There are three liver-associated enzymes in the hepatic panel: alkaline phosphatase, alanine aminotransferase, and aspartate aminotransferase. Abnormalities in these enzymes can indicate liver dysfunction or failure, which can lead to pulmonary complications such as hydrothorax, pulmonary hypertension, and hepatopulmonary syndrome.

Alkaline phosphatase (ALP) is an enzyme produced in the bile ducts that rises in response to obstruction of the duct, such as occurs in cholelithiasis. ALP also is present in bone, placenta, spleen, kidney, and intestine, where isoenzyme evaluation can often identify the source. For example, elevated bone ALP indicates increased new bone formation, as occurs in growing children.

Alanine aminotransferase (ALT) is found in high concentrations primarily in liver cells (hepatocytes). For this reason, ALT levels increase dramatically in acute liver damage, such as viral hepatitis.

Like ALT, aspartate aminotransferase (AST) is present in liver cells, but it also occurs in substantial concentrations in cardiac and skeletal muscle. As with ALT, very high AST levels occur with acute liver damage but may also indicate muscle trauma. Indeed, high levels of AST in the presence of normal levels of ALT suggest extrahepatic injury. At one time, AST also was used as a biomarker for acute myocardial infarction (AMI). However, this test has been replaced by more sensitive and specific indicators of myocardial damage (discussed subsequently).

Bilirubin

Bilirubin is a by-product of the spleen's normal breakdown of hemoglobin. This unconjugated form of bilirubin is bound to albumin and cleared from the blood by the liver. Hepatocytes process the bilirubin into a water-soluble form called *conjugated bilirubin* that is excreted into the bile and thus eliminated through stool in the lower gastrointestinal tract. An increase in total blood levels of bilirubin (hyperbilirubinemia) can be due to (1) increased production (e.g., hemolytic anemia), (2) liver damage (e.g., cirrhosis, hepatitis), or (3) impaired excretion (e.g., bile duct obstruction). If the total bilirubin is increased, knowledge of the conjugated portion can help reveal the cause of the hyperbilirubinemia. An increased total bilirubin with a normal proportion of conjugated bilirubin indicates either an increase in RBC hemolysis or failure

of the liver to process the bilirubin load (previously cited causes 1 and 2). On the other hand, if the total bilirubin and conjugated portion are both elevated, the likely cause is bile duct obstruction.

Lipid Panel

Lipids are organic compounds used throughout the body as a fuel source, as building blocks for cell structure, and in many other important biologic functions. The lipid panel includes measurement of cholesterol, lipoproteins, and triglycerides.

Cholesterol is a steroid that is essential for the function of cells, tissues, and organs and is used to make hormones and bile. The body produces cholesterol, but it is also found in certain food sources, particularly those with high saturated fat content such as eggs and fatty meats. Unlike tests intended to diagnose disease states, cholesterol testing is used to estimate the risk for atherosclerosis and heart disease. As such, this test is an important component of preventive health care management.

Lipoproteins are complex combinations of both proteins and lipids. There are four major groups of lipoproteins, of which two are routinely tested: high-density lipoproteins (HDLs) and low-density lipoproteins (LDLs). HDL is referred to as the "good cholesterol" because it removes excess cholesterol from the circulation. LDL is referred to as the "bad cholesterol" because it deposits cholesterol on blood vessel walls, which can then lead to atherosclerosis.

Triglycerides are the main storage form of fat in humans, and fatty tissue is primarily made up of these substances. Accurate results require that patients follow a stable diet 2 weeks before the testing, avoid drinking alcohol for several days, and fast 12 to 24 hours before blood collection. Although very high levels are associated with a risk for pancreatitis, triglycerides are best assessed in combination with cholesterol and lipoproteins. Table 7-5 outlines the interpretation of these lipid panel measures by their common reference ranges.

TABLE 7-5	
Lipid Profile Interpretation	
Test Result	**Interpretation**
Total Cholesterol	
<200 mg/dL	Desirable; low risk for heart disease
200-239 mg/dL	Borderline; moderate risk for heart disease
>240 mg/dL	High; high risk for heart disease
Low-Density Lipoproteins (LDLs)	
<100 mg/dL	Optimal
100-129 mg/dL	Near optimal/above optimal
130-159 mg/dL	Borderline high
160-189 mg/dL	High
>190 mg/dL	Very high
High-Density Lipoproteins (HDLs)	
<40 mg/dL (men)	Low
<50 mg/dL (women)	Low
>60 mg/dL	Optimal

Cardiac Biomarkers

Cardiac biomarkers are chemicals that appear in the blood as a result of either ischemic myocardial damage or stress. They are helpful in diagnosing and monitoring patients with either acute coronary syndrome or congestive heat failure. Biomarkers of ischemic myocardial damage include total creatine kinase (CK) and its heart-specific isoenzyme CK-MB, myoglobin, and troponin. The current biomarker used to help diagnose congestive heart failure is B-type natriuretic peptide (BNP).

CK is primarily contained in skeletal muscle, myocardium, and brain tissue. Total CK values are elevated in acute myocardial infarction (AMI) and various skeletal muscle diseases. Because high total CK levels are not very specific, testing for the more heart-specific CK-MB isoenzyme is needed to distinguish myocardial from general muscle damage. In AMI, CK-MB is elevated 4 to 6 hours after onset of symptoms, peaks at 24 hours, and returns to normal in 2 to 3 days (Fig. 7-2).

Myoglobin is a heme protein present in cardiac and skeletal muscle. Whenever there is significant muscle damage, myoglobin is elevated and can be measured. Although it is not specific for AMI, it is useful as an early biomarker because it is released from damaged myocardium or skeletal muscle within 2 to 4 hours after onset of infarction, peaks at 6 to 12 hours, and returns to normal within 24 to 36 hours (see Fig. 7-2)

Troponin is a complex of three proteins (troponin T, troponin I, troponin C) that helps regulate muscle contraction and normally is present in very small quantities in the blood. Only troponins I and T are found in the heart. Troponin I is considered the more specific of the two for the diagnosis of AMI and is considered the single best marker

for acute coronary syndrome. Troponin I can be detected in the serum 3 to 6 hours after an AMI, peaks in about 12 hours, and can persists for 7 days or more (see Fig. 7-2). Troponin T is useful in patients who do not seek immediate medical attention for their symptoms because it peaks later (2 days) and remains elevated longer (7 to 10 days) than troponin I.

BNP is a cardiac neurohormone secreted from membrane granules in the cardiac ventricles as a response to ventricular volume expansion and pressure overload. BNP levels lower than 100 pg/mL have a 90% negative predictive value and are thus useful in ruling out congestive heart failure (CHF). A comparable positive predictive value for ruling in the diagnosis of CHF occurs with BNP levels greater than 500 pg/mL. Intermediate values are less helpful and may occur in conditions with similar symptoms, including renal insufficiency, cor pulmonale, and acute pulmonary embolism. As with all laboratory tests, BNP is not recommended as a stand-alone test, and clinical presentation and other laboratory test results should be considered in the patient assessment.

SIMPLY STATED

Troponin I is the single best marker for diagnosis of acute coronary syndrome. As with all laboratory tests, the clinical presentation and other test results (e.g., ECG) should be considered in patient assessment.

Microbiology

Clinical microbiology includes routine bacteriology and the subspecialties of mycology, parasitology, virology, and mycobacteriology. Laboratory scientists specializing in

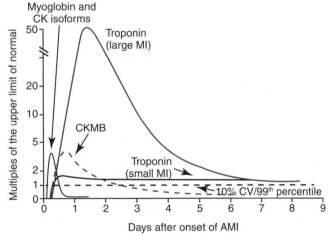

FIGURE 7-2 Cardiac biomarkers plotted showing the multiples of the cutoff for acute myocardial infarction (AMI) over time. The *dashed horizontal line* shows the upper limit of normal, defined as the 99th percentile from a normal healthy reference population. (Reprinted with permission from Anderson JL, Adams CD, Antman EM, et al: ACC/AHA 2007 guidelines for the management of patients with unstable angina/non-ST-Elevation myocardial infarction: a report of the American College of Cardiology/American Heart Association Task Force on Practice Guidelines. *J Am Coll Cardiol* 50:e1-e157, 2007.)

microbiology isolate and identify microorganisms from body tissues and fluids and perform antimicrobial susceptibility testing on pathogens to determine which antibiotics will be most effective. Although bacteria are the most common organisms isolated, most microbiology laboratories also can identify fungi, parasites, mycobacteria (tuberculosis [TB]), rickettsia, and viruses. If an institution's microbiology laboratory does not have the ability to isolate these rarer organisms, specimens can be sent to a referral laboratory for identification.

Pre-analytical Phase: Specimen Selection, Collection, and Transport

The pre-analytical phase of analysis, specimen selection, collection, and transport is critical to producing quality results. All specimens for microbiologic analysis should be collected as soon as possible on onset of symptoms and before administration of antimicrobial therapy. Specimens should be transported in appropriate transport devices, containers, or special media to preserve the integrity and viability of organisms. After specimen collection, timely transport to the laboratory for processing and testing is also critical.

Specific guidelines have been established for collection and transport of specimens by health care providers who gather microbiologic samples. Specimen selection is determined by the site of infection and organism suspected as causing the infection or disease. Patient history and clinical information are vital in directing the appropriate management of microbiologic specimens.

Many body sites are normally sterile, and the isolation of any organisms from these sites may be significant. Normally, blood, pleural fluid, ascitic fluid, urine, and tissue samples do not contain microorganisms and, if collected in a sterile manner, will not grow organisms when cultured. Other samples, such as stool and sputum, regularly contain normal flora. Normal flora refers to nonpathogenic organisms that colonize a body site and may contaminate a specimen during the collection process. Precautions should be taken during specimen collection to minimize the amount of normal flora. Another important consideration is antibiotic therapy. In general, specimens for microbiology analysis should be collected *before* use of antibiotics. If a patient has been receiving antibiotics, the organism causing the infection may not grow in culture, causing an invalid test result.

Microscopic Examination of Specimens

Initial screening of a specimen is accomplished using a direct smear. Various stains are used, with the laboratory scientist selecting staining methods based on the type of organism suspected.

The most common stain is the Gram stain, which separates bacteria into either gram-positive (purple) or gram-negative (red) groupings. Based on the stained smear,

the basic morphologic form of the organisms also can be identified as being predominantly spherical (cocci) or rod-shaped (bacilli). For example, *Streptococcus pneumoniae* (the most common cause of bacterial pneumonia) appears as encapsulated, lancet-shaped, gram-positive diplococci. *Staphylococcus aureus* appears as intensely staining gram-positive cocci in clusters. *Klebsiella pneumoniae* appears as short, fat, encapsulated gram-negative rods, and *Haemophilus influenzae* as very short gram-negative rods often described as coccobacilli. For pulmonary specimens such as sputum, and other specimens where mycobacteria (TB) are suspected, an acid-fast stain also may be performed.

In combination with relevant clinical information, the Gram stain report provides the physician with preliminary information helpful in making a proper diagnosis. In addition, antibiotic treatment may be initiated based on this preliminary information.

Culture and Sensitivity

Most specimens sent to the microbiology laboratory are for culture and sensitivity. Specimens are inoculated onto nutrient, selective, and differential agar or media that support the growth of various organisms. Although most organisms grow in 24 to 48 hours, some (e.g. mycobacteria, fungi) may require up to 6 weeks. The laboratory scientist observes the morphology of organisms growing on the media and determines whether potential pathogens are present. Definitive organism identification is accomplished through biochemical and enzymatic reactions, or molecular diagnostic tests. Traditional biochemical tests may require an additional 24 to 48 hours for full identification. Faster identification can occur using molecular methods such as polymerase chain reaction (PCR) tests. Molecular methods are useful in the rapid diagnosis of TB and other organisms that may be difficult to grow on culture media or require a lengthy time for conventional identification.

Along with the culture, a sensitivity test often is performed. The bacteria are grown in the presence of various antibiotics, thereby determining whether an organism is sensitive to a particular drug. This information is clinically important in selecting the proper antibiotic therapy.

Examination of Pulmonary Secretions

Three types of pulmonary specimens are acceptable for assessment of lower respiratory infections: (1) bronchoalveolar specimens (includes lavage fluid, brush sample, washing, and endotracheal aspirates); (2) expectorated sputum; and (3) induced sputum. Table 7-6 provides general guidelines for collection, transport, and storage of respiratory specimens.

Sputum Collection

Expectorated sputum is the preferred specimen for diagnosis of pneumonia. The goal of sputum collection is to

TABLE 7-6

Respiratory Specimen Collection, Transport, and Storage Guidelines

Specimen Type	Collection Procedure	Transport/Storage
Sputum expectorated or induced	No food for 1-2 hr before collection Brush teeth, gums, tongue Rinse/gargle with water Deep cough Collect in sterile container Minimize contamination with saliva	Sterile container, >1 mL, room temperature if transported to lab within 2 hr Refrigerate if delay in transport to lab up to 24 hr
Bronchoalveolar (BAL, bronchial brushings/washings, tracheal aspirates	Collect liquids in sterile sputum trap Place brush in sterile container with 1 mL sterile saline	Sterile container, >1 mL, room temperature, if transported to lab within 2 hr Refrigerate if delay in transport to lab up to 24 hr

obtain fresh, uncontaminated secretions from the tracheobronchial tree. This goal is readily achieved when the alert patient is carefully instructed by a trained health care provider, such as an RT, on the proper collection procedure (Table 7-6). If tuberculosis is suspected, three sputum specimens are recommended to ensure recovery of mycobacteria. An early-morning specimen is optimum and will have the highest yield of mycobacteria (AFB bacilli). The minimum quantity is 3 to 5 mL.

Occasionally, sputum induction is needed to obtain an adequate sample. Sputum induction is accomplished by having the patient breathe a slightly irritating mist, usually hypertonic saline. The mist increases flow of bronchial secretions (bronchorrhea) and stimulates a cough, which usually results in a specimen of adequate volume. Patient preparation for and transport of induced sputum samples is the same as for expectorated sputum.

If a culture is required but the patient is unwilling or unable to produce a sputum specimen (such as a young child or unconscious adult), either tracheobronchial suctioning or bronchoscopic lavage may be needed. Bronchoscopic lavage is performed by a physician during a bronchoscopy, usually with the assistance of an RT (see Chapter 17).

Sputum Examination

Macroscopic Examination. Gross examination of the sample should be conducted at the bedside to determine its origin. Appropriate sputum samples from the tracheobronchial tree typically are more viscous and purulent than saliva. A specimen obviously containing mostly saliva usually is discarded. Macroscopic examination of the sputum also identifies such characteristics as color, presence of blood, general viscosity, and odor, which can provide a presumptive diagnosis (see Chapter 3).

Microscopic Examination. On receipt of the sputum specimen in the microbiology laboratory, the laboratory scientist performs a Gram stain. This examination assesses specimen quality and provides information about microorganisms present in the sample. A good specimen will have few squamous epithelial cells and numerous polymorphonuclear leukocytes. A high number of epithelial cells suggests oral contamination. Depending on the laboratory protocol, this type of specimen may be rejected, and no further testing will be performed.

If the specimen is deemed acceptable, the microscopic examination will also provide a preliminary report of the microbial composition of the sputum along with quantitation. For example, the report may indicate numerous gram-positive cocci in pairs (diplococcic) suggestive of pneumococci, or numerous gram-negative diplococcic suggestive of *H. influenzae*. This preliminary screening information provides a quick presumptive organism identification that will aid in diagnosis and early initiation of antibiotic treatment.

The specimen is then set up for culture on agar plates. The purposes of specimen culturing are to (1) determine whether a pathogen actually is present, (2) definitively identify it, and (3) assess its susceptibility to antimicrobial agents. Typically, culture results are provided within 24 to 48 hours.

After a patient has been on a regime of antimicrobial therapy, the Gram stain and culture results can change. If the antibiotic is effective against the pathogen causing the infection, the Gram stain and culture will no longer demonstrate the pathogen, but instead will reveal organisms consistent with normal flora. If, on the other hand, the antibiotic is not effective against the organism responsible for the patient's infection, the Gram stain and culture will continue to demonstrate the pathogen.

SIMPLY STATED

Sputum Gram stain, culture, and antimicrobial sensitivity can be useful in determining the organism responsible for the respiratory infection and the appropriate antimicrobial therapy to treat the infection; use of antibiotics by the patient before collecting the specimen can influence results of the Gram stain, culture, and antimicrobial susceptibility results.

Additional microscopic examination of sputum may be performed using others stains, such as the Wright stain or Giemsa stain. These stains can be used to determine sputum eosinophil counts. If the leukocytes observed in a sputum stain are predominantly eosinophils, exposure to an allergen is likely. Sputum eosinophil counts are useful in differentiating among asthma phenotypes and monitoring the condition once therapy is discontinued. Besides asthma, eosinophilia has been associated with certain microbial infections, particularly some parasitic infections.

Bronchoalveolar Lavage

Bronchoalveolar lavage (BAL) is performed during bronchoscopy by injecting a large volume of sterile fluid into the patient's lung (see Chapter 17). This fluid mixes with the respiratory secretions within the airways and alveoli and is subsequently withdrawn for analysis in the laboratory. BAL has two main functions: (1) to evaluate the need for therapy in patients with interstitial lung disease (diseases that often cause pulmonary fibrosis) by analysis of the cells obtained in the lavage solution, and (2) to collect a quality specimen that can be analyzed for the presence of microorganisms that cause pneumonia. BAL is contraindicated in patients with severely reduced pulmonary function, hypoxemia, severe cardiovascular disease, or serious electrolyte disturbances.

After the lavage solution is recovered from the patient, the sample is sent to the laboratory for microscopic analysis. Lavage solution obtained from healthy nonsmokers is 91% to 95% macrophages, 6% to 8% lymphocytes, and 1% granulocytes (neutrophils and eosinophils). The cellular composition of this fluid shows characteristic alterations in diseases such as pulmonary sarcoidosis and hypersensitivity pneumonitis.

Pleural Fluid Examination

Normal pleural fluid is clear and pale yellow. Usually, only small amounts of fluid (3 to 20 mL) are present in the pleura. Pleural fluid (effusion, transudate, thoracentesis, empyema) is collected by percutaneous needle aspiration or surgery. A volume of at least 1 mL is required for microbiology workup; however, as much fluid as possible should be sent to the laboratory for analysis, particularly if additional testing is required. Fluid is immediately transported to the laboratory in a sterile screw-cap tube or anaerobic transport system at room temperature, and the specimen should *not* be refrigerated.

It is important to differentiate between the types of pleural fluid to aid in diagnosis of the disease or condition. A set of pleural fluid-to-serum ratios, known as *Light's criteria*, are used to distinguish between transudates and exudates. According to these criteria, the presence of any one of the following defines the fluid as an exudate:

• The ratio of pleural fluid protein to serum protein is greater than 0.5.

• The ratio of pleural fluid lactic dehydrogenase (LDH) to serum LDH is greater than 0.6.
• Pleural fluid LDH is greater than 0.6 times the normal upper limit for serum.

Additional criteria used by some laboratories to distinguish between transudates and exudates are summarized in Table 7-7.

After the type of fluid is determined, additional tests may be performed to confirm the diagnosis. Transudates usually require no further testing and are often caused by cirrhosis, CHF, and chronic renal failure. Exudates are associated with several conditions and diseases and usually require additional testing. Exudates may be caused by infections such as bacterial pneumonia or TB, pulmonary abscess, pulmonary infarction, fungal or viral infection, trauma, various cancers, and pancreatitis. Additional tests include glucose (decreased in infection and inflammation), lactate level (increased in infection and inflammation), amylase (increased in pancreatitis), triglycerides (extremely elevated in thoracic duct leakage), pH, and biomarkers for certain tumors.

Normal pleural fluid may have a few WBCs but no RBCs or microorganisms present. Pleural fluid associated with bacterial infection will be cloudy and have increased WBCs (neutrophils), and Gram or other stains will demonstrate microorganisms. A culture and sensitivity test will provide definitive identification of the pathogen and data on appropriate antibiotics to treat the patient. Pleural fluid associated with pulmonary infarction will demonstrate an increase in the RBC count.

Histology and Cytology

Biopsy of lung tissue may be done either through a bronchoscope or by means of thoracotomy or thoracoscopy. Biopsy specimens are sent to the histology or surgical pathology laboratory. The tissue is processed over a period of time and then can be cut very thin, placed on a slide, and stained so that the cells are visible when examined by a pathologist with a microscope. This can yield valuable information about infectious processes, chronic lung diseases, and benign and malignant tumors. An acid-fast (Ziehl-Neelsen) stain can be done on tissue to identify

TABLE 7-7

Criteria for Pleural Fluid Differentiation

Test	Transudate	Exudate
Physical characteristics	Clear	Cloudy
Protein	<25 g/L	>35 g/L
Fluid-to-serum protein ratio	<0.5	>0.5
Fluid-to-serum LDH ratio	<0.67	>0.67
Fluid cholesterol	<60 mg/dL	>60 mg/dL
Fluid-to-serum cholesterol ratio	<0.3	>0.3
Fluid-to-bilirubin ratio	<0.6	>0.6

mycobacteria (TB or TB-like organisms). Gomori methenamine silver (GMS) and periodic acid–Schiff (PAS) stains may be used to identify fungal organisms. GMS stains also identify *Pneumocystis* organisms, a cause of pneumonia in immunosuppressed patients, such as those with AIDS. Tissue Gram stains also may be used.

Surgical removal of lung cancer requires close cooperation between the surgeon and surgical pathologist. The surgical pathologist must provide immediate reports to the surgeon regarding the presence of cancer in the resected lung, the type of cancer present, whether the surgical margins are clear, and whether there are metastases in local or regional lymph nodes. Because there is no time during surgery to process specimens in the usual way, the tissue is frozen so that it can be immediately sectioned and reviewed under the microscope. The frozen sections are thicker and more difficult to evaluate than standard sections but are usually adequate for surgical guidance. Final histology reports are issued after surgery, when standard stains have been completed.

Tumors of the lung may be either benign or malignant. A classification of malignant lung tumors is shown in Box 7-5. Benign lung tumors are less common than malignant tumors, with hamartoma (a benign proliferation of elements normally occurring in the lung) being seen most often. The non-small cell lung cancers, squamous cell carcinoma, adenocarcinoma, and large cell carcinoma, represent 75% of the primary lung tumors, whereas small cell lung cancer represents about 15%. These tumors collectively are called *bronchogenic carcinoma*. They are usually related to smoking (with the possible exception of adenocarcinoma) and are highly malignant. Tumors consisting of a mixture of cell types and other rare types of tumors may occur. Secondary or metastatic tumors to the lung are also common. Metastases to the lung arise from squamous carcinomas originating from the gastrointestinal tract or adenocarcinomas from breast, colon, and kidney as well as hematopoietic malignancies.

Cytology is the study of fluids, secretions, or other body samples that contain cellular material but not actual fragments of intact tissue. The cells are spread on a glass slide, stained with the Papanicolaou stain, and examined by a cytotechnologist and pathologist. Often, the presence of malignancy and even the type of malignancy can be determined in this manner. Pulmonary samples that can be examined cytologically include sputum, bronchial washings, bronchial brushings, pleural fluid, and fine-needle aspiration (FNA) of lung tissue or lung masses. In FNA, a small needle is inserted into a mass, and some of the cellular material is aspirated into the needle and then expressed and spread onto a slide. The slide is then stained and examined, often yielding accurate information about the nature of the mass. FNA of lung masses is performed under radiologic guidance. For many years, this procedure has been widely used to evaluate lung masses and has proved to be a safe, simple, and effective way to diagnose malignant tumors and other processes without requiring major surgery.

Skin Testing

Over the years, skin testing was used to help diagnose selected infections (such as TB and coccidioidomycosis) and allergic disorders. The procedure involves injecting a small amount of the protein essence of the organism or allergen into the subcutaneous layer of the skin. The development of an inflammatory nodule at the location of the injection indicates an immune response to the foreign material. Unfortunately, many people develop immune unresponsiveness to foreign material, a condition called **anergy**. For this reason, many skin tests used to assess for infections and allergens have been replaced by serologic testing of the patient's immune responses.

The exception is the Mantoux tuberculin skin test for TB, also referred to as the *PPD test*. The test is performed by administering 0.1 mL of tuberculin purified protein derivative (PPD) by injection into the subcutaneous layer of skin. The test is evaluated in 48 to 72 hours. The test is positive if an intradermal or subdermal nodule develops at the site of injection. This is a cellular reaction and indicates that the patient has been infected by TB or a TB-like organism. TB causes the strongest reaction, but other nontuberculous mycobacteria can produce weakly positive reactions. Because of this cross-reactivity, there is a set of criteria for interpreting a positive PPD. A normal healthy person without risk for exposure to TB is classified as PPD skin test positive only if the skin reaction produced a 15-mm diameter welt, whereas an HIV-positive or other immunocompromised patient is classified as positive with a 5-mm diameter skin nodule.

Older patients may have had a positive skin test in the past that eventually reverts to negative. A two-step skin test with the second test performed 3 weeks after the first test often shows a true positive when the first test produced a negative result. Multiple skin tests performed on a patient who has never been exposed to TB do not cause a positive result. Bacille Calmette-Guérin (BCG) vaccination, which is common in countries with a high prevalence of TB, causes a positive PPD skin test up to 10 years after vaccination; therefore, positive PPD skin tests more than 10 years after BCG vaccination usually suggest a true TB infection.

Box 7-5	Histologic Classification of Malignant Lung Tumors

1. Non-small cell lung cancer (NSCLC)
   a. Adenocarcinoma
   b. Squamous cell carcinoma
   c. Large cell carcinoma
2. Small cell lung cancer (SCLC)

TABLE 7-8

Common Laboratory Tests Related to Respiratory Care

Patient Presentation	Recommended Tests
Evidence of tissue hypoxia but with normal Pa_{O_2}, Sp_{O_2} (e.g., fatigue, cognitive disturbances)	CBC, reticulocyte count, lactic acid, CO-oximetry (Chapter 8)
Postoperative patient with low-grade fever—possible pneumonia	CBC with differential, blood culture, sputum culture
Fluid balance disturbances	CBC, electrolytes, urinalysis
Decreased or absent urine output	Electrolytes, BUN, creatinine, GFR urinalysis
Chest pain, suspected MI or ischemia	Electrolytes, cardiac biomarkers
Hepatic disease (e.g., suspected hepatitis, history of alcohol or drug abuse)	Electrolytes, hepatic panel, acute viral hepatitis serology
Acid-base disturbances	ABGs (see Chapter 8), electrolytes, BUN, creatinine, GFR, urinalysis
PVCs or cardiac dysrhythmias without history of cardiac disease	Electrolytes, lipid panel
Uncontrolled bleeding or monitoring anticoagulation therapy	CBC and WBC differential, platelet count, PT/INR, APTT

ABGs, arterial blood gases; APTT, activated partial thromboplastin time; BUN, blood urea nitrogen; CBC, complete blood count; GFR, glomerular filtration rate; PT/INR, prothrombin time/international normalized ratio; PVCs, premature ventricular contractions; WBC, white blood cell.

An alternative to the TB skin test (PPD) is the interferon-γ release assay, or IGRA. This is a blood test that measures how the immune system reacts to the bacteria that cause TB. This test only requires one visit to have blood drawn, unlike the two-step PPD skin test. The blood test results are available in 24 to 48 hours.

Neither the TB skin test nor the TB blood test confirms a diagnosis of TB. A positive test result only indicates that a person has been infected with TB bacteria. Neither test is able to indicate whether a person has latent TB infection or active TB disease. Additional tests such as a chest radiograph and sputum AFB stain and culture are required to confirm a diagnosis of TB.

SIMPLY STATED

The PPD skin test and the IGRA blood tests for TB must be interpreted in light of the patient's medical history, and additional tests such as x-ray and sputum AFB stain and culture are required to confirm TB disease.

Recommended Laboratory Tests

Assessment of lung disease and pulmonary function is covered in detail in various chapters of this book. The clinical laboratory provides testing associated with care of patients with respiratory disorders, including analysis of arterial blood gases (see Chapter 8), CBC, various chemistry panels, pulmonary specimen culture, special stains (TB), and cytologic examination. Table 7-8 provides a brief overview of the common recommended laboratory tests based on patient presentation. Results from these tests may suggest additional diagnostic tests. The need for additional

testing depends on each individual presentation, the clinician's practice protocols, and test algorithms and protocols established by each facility. Consultation with a clinical laboratory scientist is recommended if additional advanced testing is indicated.

KEY POINTS

▶ Blood consists of two major components: plasma and the formed elements (WBCs, RBCs, and platelets).
▶ Tests that evaluate the cellular elements of the blood include the CBC, platelet count, and reticulocyte count.
▶ WBCs normally seen in the peripheral blood are neutrophils (segmented and band forms), eosinophils, basophils, lymphocytes, and monocytes.
▶ Neutrophils usually constitute 50% to 70% of the blood's WBCs and are the body's first line of defense against microbial infections.
▶ Lymphocytes are particularly important in the body's defense against viral, TB, and intracellular organism. Lymphocytes normally make up 20% to 45% of circulating WBCs.
▶ Leukocytosis is an abnormal increase in the WBC count. An abnormal decrease in the WBC count is known as leukopenia.
▶ Neutrophilia is a common response to inflammation and infection.
▶ Lymphocytosis (increase in lymphocytes) typically is seen in viral infections, especially infectious mononucleosis.
▶ Monocytosis (increase in monocytes) is characteristic of chronic infections, including TB, syphilis, typhoid fever, and subacute bacterial endocarditis.
▶ RBCs are produced in the bone marrow by maturation of nucleated cells known as normoblasts; RBCs have a life span of approximately 120 days.

KEY POINTS—cont'd

▶ Anemia is a decrease in the oxygen carrying capacity of the blood and is clinically defined by a decrease in the hemoglobin level below the reference range for the gender and age of the patient.

▶ Polycythemia is an increase in the RBC count, hemoglobin, and Hct and may be primary, secondary, or relative.

▶ Platelets are the smallest cells in the peripheral blood and play a vital role in hemostasis and clot formation at the site of an injury to a blood vessel.

▶ A decrease in the platelet count is called thrombocytopenia.

▶ The four electrolyte measured in the basic metabolic panel are Na^+, K^+, Cl^-, and total CO_2.

▶ Increased serum Na^+ concentration (hypernatremia) is seen when the body loses water without salt (e.g., profuse sweating, diarrhea, renal diseases, or prolonged hyperpnea) and if there is lack of sufficient water intake.

▶ Decreased Na^+ concentration (hyponatremia) is caused by either excess free water intake and retention or excess sodium loss.

▶ Hypokalemia (decreased serum K^+) occurs when there is increased loss of potassium or decreased intake, or when K^+ ions shift from extracellular to intracellular water space.

▶ Hyperkalemia (elevated serum K^+) can occur with increased intake, with decreased output, or when K^+ ions shift from intracellular to extracellular water space.

▶ The anion gap is the difference between the measured and unmeasured anion and cation, which can help classify the cause of metabolic acidosis.

▶ Elevated blood glucose level is called hyperglycemia. It occurs for a variety of reasons but is most often related to diabetes.

▶ The most common screening tests in assessing renal function are the BUN and creatinine.

▶ High levels of AST occur with acute hepatitis. ALP is useful in evaluating liver disease and bone disease.

▶ Troponin I is the most specific current biomarker for identifying ischemic myocardial damage.

▶ Proper specimen selection, collection, and transport are prerequisites to obtaining quality microbiology test results.

▶ Microscopic examination of sputum will assess specimen quality; a high epithelial cell count indicates oral contamination and that the specimen is not useful for diagnostic purposes.

▶ Results of the sputum Gram stain and culture normally are affected by antibiotic therapy.

▶ The most commonly used skin test is the Mantoux tuberculin skin test for TB (PPD test).

▶ An alternative to the TB skin test is the interferon-γ release assay, or IGRA, which measures how the immune system reacts to the presence of mycobacteria.

CASE STUDY 7-1

A 22-year-old woman was brought to the emergency department by her mother with chief complaints of cough, fever, and chills for the past 3 days. The patient has a history of Down syndrome and lives at home with her parents. Initial examination reveals tachycardia, tachypnea, fever, and normal blood pressure. Chest auscultation identifies bronchial breath sounds and inspiratory and expiratory crackles over the right lower lobe. The admitting physician orders a sputum Gram stain and culture, CBC, and chest film. The initial laboratory results are as follows:

CBC	Results	Reference Ranges
WBC ($\times 10^9$/L)	19.5	4.5-11.5
RBC ($\times 10^{12}$/L)	4.53	4.00-5.40
Hb (g/dL)	10.6	12.0-15.0
Hct (%)	34.9%	35-49
MCV (fL)	77.0	80.0-100.0
MCHC (g/dL)	30.4	32-36
White Blood Cell Differential (%)		
Segmented neutrophils	82	50-70
Lymphocytes	8	20-45
Monocytes	2	2-11
Eosinophils	0	1-3
Basophils	0	0-2
Bands	8	0-5

Sputum: Gram stain: 2+ gram-positive cocci in chains, pairs tetrads and groups; 1+ pus cells with many epithelial cells

Interpretation

Leukocytosis is present and is the result of an increase in the neutrophils consistent with a bacterial infection (probably pneumonia). The slight increase in immature neutrophils (bands) represents a left shift indicating stress on the bone marrow to release more neutrophils to fight the infection. The relative decrease in the percentage of lymphocytes is caused by the absolute increase in the number of neutrophils and is not an abnormality.

The RBC count is within the reference range; however, the decreases in hemoglobin, Hct, MCV, and MCHC are consistent with a mild microcytic, hypochromic anemia. Further investigation is needed to identify the cause, but iron deficiency anemia is a likely reason.

The Gram stain of the sputum revealed many epithelial cells indicating contamination with saliva. The sample should be discarded and another sputum sample obtained.

CASE STUDY 7-2

A 65-year-old woman was brought to the emergency department by her husband. The patient is complaining of severe shortness of breath, weakness, and cough. She has a long history of COPD and a 90-pack-year smoking history, currently admitting to smoking 1 pack/day. In the emergency department, she appears acutely and chronically ill and is found to be using her accessory muscles to breathe. She is cyanotic and has decreased breath sounds bilaterally. The patient is started on oxygen by nasal cannula, and the attending physician orders a CBC, electrolyte determination, and other tests. The results are as follows:

Test	Results	Reference Ranges
WBC ($\times 10^9$/L)	19.9	4.5-11.5
RBC ($\times 10^{12}$/L)	5.1	4.00-5.40
Hb (g/dL)	15.8	12.0-15.0
Hct (%)	48.5	35-49
MCV (fL)	95.1	80.0-100
MCHC (g/dL)	32.6	32-36
White Blood Cell Differential (%)		
Segmented neutrophils	76	50-70
Lymphocytes	12	20-45
Monocytes	5	2-11
Eosinophils	4	1-3
Basophils	2	0-2
Bands	1	0-5
Electrolytes (mmol/L)		
Na^+	137	135-145
K^+	4.8	3.5-5.0
Cl^-	87	98-107
Total CO_2	41	22-30

Interpretation

The increase in WBCs indicates leukocytosis and is the result of an increase in the number of circulating neutrophils. This may be in response to a bacterial infection or acute stress. The hemoglobin is slightly increased and the RBC count, Hb, and Hct are in the upper reference range. These findings are consistent with secondary polycythemia typical for patients with a chronic lung disease in which the arterial blood oxygen levels are persistently low.

The electrolyte values reveal a decreased serum Cl^- and an increased serum CO_2. This probably is related to the patient's long-term history of COPD. Some patients with COPD chronically retain CO_2 because of poor pulmonary function. To compensate for the elevated CO_2, the kidneys retain increased levels of serum HCO_3^- in an effort to maintain a near-normal serum pH. The resulting metabolic buildup of serum HCO_3^- is reflected as an increased total CO_2 in the venous blood sample. The increase in serum CO_2 (HCO_3^-) causes the kidneys to excrete more than the usual amount of Cl^- in an effort to maintain electrical neutrality. As a result, serum Cl^- levels typically are reduced in patients with chronically elevated serum CO_2.

CASE STUDY 7-3

A 27-year-old man has a CD4 count of 120 (reference range, 550-1600/μL). He is concerned about his chronic cough and sputum production. The sputum has been negative for WBCs and bacteria. A PPD skin test was placed on his right forearm 2 days ago, and a 3-cm reddened area and a 5-mm nodule have appeared at the skin test site. Initial laboratory data results are as follows:

CBC	Results	Reference Ranges
WBC ($\times 10^9$/L)	5.0	4.5-11.5
WBC Differential (%)		
Segmented neutrophils	70	50-70
Lymphocytes	20	20-45
Bands	5	0-5
Monocytes	1	2-11
Eosinophils	4	0-3
Basophils	0	0-2
Hb (g/dL)	14	14.0-18.0
Hct	42	40-54
Normal Red Cell Indices		
Sedimentation rate (mm/hr)	40 (elevated)	0-15

Interpretation

The low CD4 count suggests the patient is moderately immunocompromised, possibly caused by HIV. The elevated sedimentation rate suggests inflammation, which could be caused by TB or other infection. The large area of redness around the skin test site is not significant. The 5-mm nodule in this immunocompromised patient indicates TB infection. It is anticipated that sputum cultures will be positive in 6 weeks. A PCR test for TB bacilli in the patient's sputum is likely to be positive. This patient's normal CBC is expected despite his chronic infection because TB does not usually cause an elevated WBC count.

CASE STUDY 7-4

A 20-year-old man was brought to the emergency department by ambulance following a motor vehicle crash. He was driving in a local canyon when a deer ran out in front of his car and caused him to lose control. The vehicle left the road and rolled over in the canyon. He complains of a stiff neck and left leg pain. Although very upset and scared, he is conscious and able to move all extremities. Vital signs are normal except for a heart rate of 110 beats/minute. His initial CBC reveals the following:

Test	Results	Reference Range
WBC ($\times 10^9$/L)	14.9	4.5-11.5
RBC ($\times 10^{12}$/L)	5.1	4.60-6.00
Hb (g/dL)	15.0	14.0-18.0

CASE STUDY 7-4—cont'd

Test	Results	Reference Range
Hct (%)	45.5	40-54
MCV (fL)	89.2	80.0-100.0
MCHC (g/dL)	33.0	32-36
WBC Differential (%)		
Segmented neutrophils	76	50-70
Lymphocytes	12	20-45
Monocytes	5	2-11
Eosinophils	4	1-3
Basophils	2	0-2
Bands	1	0-5

Interpretation

The RBC count, hemoglobin, Hct, and indices are all within their reference ranges. The elevated WBC count suggests possible infection; however, the lack of fever and minimal presence of bands on the white cell differential suggest otherwise. This is most likely a case of pseudoneutrophilia, in which marginated neutrophils are released into circulation as a result of sudden stress (the accident). This type of neutrophilia is usually transient and resolves spontaneously in a matter of hours.

ASSESSMENT QUESTIONS

See Appendix for answers.

1. Which of the following is not a component of the formed elements of the blood?
   a. RBCs
   b. Lipids
   c. WBCs
   d. Platelets
2. What is the medical name for platelets?
   a. Leukocytes
   b. Thrombocytes
   c. Reticulocytes
   d. Erythrocytes
3. What is the primary role of white blood cells?
   a. Carry oxygen
   b. Promote blood clotting
   c. Fight infection
   d. Boost metabolism
4. What is the normal reference range for WBCs?
   a. 1000-3000/mm^3
   b. 3000-5000/mm^3
   c. 4500-10,000/mm^3
   d. 600-14,000/mm^3
5. Which of the following white cell types normally represents the largest percent in the WBC differential?
   a. Neutrophils
   b. Eosinophils
   c. Basophils
   d. Lymphocytes
6. A left-shifted white cell differential is evidenced by which of the following findings?
   a. An increase in the number of eosinophils
   b. A decrease in the number of segmented neutrophils
   c. An increase in the number of bands (immature neutrophils)
   d. A decrease in the number of lymphocytes
7. Which of the following is a common finding in patients with bacterial pneumonia?
   a. Neutrophilia
   b. Leukopenia
   c. Lymphocytopenia
   d. Eosinophilia
8. Which of the following is a common finding in a patient with an allergic reaction?
   a. Neutropenia
   b. Leukopenia
   c. Eosinophilia
   d. Monocytosis
9. Viral infections typically produce which of the following abnormalities?
   a. Lymphocytosis
   b. Eosinophilia
   c. Basophilia
   d. Monocytosis
10. Your patient has AIDS. The most useful test to identify the prognosis of AIDS is:
    a. Leukocyte count
    b. CD4 count
    c. Monocyte count
    d. Hemoglobin A1c
11. Chemotherapy used to treat cancer can cause a suppression of blood counts for which of the following cells?
    a. Neutrophils
    b. Erythrocytes
    c. Thrombocytes
    d. All of the above
12. Your patient may have active TB. What laboratory finding is most consistent with this suspicion?
    a. Lymphocytosis
    b. Anemia
    c. Monocytosis
    d. Eosinophilia
13. Which of the following statements is (are) true regarding Hb?
    a. It functions in oxygen transport.
    b. It is the main component of RBCs.
    c. It functions in CO_2 transport.
    d. All of the above
14. Which of the following is the most common cause of anemia?
    a. Drug-induced RBC lysis
    b. Acute blood loss
    c. Iron deficiency
    d. None of the above

15. Which of the following is not true regarding polycythemia?
    a. It can be caused by chronic hypoxemia.
    b. It is defined as an increase in RBC, Hb, and Hct.
    c. It increases the oxygen-carrying capacity of the blood.
    d. It decreases the workload on the heart.
16. Which of the following tests is used to assess the patient's blood-clotting ability?
    a. RBC count
    b. Hemoglobin
    c. Hct
    d. Prothrombin time
17. Which of the following electrolytes closely affects muscle function?
    a. Sodium
    b. Potassium
    c. Chloride
    d. Phosphorus
18. Which of the following electrolytes is mainly responsible for extracellular water balance?
    a. Calcium
    b. Sodium
    c. Magnesium
    d. Potassium
19. Anion gap is useful in assessing the cause of:
    a. Metabolic alkalosis
    b. Metabolic acidosis
    c. Respiratory acidosis
    d. Respiratory alkalosis
20. An increase in the sweat electrolyte concentration is seen in:
    a. Cystic fibrosis
    b. Patent ductus arteriosus
    c. Bronchiectasis
    d. Epiglottitis
21. Which of the following tests is (are) a measure of kidney function?
    a. BUN
    b. Creatine kinase
    c. Creatinine
    d. a and c
22. The recommend test for early detection of myocardial infarction is:
    a. AST
    b. LDH
    c. CPK
    d. Troponin
23. Which of the following bacteriologic tests is used to determine the effectiveness of antibiotics on a particular organism?
    a. Gram stain
    b. Culture
    c. Sensitivity
    d. Acid-fast stain
24. A Ziehl-Neelsen stain is used to identify which of the following organisms?
    a. *Staphylococcus aureus*
    b. *Pseudomonas aeruginosa*
    c. *Streptococcus pneumoniae*
    d. *Mycobacterium tuberculosis*
25. Which of the following items are evaluated during a macroscopic (gross) sputum examination?
    a. Color
    b. Consistency
    c. Volume
    d. All of the above
26. Which of the following is the most common cause of bacterial pneumonia?
    a. *Streptococcus pneumoniae*
    b. *Pseudomonas aeruginosa*
    c. *Haemophilus influenzae*
    d. *Klebsiella pneumoniae*
27. Which of the following findings is (are) consistent with pleural infection?
    a. Bloody pleural fluid
    b. Low pleural fluid protein levels
    c. Opaque or turbid pleural fluid
    d. All of the above
28. Which of the following tests performed during urinalysis could be helpful in diagnosing diabetes mellitus?
    a. Glucose
    b. pH
    c. Ketones
    d. All of the above
29. Proteinuria usually is indicative of which of the following?
    a. COPD
    b. Kidney disease
    c. Cardiovascular disease
    d. Spinal meningitis
30. Which of the following may cause a patient to have a negative reaction to a skin test?
    a. He/she does not have the disease.
    b. He/she is anergic.
    c. The disease has progressed to a point beyond treatment.
    d. a and b
31. Which of the following is true regarding a PPD?
    a. It is positive with coccidioidomycosis infection.
    b. It is often positive if the patient has previously had a BCG vaccination.
    c. It is negative if the induration produced is 12 mm in diameter.
    d. None of the above

Bibliography

Amodio G, Antonelli G, Di Serio F. Cardiac biomarkers in acute coronary syndromes: a review. *Curr Vasc Pharmacol* 2010;**8**: 388–93.

Arneson W, Brickell J. *Clinical chemistry a laboratory perspective.* Philadelphia: FA Davis; 2007.

Bishop ML, Fody EP, Schoeff LE. *Clinical chemistry techniques, principles, correlations.* 6th ed. Philadelphia: Lippincott Williams & Wilkins; 2010.

Chung KF. Inflammatory biomarkers in severe asthma. *Curr Opin Pulm Med* 2012;**18**:35–41.

Forbes BA, Sahm DF, Weissfeld AS, editors. *Bailey & Scott's diagnostic microbiology.* 12th ed. St Louis: Mosby Elsevier; 2007.

Laposata M. *Laboratory medicine: the diagnosis of disease in the clinical laboratory.* New York: McGraw-Hill; 2010.

McKenzie SB, Williams JL, editors. *Clinical laboratory hematology.* 2nd ed. Boston: Pearson; 2010.

Miller JM. *A guide to specimen management in clinical microbiology.* 2nd ed. Washington, DC: ASM Press; 1999.

Rodak BF, Fritsma GA, Keohane EM, editors. *Hematology: clinical principles and applications.* 4th ed. St Louis: Elsevier; 2012.

Strasinger SK, Di Lorenzo MS. *Urinalysis and body fluids.* 5th ed. Philadelphia: FA Davis; 2008.

Travis WD. Classification of lung cancer. *Semin Roentgenol* 2011;**46**:178–86.

Versalovic J, Carroll KC, Funke G, editors. *Manual of clinical microbiology.* 10th ed. Washington, DC: ASM Press; 2011.

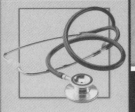

Chapter 8

Interpretation of Blood Gases

CRAIG L. SCANLAN*

CHAPTER OUTLINE

LEARNING OBJECTIVES

After reading this chapter, you will be able to:
1. Identify the reference ranges for both arterial blood gas and oximetry parameters.
2. Identify the indications for blood gas and oximetry analysis.
3. Differentiate between invasive and noninvasive methods for measuring blood gas and oximetry parameters.
4. Outline and explain the key procedural elements in obtaining arterial blood samples by means of puncture and indwelling arterial line.
5. Apply knowledge of the factors affecting hemoglobin saturation to interpretation of oximetry data.
6. Apply common indices of oxygenation to assess the cause and severity of hypoxemia.
7. Employ the Henderson-Hasselbalch equation to relate changes in P_{CO_2} and HCO_3^- to pH.
8. Describe the common causes, compensatory mechanisms, and expected blood gas findings seen in simple respiratory and metabolic acid-base disorders.
9. Describe the common causes and expected blood gas findings seen in combined and mixed acid-base disorders.
10. Identify the common pre-analytic, analytic and post-analytic errors in blood gas analysis.
11. Specify methods used to assuring valid measurement and use of blood gas data.
12. Accurately interpret arterial blood gas and/or oximetry data.

---

*Richard Wettstein BS, RRT and Robert L. Wilkins PhD, RRT contributed some of the content for this chapter as coeditors of prior editions. Portions were adapted from Narins RG, Emmett M. Simple and mixed acid-base disorders: a practical approach. *Medicine* (Baltimore) 1980;**59**:161–87.

KEY TERMS

acidemia	hypercapnia	metabolic acidosis
alkalemia	hyperoxemia	metabolic alkalosis
analytic error	hyperventilation	pre-analytic error
anemia	hypocapnia	post-analytic error
anion gap	hypoventilation	respiratory acidosis
calibration	hypoxemia	respiratory alkalosis
dead space ventilation	hypoxia	
dyshemoglobin	iatrogenic alkalosis	

Care of patients with cardiopulmonary disorders often requires precise knowledge of their oxygenation, ventilatory, and acid-base status. This information is obtained by blood gas and oximetry analysis, mainly of arterial blood samples. To assure comprehensive patient assessment and support good clinical decision making, respiratory therapists (RTs) must know when and how to obtain these measurements and be able to accurately interpret them.

This chapter focuses on the interpretation of arterial blood gas parameters because these measures best reflect the lung's ability to exchange O_2 and CO_2 with the blood, the blood's O_2 carrying capacity, and its acid-base status. Table 8-1 outlines the common reference ranges for arterial blood gas measurements.

Peripheral venous blood has passed through the tissue vascular beds, so it reflects local metabolism and is of no value in assessing lung function. On the other hand, mixed venous blood samples from the pulmonary artery can be used to evaluate overall tissue oxygenation. Use of mixed venous blood for this purpose is discussed in Chapter 14.

Indications for Blood Gas and Oximetry Analysis

Blood gas analysis is indicated if the patient's symptoms, medical history, physical examination, or laboratory data suggest abnormalities in respiratory or acid-base status. Blood gas analysis also can help evaluate treatment effects and thus be used whenever significant changes occur in therapy that affect oxygenation, ventilation, or acid-base balance.

Blood oxygenation can be assessed by arterial blood gas (ABG) analysis, hemoximetry, pulse oximetry, and transcutaneous Po_2 monitoring (mainly in infants and children). Ventilation can be measured by ABGs, transcutaneous Pco_2 monitoring, or capnography. An ABG is required for accurate assessment of acid-base status. Table 8-2 outlines the key indications for these various measurements, as recommended by the American Association for Respiratory Care.

Sampling and Measurement

Blood gas sampling and measurement approaches can be broadly classified as being invasive or noninvasive. Invasive approaches require sampling of blood by needle puncture or indwelling catheter. Noninvasive approaches measure blood gas parameters by external skin sensors.

Invasive Blood Sampling

If the goal is to accurately evaluate oxygenation, ventilation, and acid-base status, then analysis of an arterial blood sample is the gold standard against which all other measures are compared. Samples normally are obtained by percutaneous needle puncture of an artery or from an indwelling arterial catheter. Measurement of arterial pH, $Paco_2$, and Pao_2 typically is provided by a blood gas analyzer, which also uses programmed equations to compute the HCO_3^- and Sao_2 values. Standard blood gas analyzers do not measure actual Sao_2 or Hb content and cannot detect the presence of abnormal hemoglobins such

TABLE 8-1

Sample Reference Ranges for Arterial Blood Gas Parameters

Parameter	Symbol	Reference Ranges
Partial pressure of oxygen	Pao_2	80-100 mm Hg (room air)
Hemoglobin content	Hb	Males: 14-8 g/dL Females: 12-15 g/dL
Hemoglobin saturation	Sao_2	>95%
Carboxyhemoglobin saturation	COHb	<3% (nonsmokers)
Methemoglobin saturation	metHb	<1.5%
Oxygen content	Cao_2	16-20 mL/dL
Hydrogen ion concentration (negative log)	pH	7.35-7.45
Partial pressure of carbon dioxide	Pco_2	35-45 mm Hg
Plasma bicarbonate	HCO_3^-	22-26 mmol/L
Base excess	BE	±2 mmol /L

BE, base excess; HCO_3^-, plasma bicarbonate concentration; Pco_2, partial pressure of carbon dioxide; pH, hydrogen ion concentration in blood; Po_2, partial pressure of oxygen; SO_2 oxyhemoglobin saturation.

as carboxyhemoglobin (COHb). Measurement of normal and abnormal hemoglobin (Hb) content and actual saturation usually requires sample analysis by hemoximetry (CO-oximetry).

Arterial Puncture

An arterial blood sample may be obtained from the radial, brachial, dorsalis pedis, or femoral arteries. The radial artery is preferred because it is readily accessible, easy to stabilize, and least likely to cause loss of distal perfusion if it become obstructed (normally the ulnar artery provides collateral circulation to the hand). Box 8-1 outlines the key steps involved in obtaining an arterial blood sample via percutaneous puncture.

Fine points involved in arterial puncture include checking coagulation-related tests, applying appropriate infection control standards, and assessing for collateral circulation.

Coagulation-related laboratory tests should be checked to assess for risk for bleeding. Specifically, low platelet counts or increased bleeding times (high prothrombin time, partial thromboplastin time, or international normalized ratio values) may indicate a propensity for bleeding and the need to pressurize the puncture site longer than usual to prevent hemorrhage. See Chapter 7 for more detail on these tests.

In terms of infection control, standard precautions are a must. Given that blood splashes can occur during arterial puncture, in addition to wearing gloves, clinicians should wear a face shield and consider using a gown to protect the skin and clothing (see Chapter 1). When expelling any air bubbles from the sample, one also must avoid discharge of blood droplets into the environment. This important step is accomplished by either (1) using a filter cap on the syringe, or (2) expelling the bubble-containing portion of

---

TABLE 8-2

Indications for Blood Gas and Oximetry Analysis

Method	Indications
Arterial blood gas analysis	Evaluate ventilation (P_{CO_2}), acid-base (pH, P_{CO_2} and HCO_3^-), and oxygenation (P_{O_2}) status
	Assess the patient's response to therapy and/or diagnostic tests (e.g., O_2 therapy, exercise testing)
	Monitor the severity and progression of a disease process
Hemoximetry (CO-oximetry)	Determine actual blood O_2 saturation (as opposed to that computed with a simple blood gas analyzer)
	Measure abnormal hemoglobins levels (e.g., COHb, metHb)
Pulse oximetry	Monitor the adequacy of oxyhemoglobin saturation
	Quantify the response of oxyhemoglobin saturation to therapeutic intervention or to diagnostic procedure (e.g., bronchoscopy)
	Comply with mandated regulations or recommendations by authoritative groups (e.g., anesthesia monitoring)
	Screen infants for critical congenital heart diseases
Transcutaneous monitoring (P_{tcO_2}, P_{tcCO_2})	Continuously monitor the adequacy of arterial oxygenation and/or ventilation
	Continuously monitor for excessive arterial oxygenation (hyperoxemia)
	Quantify real-time changes in ventilation and oxygenation due to diagnostic or therapeutic interventions
	Screen infants for critical congenital heart diseases

Box 8-1	**Key Steps in Obtaining an Arterial Blood Sample by Needle Puncture**

1. Verify doctor's order.
2. Review chart for diagnosis, anticoagulant therapy, coagulation-related tests, F_{IO_2}, ventilator settings.
3. Gather, assemble, and check required equipment (arterial blood gas kit).
4. Decontaminate hands and apply standard/transmission-based precautions as appropriate.
5. Identify patient (using two identifiers); introduce self.
6. Explain procedure and confirm patient understanding.
7. Palpate pulses on both sides to select best site (use nondominant arm if possible).
8. Perform Allen test if radial artery selected; if negative, repeat on other arm.
9. Prepare the site by rubbing with a 70% isopropyl alcohol solution for at least 30 seconds. *clea circle – wax on!*
10. Position puncture site by extending wrist 30 degrees over supporting towel.
11. Slowly insert needle bevel up at 45 degrees ~~or less~~ until flash of blood is observed; readjust angle if necessary.
12. Obtain sample; remove needle and immediately apply pressure with sterile gauze. *~1mL*
13. Follow sharps procedure to shield needle, e.g., apply automatic capping device.
14. Maintain pressure on site for 3 to 5 minutes; 10 minutes or longer if patient has bleeding disorder or uses anticoagulants.
15. Check puncture site for bleeding, swelling, discoloration, return of proximal and distal pulses.
16. Use gauze pad or venting cap to expel air bubbles from sample (Occupational Safety and Health Administration guidelines).
17. Mix sample with anticoagulant by repeatedly rolling sample between hands and inverting syringe.
18. Label sample with date, time, patient ID, F_{IO_2}, ventilator settings; place in sealed container for transport (not required for point-of-care analysis).
19. Dispose of infectious waste; decontaminate hands.
20. Record pertinent data in chart and departmental records.
21. Notify appropriate personnel and make any necessary recommendations or modifications to the care plan.
22. Recheck puncture site after 20 minutes if patient is on anticoagulant therapy or has a bleeding disorder.

the sample slowly into sterile gauze pad contained in a sealable plastic bag.

When the radial artery is selected, a modified Allen test must be performed to evaluate the adequacy of collateral circulation to the hand (Fig. 8-1). To perform this test, the patient is instructed to make a tight fist. Then the RT compresses both the radial and ulnar arteries, after which the patient is told to open and relax the hand, which should reveal a blanched palm and fingers. Next, the RT releases pressure over the ulnar artery while observing the patient's hand for color changes. If collateral flow is adequate, the patient's hand will "pink up" within 10 to 15 seconds—a positive Allen test. A positive result confirms adequate collateral flow and that the radial artery is an acceptable sampling site. If the test is negative (the hand does not pink up rapidly), the radial artery is not an acceptable site for puncture. In such cases, the other wrist is evaluated, or the brachial artery is used to obtain the sample.

After the sample is obtained and the puncture site stabilized, the sample is either sent to the laboratory or analyzed at the bedside using a point-of-care analyzer. When using a point-of-care analyzer, the instrument needs to be properly prepared before obtaining the blood sample. Normally, this involves verifying its power-up operation, inserting the needed cartridge, and confirming internal calibration. After the sample is obtained, it should be thoroughly mixed and dispensed into the cartridge within 3 minutes (do not place it in ice!). If the analysis results fall outside the analyzer's reportable ranges (results "flagged"), the remaining sample should be sent to the central laboratory for analysis.

Of course, the RT should never wait for the repeat results if the findings indicate a life-threatening problem. For example, if the bedside results indicate oxygen levels below the analyzer's reportable ranges and the patient is cyanotic, the RT should immediately start oxygen administration or raise the F_IO_2 while awaiting test results from the central laboratory.

Indwelling Catheter (A-Line)

Arterial puncture causes trauma, so an indwelling arterial catheter, or A-line, should be used when frequent sampling is necessary. As a result of the potential hazards of hemorrhage and bloodstream infection, A-lines require careful management, and their use generally is limited to patients undergoing intensive care.

An A-line system consists of a pressurized infusion set connected to a pressure transducer, intraflow flush device, and sampling port. Two different approaches are used for blood sampling: a three-way stopcock and a closed reservoir. Figure 8-2 depicts the design and operation of a typical three-way stopcock sampling port.

The preparatory and follow-up steps for obtaining and processing a blood sample from an A-line are similar to those for radial arterial puncture, and an Allen test is obviously not needed. Instead, to confirm perfusion at the site of cannulation and proper continuous blood pressure measurement, one should observe the monitor and verify a satisfactory arterial waveform (see Chapter 15 for details on assessing arterial pressure waveforms). After gathering the needed equipment, the RT can proceed to obtain the sample using the applicable procedure, as outlined in Table 8-3.

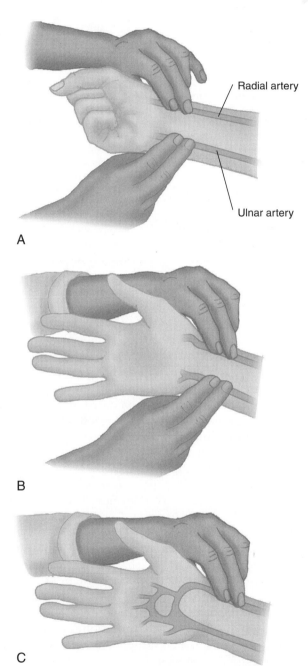

Radial artery

Ulnar artery

A

B

C

FIGURE 8-1 Assessment of collateral circulation before radial artery sampling. **A,** Patient clenches fist while examiner obstructs radial and ulnar arteries. **B,** Patient gently opens hand while pressure is maintained over both arteries. **C,** Pressure over ulnar artery is released, and changes in color of patient's palm are noted. (From Kacmarek RM, Stoller JK, Heuer, AJ: *Egan's fundamentals of respiratory care*, ed 10, St. Louis, 2013, Mosby-Elsevier).

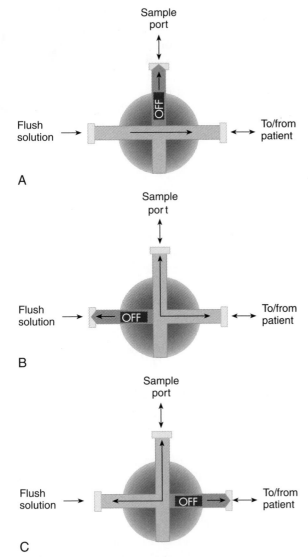

Sample port

OFF

Flush solution → ← To/from patient

A

Sample port

OFF

Flush solution → ← To/from patient

B

Sample port

OFF

Flush solution → ← To/from patient

C

FIGURE 8-2 A three-way stopcock in a vascular line system showing the various positions used. **A,** Normal operating position with flush solution going to the patient and the sample port closed. **B,** Position to draw a blood sample from the vascular line (closed to flush solution). **C,** Position to flush sampling port (closed to patient). In any intermediate position, all ports are closed. (From Kacmarek RM, Stoller JK, Heuer, AJ: *Egan's fundamentals of respiratory care,* ed 10, St. Louis, 2013, Mosby-Elsevier).

TABLE 8-3	
Procedures for Obtaining Blood Samples from an Arterial Line (Adult Patient)	
Three-Way Stopcock Sampling	**In-line Closed Reservoir Sampling**
Swab sample port with alcohol	Slowly draw blood into the reservoir to the needed fill volume
Attach waste syringe and turn stopcock off to flush solution/bag	Close the reservoir shut-off valve
Aspirate 5-6 mL blood (at least 6 times the system "dead" volume)	Swab sample port with alcohol
Turn stopcock off to port	Attach the blunt/needleless sampling syringe to the valved sampling port
Remove waste syringe, properly discard	Aspirate the needed volume of blood
Secure heparinized syringe to port, reopen stopcock, collect sample	Open the reservoir shut-off valve
Turn stopcock off to port, remove syringe	Slowly depress reservoir plunger to reinfuse blood into patient
Flush line until clear	Reswab port and flush line until clear
Turn stopcock off to patient, briefly flush sampling port, reswab with alcohol	Confirm restoration of arterial pulse pressure waveform
Turn stopcock off to port and confirm restoration of arterial pulse pressure waveform	

Po_2/Pco_2 monitoring, is used mainly with infants and children.

Pulse Oximetry

Pulse oximetry is a noninvasive technique for measuring oxygen saturation of hemoglobin (Hb) in the blood, with the reported measure being abbreviated as Spo_2. When compared with analysis of arterial blood Hb saturation by invasive sampling and hemoximetry (Sao_2) among patients with good perfusion, pulse oximeters exhibit an overall accuracy in the 2% to 4% range.

As the "fifth vital sign," pulse oximetry commonly is used in intensive care units, the emergency department, operating rooms, during patient transport, and during special procedures such as bronchoscopy, computed tomography scanning, sleep studies, exercise testing, and weaning from supplemental O_2 and mechanical ventilation. Pulse oximetry also provides the basis for prescribing and adjusting O_2 therapy in both the hospital and home care settings.

Proper use of pulse oximeters and the data they provide requires basic knowledge of their operation and limitations. Pulse oximeters use the spectrophotometric principle of light absorption. The standard device probe transmits two wavelengths of light—red and infrared—through capillary beds such as the earlobe or digit. A more or less constant level of light is absorbed by the tissues and venous blood. However, a portion of the light is absorbed by the pulsatile flow of arterial blood, yielding variable rates of absorption for oxygenated Hb (HbO_2) and reduced Hb (HHb). The

Given that closed reservoir sampling minimizes blood waste, reduces the potential for line contamination, and better protects against exposure to bloodborne pathogens than the stopcock method, it is becoming the standard approach in many intensive care units.

Noninvasive Measurements

Noninvasive blood gas analysis uses external skin sensors to measure relevant parameters. By far, pulse oximetry is the most common noninvasive method for ABG-related measurements. An alternative approach, transcutaneous

TABLE 8-4

Common Factors Causing Erroneous Sp_{O_2} Readings (Compared with CO-Oximetry)

Factor	Potential Error
Presence of COHb	Falsely high Sp_{O_2}
Presence of metHb	Falsely low Sp_{O_2} if $Sa_{O_2} > 85\%$
	Falsely high Sp_{O_2} if $Sp_{O_2} < 85\%$
Vascular dyes (e.g., methylene blue)	Falsely low Sp_{O_2}
Dark skin pigmentation	Falsely high Sp_{O_2} (3%-5%)
Nail polish	Falsely high Sp_{O_2} (especially black)
Poor local perfusion (vasoconstriction and/or hypothermia)	Possible loss of signal, falsely low Sp_{O_2} (may be falsely high is sepsis)
Motion artifact	Unpredictable spurious readings or false alarms
Ambient light	Varies (e.g., falsely high Sp_{O_2} in sunlight); may also cause falsely high pulse reading

oximeter circuitry then compares these differences in light absorption and computes the Sp_{O_2} as follows:

$$\text{Pulse saturation } (Sp_{O_2} \text{ as \%}) = \frac{HbO_2}{HbO_2 + HHb} \times 100$$

Computed in this manner, the Sp_{O_2} often is called the *functional saturation* because it is based solely on the presence of normal Hb, that is, the amount available for binding with oxygen.

Abnormal hemoglobin combinations or **dyshemoglobins** such as carboxyhemoglobin (Hbco) cannot be measured by standard pulse oximeters that emit only two wavelengths of light. To measure dyshemoglobins requires at least four wavelengths of light, as provided by bench-top hemoximeters (CO-oximeters) and some multifunction blood gas analyzers. The Sa_{O_2} measured by a CO-oximeter is called the *fractional saturation* because it compares the proportion of Hb saturated with oxygen with the total amount of Hb present, including any dyshemoglobins:

$$\text{CO-oximeter } Sa_{O_2} = \frac{HbO_2}{HbO_2 + HHb + \text{Dyshemoglobins}} \times 100$$

Thus, because CO-oximeters measure the total complement of Hb and standard pulse oximeters do not, *in the presence of dyshemoglobins, pulse oximetry will overestimate the true* Sa_{O_2}. Other factors that can result in erroneous estimation of Sa_{O_2} using pulse oximetry are summarized in Table 8-4. Pulse oximeter accuracy also is affected by the Sa_{O_2} level, with the range of error increasing substantially when saturations drop below 65% to 70%.

To overcome errors associated with the presence of dyshemoglobins (such as a patient with suspected CO poisoning), one normally would obtain an arterial blood sample and analyze it using a laboratory hemoximeter. More recently, portable multiwavelength pulse oximeters

have become available that can provide relatively accurate noninvasive measurement of common dyshemoglobins at the bedside. Likewise, technological advances in sensor design and circuitry have helped decrease the spurious readings and false alarms associated with motion artifact. Simply shielding the sensor from ambient light can eliminate that source of error. More problematic are the errors that occur with poor perfusion at a peripheral sampling site. In these cases, placement of a reflectance (as opposed to an absorption-type) probe on a core body site such as the forehead or chest will provide more accurate estimates of Hb saturation.

When accuracy is essential (as in some critically ill patients), Sp_{O_2} should be compared to simultaneous hemoximetry analysis. The discrepancy between the Sa_{O_2} and Sp_{O_2} can then be used to "calibrate" the pulse oximetry reading. For example, if the Sp_{O_2} reading is 93% and hemoximetry analysis reveals an Sa_{O_2} of 90%, subtracting 3% from the subsequent Sp_{O_2} measurements will provide a more valid estimate of arterial oxygen saturation.

Pulse oximetry has dramatically reduced the need for invasive sampling of arterial blood. However, it should never be substituted for actual blood sample analysis when the clinical situation demands accurate and complete assessment of oxygenation. In addition, because pulse oximeters only provide oxygenation data, abnormalities in ventilation (Pco_2) or acid-base balance (pH/HCO_3^-) can go undetected unless they, too, are measured. Standard pulse oximetry only measures the relative proportion of O_2Hb and not the actual amount of circulating Hb in the blood, so anemia also can be missed if not separately assessed. Finally, as a result of the relationship between Hb saturation and O_2 partial pressures, pulse oximetry is of limited utility for detecting abnormally high Po_2 values (**hyperoxemia**). For this reason, RTs should be extra careful when using pulse oximetry to monitor oxygenation in newborn infants at risk for retinopathy of prematurity, one cause of which is hyperoxemia. In these cases, the upper limit for Sp_{O_2} should be in the 93% to 95% range, with higher values the basis for lowering the F_IO_2.

Transcutaneous Analysis

As a noninvasive measure of blood gas tensions, the transcutaneous measurement of oxygen (Ptc_{O_2}) and carbon dioxide (Ptc_{CO_2}) partial pressures has been available for more than 30 years. A typical transcutaneous blood gas sensor includes an O_2 and CO_2 electrode and a heating element. These electrodes measure gas pressures using the same electrochemical principles used in bench-top blood gas analyzers. However, instead of measuring the gas partial pressures in a blood sample, the electrodes measure the Po_2 and Pco_2 in an electrolyte gel at the skin surface. The heating element warms the underlying skin to 40°C to 42°C, which increases blood flow and thus "arterializes" the blood. Warming also increases skin permeability and enhances diffusion of O_2 and CO_2 from the capillaries into the electrolyte gel under the sensor.

Transcutaneous blood gas analysis generally has been limited to use with infants and small children in need of continuous monitoring of oxygenation and ventilation (see Chapter 12 for details). However, with the notable exception of monitoring for hyperoxemia, $Ptco_2$ monitoring been replaced by pulse oximetry. This is because the accuracy of $Ptco_2$ measures is highly dependent on the adequacy of perfusion. Low cardiac output, peripheral vasoconstriction, and dehydration all decrease capillary flow, which lowers $Ptco_2$. And as with Pao_2, $Ptco_2$ does not fully reflect total oxygen content of the blood. As discussed subsequently, complete assessment of blood oxygen content also requires knowledge of Hb content and saturation.

On the other hand, the $Ptcco_2$ can be reliably measured in patients in most age groups, making it a good choice for the continuous noninvasive monitoring of ventilation. $Ptcco_2$ monitoring is particularly useful when capnography is unavailable or impractical, such as during noninvasive ventilation. In general, in properly calibrated systems with good sensor placement, $Ptcco_2$ values will fall within 3 to 5 mm Hg of the measured $Paco_2$.

As a result of the lengthy set-up, calibration, and stabilization times needed by transcutaneous monitors, they have no place in assessing patients during emergencies. In these cases, pulse oximetry is a better choice for assessing oxygenation, with arterial sampling and point-of-care ABG analysis used to obtain a quick but complete picture of oxygenation, ventilation, and acid-base balance.

Capnography

Capnography involves the measurement of CO_2 concentrations or partial pressures in the respired gases and their real-time graphic display during breathing. Measurement is based on the fact that CO_2 gas absorbs light in the infrared spectrum in proportion to its concentration. Using this principle, a capnograph employs a photodetector that measures changes in the intensity of infrared light passed through an analysis chamber.

The primary application of capnography is to monitor patients during general anesthesia, mechanical ventilation, or resuscitation. As a noninvasive substitute for $Paco_2$ to assess ventilation, we use the end-tidal level of CO_2, either its partial pressure ($Petco_2$) or %CO_2. Normally, the $Petco_2$ averages about 2 to 5 mm Hg less than the $Paco_2$, or between 30 and 43 mm Hg (about 4.0% to 5.6%). Ventilation-perfusion imbalances can alter the difference between the $Paco_2$ and $Petco_2$, and these imbalances are common in patients with respiratory disorders; therefore, we normally focus on trending of the end-tidal CO_2 levels when using capnography for continuous monitoring. On the other hand, discrete breath analysis can be used to identify abnormal events such as extubation or rebreathing. Chapter 14 provides more detail on the use of capnography to monitor patients in intensive care.

Assessment of Oxygenation

A complete assessment of arterial blood gas parameters indicating the state of patient oxygenation includes the arterial partial pressure of oxygen (Pao_2), hemoglobin content (Hb) and Hb saturation (Sao_2, Spo_2), and arterial O_2 content (Cao_2).

Partial Pressure of Oxygen (Pao_2)

REFERENCE RANGE : 80 to100 mm Hg breathing room air

The Pao_2 is the pressure exerted by dissolved oxygen in the arterial blood. The Pao_2 reflects the lung's ability to transfer O_2 from the inspired gas into the circulating blood. Thus, the Pao_2 depends on both environmental factors (O_2 concentration and barometric pressure) and lung function, as determined by both age and the presence of disease.

Alveolar Air Equation

Assuming normal lung function and taking into account the environmental factors, we can compute the partial pressure of oxygen in the alveoli ($P_{A}O_2$) using the alveolar air equation:

$$P_{A}O_2 = F_{I}O_2 (P_B - P_{H_2O}) - (Paco_2 \times 1.25)$$

where $P_{A}O_2$ = partial pressure of oxygen in the alveoli; $F_{I}O_2$ = fraction of inhaled oxygen; P_B = barometric pressure; P_{H_2O} = water vapor pressure in alveoli, 47 mm Hg at BTPS; $Paco_2$ = arterial partial pressure of CO_2 (assumed to approximate the alveolar Pco_2); and 1.25 = factor based on the ratio of CO_2 production to O_2 consumption (respiratory quotient). For example, the $P_{A}O_2$ of a patient breathing room air ($F_{I}O_2$ = 0.21) at sea level (P_B = 760 mm Hg) with a $Paco_2$ of 40 mm Hg would be computed as follows:

$$P_{A}O_2 = 0.21(760 \text{ mm Hg} - 47 \text{ mm Hg}) - (40 \times 1.25)$$
$$= (0.21 \times 713 \text{ mm Hg}) - 50 \text{ mm Hg}$$
$$= 149.7 \text{ mm Hg} - 50 \text{ mm Hg}$$
$$= 99.7 \text{ mm Hg} \approx 100 \text{ mm Hg}$$

Even in healthy lungs gas transfer is imperfect, so not all of the O_2 in the alveoli diffuses into the pulmonary capillaries. How much of the O_2 in the lungs actually diffuses into the blood depends on both age and the presence of disease. In children and young adults with normal lungs breathing at sea level, there exists on average a 10 mm Hg gradient between the $P_{A}O_2$ and Pao_2, yielding a normal Pao_2 in the 90- to 100 mm Hg range. This difference—called the alveolar-arterial oxygen tension gradient and abbreviated as $P(A-a)O_2$—increases with increasing age, owing to a progressive decline in lung function. For patients breathing room air, this increase in $P(A-a)O_2$ is estimated by multiplying their age by 0.3. For example, we would estimate the $P(A-a)O_2$ of an otherwise healthy 70-year-old patient as being 0.3×70, or about 20 mm Hg. This would yield an expected Pao_2 for this patient of about $100 - 20 = 80$ mm Hg. Note that recent epidemiologic studies suggest that the age-associated increase in $P(A-a)_{O_2}$ levels off at about 70 years of age, making about 80 mm Hg the lower limit of the Pa_{O_2} reference range for essentially all age groups breathing air at sea level. Of course, the lower bound of the reference range for Pa_{O_2} decreases for individuals living at high altitudes in direct proportion to the decrease in barometric pressure.

Hypoxemia: Severity and Causes

When the Pa_{O_2} is below 80 mm Hg, a condition of **hypoxemia** exists. As indicated in Table 8-5, the Pa_{O_2} level determines whether hypoxemia is classified as mild, moderate, or severe.

Causes of hypoxemia include hypoventilation, ventilation-perfusion ($\dot{V}/\dot{Q}$) mismatch, pulmonary shunting, diffusion defect, and breathing gas with a low partial pressure of oxygen ($P_{I_{O_2}}$). Table 8-6 summarizes these causes, identifies some example conditions, and specifies how to differentiate among them. The $\dot{V}/\dot{Q}$ mismatch is the most common cause of hypoxemia seen by RTs, with pure diffusion defects being relatively rare in general clinical practice.

The clinical recognition of hypoxemia often is first suggested by the patient complaining of shortness of breath, especially with exertion. Additional common clinical manifestations of hypoxemia include mental confusion, tachycardia, tachypnea, hypertension, and cyanosis.

Although universally used as a measure of pulmonary gas exchange, the Pa_{O_2} provides only a limited picture of patient oxygenation. Indeed, dissolved oxygen represents only 1% to 2% of the total normally transported to the tissues. A full picture of patient oxygenation requires assessment of Hb content and saturation, total O_2 content, and actual O_2 transport and delivery to the tissues.

Hemoglobin (Hb) and Hb Saturation (Sa_{O_2}, Sp_{O_2})

REFERENCE RANGES : Hb males , 14-18 g/dL ;
females , 12-15 g/dL ; $Sa_{O_2}/Sp_{O_2} > 95\%$

Normally, more than 98% of the O_2 in arterial blood is chemically bound to hemoglobin. How much oxygen Hb carries in a given volume of blood depends on (1) the total hemoglobin concentration and (2) the proportion of oxygen bound to it (the Hb saturation or Sa_{O_2}). The Sa_{O_2} in

TABLE 8-5

Classification of Hypoxemia

Pa_{O_2} (mm Hg)	Relative Severity
60-79	Mild
40-59	Moderate
<40	Severe

TABLE 8-6

Causes of Hypoxemia

Type of Hypoxemia	Underlying Cause	Clinical Examples	Differential Assessment	
			$P(A-a)_{O_2}$	Response to O_2 therapy
Hypoventilation	Rise in $P_{A_{CO_2}}$ reduces $P_{A_{O_2}}$ (alveolar air equation)	Drug overdose Neuromuscular disorders	Normal*	Marked
$\dot{V}/\dot{Q}$ mismatch	Blood flows through under-ventilated regions of the lung	COPD Asthma	Increased	Marked
Pulmonary shunting	Blood flows by alveoli that are not ventilated, does not pick up any oxygen	Atelectasis Pneumonia Pulmonary edema ARDS	Increased	Minimal
Diffusion defect	Impaired gas transfer across alveolar-capillary membrane	Interstitial lung diseases (e.g., pulmonary fibrosis, sarcoidosis)	Increased	Marked
Low $P_{I_{O_2}}$	Decreased $P_{I_{O_2}}$ lowers $P_{A_{O_2}}$	Altitude sickness Equipment failure	Normal	Marked

*Normal $P(A-a)_{O_2}$ but $P_{A_{O_2}}$ decreased in proportion to rise in $P_{A_{CO_2}}$. Breathing room air, the two gas partial pressures normally sum to about 140 mm Hg. Thus, with pure hypoventilation, if the $P_{A_{CO_2}}$ rises from 40 to 70 mm Hg (+30 mm Hg), the $P_{A_{O_2}}$ should fall by a roughly comparable amount, that is, from 100 to 70 mm Hg.
ARDS, acute respiratory distress syndrome; COPD, chronic obstructive pulmonary disease.

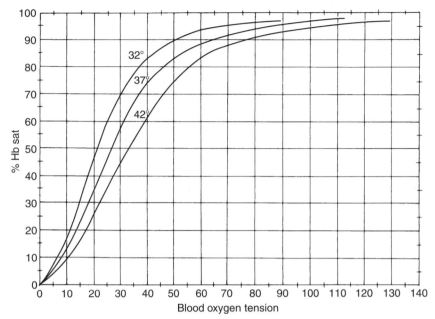

FIGURE 8-3 Oxygen dissociation curve of blood at a pH of 7.40, showing variations at three temperatures. For a given oxygen tension, the lower the blood temperature, the more the hemoglobin holds onto oxygen, maintaining higher saturation. (From Kacmarek RM, Stoller JK, Heuer, AJ: *Egan's fundamentals of respiratory care*, ed 10, St. Louis, 2013, Mosby-Elsevier).

turn depends on the Pa_{O_2} and a number of other factors affecting O_2 binding with hemoglobin.

It is important to note that the Sa_{O_2} reported by standard ABG analysis is a calculated value and that the Sp_{O_2} represents only the functional saturation of normal Hb with O_2. For this reason, to obtain true Sa_{O_2} values (as well as measures of common dyshemoglobins) requires that blood samples undergo hemoximetry analysis.

Each gram of normal hemoglobin has the capacity to bind with 1.34 mL O_2. With an average Hb content of 15 g/dL, this means that each 100 mL of blood has the potential for carrying about 20 mL O_2 (1.34 mL/g × 15 g/dL = 20.1 mL/dL). If the Hb content is lower than normal (as in anemia), the maximal O_2 carried is reduced proportionately. For example, if a patient's Hb were to drop by 50% from 15 g/dL to 7.5 g/dL, the O_2 carrying capacity of Hb would also be reduced in half, from about 20 mL/dL to about 10 mL/dL. For this reason, a complete assessment of patient oxygenation must include knowledge of Hb content, as determined by either CO-oximetry or a complete blood cell count (CBC).

Sa_{O_2} is a measure of how well Hb molecules are "filled" with O_2. The primary factor determining Sa_{O_2} is the blood Pa_{O_2}. The oxyhemoglobin dissociation curve quantifies the relationship between Pa_{O_2} and Sa_{O_2} (Fig. 8-3). This curve is composed of an upper flat portion and a lower steep portion, with a Pa_{O_2} of 60 mm Hg and Sa_{O_2} of 90% marking the dividing point between the two. Looking at the upper flat portion, as the Pa_{O_2} drops 40 mm Hg from 100 mm Hg down to 60 mm Hg, the Sa_{O_2} decreases very little, by only about 5% to 7%. On the other hand, when the Pa_{O_2} falls below 60 mm Hg onto the steep portion of the curve, the

Sa_{O_2} decrease is much more precipitous. For example, on this portion of the curve, a decrease in Pa_{O_2} of only 20 mm Hg (from 60 to 40 mm Hg) causes a 15% to 20% drop in Sa_{O_2}.

In patients with normal Hb content, if the Sa_{O_2} drops below 80% (equivalent to a Pa_{O_2} of about 50 mm Hg), the amount of desaturated Hb in the capillaries is sufficient to cause central cyanosis, the bluish discoloration of the capillary beds observed most easily around the lips and oral mucosa. However, because cyanosis requires an absolute quantity of desaturated Hb (about 5 g/dL HHb), if the total Hb content is low (**anemia**), this sign may not be apparent, even if the hypoxemia is severe.

> **SIMPLY STATED**
>
> To relate Pa_{O_2} to Sa_{O_2}, use the "40-50-60/70-80-90" rule: Hb saturations of 70%, 80%, and 90% are approximately equivalent to P_{O_2} values of 40, 50, and 60 mm Hg, respectively. Hb saturations must always be interpreted with knowledge of Hb content. With normal Hb content, the goal is to keep the Sa_{O_2} at or above 90%, which corresponds to a Pa_{O_2} of 60 mm Hg or higher.

In addition to Pa_{O_2}, Sa_{O_2} is affected by a number of other factors, the most important of which are body temperature, blood pH, and Pa_{CO_2} (Box 8-2). Alkalosis, hypocapnia, hypothermia, and the presence of fetal Hb and carboxyhemoglobin shift the oxyhemoglobin dissociation curve to the left, resulting in a higher Sa_{O_2} for a given Pa_{O_2}. Shifts to the left cause oxygen to bind more tightly to Hb, which facilitates O_2 uptake in the lungs but can impair unloading at the tissues. Conversely, acidosis, hypercapnia,

| Box 8-2 | Factors Influencing the Oxyhemoglobin Dissociation Curve |

SHIFT TO LEFT (INCREASE IN HEMOGLOBIN-OXYGEN AFFINITY)
Alkalosis
Hypocapnia
Hypothermia
Fetal hemoglobin
Carboxyhemoglobin

SHIFT TO RIGHT (DECREASE IN HEMOGLOBIN-OXYGEN AFFINITY)
Acidosis
Hypercapnia
Fever

and fever shift the curve to the right and result in lower Sao_2 values for the same Pao_2. Shifts to the right have the opposite effect, resulting in decreased oxygen affinity for Hb. Although this facilitates unloading of O_2 at the tissues, it can impair uptake in the pulmonary capillaries.

Dyshemoglobins

REFERENCE RANGES : COHb < 3 % (nonsmokers); metHb < 1.5 %

Dyshemoglobins such as COHb and metHb affect oxygenation in much the same way as anemia. Every gram of Hb chemically bound to a molecule other than O_2 is equivalent to an absolute reduction of 1 g/dL of circulating Hb. For example, if a smoke inhalation patient with normal Hb content has a COHb saturation of 40%, it would be as if he had only 9 g/dL circulating Hb, instead of 15 g/dL.

As already noted, the presence of carboxyhemoglobin also shifts the oxyhemoglobin dissociation curve to the left, which further impairs oxygenation by inhibiting the unloading of oxygen at the tissues. Normal COHb levels for nonsmokers are less than 3% and have a minimal impact on oxygenation. Smokers typically exhibit COHb levels in the 5% to 10% range. Higher levels of COHb occur with inhalation of fire smoke or engine exhaust, typically in enclosed spaces. In such cases, the Sao_2 (but not necessarily Pao_2) will be significantly reduced; the conscious patient may complain of headache, dyspnea, and nausea; and signs of hypoxemia such as tachypnea and tachycardia may be present. However, because carboxyhemoglobin is cherry red in color, cyanosis does not occur. At COHb levels above 40%, visual disturbance, myocardial damage, coma, and eventually, death may occur.

Another common dyshemoglobin is methemoglobin (metHb). metHb is a variant of hemoglobin in which the iron in the heme group has been oxidized from its normal Fe^{2+} (ferrous) state to the Fe^{3+} (ferric) state, which is incapable of binding with O_2. As with CO poisoning, increased levels of metHb have the same effect as an absolute anemia, causing a reduction in Cao_2 called methemoglobinemia.

Patients with high metHb levels can be found in every clinical service department of the hospital. Indeed, as many as one in five of all patients evaluated with traditional CO-oximetry exhibit a metHb above the reference range. Methemoglobinemia can be inherited (cytochrome reductase deficiency, hemoglobin M disease) or acquired by exposure to Hb-oxidizing agents. Environmental exposure to nitrates, nitrites, aniline, or benzene can induce methemoglobinemia, as can inhaling fumes containing nitric oxide (NO). More common is methemoglobinemia caused by the administration of nitrogen-based cardiac medications (e.g., nitroglycerin, nitroprusside), local anesthetic agents (e.g., benzocaine, prilocaine, lidocaine, EMLA creams), and selected antibiotics (e.g., dapsone, sulfonamides). Also, patients treated with inhaled NO are susceptible to acquired methemoglobinemia.

The Pao_2 in patients with methemoglobinemia generally is normal, and standard pulse oximetry cannot measure metHb; therefore, detection requires either laboratory CO-oximetry or multiwavelength pulse oximetry. As a result of its dark reddish brown color, metHb levels as low as 15% can cause cyanosis. Indeed, the presence of central cyanosis in patients with normal Pao_2 strongly suggests methemoglobinemia. Signs and symptoms like those due to CO poisoning occur at metHb levels in the 25% to 50% range. Above 50%, metHb cardiac dysrhythmias, severe central nervous system (CNS) depression, and profound metabolic acidosis can develop, leading to death if not treated. Treatment involves removing the causative factors and administering a reducing agent such as methylene blue. Supplemental O_2 therapy is commonly used to maximize the O_2 carrying capacity of the remaining normal hemoglobin but is of little value until the normal state of the Hb molecule is restored.

SIMPLY STATED

CO poisoning represents double trouble for tissue oxygenation. It reduces the oxygen-carrying capacity of the Hb and inhibits unloading of oxygen at the tissues.

Arterial O_2 Content (Cao_2)

REFERENCE RANGE : 16 to 20 mL/dL

Cao_2 represents the total oxygen content in the arterial blood, measured in mL/dL. It consists of both physically dissolved O_2 and that chemically bound to Hb. The vast proportion of the O_2 carried in the blood is bound to Hb; therefore, a normal Cao_2 requires a normal volume of circulating red blood cells containing normal quantities of Hb.

Cao_2 is calculated by summing its component parts, that is, dissolved O_2 and O_2 chemically bound to Hb. Dissolved O_2 is computed by multiplying the solubility coefficient of O_2 in plasma at 37°C (0.003 mL/dL/mm Hg) times the Pao_2. At a normal Pao_2 of 100 mm Hg, the dissolved O_2 would therefore be calculated as follows:

Dissolved O_2 = 0.003 mL/dL/mm Hg × 100 mm Hg = 0.3 mL/dL

The volume of O_2 chemically bound to Hb is computed by multiplying the Hb content by its carrying capacity (1.34 mL/g) by the Sa_{O_2}. With 15 g/dL Hb normally saturated to 97%, the amount of chemically bound O_2 would therefore be calculated as follows:

Chemically bound O_2 = 15 g/dL × 1.34 mL/g × 0.97 = 19.5 mL/dL

Summing the two yields the "normal" total O_2 content:

Ca_{O_2} = 0.3 mL/dL + 19.5 mL/dL = 19.8 mL/dL

Knowledge of Ca_{O_2} is critical because it is one of two major factors affecting delivery of O_2 to the tissues. Thus, anything that lowers the Ca_{O_2} potentially decreases the availability of O_2 to the body's cells. As previously discussed, a reduction in the availability of Hb, either absolute (anemia) or relative (dyshemoglobinemias), is a primary culprit in lowering Ca_{O_2}. A reduction in Pa_{O_2} will also lower Ca_{O_2}, but mainly by its effect on Sa_{O_2}, and then mostly when it falls below 60 mm Hg.

O_2 Delivery and Hypoxia

In addition to Ca_{O_2}, O_2 delivery to the tissues depends on blood flow or cardiac output (CO). Indeed, we can easily compute O_2 delivery to the tissues (D_{O_2}) as the product of the two:

$$D_{O_2} = Ca_{O_2} \times CO$$

With average cardiac output for a normal adult being about 5 L/minute, a normal O_2 delivery would be computed as follows:

$$D_{O_2} = 200 \text{ mL/L} \times 5 \text{ L/min} = 1000 \text{ mL/min}$$

Given a normal resting O_2 consumption of about 250 mL/min, the delivery of 1000 mL/min O_2 provides a reserve sufficient to accommodate differences in metabolism across organ systems and protect against a reduction in the availability of O_2 to the tissues, at least for a short time.

When the amount of oxygen available to the tissues falls short of metabolic needs, a condition of **hypoxia** exists. Adequate O_2 delivery depends on both adequate Ca_{O_2} and cardiac output; therefore, a complete assessment of patient oxygenation must take into account the adequacy of blood flow. Clinical signs of an inadequate cardiac output include hypotension, cool extremities, weak or absent peripheral pulses, reduced urine output, and depressed levels of consciousness. More details on the basic assessment of a patient's state of perfusion are provided by physical examination (see Chapter 5) and measurement of blood pressure (see Chapter 4). For critically ill patients, advanced monitoring techniques can provide quantitative assessment of both cardiac output (see Chapter 16) and tissue oxygenation (see Chapter 14).

SIMPLY STATED

The single most important parameter that reflects the quantity of oxygen carried in the arterial blood is the Ca_{O_2}. An adequate Hb concentration must be present for this parameter to be normal.

Assessment of Acid-Base Balance

The average adult produces about 12,000 mmol of acid each day. In combination, the lungs and kidneys ensure proper excretion of this daily acid load, maintaining appropriate acid-base balance. The lungs remove the bulk of the acid load through ventilation and CO_2 excretion. The kidneys remove a smaller quantity of acid but help restore the buffer capacity of the body fluids by replenishing HCO_3^- levels. Failure of either system can disrupt normal acid-base balance.

Accurate assessment of a patient's acid-base balance is based mainly on interpretation of the arterial pH, partial pressure of carbon dioxide (Pa_{CO_2}), bicarbonate concentration (HCO_3^-), and base excess (BE).

pH

REFERENCE RANGE : 7.35 to 7.45

The arterial blood pH is a measurement of the hydrogen ion concentration in the plasma, abbreviated as H^+. The actual arterial blood H^+ is very low, about 0.00004 mol/L (40 nm/L). Instead of dealing with such small numbers, we convert the H^+ to equivalent units on the pH scale. This is a negative logarithmic conversion; therefore, H^+ and pH changes are inversely related by a power of 10. For example, a 1-unit decrease in pH from 7.40 to 6.40 represents a tenfold increase in blood H^+. A 0.3-unit change in pH alters the H^+ by a factor of 2 (e.g., a 0.3 decrease in pH coincides with a doubling of the H^+, whereas a 0.3 increase in pH halves the H^+).

The arterial pH is important to monitor because the majority of body functions occur optimally at or near a pH of 7.40. Alterations in pH above or below normal can have profound effects on many body systems, especially the CNS.

pH values below 7.35 indicate an abnormally high blood H^+ or **acidemia**. Acidosis tends to depress CNS function. For this reason, patients with acidosis may appear lethargic and disoriented. As the acidosis worsens, coma may develop. Significant acidosis also may reduce myocardial contractility and reduce blood flow throughout the body.

pH values above 7.45 indicate an abnormally low blood H^+ or **alkalemia**. The major effect of alkalosis is overexcitability of the CNS and peripheral nerves. Nerves can become so responsive that they automatically and repetitively depolarize, resulting in tetany. Extreme alkalosis also may cause muscular spasms of the extremities, face, and body and cardiac dysrhythmias. Respiratory failure may occur if the nerves and muscles of ventilation are involved.

Partial Pressure of Carbon Dioxide (Pa_{CO_2})

REFERENCE RANGE : 35 to 45 mm Hg

The Pa_{CO_2} measures the adequacy of ventilation relative to the metabolic production of CO_2 by the tissues. The presence of a $Paco_2$ above 45 mm Hg is termed **hypercapnia**. Hypercapnia occurs when the level of alveolar ventilation is not sufficient to remove CO_2 at an acceptable rate (**hypoventilation**). The presence of a $Paco_2$ below 35 mm Hg is termed **hypocapnia**. Hypocapnia occurs when alveolar ventilation is excessive relative to metabolic needs (**hyperventilation**).

As an excretion mechanism for a by-product of metabolism, the $Paco_2$ also plays a major role in acid-base balance. $Paco_2$ alters H^+ and pH according to the following hydration/dissociation equation for carbonic acid (H_2CO_3):

$$CO_2 + H_2O \rightleftharpoons H_2CO_3 \rightleftharpoons HCO_3^- + H^+$$

An increase in $Paco_2$ (hypercapnia) shifts the equilibrium equation to the right, resulting in an increase in H^+ production and a decrease in pH. Acidemia due to an increase in $Paco_2$ is called **respiratory acidosis**. A decrease in $Paco_2$ (hypocapnia) shifts the equation to the left, lowers H^+ production and causes a rise in pH. Alkalemia due to a decrease in $Paco_2$ is called **respiratory alkalosis**. Adjustments in the plasma concentration by the kidneys can compensate for these respiratory acid-base disorders, which are discussed subsequently.

The $Paco_2$ is the best measure for evaluating the effectiveness of ventilation and should be interpreted in light of the patient's minute ventilation ($\dot{V}_E$). A normal $Paco_2$ should be accompanied by a normal $\dot{V}_E$ (5 to 10 L/min in adults). With a normal metabolic rate, an increased $\dot{V}_E$ normally results in hypocapnia. A normal $Paco_2$ in the presence of a higher than normal $\dot{V}_E$ indicates either an increased metabolic rate (as with exercise) or increased **dead space ventilation**. Increased dead space ventilation occurs when perfusion to well-ventilated areas of the lungs is reduced, as may occur with a pulmonary embolism. With a normal metabolic rate, any reduction in $\dot{V}_E$ below normal usually produces hypercapnia. A normal $Paco_2$ in the presence of a lower than normal $\dot{V}_E$ usually indicates a decreased metabolic rate.

SIMPLY STATED

The best parameter for evaluating the adequacy of ventilation is the $Paco_2$. Proper assessment of $Paco_2$ should take into account the patient's minute ventilation ($\dot{V}_E$).

Plasma Bicarbonate

REFERENCE RANGE : 22 to 26 mmol/L

The plasma HCO_3^- primarily reflects the metabolic component of acid-base balance and is regulated by the renal system. Since HCO_3^- functions chemically as base, changes in its concentration will cause equivalent directional changes

in pH; that is, if the HCO_3^- increases, the pH will rise, and if the HCO_3^- decreases, the pH will fall.

A primary increase in HCO_3^- that causes alkalemia (pH > 7.45) is termed **metabolic alkalosis**. A primary decrease in HCO_3^- that causes acidemia (pH < 7.35) is termed **metabolic acidosis**. HCO_3^- levels may also change as a compensatory or secondary response to primary changes in $Paco_2$ levels; this usually requires at least 12 to 24 hours to occur, with full compensation taking as long as 3 days or more.

The previously described carbonic acid hydration/dissociation equation indicates that changes in dissolved CO_2 levels affect HCO_3^- concentrations. Thus, because the HCO_3^- concentration depends in part on $Paco_2$ levels, it is not considered a pure measure of metabolic activity.

Base Excess (BE)

REFERENCE RANGE : ± 2 mmol/L $\left(mEq/L \right)$

BE measures changes in total blood buffer base above or below normal. The total quantity of buffer anions in the blood is 45 to 50 mmol/L, or approximately twice that of HCO_3^-. Thus, HCO_3^- accounts for only about half of the total buffering capacity of the blood. Therefore, BE provides a more complete picture of blood buffering. Moreover, unlike HCO_3^-, acute changes in $Paco_2$ do not affect BE. For this reason, BE is considered a pure measure of the metabolic component of acid-base balance.

The calculation of BE requires measurements of pH, $Paco_2$, HCO_3^-, and hemoglobin content. Hemoglobin is required in the calculation because in its unsaturated form (HHb), it can reversibly bind with H^+, thus serving as a blood buffer.

BE is reported as a positive or negative value depending on the direction of buffer base deviation from normal. The larger the value, the more severe the deviation in the metabolic component. A positive BE indicates either the presence of excess base or excessive loss of acid. A negative BE (sometimes call a *base deficit*) indicates either the presence of excess acid or excessive loss of base.

Henderson-Hasselbalch Equation

There are two basic types of acid-base disorders: metabolic and respiratory. Metabolic disorders are recognized by abnormalities in plasma HCO_3^-, whereas respiratory disorders alter $Paco_2$. The relationship between these two measures and blood pH are defined in the Henderson-Hasselbalch equation:

$$pH = pK + \log_{10}\left(\frac{HCO_3^- \; (renal/metabolic/base)}{Paco_2 \times 0.03 \; (lungs/respiratory/acid)} \right)$$

where pK = 6.1 (an ionization constant) and 0.03 = factor to convert $Paco_2$ to mmol/L (concentration of dissolved CO_2).

Assuming a normal and Pa_{CO_2}, we compute a normal pH as follows:

$$pH = 6.1 + \log\left(\frac{24}{40 \times 0.03}\right)$$

$$pH = 6.1 + \log\left(\frac{24}{1.2}\right)$$

$$pH = 6.1 + \log(20)$$

$$pH = 6.1 + 1.30$$

$$pH = 7.40$$

Note that for a normal pH, the ratio of HCO_3^- to dissolved CO_2 must be 20:1. Any major change in this ratio will result in an abnormal pH. For example, an increase in Pa_{CO_2} from 40 to 60 mm Hg increases the concentration of dissolved CO_2 to 1.8 mmol/L, decreasing this ratio from 20:1 to about 13:1. Based on this decreased ratio of base to acid (due to more acid), we compute a lower pH of 7.23:

$$pH = 6.1 + \log\left(\frac{24}{60 \times 0.03}\right)$$

$$pH = 6.1 + \log\left(\frac{24}{1.8}\right)$$

$$pH = 6.1 + \log(13.33)$$

$$pH = 6.1 + 1.13$$

$$pH = 7.23$$

Clearly, return of the Pa_{CO_2} to 40 mm Hg (dissolved CO_2 = 1.2 mmol/L) would restore the ratio to 20:1 and the pH to 7.4. However, restoration of the pH back to normal could also occur by increasing the HCO_3^- concentration to 36 mmol/L (36:1.8 = 20:1). Thus, a pH change due to alteration in one component of acid-base balance can be corrected by a compensatory change in the other component. This example reinforces the concept that pH is not determined by the absolute values of Pa_{CO_2} and HCO_3^- but by the ratio of the two.

Simple Acid-Base Imbalances

Most acid-base abnormalities occur as simple disorders. Simple disorders involve a primary abnormality in one component of acid-base balance, either Pa_{CO_2} or HCO_3^-. Simple acid-base disorders also can involve compensatory responses by which the component not primarily affected is altered to restore the pH back toward normal. Thus, the presence of a near-normal pH does not rule out the possibility of a primary acid-base disorder, but instead may indicate the presence of a compensatory response.

Respiratory Acidosis

Simple respiratory acidosis is an abnormal condition in which there is a primary reduction in alveolar ventilation relative to the rate of CO_2 production, that is, inadequate ventilation. The hallmark of acute respiratory acidosis is an elevated Pa_{CO_2} in association with a decreased pH and normal HCO_3^- and BE. Acute respiratory acidosis also is termed *uncompensated respiratory acidosis* because the kidney's compensatory response (increased HCO_3^-) has not occurred.

Respiratory acidosis can occur in a variety of respiratory and nonrespiratory abnormalities. Examples include the following:

- Respiratory
  - Acute upper airway obstruction
  - Severe diffuse airway obstruction (acute or chronic)
  - Massive pulmonary edema
- Nonrespiratory
  - Drug overdose
  - Spinal cord trauma
  - Neuromuscular disease
  - Head trauma
  - Thoracic trauma
  - Gross obesity

Compensation for respiratory acidosis occurs through renal reabsorption of HCO_3^-. Partial compensation occurs when the plasma HCO_3^- is above normal, but the pH is not yet within normal limits. If the plasma HCO_3^- is elevated enough to return the pH to within normal range, it is called *fully compensated respiratory acidosis*. Once full compensation occurs, HCO_3^- levels do not rise further, and the pH levels typically remains in the 7.35 to 7.40 range. As a result of the time needed to change HCO_3^- levels, compensated respiratory acidosis also is referred to as *chronic respiratory acidosis* or *chronic ventilatory failure*.

Identifying the expected change in HCO_3^- is useful in determining the degree of compensation. For acute respiratory acidosis, for each 10 to 15 mm Hg increase in Pa_{CO_2}, the plasma HCO_3^- increases by 1 mmol/L. Proportionately greater increases in HCO_3^- indicate a compensatory response, usually about 5 mmol/L for each 10 mm Hg increase in Pa_{CO_2}. If the expected compensation is not occurring, a complicating metabolic disorder may be present.

The combination of an acutely elevated Pa_{CO_2} and acidosis usually has a significant effect on the clinical findings. Patients with an intact respiratory drive may exhibit dyspnea and tachypnea. In contrast, if the respiratory center is impaired (e.g., narcotic drug overdose), the respiratory rate will be reduced. Since patients with acute hypercapnia breathing room also are subject to a reduction in Pa_{O_2}, clinical manifestations of hypoxemia may be apparent. Acidosis causes CNS depression, so patients with acute hypercapnia often are confused, semiconscious, and—at Pa_{CO_2} levels higher than 70 mm Hg—may become comatose. CNS depression may not be evident, however, because of normalization of the pH in chronic respiratory acidosis.

High Pa_{CO_2} levels cause systemic vasodilation; therefore cardiovascular manifestations also may be observed. Peripheral vasodilation and an increased cardiac output promote warm flushed skin and a bounding pulse. Dysrhythmias are occasionally observed. Cerebral vasodilation also occurs, resulting in elevated intracranial pressures, retinal venous distention, papilledema, and headache. Finally, increases in HCO_3^- levels as a result of renal compensation are accompanied by decreased chloride levels (hypochloremia).

> **SIMPLY STATED**
>
> Respiratory acidosis is present when the $Paco_2$ exceeds the upper limit of the reference range (45 mm Hg) and is causing a primary reduction in the blood pH.

Respiratory Alkalosis

Simple respiratory alkalosis is an abnormal condition in which there is a primary increase in alveolar ventilation relative to the rate of CO_2 production (i.e., hyperventilation.) The hallmark of acute or uncompensated respiratory alkalosis is a reduction in $Paco_2$ in association with an elevated pH and normal HCO_3^- and BE. Hyperventilation usually is the result of an increased stimulus or drive to breathe. This occurs with pain, anxiety, and hypoxemia (Pao_2 <60 mm Hg) and as a compensatory response to metabolic acidosis. Respiratory alkalosis also may be induced accidentally in patients receiving positive-pressure ventilation. Clinical signs and symptoms associated with acute respiratory alkalosis include tachypnea, dizziness, sweating, tingling in the fingers and toes (paresthesia), and muscle weakness or spasm.

The kidneys compensate for respiratory alkalosis by increasing HCO_3^- excretion. Partial compensation occurs when the plasma HCO_3^- falls below normal, but the pH remains above 7.45. Full compensation occurs when the plasma HCO_3^- decreases enough to return the pH to the high end of the reference range (7.40 to 7.45).

The expected compensatory change in plasma HCO_3^- with respiratory alkalosis depends on the severity and duration of hyperventilation. In acute respiratory alkalosis, for every for every 5 mm Hg decrease in $Paco_2$, the HCO_3^- decreases only by about 1 mmol/L. Proportionately greater decreases in HCO_3^- indicate a compensatory response, usually about 5 mmol/L for each 10 mm Hg decrease in $Paco_2$. If the expected compensation is not present, a complicating metabolic disorder may be present.

Metabolic Acidosis

Simple metabolic acidosis is an abnormal condition resulting from a net gain in fixed blood acids or reduction in buffer base. The hallmark of metabolic acidosis is a reduced pH associated with a primary decrease in blood buffers, as indicated by a fall in HCO_3^- or BE. Gains in fixed acid load can result from increased metabolic acid production or decreased renal excretion. A reduction in base normally is associated with excessive loss of HCO_3^-. Common causes of these two types of metabolic acidosis include the following:

Increase in fixed acids:
- Ketoacidosis (e.g., diabetes/starvation)
- Renal failure (distal tubules/retention of H^+)
- Lactic acidosis (shock/anaerobic metabolism)
- Ingestion of acids (e.g., methanol)

Loss of base (HCO_3^-):
- Diarrhea
- Pancreatic fistula
- Renal failure (proximal tubules/loss of HCO_3^-)
- Hyperalimentation

To differentiate between metabolic acidosis due to acid gain versus that associated with loss of base, we use a measure called the **anion gap**. The anion gap is the difference between the concentration of the major serum cations and major anions (the difference being due to unmeasured ions). The most commonly used formula to compute the anion gap is:

$$Anion\ gap = [Na^+] - ([Cl^-] + [HCO_3^-])$$

A frequently cited reference range for the anion gap is 8 to 16 mmol/L. It is important to note that the reference range differs according to whether K^+ is included in the formula and the methods used to measure the electrolytes. *For this reason, it is essential that clinicians know the anion gap reference range used in their institution.*

Metabolic acidosis caused by an increase in fixed acids depletes stores and increases the anion gap. On the other hand, when metabolic acidosis is caused by loss of bicarbonate, the anion gap usually remains within the reference range. This is because bicarbonate loss is offset by a gain in chloride. For this reason, metabolic acidosis with a normal anion gap is often termed *hyperchloremic acidosis.*

Acute or uncompensated metabolic acidosis is rarely seen because the compensatory response—a reduction in $Paco_2$ through hyperventilation—tends to occur as the acidosis develops. Indeed, the most common sign of metabolic acidosis is rapid and deep breathing, called *Kussmaul respirations.* The following equation can be used to predict the $Paco_2$ level needed to fully compensate for metabolic acidosis:

$$Paco_2 = [(1.5 \times HCO_3^-) + 8] \pm 2$$

When the $Paco_2$ is higher than predicted, the patient may not have the ability to hyperventilate, which suggest the presence of a concurrent respiratory abnormality.

As metabolic acidosis worsens, the patient may complain of dyspnea, headache, nausea, and vomiting. Confusion and stupor may follow. Constriction of the venous blood vessels may shift blood flow to the lungs and cause pulmonary edema. Dysrhythmias can occur with severe acidosis.

> **SIMPLY STATED**
>
> Metabolic acidosis puts extra stress on the respiratory system to reduce $Paco_2$ as a compensatory response. This may precipitate respiratory failure in patients with limited respiratory reserves, that is, those with lung disease.

Metabolic Alkalosis

Simple metabolic alkalosis is an abnormal condition resulting from a net gain in buffer base or loss in fixed acids. The hallmark of metabolic alkalosis is an elevated pH accompanied by an increase in blood buffers, as indicated by a rise in HCO_3^- or BE. Common causes of metabolic alkalosis include the following:

- Hypokalemia or hypochloremia
- Nasogastric suction (loss of stomach acid)
- Persistent vomiting (loss of stomach acid)
- Diuretic therapy
- Steroid therapy
- Excessive administration of sodium bicarbonate

Certain electrolyte imbalances can lower H^+ or increase HCO_3^-. Hypokalemia promotes migration of H^+ ions into the intracellular fluids in exchange for K^+. Hypokalemia also increases renal excretion of H^+ ions, further increasing buffer base.

As previously described, to maintain electrolytic balance, chloride and bicarbonate ion concentrations tend to vary inversely with each other. For this reason, when hypochloremia is present, the concentration of HCO_3^- usually rises, causing metabolic alkalosis.

Direct loss of acid can occur through gastric suction or vomiting, both of which cause loss of stomach acid (HCl). In this case, the loss of both H^+ and Cl^- ions leads to a proportionate increase in the blood buffer base.

Excessive administration of bicarbonate can lead to metabolic alkalosis, which used to be a common occurrence during cardiopulmonary resuscitation. However, the routine use of sodium bicarbonate no longer is recommended for patients in cardiac arrest, in part because it can produce hypernatremia, elevate CO_2 levels, and impair O_2 unloading at the tissues.

The expected compensatory response for metabolic alkalosis is an elevation in Pa_{CO_2}, that is, hypoventilation. However, significant hypoventilation tends not to occur in most patients, in part because the hypoxic ventilatory stimulus may supervene. On the other hand, a patient with metabolic alkalosis and CNS depression may hypoventilate. In such cases, the hypercapnia can cause hypoxemia unless supplemental O_2 is provided.

SIMPLY STATED

A patient with metabolic alkalosis may tend to hypoventilate, so this acid-base imbalance should be corrected before any attempt to wean from mechanical ventilation is initiated.

Table 8-7 summarizes the anticipated pH, Pa_{CO_2}, and HCO_3^- changes seen in the four simple acid-base imbalances, including the expected compensatory responses.

TABLE 8-7

Summary of Simple Acid-Base Disorders and Expected Compensatory Responses

Acid-Base Imbalance	pH	Pa_{CO_2}	HCO_3^-	Expected Compensatory Response
Respiratory Alkalosis				
Uncompensated/acute	↑	↓	N	For each 10- to 15-mm Hg increase in Pa_{CO_2}, the HCO_3^- increases by about 1 mmol/L
Partially compensated	↑	↓	↓	For every 10-mm Hg increase in Pa_{CO_2}, the HCO_3^-
Fully compensated/chronic	N	↓	↓	increases by 5 mmol/L; partial compensation becomes apparent within 12-24 hr, with a full response taking up to 72 hr or more
Respiratory Acidosis				
Uncompensated/acute	↓	↑	N	For every 5-mm Hg decrease in Pa_{CO_2}, HCO_3^- decreases 1 mmol/L
Partially compensated	↓	↑	↑	HCO_3^- falls 5 mmol/L for every 10 mm Hg fall in
Fully compensated/chronic	N	↑	↑	Pa_{CO_2}; partial compensation becomes apparent within 12-24 hr, with a full response taking up to 72 hr or more
Metabolic Acidosis				
Uncompensated/acute	↓	N	↓	Lack of compensation indicates respiratory abnormality
Partially compensated	↓	↓	↓	Compensation normally occurs simultaneously with
Fully compensated/chronic	N	↓	↓	acidosis; expected $Pa_{CO_2} = [(1.5 \times HCO_3^-) + 8] \pm 2$
Metabolic Alkalosis				
Uncompensated/acute	↑	N	↑	Compensation via hypoventilation uncommon;
Partially compensated	↑	↑	↑	if present Pa_{CO_2} usually does not rise above
Fully compensated/chronic	N	↑	↑	50-55 mm Hg

HCO_3^-, plasma bicarbonate concentration; N, within reference range; pH, hydrogen ion concentration in blood; Pa_{CO_2}, partial pressure of CO_2 in arterial blood; ↑, above reference range; ↓, below reference range.

Combined Acid-Base Disturbances

Combined acid-base disorders are identified easily because the derangements in Pa_{CO_2} and HCO_3^- both drive the pH in the same direction—either low (combined respiratory and metabolic acidosis) or high (combined respiratory and metabolic alkalosis)

Respiratory and Metabolic Acidosis

The hallmark of combined respiratory and metabolic acidosis is the simultaneous presence of an elevated Pa_{CO_2} and a reduced HCO_3^-, which together can dramatically reduce the pH. Even mild hypercapnia (Pa_{CO_2} = 50 mm Hg) occurring with a moderate reduction in HCO_3^- (15 to 17 mmol/L) results in profound acidosis (pH < 7.15). This combined disorder occurs in a variety of situations, including the following.

Cardiac Arrest

During cardiac arrest, both blood flow and ventilation cease. The lack of blood flow causes tissue hypoxia, which leads to anaerobic metabolism and lactic acidosis. Inadequate ventilation causes CO_2 retention and respiratory acidosis.

Chronic Obstructive Pulmonary Disease

Many patients with chronic obstructive pulmonary disease (COPD) have chronically elevated Pa_{CO_2} levels. In these patients, severe electrolyte disturbances, sudden hypotension, renal failure, or anemia can cause a metabolic acidosis to develop "on top" of their chronic respiratory acidosis. The reduction in plasma HCO_3^- on top of the elevated Pa_{CO_2} can result in a significant fall in pH.

Poisoning and Drug Overdose

Many cases of poisoning and drug overdose result in depression of the respiratory center and respiratory acidosis. The poisons or drugs also may be metabolized to strong acids and produce a concurrent metabolic acidosis.

Metabolic and Respiratory Alkalosis

The hallmark of combined respiratory and metabolic alkalosis is the simultaneous presence of an elevated HCO_3^- and low Pa_{CO_2}, which together will cause a large rise in pH. Two clinical situations causing combined respiratory and metabolic alkalosis are noteworthy.

Critically Ill Patients

Respiratory alkalosis is common among patients undergoing critical care. Causes include anxiety, pain, hypoxemia, hypotension, and neurologic damage. Concurrent metabolic alkalosis may develop as a result of nasogastric suctioning, vomiting, blood transfusions, or antacid therapy. The resulting combined alkalosis can be severe and can result in serious complications such as life-threatening cardiac dysrhythmias.

Ventilator-Induced Alkalosis

Ventilator-induced alkalosis (also called **iatrogenic alkalosis**) can occur when patients with compensated respiratory acidosis undergo mechanical ventilation. Typically, these are patients with COPD who have chronically elevated Pa_{CO_2} levels and develop acute-on-chronic respiratory failure. Their "normal" acid-base state is a compensated respiratory acidosis, and delivery of inappropriately high volumes may cause a precipitous drop in the Pa_{CO_2} and a respiratory alkalosis. At the same time, the HCO_3^-—already high because of renal compensation—remains elevated, yielding the combined alkalosis. This problem can be avoided if initial ventilator settings target a Pa_{CO_2} that is consistent with the patient's elevated "normal" or if the ventilator is adjusted to lower Pa_{CO_2} slowly.

Mixed Acid-Base Disturbances

Mixed acid-base disorders occur when two primary imbalances coexist, with each driving the pH in the opposite direction. These disorders are most common among critically ill patients and generally indicate a poor prognosis. Box 8-3 outlines some of the common causes of mixed acid-base disorders.

> **SIMPLY STATED**
>
> A normal or near-normal pH in the presence of severe abnormalities in HCO_3^- or Pa_{CO_2} suggests a mixed acid-base disorder.

Mixed imbalances are difficult to recognize because they can be confused with secondary compensation for a primary disorder. However, in most mixed imbalances, the degree of compensation for what is the presumed a primary disorder is greater than the expected response, as previously outlined in Table 8-7.

Box 8-3	Common Causes of Mixed Acid-Base Disorders

- Chronic respiratory acidosis and metabolic acidosis
  - Chronic obstructive pulmonary disease (COPD) patient who develops shock and lactic acidosis
- Chronic respiratory acidosis and metabolic alkalosis
  - Pulmonary insufficiency and diuretic therapy
  - COPD patient treated with steroids or ventilation
- Respiratory alkalosis and metabolic acidosis
  - Salicylate intoxication
  - Gram-negative sepsis
  - Severe pulmonary edema

Mixed Metabolic Acidosis and Respiratory Alkalosis

Most often, metabolic acidosis occurs as the primary disorder, with a predictable decrease in $Paco_2$ compensating for the acidemia (see Table 8-7). When metabolic acidosis is accompanied by a lower than predicted $Paco_2$, a concurrent respiratory alkalosis is present. In this situation, the pH may be elevated slightly above 7.40 and give the appearance of a compensated respiratory alkalosis. Conversely, this mixed disorder may be diagnosed in a patient with primary respiratory alkalosis when the reduction in plasma HCO_3^- exceeds the predicted amount (see Table 8-7). Generally, the primary problem can be ascertained by determining on which side of normal the pH falls. For example, if the pH is less than 7.40, the primary problem likely is the one causing acidosis. Sometimes, however, knowledge of the patient's underlying pathology is needed to determine which imbalance is the primary one.

Mixed Metabolic Alkalosis and Respiratory Acidosis

When a patient with respiratory acidosis has a greater than predicted HCO_3^- level (see Table 8-7), a mixed metabolic alkalosis and respiratory acidosis is likely. Conversely, when a patient with a known metabolic alkalosis has $Paco_2$ above 50 to 55 mm Hg (see Table 8-7), a complicating respiratory acidosis is occurring. The pH in such situations is determined by the severity of each simple disorder and may be lower than, higher than, or within the normal reference range. A pH of 7.40 occurring simultaneously with significant abnormalities in $Paco_2$ and HCO_3^- suggests a mixed disorder because normal compensation seldom returns the pH to 7.40.

A typical clinical situation in which mixed metabolic alkalosis and respiratory acidosis may occur is treatment of the patient with COPD who has chronic respiratory acidosis. This type of patient often is treated with diuretics and steroid therapy, which can induce metabolic alkalosis. The complicating metabolic alkalosis may promote further hypoventilation and worsen the clinical picture. Metabolic alkalosis can make weaning patients from mechanical ventilation difficult because it decreases the patient's ventilatory drive. Recognition and treatment of the metabolic alkalosis is vital to optimizing the patient's respiratory function and often results in a significant reduction in $Paco_2$.

Assuring Valid Measurement and Use of Blood Gas Data

Blood gas results are used to make critical decisions, so measurements must be accurate, their interpretation valid, and their application to patient care correct. Errors in any of these areas can result in poor patient management and unsatisfactory outcomes.

To avoid errors in the measurement and use of blood gas data requires a comprehensive quality assurance program. Such programs are designed to assure quality in sample acquisition and handling (pre-analytic phase: **pre-analytic errors**); calibration, use, and maintenance of the measurement device (analysis phase: **analytic errors**); and post-analytic reporting (**post-analytic errors**), interpretation, and use of test results.

Pre-analytic Errors

Blood samples obtained by invasive sampling are analyzed either at the bedside using a point-of-care device or in a central laboratory using a bench-top analyzer. In either case, it is essential that the sample provided for analysis be free of pre-analytic errors. Table 8-8 summarizes the common pre-analytic errors associated with arterial blood sampling, their effect on measurement, and how to recognize and avoid them.

Analytic Errors

Blood gas quality control measures help avoid errors during sample analysis. To minimize analytic errors requires regular calibration of the measurement device. **Calibration** involves exposing the analyzer to calibration media at two or more known levels of measurement. For example, the calibrating media for a standard blood gas analyzer includes precision mixtures of O_2 and CO_2 gas (to calibrate the O_2 and CO_2 electrodes) and buffer solutions with known pH values (to calibrate the pH electrode). During this automated or semi-automated process, the analyzer adjusts its output to correspond exactly to the calibration media's known values. Note that because pulse oximeters measure relative and not absolute concentrations of Hb, they do not require calibration using known media. However, empirical calibration can be performed using "biologic controls," that is, healthy subjects with known saturation levels.

In addition to automated calibration, analyzers should be subject to regular calibration verification. Calibration verification involves analyzing control media representing at least three levels of the measured analyte. By plotting these data on a chart and using statistical analysis to identify outlier measurements or inappropriate trends, potential malfunctions of the analyzer can be identified and corrected before they affect the accuracy of reported results from patient samples.

An additional component of laboratory quality control is proficiency testing. Proficiency testing involves blind testing of samples distributed by a central site. Once analyzed, results are returned for review and validation. The central site then sends a report back to participating laboratories for inclusion in their quality assurance documentation. Proficiency testing is required to maintain accreditation of laboratories, including blood gas laboratories.

Post-analytic Errors

In the post-analytical phase, results are provided to the clinician, who interprets them and makes patient management

TABLE 8-8

Pre-analytic Errors Associated with Arterial Blood Sampling

Error	Effect(s)	How to Recognize	How to Avoid
Air in sample	Lowers P_{CO_2} Raises pH Raises low P_{O_2} Lowers high P_{O_2}	Visible bubbles or froth Low P_{CO_2} inconsistent with patient status	Discard frothy samples Fully expel bubbles Mix only after air expelled Cap syringe quickly
Venous blood or venous admixture	Raises P_{CO_2} Lowers pH Can greatly lower P_{O_2}	Failure of syringe to fill by pulsations Patient has no symptoms of hypoxemia	Avoid femoral site Do not aspirate sample Use short-bevel needles Avoid artery "overshoot" Cross-check with Sp_{O_2}
Excess liquid heparin (dilution)*	Lowers P_{CO_2} Raises pH Raises low P_{O_2} Lowers high P_{O_2}	Visible liquid heparin remains in syringe before sampling	Fill dead space only Collect > 2 mL (adults) Use dry heparin
Metabolic effects	Raises P_{CO_2} Lowers pH Lowers P_{O_2}	Excessive time lag since sample collection Values inconsistent with patient status	Analyze within 30 minutes If analysis cannot occur with 30 minutes, place sample in ice slush

*Rare occurrence, with most arterial blood gas kits now using dry lyophilized heparin.
Modified from Scanlan CL: Analysis and monitoring of gas exchange. In Scanlan CL, Wilkins RL, Stoller JK, editors: *Egan's fundamentals of respiratory care,* ed 7, St. Louis, 1999, Mosby.

decisions accordingly. Errors in this phase can include incorrect reporting and improper interpretation or use of results. Proper interpretation and use of blood gas results is covered in subsequent sections. However, before results are interpreted and applied to patient management, clinicians should perform both internal and external validity checks on the results reported to them.

Internal Validity Checks

Application of the Henderson-Hasselbalch equation makes it easy to identify gross errors in blood gas analysis reports. For example, when the pH is greater than 7.45 (alkalemia), either the CO_2 must be low or the HCO_3^- high. Likewise, in the presence of elevated CO_2 and a decreased HCO_3^-, acidemia must be present. If results are not consistent with the relationship established in the Henderson-Hasselbalch equation, they should be deemed inaccurate and not be acted on. Instead, reanalysis should be undertaken.

External Validity Checks

An important question to ask before making any decisions based on blood gas results is whether the patient's condition is consistent with the results. For example, if a patient presents without cyanosis and is well oriented and in no respiratory distress, a reported Pa_{O_2} of less than 50 mm Hg should be suspect (in this case, likely a venous blood sample).

Another validity check is to assess whether the reported Pa_{O_2} is attainable on the stated F_IO_2. If a patient is breathing room air and the sum of the Pa_{O_2} and Pa_{CO_2} exceeds 150 mm Hg, then either a measurement or reporting error has occurred. Also, any time the Pa_{O_2} is more than five times the O_2 percentage, the results are suspect (the "rule

of 5"). Most likely, the F_IO_2 is higher than reported, or the Pa_{O_2} is inaccurate. For greater accuracy, use the alveolar air equation to determine the $P_{A}O_2$. Any Pa_{O_2} that is equal to or greater than the $P_{A}O_2$ is inaccurate.

Discrepancies between measures made by different devices also can occur. For example, a pulse oximeter may indicate a saturation of 85%, but analysis of an arterial sample with a CO-oximeter may indicate an Sa_{O_2} of 93%. Such discrepancies are best addressed first by determining which results are most consistent with the patient's condition. If this check fails to resolve the difference, generally one should rely on the most valid analysis results, in this case the CO-oximetry results.

> **SIMPLY STATED**
>
> Rule of 5: if the Pa_{O_2} is greater than 5 times the oxygen percentage, the result is suspect.

Systematic Interpretation of Blood Gases

To interpret blood gas measurements, oxygenation should be assessed first, followed by a separate evaluation of acid-base balance. This priority is based on the greater sensitivity and more rapid impact that inadequate oxygenation has on organs and tissues than that caused by acid-based imbalances.

Oxygenation Assessment
Step 1

Identify the Pa_{O_2} and determine whether it is within reference range. In doing so, be sure to account for the patient's age, F_IO_2, and barometric pressure. If hypoxemia is present, determine its cause by assessing the $P(A-a)O_2$ and patient's response to O_2 therapy.

Step 2

Identify the Hb saturation (SaO_2) and compare it to the reference range. Ideally, this assessment should include the SaO_2 obtained by CO-oximetry to determine the impact of dyshemoglobins such as COHb and metHb.

Step 3

Identify the Hb concentration and CaO_2, again ideally through CO-oximetry. Note that CaO_2 values reported from laboratories without CO-oximeters are calculated and may not be accurate. As an alternative, use a recent Hb measurement from a CBC report.

Step 4

Assess the adequacy of circulation. Remember that oxygen delivery depends on both CaO_2 and cardiac output. Basic evaluation of the adequacy of circulation involves assessment of blood pressure and palpation of the extremities for temperature, arterial pulses and capillary refill (see Chapter 5).

Acid-Base Assessment
Step 1

Identify the pH measurement. If pH is within its reference range, a normal acid-base status, a completely compensated acid-base disorder, or a mixed acid-base disorder is present. A normal acid-base status is present when both the $PaCO_2$ and HCO_3^- fall within their reference ranges. If plasma HCO_3^- and $PaCO_2$ are both abnormal with a pH in the normal range, either a fully compensated or mixed acid-base disorder is present.

If the pH is lower than 7.35, the primary imbalance must be an acidosis. Look at HCO_3^- and $PaCO_2$ to identify which one is contributing to the acidosis. An elevated $PaCO_2$ indicates a primary respiratory acidosis, whereas a decreased HCO_3^- indicates a primary metabolic acidosis.

If pH is greater than 7.45, alkalosis is present. An increase in HCO_3^- above its reference range indicates a primary metabolic alkalosis, whereas a decrease in $PaCO_2$ below 35 mm Hg indicates a primary respiratory alkalosis.

Step 2

Once the primary acid-base disorder is identified as either respiratory or metabolic, assess the degree of compensation (see Table 8-7). An elevation in HCO_3^- compensates for respiratory acidosis, and a decrease in HCO_3^- compensates for respiratory alkalosis. On the other hand, a decrease in $PaCO_2$ compensates for metabolic acidosis, and an elevation in $PaCO_2$ compensates for metabolic alkalosis.

In general, when the compensatory response is present but incomplete, the pH will remain outside its normal range. This is called *partial compensation*. On the other

hand, the imbalance is fully compensated if the secondary response restores the pH back to within the reference range. When full compensation occurs, the primary abnormality can be identified by determining on which side of the normal mean (7.4) the pH lies. If the pH is on the acid side (7.35 to 7.39), the primary disturbance is likely the one causing the acidemia. Conversely, if the pH is on the alkaline side (7.41 to 7.45), the primary disturbance is likely the one causing the alkalemia (see Table 8-7).

Compensation for a primary acid-base disturbance often occurs in a predictable manner. This is particularly true for metabolic acidosis, respiratory alkalosis, and respiratory acidosis. A mixed acid-base problem probably is present when the predicted compensation is not present.

KEY POINTS

▸ Blood gas analysis is indicated if the patient's symptoms, medical history, physical examination, or laboratory data suggest abnormalities in respiratory or acid-base status.

▸ If the goal is the most accurate evaluation of oxygenation, ventilation, and acid-base status, then invasive sampling and analysis of an arterial blood sample are required.

▸ The radial artery is the preferred puncture site for ABG sampling because it is accessible, easy to stabilize after puncture, and normally has good collateral circulation.

▸ Arterial puncture causes trauma, so an indwelling arterial catheter, or A-line, should be used when frequent sampling is necessary.

▸ Measurement of normal and abnormal Hb content and actual saturation normally requires sample analysis through hemoximetry (CO-oximetry).

▸ Pulse oximeters only provide oxygenation data; abnormalities in ventilation and/or acid-base balance can go undetected unless they too are measured.

▸ A measured PaO_2 below the predicted range for a patient breathing room air, regardless of the actual F_IO_2, is called hypoxemia; hypoxia exits when oxygen delivery to the tissues is inadequate to meet their needs.

▸ Hypoxemia occurs secondary to ventilation/perfusion ($\dot{V}/\dot{Q}$) mismatch, shunt, diffusion defect, hypoventilation, or a reduced partial pressure of oxygen in the inhaled gas (P_IO_2), with ($\dot{V}/\dot{Q}$ mismatch being the most common cause of hypoxemia.

▸ Alkalosis, hypocapnia, hypothermia, fetal Hb, and HbCO shift the oxyhemoglobin curve to the left, resulting in higher SaO_2 values at the same PaO_2 (impaired unloading at the tissues).

▸ Acidosis, hypercapnia, and fever shift the curve to the right and result in lower SaO_2 values for the same PaO_2 (improved unloading at the tissues).

▸ The pH is a reflection of the acid-base status of the arterial blood.

▸ The $PaCO_2$ is the best measure for assessing the adequacy of ventilation but should be interpreted in conjunction with knowledge of the patient's minute ventilation.

▸ The plasma HCO_3^- is primarily a reflection of the metabolic component of acid-base balance and is regulated by the renal system.

KEY POINTS—cont'd

▶ Arterial blood pH is determined by the ratio of HCO_3^- to $Paco_2$, which normally is 20:1.

▶ Respiratory acidosis is present when the pH indicates acidemia and the $Paco_2$ is elevated above its reference range; respiratory alkalosis is present when the pH indicates alkalemia and the $Paco_2$ is decreased below its reference range.

▶ Metabolic acidosis is present when the pH indicates acidemia and the HCO_3^- or BE falls below its reference range; metabolic alkalosis is present when the pH indicates alkalemia and the HCO_3^- or BE is elevated above its reference range.

▶ When metabolic acidosis is accompanied by a $Paco_2$ that is lower than the predicted level for the degree of acidosis, a respiratory alkalosis is occurring simultaneously. This is known as a *mixed acid-base disorder*.

▶ Venous admixture, air in the sample, excessive liquid anticoagulant, and ongoing cell metabolism can all lead to preanalytic errors in measurement of blood gas parameters.

▶ Analytic errors in measurement of blood gas parameters can be minimized by instrument calibration, calibration verification, and ongoing proficiency testing.

▶ Never act on a blood gas report without first performing internal and external validity checks on the data.

CASE STUDY

A 52-year-old man is admitted to the hospital after a sudden onset of chest pain and shortness of breath. Thirty minutes after admission to intensive care unit, the patient suffered cardiac arrest. Cardiopulmonary resuscitation was initiated and was successful after about 10 minutes.

Initial examination after resuscitation revealed that the patient was hypotensive with a spontaneous respiratory rate of 40 breaths/minute and a heart rate of 120 beats/minute. He was comatose, with central cyanosis, cool extremities, coarse inspiratory and expiratory crackles, and weak pulse. The initial blood gas measurements after resuscitation were as follows:

Parameter	Results
pH	7.17
$Paco_2$	40 mm Hg
Pao_2	53 mm Hg
Sao_2	85%
Cao_2	11 mL/dL
HCO_3^-	14 mmol/L
BE	−14 mmol/L
F_IO_2	1.0
$P(A-a)o_2$	610 mm Hg

Interpretation

The Pao_2 of 53 mm Hg is considered moderate hypoxemia; however, considering that the patient is breathing 100% oxygen, the Pao_2 is significantly below the value predicted by the alveolar air equation (>650 mm Hg). The high $P(A-a)O_2$ on 100% O_2 indicates that the primary cause

of the hypoxemia is shunting. The Sao_2 and Cao_2 are significantly lower than normal. Since Cao_2 is reduced proportionately more than Sao_2, the patient must be anemic.

The clinical signs of tissue hypoxia and metabolic acidosis probably are related. The lack of adequate oxygenation and circulation of the arterial blood is resulting in anaerobic metabolism and lactic acidosis. When hypoxemia and the clinical signs of inadequate perfusion occur simultaneously, metabolic acidosis from the production of lactic acid is a possibility.

The pH is well below normal, indicating acidemia. The plasma HCO_3^- is reduced, and the $Paco_2$ is normal, indicating metabolic acidosis as the primary problem. When primary metabolic acidosis is occurring, the expected compensatory change in $Paco_2$ can be calculated by using the following formula:

$$Paco_2 = [(1.5 \times HCO_3^-) + 8] \pm 2$$
$$\text{Expected } Paco_2 = [(1.5 \times 14) + 8] = 29 \pm 2$$

Since the measured $Paco_2$ is higher than this value, a ventilatory disorder also must be present. A lack of adequate pulmonary perfusion probably is resulting in an increase in wasted or dead space ventilation. A combined metabolic and respiratory acidosis is present.

CASE STUDY

A 12-year-old boy is brought to the emergency department with chief complaints of shortness of breath and cough. His past medical history was positive for allergies and atopic disorders (eczema). His family history was also positive for allergies and asthma. Physical examination revealed the following:

Pulse	124 beats/min
Respiratory rate	35 breaths/min
Blood pressure	120/76 mm Hg
Temperature	98.9° F

The boy was restless and using his accessory muscles to breathe. Bilateral expiratory wheezes were heard on auscultation. His chest appeared hyperexpanded. His expiratory phase was prolonged. The complete blood count demonstrated a slight increase in white blood cells as a result of eosinophilia. The hemoglobin and hematocrit levels were within normal limits. Arterial blood gas measurements were as follows:

Parameter	Results
pH	7.49
$Paco_2$	30 mm Hg
Pao_2	68 mm Hg
Sao_2	91.5%
Cao_2	16 mL/dL
HCO_3^-	22 mmol/L
BE	−1 mmol/L

CASE STUDY—cont'd

Parameter	Results
F_IO_2	0.21
$P(A\text{-}a)O_2$	40 mm Hg

Interpretation

The PaO_2 and SaO_2 are decreased and indicate mild hypoxemia. However, because the CaO_2 is within its reference range, anemia must not be present. The slight increase in $P(A\text{-}a)O_2$ indicates that the hypoxemia is most likely due to $\dot{V}/\dot{Q}$ mismatching. The clinical signs of hypoxemia are evident by the tachycardia and tachypnea. The hypoxemia probably would be worse if the patient were not hyperventilating.

The pH indicates alkalemia and corresponds to decreased $PaCO_2$. The HCO_3^- is within its reference range, so a simple uncompensated respiratory alkalosis is present. The respiratory alkalosis is a result of the tachypnea and shortness of breath. The patient has an increase in the work of breathing because of diffuse airway obstruction, as evidenced by the expiratory wheezing. It is important to note that, although the arterial blood gas measurements do not identify any severe abnormalities, the patient's cardiopulmonary system is working hard to maintain these borderline measurements. Without proper treatment, the patient's condition could deteriorate rapidly.

CASE STUDY

A 57-year-old man has a history of chronic cough and sputum production. He was admitted to the hospital for abdominal surgery. On admission, the patient was noted to be using his accessory muscles to breathe, and he appeared mildly short of breath at rest. He had diminished breath sounds bilaterally, increased anteroposterior chest diameter, and increased resonance to percussion. He has an 80-pack-year smoking history. As part of the preoperative evaluation, blood gases were drawn and revealed the following:

Parameter	Results
pH	7.41
$PaCO_2$	60 mm Hg
PaO_2	66 mm Hg
SaO_2	91.4%
CaO_2	12.2 mL/dL
HCO_3^-	37 mmol/L
BE	+11 mmol/L
F_IO_2	2 L/min via cannula

Interpretation

Mild hypoxemia is present even though the patient is breathing supplemental oxygen through a nasal cannula. The hypoxemia probably is a result of hypoventilation and mismatching. With an SaO_2 above 90%, the CaO_2 should be closer to 20 mL/dL. Since it is lower than normal, anemia is likely.

The pH is within normal range; however, the $PaCO_2$ and HCO_3^- are elevated above normal. The initial temptation is to interpret the acid-base status as completely compensated metabolic alkalosis because the pH is on the alkaline side of 7.40. However, in light of the patient's history and physical examination findings and because patients with normal respiratory systems usually do not hypoventilate significantly to compensate for metabolic alkalosis, the correct interpretation probably is respiratory acidosis and metabolic alkalosis. A mixed acid-base disorder is present. A cause for metabolic alkalosis must be sought to optimize respiratory function before surgery.

CASE STUDY

A 25-year-old woman has no previous history of cardiopulmonary disease. She was admitted to the hospital complaining of frequent urination, excessive thirst, and nausea for the past 3 days. At the time of admission, she was drowsy but coherent, her skin was warm and dry, and her breathing was extremely deep and rapid. Blood gas and chemistry results were as follows:

Parameter	Results
pH	7.13
$PaCO_2$	17 mm Hg
PaO_2	110 mm Hg
SaO_2	99%
CaO_2	19 mL/dL
HCO_3^-	5.5 mmol/L
BE	−21 mmol/L
F_IO_2	Room air
Na^+	142 mmol/L
Cl^-	106 mmol/L

Interpretation

The patient's oxygenation status is normal, with the PaO_2 actually higher than predicted on room air. This is due to the profound hyperventilation (likely Kussmaul respirations), which in reducing the $PaCO_2$ has simultaneously elevated the PaO_2.

The pH is well below its reference range (acidemia) and corresponds to the large decrease in HCO_3^- and BE. The $PaCO_2$ is significantly reduced, indicating that the respiratory system is attempting to compensate for the severe metabolic acidosis.

The expected compensation for the metabolic acidosis can be calculated as follows:

$$PaCO_2 = [(1.5 \times 5.5) + 8] \pm 2$$
$$PaCO_2 = [(8.25) + 8] \pm 2$$
$$PaCO_2 = 16.25 \pm 2$$

The measured $PaCO_2$ (17 mm Hg) is consistent with the expected compensatory response. However, the metabolic acidosis remains only partially compensated owing its severity and the limited ability of the patient to further increase her ventilation. The anion gap (Na^+ − [Cl^- + HCO_3^-]) is 30.5 mmol/L. This result is well above the common reference range of 8 to 16 mmol/L and indicates that the metabolic acidosis is due to acid gain, consistent with a severe diabetic ketoacidosis.

CASE STUDY

A 38-year-old woman has a positive smoking history but no history of cardiopulmonary disease. She came to the emergency department complaining of right lower quadrant abdominal pain. She is quickly diagnosed with acute appendicitis and taken to the operating room for an emergency appendectomy. The surgery went well. She is brought to the surgical intensive care unit because she is slow waking up from anesthesia. After extubation, she is breathing spontaneously on a 35% air entrainment mask. The attending physician ordered arterial blood gas studies. The results revealed the following:

Parameter	Results
pH	7.55
$Paco_2$	44 mm Hg
Pao_2	210 mm Hg
Sao_2	100%
Cao_2	17.5 mL/dL
HCO_3^-	22 mmol/L
BE	−4 mmol/L
F_Io_2	0.35

Interpretation

Regarding the patient's oxygenation status, her Pao_2 is 210 mm Hg and Sao_2 is 100%. Although these values look very good, a quick check should be performed before taking action. The Rule of 5 should be applied as follows:

$$\% \ O_2 \times 5 = \text{estimated maximum } PaO_2$$
$$35\% \ \times 5 = 175 \text{ mm Hg}$$

That the patient's Pao_2 is higher than the maximum suggests an error. To confirm that this is an error, the Pao_2 should be computed:

$$Pao_2 = F_Io_2(PB - PH_2O) - (Paco_2 \times 1.25)$$
$$Pao_2 = 0.35(760 - 47) - (44 \times 1.25)$$
$$Pao_2 = 0.35(713) - (55)$$
$$Pao_2 = 250 - 55$$
$$Pao_2 = 195 \text{ mm Hg}$$

Thus, the reported Pao_2 has to be inaccurate if the patient is breathing 35% O_2. There are two possible explanations: either the patient was receiving more than 35% O_2, or the reported Pao_2 is incorrect. If oxygen analysis confirms that the patient is breathing 35%, then the laboratory should be called and informed that an error has occurred.

In terms of acid-base balance, the pH is well above the normal range (alkalemia). The $Paco_2$ is at the high end of its reference range, which would tend to slightly lower the pH. This suggests that alkalosis is not of respiratory origin. The HCO_3^- is on the low end of its reference range, which would also decrease the pH. Thus, considering the combination of slightly elevated $Paco_2$ and a mildly decreased HCO_3^-, the pH should be on the acid side of normal. To confirm whether an error has occurred, the $Paco_2$ and HCO_3^- should be entered into the Henderson-Hasselbalch equation:

$$pH = 6.1 + \log [HCO_3^- / Paco_2 \times 0.03]$$
$$pH = 6.1 + \log [22/44 \times 0.03]$$
$$pH = 6.1 + \log 16.67$$
$$pH = 7.32$$

This confirms another potential laboratory error. Based on these validity checks, no patient management decisions should be made on these data until another arterial sample is obtained and sent to the laboratory for retesting.

ASSESSMENT QUESTIONS

See Appendix for answers.

1. What is the common reference range for arterial pH?
   a. 7.25-7.35
   b. 7.35-7.45
   c. 7.45-7.55
   d. 7.55-7.65
2. What is the common reference range for Pao_2 breathing air at sea level?
   a. 50-60 mm Hg
   b. 60-70 mm Hg
   c. 70-80 mm Hg
   d. 80-100 mm Hg
3. What is the common reference range for CaO_2?
   a. 16-20 mL/dL
   b. 12-16 mL/dL
   c. 8-12 mL/dL
   d. 4-8 mL/dL
4. To evaluate a patient's acid-base status, you would recommend which of the following?
   a. Transcutaneous Pco_2
   b. Pulse oximetry
   c. Arterial blood gas
   d. CO-oximetry
5. To measure actual blood O_2 saturation, you would recommend:
   a. Transcutaneous Po_2
   b. Pulse oximetry
   c. Arterial blood gas
   d. CO-oximetry

6. Which of the following could you use to assess the adequacy of ventilation in an intubated child receiving mechanical ventilation?
   1. Transcutaneous P_{CO_2}
   2. Capnography
   3. Pulse oximetry
   4. Arterial blood gas
      a. 1 and 2 only
      b. 1, 2, and 4
      c. 4 only
      d. 1, 2, and 3

7. Continuous noninvasive assessment of patient oxygenation can be provided by which of the following methods?
   1. Transcutaneous P_{O_2}
   2. Capnography
   3. Pulse oximetry
   4. Indwelling arterial line
      a. 1 and 3 only
      b. 1 and 2 only
      c. 3 and 4 only
      d. 1, 3, and 4

8. A patient receiving mechanical ventilation requires frequent assessment of oxygenation, ventilation, and acid-base balance. Which of the following would you recommend?
   a. $Ptco_2/Ptcco_2$ monitoring
   b. Continuous pulse oximetry
   c. Continuous capnography
   d. Arterial blood gas sampling through an A-line

9. Before an arterial blood gas sample is obtained, the patient's clotting parameters should be evaluated because:
   a. They may affect the accuracy of the sample Pao_2
   b. If reduced, they may hinder filling of the syringe
   c. Bleeding time may be prolonged if they are abnormal
   d. They may impact the accuracy of sample pH

10. Which of the following is the preferred site for arterial puncture?
    a. Radial artery
    b. Femoral artery
    c. Dorsalis pedis
    d. Brachial artery

11. In performing an Allen test on a patient's left wrist before drawing an arterial sample, you note that her hand remains blanched for more than 25 seconds after releasing pressure on the ulnar artery. Which of the following actions would you take at this time?
    a. Insert a catheter into the brachial artery
    b. Repeat the test on the opposite wrist
    c. Report that the sample cannot be obtained
    d. Proceed with sampling through left radial artery

12. Which of the following infection control precautions would you apply when obtaining an arterial blood gas sample?
    a. Standard precautions plus face shield
    b. Contact precautions plus gown
    c. Droplet precautions plus surgical mask
    d. Airborne precautions plus N95 respirator

13. A patient has a measured Sao_2 of 82%. What is his approximate Pao_2?
    a. 50 mm Hg
    b. 60 mm Hg
    c. 70 mm Hg
    d. 80 mm Hg

14. Which of the following is TRUE regarding standard pulse oximeters?
    a. They measure the fractional saturation of Hb (O_2 Hb to total Hb)
    b. In patients with good perfusion, their accuracy is in the 2% to 4% range
    c. Their accuracy increases when the Hb saturation drops below 65% to 70%
    d. In the presence of dyshemoglobins, they tend to underestimate the true Sao_2

15. A 5-year-old patient is admitted to the emergency department with suspected smoke inhalation. To assess the oxygenation status, you would recommend:
    a. Standard pulse oximetry
    b. Arterial sample plus arterial blood gas analysis
    c. Trancutaneous P_{O_2}
    d. Arterial sample + CO-oximetry

16. Which of the following represents a normal $P(A-a)o_2$ for a 50-year-old woman breathing room air?
    a. 105 mm Hg
    b. 75 mm Hg
    c. 45 mm Hg
    d. 15 mm Hg

17. An 80-year-old patient has a Pao_2 of 71 mm Hg. How would you describe this finding?
    a. Normal for his age
    b. Mild hypoxemia
    c. Moderate hypoxemia
    d. Severe hypoxemia

18. A patient breathing 40% O_2 has a markedly higher than normal $P(A-a)o_2$, which does not improve when the O_2 concentration is increased to 50%. What is the most likely cause of her hypoxemia?
    a. $\dot{V}/\dot{Q}$ imbalance
    b. Pulmonary shunting
    c. Hypoventilation
    d. Diffusion defect

19. Which of the following parameters represents the respiratory component of acid-base status?
    a. $Paco_2$
    b. HCO_3^-
    c. Pao_2
    d. BE

20. Which of the following is the best indicator of metabolic acid-base status?
    a. Plasma HCO_3^-
    b. Base excess
    c. Standard HCO_3^-
    d. T40 HCO_3^-

21. Which of the following ratios of $HCO_3^-/Paco_2$ would result in a pH of 7.40?
    a. 24:1
    b. 10:0.5
    c. 6:0.82
    d. 15:1

22. Which of the arterial blood gas acid-base reports represents an error?
    a. pH = 7.30, $Paco_2$ = 60 mm Hg, HCO_3^- = 29 mmol/L
    b. pH = 7.40, $Paco_2$ = 25 mm Hg, HCO_3^- = 15 mmol/L
    c. pH = 7.50, $Paco_2$ = 50 mm Hg, HCO_3^- = 20 mmol/L
    d. pH = 7.60, $Paco_2$ = 35 mm Hg, HCO_3^- = 33 mmol/L

23. Which of the following is TRUE regarding respiratory alkalosis?
    a. The $Paco_2$ is less than 35 mm Hg
    b. An increase in HCO_3^- compensates for respiratory alkalosis
    c. It is called completely compensated if the pH is 7.52
    d. It is called partially compensated if the pH is in the normal range

24. A patient has the following arterial blood gas results: pH 7.33, $Paco_2$ 35 mm Hg, 18 mmol/L, BE −7 mmol/L. Based on these findings, the patient has which of the following?
    a. Compensated metabolic acidosis
    b. Uncompensated respiratory acidosis
    c. Uncompensated metabolic acidosis
    d. Compensated respiratory acidosis

25. A 35-year-old, 54-kg woman with congestive heart failure enters the emergency department short of breath. An arterial blood gas sample shows the following results: pH 7.51, $Paco_2$ 30 mm Hg, HCO_3^- 23 mmol/L, BE +1 mmol/L. These results indicate which of the following?
    a. Uncompensated respiratory alkalosis
    b. Compensated respiratory acidosis
    c. Uncompensated metabolic alkalosis
    d. Uncompensated metabolic acidosis

26. Given the following arterial blood gas results, interpret the acid-base status: pH 7.45, $Paco_2$ 25 mm Hg, HCO_3^- 17 mmol/L, BE −6 mmol/L.
    a. Compensated metabolic acidosis
    b. Uncompensated respiratory alkalosis
    c. Uncompensated respiratory acidosis
    d. Compensated respiratory alkalosis

27. A 17-year-old man is brought into the emergency department. Vitals are as follows: pulse, 100 beats/minute; respiratory rate, 4 breaths/minute; and blood pressure, 100/65 mm Hg. The patient was at a party where he was discovered by his friends to be slumped in a chair and unresponsive. Arterial blood gas results are as follows: pH 7.24, $Paco_2$ 68 mm Hg, HCO_3^- 28 mmol/L, BE +1 mmol/L. The patient's acid-base status is classified as which of the following?
    a. Uncompensated respiratory acidosis
    b. Partially compensated respiratory acidosis
    c. Compensated respiratory alkalosis
    d. Uncompensated metabolic acidosis

28. An acute increase in $Paco_2$ of 10 to 15 mm Hg causes a corresponding increase in plasma HCO_3^- of how much?
    a. 1 mmol/L
    b. 2 mmol/L
    c. 3 mmol/L
    d. 4 mmol/L

29. Which of the following causes metabolic acidosis?
    a. Hyperventilation
    b. Renal disease
    c. Hypokalemia
    d. Vomiting

30. Given the following arterial blood gas results, interpret the acid-base status: pH 7.14, $Paco_2$ 55 mm Hg, HCO_3^- 18 mmol/L.
    a. Combined respiratory and metabolic acidosis
    b. Partially compensated respiratory acidosis
    c. Mixed respiratory acidosis and metabolic alkalosis
    d. Uncompensated metabolic acidosis

31. Given the following arterial blood gas results, interpret the acid-base status: pH 7.62, $Paco_2$ 30 mm Hg, HCO_3^- 30 mmol/L.
    a. Partially compensated metabolic alkalosis
    b. Mixed respiratory alkalosis and metabolic acidosis
    c. Combined respiratory and metabolic alkalosis
    d. Uncompensated metabolic alkalosis

32. A mixed metabolic acidosis and respiratory alkalosis is likely when the pH and HCO_3^- are low and the $Paco_2$ is:
    a. Higher than the predicted
    b. Within its reference range
    c. Lower than the predicted
    d. 20 times the concentration

33. Given the following arterial blood gas results, interpret the acid-base status: pH 7.42, $Paco_2$ 56 mm Hg, HCO_3^- 35 mmol/L.
    a. Partially compensated metabolic alkalosis
    b. Mixed metabolic alkalosis and respiratory acidosis
    c. Combined respiratory and metabolic alkalosis
    d. Fully compensated respiratory acidosis

34. The best way to minimize the impact of cell metabolism on analysis of an arterial blood gas sample is to:
    a. Use extra heparin in the syringe
    b. Analyze the sample within 30 minutes
    c. Immediately place the sample in ice
    d. Fully expel all air bubbles

35. The procedure whereby a blood-measuring instrument is exposed to samples at two or more known levels to ensure accuracy is termed:
    a. Proficiency testing
    b. Analyzer calibration
    c. Pre-analytic validation
    d. Preventive maintenance

36. The blood gas results from a patient breathing a confirmed O_2 concentration of 30% indicates a Pa_{O_2} of 250 mm Hg. Based on these data, it can be conclude that the:
    a. Patient has a large pulmonary shunt
    b. Pa_{O_2} is in the expected range for this % O_2
    c. Patient must be at high altitude
    d. Pa_{O_2} is in error and should be re-measured

Answer Questions 37 to 40 based on the following blood gas data:

pH	7.21
Pa_{CO_2}	67 mm Hg
HCO_3^-	26 mmol/L
BE	+2 mmol/L
Pa_{O_2}	49 mm Hg
Sa_{O_2}	78%
Hb	10.1 g/dL
Ca_{O_2}	10.4 mL/dL
Respiratory rate	25 breaths/min
$F_{I}O_2$	0.70

37. Which of the following is TRUE regarding the patient's Pa_{O_2}?
    a. It is adequate
    b. It shows mild hypoxemia
    c. It shows moderate hypoxemia
    d. It shows severe hypoxemia

38. Which of the following is TRUE regarding the patient's oxygen-carrying capacity?
    a. It is normal
    b. It is increased
    c. It is decreased
    d. Unable to determine

39. The acid-base status is classified as:
    a. Uncompensated metabolic alkalosis
    b. Partially compensated metabolic alkalosis
    c. Uncompensated respiratory acidosis
    d. Partially compensated respiratory acidosis

40. Which of the following could cause this patient's problem?
    a. Anxiety and fear
    b. Acute airway obstruction

    c. Lactic acid production
    d. Renal failure

Bibliography

Adrogue HJ. Mixed acid-base disturbances. *J Nephrol* 2006; **19**(Suppl. 9):S97–103.

American Association for Respiratory Care. Clinical practice guideline. Pulse oximetry. *Respir Care* 1991;**36**(12):1406–9.

American Association for Respiratory Care. Clinical practice guideline. Sampling for arterial blood gas analysis. *Respir Care* 1992;**37**(8):891–7.

American Association for Respiratory Care. Clinical practice guideline. Blood gas analysis and hemoximetry: 2001 revision and update. *Respir Care* 2001;**46**(5):498–505.

American Association for Respiratory Care. Clinical practice guideline. Transcutaneous blood gas monitoring for neonatal and pediatric patients: 2004 revision and update. *Respir Care* 2004;**49**(9):1070–2.

Barker SJ, Badal JJ. The measurement of dyshemoglobins and total hemoglobin by pulse oximetry. *Curr Opin Anaesthesiol* 2008;**21**(6):805–10.

Breen PH. Arterial blood gas and pH analysis: clinical approach and interpretation. *Anesthesiol Clin North Am* 2001;**19**(4):885–906.

Casaletto JJ. Differential diagnosis of metabolic acidosis. *Emerg Med Clin North Am* 2005;**23**(3):771–87:ix.

Clinical and Laboratory Standards Institute. *Blood gas and pH analysis and related measurements: approved guideline.* CLSI document C46-A2, 2nd ed. Wayne, PA: Clinical and Laboratory Standards Institute; 2009.

Edwards SL. Pathophysiology of acid base balance: the theory practice relationship. *Intensive Crit Care Nurs* 2008;**24**(1):28–38:quiz 38-40.

Fouzas S, Priftis KN, Anthracopoulos MB. Pulse oximetry in pediatric practice. *Pediatrics* 2011;**128**(4):740–52.

Hardie JA, Vollmer WM, Buist AS, et al. Reference values for arterial blood gases in the elderly. *Chest* 2004;**125**(6): 2053–60.

Jones MB. Basic interpretation of metabolic acidosis. *Crit Care Nurse* 2010;**30**(5):63–9.

Kacmarek R, Stoller JL, Heuer AJ. *Egan's fundamentals of respiratory care.* 10th ed. St Louis: Mosby-Elsevier; 2013.

Kellum JA. Disorders of acid-base balance. *Crit Care Med* 2007;**35**(11):2630–6.

Kemper AR, Mahle WT, Martin GR, et al. Strategies for implementing screening for critical congenital heart disease. *Pediatrics* 2011;**128**(5):e1259–67.

Khanna A, Kurtzman NA. Metabolic alkalosis. *J Nephrol* 2006;**19**(Suppl. 9):S86–96.

Mahle WT, Newburger JW, Matherne GP, et al. Role of pulse oximetry in examining newborns for congenital heart disease: a scientific statement from the American Heart Association and American Academy of Pediatrics. *Circulation* 2009;**120**(5): 447–58.

Malley WJ. *Clinical blood gases: assessment and intervention.* 2nd ed. St Louis: Saunders; 2005.

Pullen Jr RL. Using pulse oximetry accurately. *Nursing* 2010; **40**(4):63.

Reddy P, Mooradian AD. Clinical utility of anion gap in deciphering acid-base disorders. *Int J Clin Pract* 2009;**63**(10):1516–25.

Ruckman JS. CO-oximeters. *Biomed Instrum Technol* 2012;**46**(1): 61–3.

Sandberg KL, Brynjarsson H, Hjalmarson O. Transcutaneous blood gas monitoring during neonatal intensive care. *Acta Paediatr* 2011;**100**(5):676–9.

Storre JH, Magnet FS, Dreher M, et al. Transcutaneous monitoring as a replacement for arterial P_{CO_2} monitoring during nocturnal non-invasive ventilation. *Respir Med* 2011;**105**(1):143–50.

Walsh BK, Crotwell DN, Restrepo RD. Capnography/capnometry during mechanical ventilation: 2011 (American Association for Respiratory Care clinical practice guideline). *Respir Care* 2011;**56**(4):503–9.

Woodrow P. Essential principles: blood gas analysis. *Nurs Crit Care* 2010;**15**(3):152–6.

Yucha C. Renal regulation of acid-base balance. *Nephrol Nurs J* 2004;**31**(2):201–6.

Zijlstra WG. Clinical assessment of oxygen transport-related quantities. *Clin Chem* 2005;**51**(2):291–2.

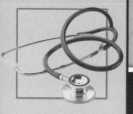

Chapter 9

Pulmonary Function Testing

CRAIG L. SCANLAN*

CHAPTER OUTLINE

Lung Volumes and Capacities
Spirometry
   Indications and Contraindications
   Forced Vital Capacity
   Flow-Volume Loops
   Maximal Voluntary Ventilation
   Spirometry Quality Assurance
   Interpretation of Spirometry Test Results
Static Lung Volumes
   Indications and Contraindications
   Methods
   Interpretation

Diffusing Capacity of the Lung (D_{LCO})
   Indications
   Equipment and Quality Assurance
   Test Procedure and Calculations
   Interpretation
Specialized Tests
   Airway Resistance
   Lung and Chest Wall Compliance
   Airway Hyperresponsiveness and Inflammation
   Exercise Tests
Infection Control

LEARNING OBJECTIVES

After reading this chapter, you will be able to:
1. Define and cite typical values for and differentiate among the lung volumes and capacities.
2. Compute any lung capacity based its constituent parts.
3. Specify the indications and contraindications for basic spirometry.
4. Differentiate between the measurement and use of the slow and forced vital capacity.
5. Define the parameters typically derived from a forced vital capacity (FVC) maneuver, plotted as volume versus time.
6. Describe the appropriate use of the peak expiratory flow measure.
7. Define the parameters typically derived from the maximal inspiratory-expiratory flow-volume curves and their use in identifying patterns of ventilatory impairment.
8. Define, describe the utility, and specify how to estimate the maximal voluntary ventilation.
9. Identify the necessary calibration tests and accuracy standards for spirometry equipment.
10. Outline the key procedural elements required to obtain accurate spirometry data.
11. Specify the acceptability and repeatability criteria for FVC measurements.
12. Apply the concept of reference ranges and upper and lower limits of normal to the interpretation of spirometry data.
13. Given a subject's basic spirometry test parameters, classify the results as representing normal function or an obstructive or restrictive ventilatory impairment.
14. Describe how to use basic spirometry to assess for reversibility of an obstructive ventilatory impairment.
15. Specify the indications and contraindications for static lung volume determination.
16. Differentiate among the principles employed, equipment used, and quality assurance standards associated with the three primary methods for measuring functional residual capacity.
17. Compare and contrast the patterns of lung volumes and capacities in normal subjects and those with either an obstructive or restrictive ventilatory impairment.
18. Specify the indications for measuring the diffusing capacity of the lung (D_{LCO}).
19. Identify the equipment needed and test and quality assurance procedures used to measure D_{LCO}.

---

*Dr. Robert Wilkins and James Dexter contributed some of the content for this chapter as coeditors of the prior edition of this text.

LEARNING OBJECTIVES—cont'd

20. In combination with spirometry and lung volume values, apply DLCO measurements to differentiate among blood/pulmonary vascular disorders and potential causes of restrictive and obstructive ventilatory impairments.
21. Describe three methods used to measure airway resistance and its commonly cited normal reference range.
22. Describe how lung compliance is measured and the commonly cited normal values for lung, thorax/chest wall, and total compliance.
23. Identify the indications for methacholine bronchoprovocation testing, the basic procedure used, and how results are interpreted to classify airway responsiveness.
24. Describe the indications, equipment needed, and quality assurance procedures for measuring expired nitric oxide (F_ENO).
25. Apply recommended F_ENO cut-off points to the diagnosis and management of patients with asthma.
26. Outline the basic steps in the 6-Minute Walk Test, specify the cut-off points associated with abnormal functional capacity, and stipulate the percentage change needed to indicate improvement due to medical or surgical interventions.
27. Specify the indications and contraindications for cardiopulmonary exercise testing.
28. Define the measurements made when assessing exercise capacity and their typical values at peak capacity.
29. Apply the results of exercise testing to differentiate among patients with poor conditioning and those with cardiovascular or pulmonary limitations to exercise.
30. Outline the key infection control standards that apply to pulmonary function testing

KEY TERMS

6MWD	HRmax	obstructive ventilatory impairment
acceptability	inspiratory capacity (IC)	
airway hyperresponsiveness (AHR)	inspiratory reserve volume (IRV)	PC_{20}
airway resistance	interstitial lung disease (IDL)	peak expiratory flow (PEF)
anaerobic threshold	linearity (volume, flow)	reference range
back-extrapolated volume	lower/upper limit of normal (LLN/ULN)	repeatability
biologic control		residual volume (RV)
breathing reserve	maximal expiratory flow-volume curve (MEFV)	respirometer
bronchoprovocation testing	maximal inspiratory flow-volume curve (MIFV)	restrictive ventilatory impairment.
calibration	maximal midexpiratory flow ($FEF_{25-75\%}$)	slow vital capacity (SVC)
compliance		specific conductance (G_{aw}/TGV)
diffusing capacity	maximal voluntary ventilation (MVV)	spirogram
expiratory reserve volume (ERV)	metabolic equivalent of task (MET)	switch-in error
F_ENO	minute volume ($\dot{V}_E$)	thoracic gas volume (TGV)
flow-volume loop	nitrogen washout	tidal volume (V_T)
forced vital capacity (FVC)	O_2 pulse	total lung capacity (TLC)
functional lung volume		vital capacity (VC)
functional residual capacity (FRC)		$\dot{V}_{O_2}$max
		volumeter

Pulmonary function testing commonly includes spirometry, static lung volume measurements, and diffusing capacity studies. Pulmonary function testing may also involve measurement of the mechanical properties of the lungs and thorax, such as airway resistance and compliance. Some pulmonary function laboratories also may assess airway hyperresponsiveness using bronchoprovocation testing or exhaled nitric oxide measurements and perform exercise testing.

Because spirometry is commonly performed by respiratory therapists (RTs) at the bedside, this chapter emphasizes the measurement and interpretation of parameters obtained using this assessment method. However, because full comprehension of the role of pulmonary function testing in diagnosis requires some knowledge of the more advanced tests, they will be discussed in brief. Also covered are basic equipment needs, quality assurance procedures, and infection control considerations. This chapter ends with a selection of case studies designed to assist the learner in interpreting pulmonary function data.

Lung Volumes and Capacities

Fundamental to understanding pulmonary function testing is knowledge of the lung's volumes and capacities. Figure 9-1 portrays the four lung volumes and four lung

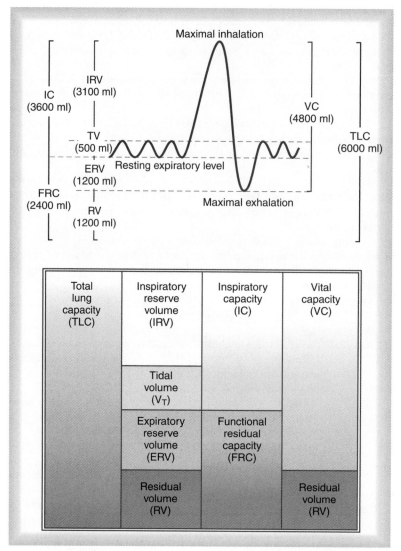

FIGURE 9-1 Lung volumes and capacities. Representation of a simple spirogram and divisions of lung volumes and capacities. (From Kacmarek RM, Stoller JK, Heuer AJ: *Egan's fundamentals of respiratory care,* ed 10, St Louis, 2013, Mosby.)

capacities both as a graphic plot of inspired and expired volumes over time (called a **spirogram**) and as a block diagram. Each measure includes its standard abbreviation, with the spirogram also providing average values for the lung volumes and capacities for a healthy young 70-kg adult male. **Reference ranges** for these measures vary primarily with the height of the individual but are also affected by gender, age, and race.

As indicated in Figure 9-1, the four lung volumes (inspiratory reserve volume [IRV], tidal volume [V_T], expiratory reserve volume [ERV], and residual volume [RV]) are separate from each other and do not overlap. On the other hand, a lung capacity consists of two or more lung volumes. For example, the total lung capacity (TLC) represents the sum of all four lung volumes. As such, lung capacities do overlap with each other. Note that the **residual volume (RV)** and the capacities that include it (functional residual capacity and total lung capacity) are not recorded on the

spirogram plot in Figure 9-1. This is because the residual volume remains in the lungs at all times.

Table 9-1 provides functional definitions for each of these volume and capacities.

> **SIMPLY STATED**
>
> The residual volume and the capacities that include it (FRC and TLC) are not recorded on a simple spirogram because this volume remains in the lungs at all times.

Knowing the tidal volume and rate of breathing (f) allows computation of the volume of gas inhaled or exhaled over 1 minute, called the **minute volume** or *minute ventilation* and abbreviated as $\dot{V}_E$:

$$\dot{V}_E = f \times V_T$$

Minute volume is commonly measured at the bedside using a simple mechanical or electronic **respirometer**. For

TABLE 9-1

Lung Volumes and Capacities

Measure	Abbreviation	Functional Definition
Volumes		
Tidal volume	V_T	Volume of air inhaled or exhaled during each normal breath
Inspiratory reserve volume	IRV	Maximal volume of air that can be inhaled over and above the inspired tidal volume
Expiratory reserve volume	ERV	Maximal volume of air that can be exhaled after exhaling a normal tidal breath
Residual volume	RV	Volume of air remaining in the lungs after a maximal exhalation
Capacities		
Total lung capacity	TLC	Maximal volume of air in the lungs at the end of a maximal inhalation (sum of RV + V_T + ERV + RV)
Functional residual capacity	FRC	Volume of air present in the lung at end-expiration during tidal breathing (sum of RV + ERV)
Inspiratory capacity	IC	Maximal volume of air that can be inhaled from the resting end-expiratory level (sum of IRV + V_T)
Vital capacity	VC	Maximal volume of air that can be exhaled after a maximal inhalation (sum of IC + V_T + ERV)

a typical adult breathing at a frequency of 12 breaths/minute with an average tidal volume of 500 mL, the minute volume would be computed as:

$$\dot{V}_E = 12 \text{ breaths/min} \times 500 \text{ mL/breath}$$
$$= 6000 \text{ mL/min} = 6 \text{ L/min}$$

Normal minute volumes range between 5 and 10 L/minute, depending primarily on the size of the subject. The minute volume increases with fever, pain, hypoxia, acidosis, and increased metabolic rate. It can rise to 60 L/minute or more during strenuous exercise.

Also commonly measured at the bedside is the vital capacity. Two different procedures are used, resulting in different measures. If the patient gently but fully exhales from a maximal inspiration, the resulting measure is called a **slow vital capacity (SVC).** If the patient forcefully empties the lungs from a maximal inspiration, the measure is called the **forced vital capacity (FVC).**

Typically, the SVC is measured using a respirometer. The SVC measurement can help in assessing perioperative risk because it reflects the patient's ability to take a deep breath, cough, and clear the airways of excess secretions. In general, SVC values lower than 20 mL/kg of predicted body weight indicate an increased risk for postoperative respiratory complications. The SVC also has been used as one of many measures to evaluate a patient's need for mechanical ventilation or readiness to wean. The most commonly cited threshold is 15 mL/kg, with lower values indicating inadequate ventilatory reserve and the need for mechanical ventilatory support.

Measurement of the FVC requires more sophisticated instrumentation capable of nearly instantaneous measurement of airflow. The measurement of FVC and its components is the basis for clinical spirometry.

Spirometry

Spirometry is the most commonly performed pulmonary function test. Spirometry testing can be conducted in the pulmonary function laboratory, at a patient's bedside, or in an outpatient clinic or doctor's office. Spirometry primarily involves measurement of parameters during patient performance of an FVC maneuver. Spirometry may also include measurement of a patient's **maximal voluntary ventilation (MVV).**

Indications and Contraindications

Spirometry is indicated to:

- Detect abnormalities in the lung function suggested by patient history, physical examination, or related diagnostic tests such as chest radiograph.
- Quantify the severity or stage of a known lung disease.
- Follow the course of a patient's disease and response to treatment.
- Assess the risk for perioperative pulmonary complications.
- Evaluate patients for the presence of pulmonary-related disabilities.
- Monitor the effects of exposure to drugs or toxins affecting the lungs.

Relative contraindications for performing spirometry include unstable cardiovascular status, hemoptysis, pneumothorax, and any acute condition that might hinder test performance, such as nausea or vomiting.

Forced Vital Capacity

The most common spirometry test is the FVC. Table 9-2 summarizes the parameters typically measured and evaluated during this test.

Figure 9-2 illustrates these parameters on a typical volume-versus-time spirogram. Note that the forced expiratory

TABLE 9-2

Parameters Typically Measured During Spirometry

Parameter	Abbreviation	Definition
Forced vital capacity	FVC	Total volume of air that can be exhaled during a maximal forced expiration effort
Forced expiratory volume in 1 second	FEV_1	Volume of air exhaled in the first second after a maximal forced inhalation
Ratio of FEV_1 to FVC	FEV_1/FVC	Proportion or percentage of the FVC expired during the first second of the maneuver
Forced expiratory volume in 3 seconds	FEV_3	Volume of air exhaled in 3 seconds after a forced maximal inhalation
Forced expiratory volume in 6 seconds	FEV_6	Volume of air exhaled in 6 seconds after a forced maximal inhalation
Peak expiratory flow	PEF	Maximal expiratory flow, typically achieved within 120 msec of the start of the forced exhalation
Maximal midexpiratory flow	$FEF_{25-75\%}$	Average flow occurring between 25% and 75% of the FVC

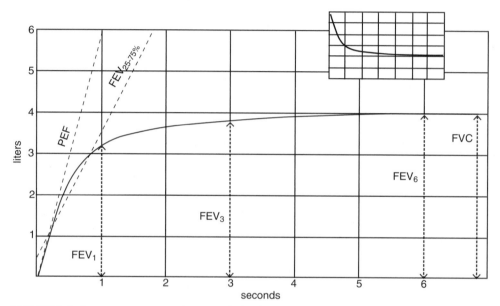

FIGURE 9-2 Parameters measured on a typical volume vs. time spirogram. FEV_1, FEV_3, and FEV_6 are all volumes measured at specific times during the forced exhalation. The PEF and $FEF_{25-75\%}$ are flow measures, computed as slopes on the spirogram ($\Delta V/\Delta T$). The *inset* shows an inverted mirror image of the same curve as produced on some spirometers. (Courtesy of Strategic Learning Associates, LLC, Little Silver, NJ)

volume in 1, 3, and 6 seconds (FEV_1, FEV_3, and FEV_6) are all volumes measured at specific times during the forced exhalation. Note also that a normal individual is able to exhale more than 75% of the FVC in 1 second and generally 95% or more in 3 seconds. However, the minimal time needed to assure a valid FVC measurement is 6 seconds, with some patients requiring more than 10 seconds to fully empty their lungs.

SIMPLY STATED

A normal individual is able to exhale at least 75% of FVC in 1 second and generally 95% or more in 3 seconds.

Unlike the volume measures, the **peak expiratory flow (PEF)** and forced expiratory flow ($FEF_{25-75\%}$) are represented as sloped lines on the graph. The slope of any line on a graph of volume versus time is flow. The line representing

PEF corresponds to the steepest slope of the FVC curve and thus the highest generated flow. The $FEF_{25-75\%}$ line is drawn by connecting the two points corresponding to the 25th and 75th percentiles of the FVC. In this example, the FVC is 4 L, so the 25th percentile is reached at 1 L and the 75th percentile occurs at 3 L. Also in this example, as always should be the case, the slope of the $FEF_{25-75\%}$ line is less than that plotted for the PEF, signifying what is a progressive decrease in flow throughout the maneuver after the initial PEF blast.

In general, the volume measures obtained by spirometry, including the FEV_1/FVC ratio, are more reproducible than the flow measures. In particular, PEF is very effort dependent. For this reason, it is not given much weight in the overall assessment of pulmonary function.

On the other hand, the PEF is often used by patients with asthma to monitor for evidence of bronchospasm.

The test is performed regularly using an inexpensive hand-held peak flowmeter. Results are used to help make self-management decisions and incorporated into personal action plans. Typically, these action plans identify 80% to 100% of the patient's personal best peak flow as the green zone, or normal (no special action required); 50% to 80% of the patient's personal best as the yellow zone (requiring self-administration of bronchodilator plus possibly oral steroids); and below 50% of the patient's personal best as the red zone (requiring self-administration of bronchodilator, contacting the doctor, and calling 9-1-1).

> ### SIMPLY STATED
>
> PEF is a highly effort-dependent measure and is not particularly useful in diagnosing pulmonary dysfunction. However, it is commonly used by patients with asthma to monitor the severity of bronchospasm and its response to treatment.

Flow-Volume Loops

Most electronic spirometers also can display and record the FVC maneuver as a plot of flow versus volume, typically referred to as a **flow-volume loop** (Fig. 9-3). To produce a complete flow-volume loop, the patient must be instructed to take a full forced inspiration to TLC before *and* after the forced exhalation maneuver. The spirometer then records *both* the inspiratory and expiratory efforts. The expiratory component of the maneuver, called the **maximal expiratory flow-volume curve (MEFV)**, is plotted above the horizontal zero flow line, with the **maximal inspiratory flow-volume curve (MIFV)** recorded below the zero flow line. The FVC equals the maximal width of the loop along the zero flow line. The PEF equals the maximal positive deflection on the flow axis, with the peak inspiratory flow (PIF) represented as maximal negative deflection on this axis. The FEF at any point in the FVC can also be measured directly. Typically, spirometers record the FEF at 25%, 50%, and 75% of the FVC. For example, the $FEF_{50\%}$ mark on the flow-volume loop in Figure 9-3 represents the instantaneous forced expiratory flow at 50% of the FVC. Differences in flow between any of these points can also be computed, with the most common being the $FEF_{25-75\%}$, which is equivalent to the same measure plotted on a volume-versus-time spirogram.

None of the expiratory measures obtained from a flow-volume loop have proved superior to the FEV_1, FVC, $FEV_1/$ FVC and $FEF_{25-75\%}$ obtained by volume-versus-time plots. On the other hand, the shape of the MEFV and MIFV curves can be helpful in detecting certain patterns of disease, as discussed subsequently.

Maximal Voluntary Ventilation

The MVV is the maximal volume of air a subject can breathe over a specified period of time, usually 12 seconds. The 12-second volume then is multiplied by 5 to extrapolate what could be achieved in 1 minute, with the

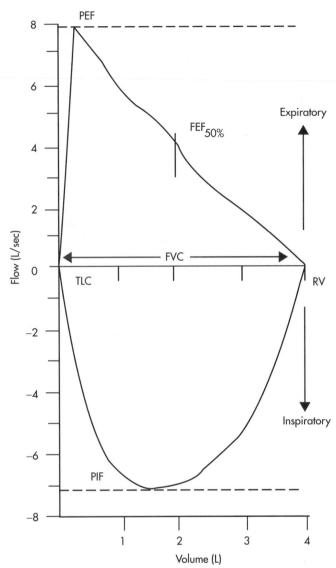

FIGURE 9-3 Example flow-volume loop. Flow in L/sec is plotted on the Y-axis and volume in liters on the X-axis. By convention, expiratory flow is plotted upward (positive), and inspiratory flow is plotted downward (negative). (From Mottram C: *Ruppel's manual of pulmonary function testing*, ed 10, St. Louis, 2013, Mosby.)

value expressed in liters per minute. The MVV is affected by the strength of the respiratory muscles, compliance of the lungs and thorax, inspiratory and expiratory airway resistance, and patient motivation and effort. Reference values vary widely, ranging from more than 170 L/minute for young adult males to less than 90 L/minute for elderly females.

Because one can estimate a patient's MVV by multiplying the measured FEV_1 by a factor of 40, this demanding test is no longer included in most standard spirometry protocols. However, the MVV is still used to assess conditions in which ventilatory capacity may be impaired by mechanisms different from those affecting FEV_1. For example, some patients with neuromuscular disorders exhibit much larger than expected decreases in their MVV relative to that predicted from their FEV_1. The MVV also is used in exercise testing to estimate a subject's breathing reserve (discussed later in this chapter).

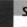 **SIMPLY STATED**

To estimate a patient's MVV, multiply the measured FEV_1 by 40.

Spirometry Quality Assurance

To obtain valid spirometry data requires accurate instrumentation. However, because FVC maneuvers are technique dependent, obtaining accurate data also depends on the subject being able to perform the maneuvers in an acceptable and reproducible way. Thus, there are two major components to spirometry quality assurance: equipment calibration and technique validation.

Equipment Calibration

The American Thoracic Society (ATS) guidelines specify that spirometers should be capable of measuring volumes of 8 L or more and capturing exhalation maneuvers for at least 15 seconds. Volume accuracy should be at least ±3.5% or ±0.065 L, with the measured flow range between 0 and 14 L/second (−14 to + 14 L/second for flow-volume loops). Flow measurements should be accurate within ±5% of the true value over a range of −14 to +14 L/second with a sensitivity (minimal detectable flow) of 0.025 L/second. Spirometers should be able to produce printouts of both volume-time and flow-volume plots.

To assure spirometry accuracy, regular **calibration** tests are required. Table 9-3 summarizes these tests as recommended by the ATS and European Respiratory Society (ERS).

Volume calibration should be performed daily using a calibrated 3-L syringe. The syringe itself must have an accuracy of ±0.5% (±15 mL for a 3-L syringe), which is incorporated into the volume accuracy standard (3.0% + 0.5% = 3.5%). To assess **volume linearity**, the syringe should be discharged in three 1-L steps, with each successive volume meeting the 3.5% accuracy standard. To assess **flow linearity**, the syringe volume should be injected at three different flows, ranging between 0.5 and 12 L/second. With a 3-L syringe, this would equate to injection times between 6 seconds and 0.5 second. The volume at each flow should meet the accuracy standard of ±3.5%.

Regular testing using biologic controls also is recommended to assess spirometer performance and accuracy of software computations. A **biologic control** is a healthy subject for whom quality control data are available. Such data typically include the mean and standard deviation of 8 to 10 reproducible FVC maneuvers measured at different times.

If volume or flow inaccuracy is detected, no tests should be conducted until the cause of the measurement error is corrected. As with any quality assurance program, logs should be maintained to document spirometer calibration, maintenance, and any corrective actions taken.

TABLE 9-3

Calibration Tests for Spirometry Equipment

Test	Minimum Interval	Action
Volume	Daily	Calibration check with a calibrated 3-L syringe
Volume linearity	Quarterly	1-L increments with a calibrated syringe over entire volume range
Flow linearity	Weekly	Test at least three different flow ranges
Software	New versions	Log installation date and perform test using biologic controls and known subject

Technique Validation

FVC maneuvers are highly technique dependent. For this reason, accurate measurements require proper patient performance of the procedure. Providing clear instructions and eliciting a maximal effort are the keys to assuring a valid FVC maneuver. In addition, the clinician must be able to recognize and correct any observed errors in technique.

Box 9-1 outlines the key elements in the measurement of FVC using an electronic bedside spirometer. Most elements also pertain to spirometry measurement in the pulmonary function laboratory.

The goal is to obtain at least three acceptable and error-free maneuvers that are repeatable. An acceptable maneuver must be free from artifacts, exhibit a good and forceful start, and achieve complete exhalation. To assure **repeatability**, the therapist must confirm that the key volume measures (FVC and FEV_1) are free of significant variability. Although many computerized spirometers automatically perform validity checks on each FVC maneuver, the clinician still must manually inspect each plot to confirm that it is acceptable and that the multiple measures are repeatable. A summary of the **acceptability** and repeatability criteria recommended by the ATS/ERS for FVC maneuvers (plotted as volume vs. time) appear in Box 9-2.

The most common error in obtaining an acceptable FVC is failure to achieve a rapid start to the forced exhalation. This typically is evident when the plotted FVC-versus-time curve is S shaped (like the oxyhemoglobin curve). Alternatively, one can change the spirometer display from volume versus time to flow versus volume and inspect the expiratory curve to determine whether the start of test was satisfactory. On a flow-volume curve, the PEF should be achieved with a sharp rise and occur close to the point of maximal inflation.

Spirometry software programs typically identify a slow start to forced exhalation by detecting a delay in time to peak flow (>120 msec) or by calculating the **back-extrapolated volume**. Figure 9-4 demonstrates how the back-extrapolated volume is calculated, normally by the

Box 9-1	Key Elements in Performance of Forced Vital Capacity Maneuver

- Turn device on, insert mouthpiece/sensor, input sensor data, perform start-up test.
- Accurately input all required patient information (height, age, gender race).
- Have the patient remove candy, gum, and dentures from the mouth.
- Have the patient sit upright or stand with good posture and head slightly elevated (be consistent and record position).
- Demonstrate the procedure using your own mouthpiece/sensor, being sure to show:
  - How to hold the sensor steady and avoid jerky motions.
  - How deeply to inhale (completely).
  - How to correctly place the mouthpiece on top of the tongue.
  - How to blast out the breath for as long as possible.
- Use nose clips to prevent patient leaks.
- Have the patient inhale completely and rapidly with a pause of >1 second at TLC.*
- Have the patient place mouthpiece/sensor in mouth and obtain tight seal with lips.
- Have the patient perform the FVC maneuver while you observe.
- Have the patient BLAST the breath out, as fast and long as possible.
- Loudly prompt MORE, MORE, MORE, until the subject has exhaled for at least 6 seconds.
- Carefully observe the patient for poor technique and correct as needed.
- Repeat instructions as necessary, coaching vigorously.
- Repeat the procedure until you have three acceptable maneuvers.
- Document the quality of the results, including any validity issues.

*To produce a complete flow-volume loop (MEFV + MIFV curves), the patient places the mouthpiece/sensor in mouth before inhalation and must be instructed to take a full forced inspiration to TLC before and after the forced exhalation maneuver.

Box 9-2	Acceptability and Repeatability Criteria for Forced Vital Capacity Maneuvers

The spirogram is *acceptable* if it is:
- Free from artifacts
  - Coughing/breathing during the maneuver
  - Early termination or cut-off
  - Submaximal effort
- Exhibits a rapid, forceful start
  - Time to peak flow <120 msec
  - Back extrapolated volume <5% of FVC or 150 mL, whichever is greater
- Achieves complete exhalation
  - Duration of at least 6 sec (COPD patients may need >10 second), *or*
  - Attainment of a plateau (<25 mL change in volume for ≥1 second)

Results are *repeatable* if after three acceptable spirograms have been obtained:
- The two largest values of FVC must be within 0.150 L of each other, *and*
- The two largest values of FEV_1 must be within 0.150 L of each other

COPD, chronic obstructive pulmonary disease; FVC, forced vital capacity; FEV_1, forced expiratory volume at 1 second.

Interpretation of Spirometry Test Results

Interpretation of spirometry test results normally is performed by a trained physician. Assessment involves comparison of the individual patient's data with reference values generated from samples of healthy subjects and review of the applicable plots.

Although other spirometry reference values are available, the preferred prediction equations for subjects 8 to 80 years of age are those established by the National Health and Nutrition Examination Survey (NHANES) III. These equations provide reference ranges for all spirometry parameters based on the subject's height, gender, age, and race.

The pulmonary function community has adopted ±2 standard deviations (SD) from the predicted mean as the normal reference range. With ±2 SD encompassing 95% of the values in a normal distribution (Fig. 9-5), one can define the boundaries of this range as cut-off points, outside of which results are abnormal. These cut-off points are called the **lower limit of normal (LLN)** and (if applicable) the **upper limit of normal (ULN).**

For interpretation of tests in which either abnormally low or high values apply, the LLN occurs at the 2.5th percentile and the ULN at the 97.5th percentile. If only abnormally low values are the focus (as with spirometry measures), then only the LLN is applicable, which corresponds to values in the distribution below the 5th percentile.

Figure 9-6 outlines the basic process for interpreting spirometry test results. After ensuring that the test results

spirometer's microprocessor. If the back-extrapolated volume is more than 5% of FVC or more than 150 mL, the FVC is unacceptable, and a repeat maneuver is required. On the other hand, if the back-extrapolated volume falls below this quality threshold, the FVC breath still can be used, but with the breath starting point adjusted to the new extrapolated zero time point.

If no acceptable maneuvers can be obtained, results should not be reported; rather, all specific errors encountered should be documented. Only if three acceptable maneuvers can be obtained, meeting both repeatability criteria, should results be reported. If the initial results are acceptable but are not repeatable, additional testing should be conducted until either the repeatability criteria are met or the patient cannot continue. All reports should contain the therapist's overall assessment of test quality.

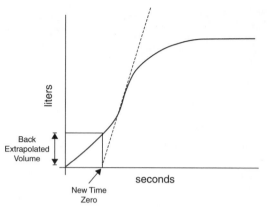

FIGURE 9-4 Calculation of back extrapolated volume (BEV). Back-extrapolation is used when the spirogram does not exhibit a sharp rise in flow at the beginning of the forced vital capacity (FVC). To compute the BEV, a straight line is drawn through the steepest part of the curve and extended to cross the volume baseline. The point of intersection is the back-extrapolated time zero. The distance from the time zero point to the FVC curve is the BEV. (Courtesy of Strategic Learning Associates, LLC, Little Silver, NJ)

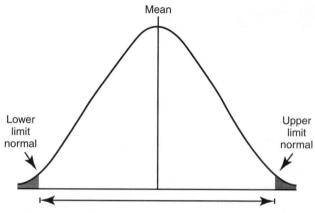

± 2 standard deviations (95% of the values)

FIGURE 9-5 Determination of upper and lower limits of normal. Ninety-five percent of all values in a normal distribution fall within ±2 standard deviations (SD) of the mean. The boundaries of this range are the lower limit of normal (LLN) and the upper limit of normal (ULN). (Courtesy of Strategic Learning Associates, LLC, Little Silver, NJ)

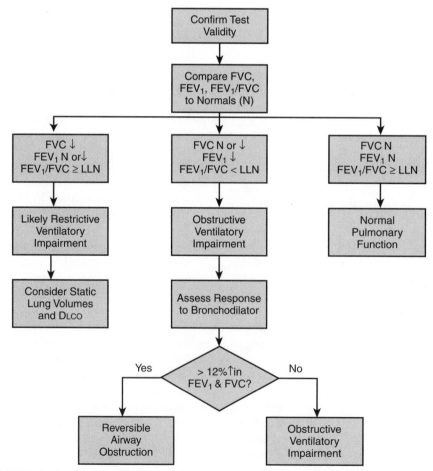

FIGURE 9-6 Algorithm for interpreting spirometry test results. D_{LCO}, diffusing capacity; FVC, forced vital capacity; LLN, lower limit of normal. (Courtesy of Strategic Learning Associates, LLC, Little Silver, NJ)

are valid (three acceptable maneuvers, with two of them being repeatable), one compares the patient's FVC, FEV_1, and FEV_1/FVC to the predicted reference ranges. If all three values fall within the reference ranges, the results are deemed normal.

If, however, the FEV_1 is reduced and the FEV_1/FVC ratio falls below its LLN (below the 5th percentile of predicted), an expiratory flow limitation exists, and the patient is classified as having an **obstructive ventilatory impairment**. Often, the severity of obstruction is quantified according to magnitude of reduction in FEV_1/FVC, as outlined in Table 9-4.

The other major possibility is a reduced FVC, normal or reduced FEV_1, and FEV_1/FVC *above* the LLN (normal or higher than normal). *An FEV_1/FVC above the LLN rules out an obstructive impairment.* However, the presence of a reduced FVC suggests that the patient may have a reduction in lung volume, which would be classified as a **restrictive ventilatory impairment**.

SIMPLY STATED

An obstructive ventilatory impairment is characterized by reduced flows, as evident by an FEV_1/FVC ratio lower than the predicted lower limit of normal. A restrictive ventilatory impairment is characterized by decreased lung volumes.

TABLE 9-4

Severity Classification of Airway Obstruction

Severity of Obstruction	FEV_1 (% Predicted)
Mild	70-74
Moderate	60-69
Moderately severe	50-59
Severe	35-49
Very severe	<35

Interpretation is enhanced by review of the graphic plots obtained by spirometry. Figure 9-7 portrays typical volume-versus-time curves for a normal subject, one with an obstructive impairment and one with a restrictive disorder. Note that the obstructive pattern is characterized by a decrease in the slope of the curve (indicating reduction in expiratory flow) and a longer time to empty the lungs. On the other hand, in the restrictive pattern, the lung empties as fast or faster than normal but to a smaller volume.

Inspection of the patient's flow-volume loop can aid in interpretation, especially in identifying the presence and location of large airway obstruction. Figure 9-8 provides six examples of flow-volume loops representing distinct patterns of abnormal function. Disorders causing generalized expiratory obstruction—like asthma and emphysema—mainly affect the MEFV curve, with both exhibiting a reduction in peak flow and $FEF_{50\%}$. Note also that the MEFV portion of the loop on the patient with emphysema is markedly concave and positioned left of the normal loop, indicating greater flow obstruction at lower lung volumes as well as air trapping and hyperinflation. On the other hand, a patient with a restrictive ventilatory impairment typically produces a flow-volume loop with the same shape as normal, but one that is markedly narrower on the volume axis, consistent with the smaller FVC.

The bottom three flow-volume loops in Figure 9-8 portray different types of *large airway obstruction*. The variable intrathoracic obstruction loop reveals a markedly reduced peak flow on expiration despite near-normal inspiratory flows. This typically is the result of expiratory flow obstruction in the large airways, as may occur with tracheomalacia or tumors of the trachea or bronchi. The opposite pattern is seen in variable extrathoracic obstruction, that is, reduced inspiratory flow and relatively normal expiratory flow. Vocal cord dysfunction and laryngeal edema are common causes of variable extrathoracic obstruction. An equal

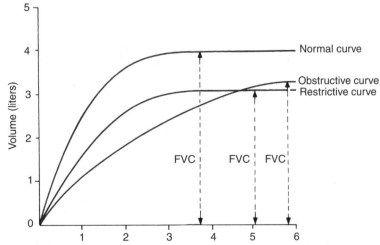

FIGURE 9-7 Forced vital capacity (FVC) curves comparing normal, obstructive, and restrictive disorders. Curves are as they appear on commonly available spirometers with tracings beginning at the bottom left corner. (From Kacmarek RM, Stoller JK, Heuer AJ: *Egan's fundamentals of respiratory care,* ed 10, St. Louis, 2013, Mosby.)

reduction in inspiratory and expiratory flows suggests a fixed large airway obstruction. Causes of fixed large airway obstruction include tracheal stenosis, tracheal tumors, and foreign body aspiration.

After the basic pattern is identified, additional testing may be indicated. If the spirometry results indicate that the patient has an expiratory obstructive impairment, the doctor typically will want to determine whether the obstruction is reversible with treatment, that is, if it responds to bronchodilator therapy (see Fig. 9-6). This is accomplished by measuring spirometry values before and after administration of the selected bronchodilator. Normally, the baseline spirometry should be conducted at least 4 hours after any prior use of a short-acting β-agonist (e.g., albuterol) and at least 12 hours after any administration of a long-acting bronchodilator (e.g., salmeterol).

Box 9-3 outlines the key elements in the procedure for assessing reversibility. If after bronchodilator administration, the FEV_1 or FVC increases by more than 12% and at least 200 mL, the obstructive impairment is considered reversible. A lesser response indicates that airflow limitation is not reversible. However, some patients who do not meet the criteria for reversibility may still experience improvement after bronchodilator therapy, such as a decrease in dyspnea. This response likely is due to a decrease in hyperinflation occurring without a significant decrease in airway resistance.

SIMPLY STATED

An obstructive ventilatory defect is considered reversible if, after bronchodilator administration, the FEV_1 or FVC increases by more than 12% and 200 mL.

As indicated in Figure 9-6, a reduced FVC in the presence of a normal or high FEV_1/FVC suggests that the

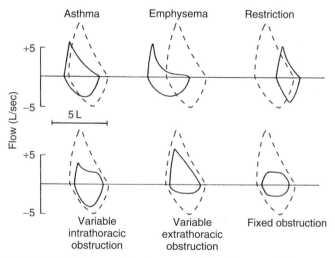

FIGURE 9-8 Patterns of pulmonary dysfunction revealed by flow-volume loops. For comparison, a normal loop is shown with each (*dashed lines*). See text for details. (From Mottram C: *Ruppel's manual of pulmonary function testing*, ed 10, St. Louis, 2013, Mosby.)

patient may have a reduction in lung volumes. However, this same pattern can occur among patients who fail to completely inhale or exhale during the maneuver. For this reason, confirmation of a reduction in lung volumes and the presence of a restrictive disorder requires measurement of static lung volumes (FRC, RV, TLC). Moreover, if it is suspected that the restrictive condition is due to an interstitial disease processes, most doctors will also request a diffusing capacity study (D_{LCO}).

Static Lung Volumes

Static lung volume determination involves measurement of the resting lung volume or FRC. If the FRC is known and the inspiratory capacity (IC) and ERV also are obtained by spirometry, both the RV (FRC − ERV) and the TLC (FRC + IC) can be computed. In general, static lung volume testing is performed in the pulmonary function laboratory.

Indications and Contraindications

Static lung volume measurements are indicated to:
- Confirm a suspected restrictive disease pattern (low FVC, normal or high FEV_1/FVC)
- Assess the impact of or response to medical or surgical interventions such as lung-volume reduction, lobectomy, lung transplantation, and radiation or chemotherapy
- Provide an index of gas trapping (requires comparison of FRC by gas dilution to plethysmographic thoracic gas volume)

Contraindications against performing static lung volume determinations are essentially the same as those previously described for basic spirometry.

Methods

There are three different methods used to measure FRC: (1) closed-circuit helium dilution, (2) open-circuit nitrogen washout, and (3) body plethysmography. Currently, there is no firm evidence to recommend any one technique over

Box 9-3	Basic Pre- and Post-Bronchodilator Test for Reversibility of Airflow Limitation

1. Ensure that the patient has not taken any bronchodilator breaths before the test.
2. Obtain three acceptable baseline FVC maneuvers.
3. Administer the prescribed β-agonist.*
4. Wait at least 10 minutes for the drug to take effect.
5. Repeat spirometry (three acceptable maneuvers).
6. Compare pre- and post-bronchodilator FVC and FEV_1.

*To standardize the test and ensure a full patient response, the American Thoracic Society recommends that four separate 100-mg doses of albuterol (total dose, 400 mg) be delivered by metered-dose inhaler and spacer at 30-second intervals. Lower doses may be considered if side effects are a concern.

FVC, forced vital capacity; FEV_1, forced expiratory volume at 1 second.

the others. In most cases, the method used will be based on the available equipment and personnel.

Closed-Circuit Helium Dilution

The closed-circuit helium dilution test is based on the principle that if a known volume and concentration of a gas is added to the patient's respiratory system, it will be diluted in proportion to the lung volume to which it is added (Fig. 9-9). Helium is used because it is an inert gas and is not significantly absorbed from the lungs by the blood. In normal subjects, equilibrium takes about 7 minutes so that oxygen must be added and carbon dioxide (CO_2) removed from the system to keep the gas concentrations constant and prevent hypercapnia. After equilibrium is reached, the FRC is calculated as follows:

$$FRC = \frac{(\text{initial He\%} - \text{final He\%}) \times Vapp}{\text{final He\%}} - V_{Dmech}$$

where Vapp = apparatus volume (volume in the spirometer and connecting tubing) and V_{Dmech} = dead space of the mouthpiece/breathing valve, with the results corrected for BTPS (body temperature and pressure) conditions.

Because helium does not reach areas of the lung distal to any obstruction, the measured FRC reflects only **functional lung volume**, that is, that in open communication with the airways. The volume of any air trapped in the lungs is not measured.

Measurements normally are made using a volume-displacement (bell or bellows) spirometer. To ensure accuracy, the spirometer capacity should be at least 7 L, and be tested daily for leaks. Ideally, the volume in the empty spirometer and connecting tubing should be ≤4.5 L because the smaller the apparatus volume, the more accurate the measurement. In addition, the breathing valve and mouthpiece should together add less than 100 mL dead space to the system (which is adjusted for in the FRC computation). It is also essential that the test be initiated immediately after the patient normally exhales to FRC. Errors in measurement—called **switch-in errors**—will occur if the test is initiated at a point either above or below the resting end-expiratory level.

Included with the spirometer should be a helium analyzer with water vapor absorber, a mixing fan, CO_2 absorber, and O_2 and helium supplies. The helium analyzer should have a range of 0% to 10% with an accuracy of 0.5% of full scale (0.05% for 10% He). Linearity should be checked weekly by two-point calibration with a low gas (room air/0% He) and a known "high" concentration of He (~10%). As with spirometry, regular testing of biologic controls should be part of the quality control program. Biologic control testing has the advantage over standard equipment calibration methods in that it also helps assess the repeatability of the actual procedure used.

Open-Circuit Nitrogen Washout

Figure 9-10 depicts the basic principle underlying the **nitrogen washout** method for measuring FRC. The patient breathes 100% O_2, with the expired N_2 concentration continuously monitored. The test continues for at least 7 minutes or until all the N_2 is washed out of the patient's lungs. Washout is judged complete when the N_2 concentration is less than 1.5% for at least three consecutive breaths.

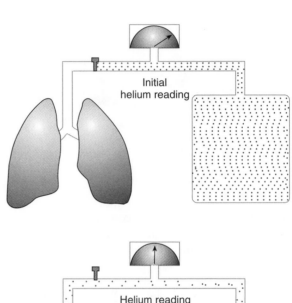

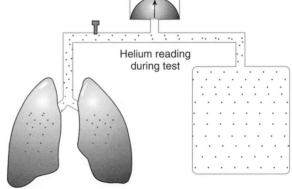

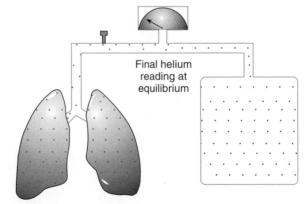

FIGURE 9-9 Closed-circuit helium dilution method for measuring functional residual capacity. Before measurement, enough 100% helium should be added to the system to give a helium reading of about 10%. (From Kacmarek RM, Stoller JK, Heuer AJ: *Egan's fundamentals of respiratory care*, ed 10, St Louis, 2013, Mosby.)

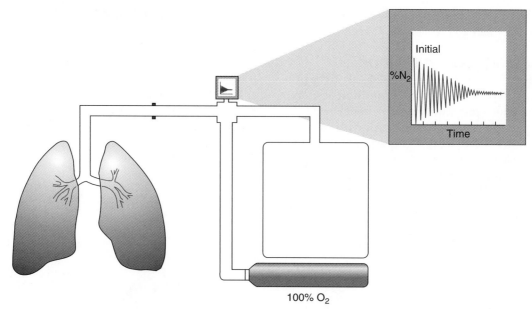

FIGURE 9-10 Open-circuit nitrogen washout method for determining functional residual capacity. (From Kacmarek RM, Stoller JK, Heuer AJ: *Egan's fundamentals of respiratory care*, ed 10, St Louis, 2013, Mosby.)

With the total volume and concentration of exhaled N_2 known and the knowledge that the air originally in the patient's lungs contained 78% N_2, the patient's FRC is computed as follows:

$$\text{FRC} = \frac{\text{vol } N_2 \text{ washed out} - \text{vol } N_2 \text{ from tissues}}{\text{starting } N_2 \% - \text{ending } N_2 \%}$$

The volume of nitrogen washed out during the test is determined either by collecting the entire volume of expired gas and measuring its $N_2\%$ or by computer compilation of the breath-by-breath volume and $N_2\%$. The volume of N_2 excreted from the tissues is estimated by equation based on the patient's body surface area.

As with the helium dilution method, accuracy of FRC determination by N_2 washout requires an accurate and properly calibrated gas analyzer. The N_2 analyzer should have a range of 0% to 100%, with an accuracy of ±0.2% and a rapid response time (<60 msec to a 10% change in $N_2\%$). A two-point calibration should be performed before each patient is tested, with the low gas 100% O_2 and the high gas room air (79% N_2).

Because a nitrogen washout system simultaneously measures breath-by-breath volumes, the accuracy of volume measurements also must be confirmed daily. Typically, this is done by pumping a calibrated syringe at about the same rates and volumes as expected during patient testing. As with helium dilution, regular (monthly) testing of biologic controls can be used to confirm both equipment function and repeatability of the testing procedure.

Also as with helium dilution, the volume measured by N_2 washout is limited to that in open communication with the airways. For this reason, in the presence of significant air trapping, the N_2 washout technique will tend to underestimate the actual FRC.

Body Plethysmography

Figure 9-11 depicts the concept used to measure lung volumes using a body plethysmograph. The patient sits inside a rigid boxlike enclosure and breathes through a pneumotachometer equipped with a pressure transducer that measures pressure changes at the mouth. The internal box pressure also is measured by a sensitive pressure transducer, calibrated to reflect volume changes inside the enclosure. After the patient completes a normal exhalation, a shutter in the pneumotachometer closes, occluding the airway. At the same time, the patient gently pants about once per second against the occlusion for 2 to 3 seconds. During the panting maneuver, changes in mouth pressure (ΔP) are recorded by the pneumotachometer's pressure transducer, with the pressure at times of zero flow equivalent to alveolar pressure (P_{alv}). Simultaneously, as the patient compresses and decompresses the gas in the lungs while panting, the box pressure transducer measures the corresponding volume changes as the thorax expands and contracts (ΔV).

Thus, we have a starting volume (the *unknown* FRC = V_1) and starting pressure (alveolar pressure before inspiratory phase of pant = P_1), as well as an ending volume (FRC + ΔV = V_2) and ending pressure (alveolar pressure at end-inspiratory phase of pant = P_2). According to Boyle's law:

$$P_1 \times V_1 = P_2 \times V_2$$

Based on this formula, V_1 (the unknown FRC) can be computed as:

$$V_1 = \frac{V_2 \times P_2}{P_1}$$

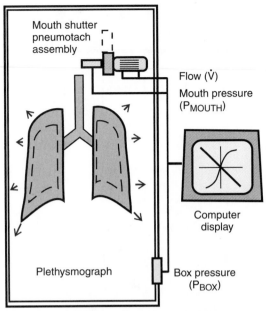

FIGURE 9-11 Body plethysmography method for measuring thoracic gas volume. See text for details. (From Mottram C: *Ruppel's manual of pulmonary function testing*, ed 10, St. Louis, 2013, Mosby.)

Expressing pressure and volume as *changes* from baseline:

$$FRC = \frac{\Delta V}{\Delta P} \times P_2$$

Since the panting creates only small pressure changes around barometric pressure, P_2 is assumed to equal P_B:

$$FRC = \frac{\Delta V}{\Delta P} \times P_B$$

Thus, the FRC equals the slope of the changes in thoracic volume (measured as changes in box pressure) versus the change in mouth pressure during the panting maneuver, as portrayed on the computer display (see Fig. 9-11).

Unlike the helium dilution and nitrogen washout methods, body plethysmography measures the total compressible gas volume in the thorax, whether or not it is in communication with open airways. When not referenced to any starting point, this volume is called the **thoracic gas volume (TGV)**. When measured from a normal end-inspiratory level, the abbreviation FRC_{pleth} should be used.

In terms of equipment performance, the flow sensor should meet the same accuracy standards as those previously described for spirometers, with the box pressure transducer being accurate to ± 0.2 cm H_2O, and calibrated daily using volume changes similar in size and frequency to patient panting (usually by a small piston pump delivering 20- to 50-mL stroke volumes). Likewise, the mouth pressure transducer and pneumotachometer should be calibrated daily using a both a calibrating manometer (pressure) and syringe (volume).

In regard to procedural quality assurance, sufficient time should be allowed after the patient enters the plethysmograph for the temperature to stabilize. During the panting maneuver, the patient should wear a nose clip (to prevent leaks) and hold the flat of both hands against the cheeks (to prevent error due to oral gas compression and expansion). Typically, the patient is asked to repeat the panting maneuver until at least three FRC_{pleth} measurements can be obtained that are within $\pm 5\%$ of each other. After the FRC_{pleth} measurements, the shutter is opened, and the patient performs an ERV maneuver, followed by an inspiratory **vital capacity (VC)**, or maximal inhalation from a maximal exhalation.

Overall accuracy (equipment plus procedure) should be assessed at least monthly. One approach is to use a 3- to 4-L glass flask connected both to the pneumotachometer and a large squeeze bulb. Squeezing the bulb simulates the panting maneuver. The average of five such maneuvers should be within ± 50 mL or 3% of the known flask volume. Alternatively, two biologic controls should undergo FRC_{pleth} measurement. Values that differ significantly (more than $\pm 10\%$) from their previously established means indicate either equipment or procedural error.

Interpretation

Static lung volume measurements are used primarily to confirm the presence of a restrictive ventilatory impairment suggested by spirometry results (low FVC, FEV_1/FVC ratio > LLN). As with spirometry, a patient's lung volumes are compared with reference values generated using equations derived from normal subjects, with values outside the 95% prediction interval considered abnormal. Thus, an abnormally low FRC, RV, or TLC would be below its LLN, or below the 5th percentile of its predicted value. Based on this interpretation framework, *a patient has a purely restrictive ventilatory impairment if the TLC is lower than its LLN but the FEV_1/FVC ratio exceeds its LLN.*

Static lung volumes also have been used to assess for air trapping and hyperinflation in patients with obstructive ventilatory impairments. These abnormalities are associated with an increase in the RV and FRC, with or without an increase in TLC. An increase in the RV occurring *with* an increase in the TLC (RV/TLC ratio < 35%) is the classic pattern of hyperinflation, sometimes seen in emphysema. An increase in the RV *without* an increase in the TLC (RV/TLC ratio > 35%) is more consistent with air trapping, as may occur during an exacerbation of asthma. Unfortunately, these patterns often are not so clear-cut, in part because air trapping and hyperinflation are not well-distinguished phenomenon. Nonetheless, measurement of the RV in patients with obstructive impairments is potentially useful for monitoring response to therapy (e.g., bronchodilator treatment) and disease progression.

Moreover, knowledge of how lung volumes in restrictive and obstructive disorders differ from normal can be helpful in understanding the nature of these impairments and their differential diagnosis. Figure 9-12 depicts these patterns compared with normal.

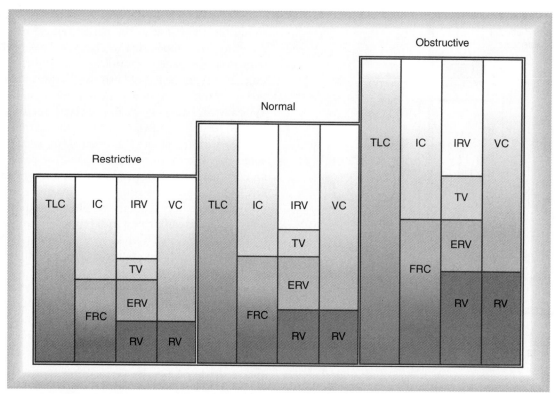

FIGURE 9-12 Changes in lung volumes and capacities characteristic of restrictive and obstructive ventilatory impairments compared with normal. ERV, expiratory reserve volume; FRC, functional residual capacity; IC, inspiratory capacity; IRV, inspiratory reserve volume; RV, residual volume; TLC, total lung capacity; TV, tidal volume; VC, vital capacity. (From Kacmarek RM, Stoller JK, Heuer AJ: *Egan's fundamentals of respiratory care*, ed 10, St. Louis, 2013, Mosby.)

Diffusing Capacity of the Lung (DLCO)

The **diffusing capacity** (also called the *transfer factor*) is a measure of the lung's ability to exchange oxygen with the mixed venous blood. Because all methods use low concentrations of carbon monoxide (CO) gas, the abbreviation DLCO is used to refer to this measurement. Several methods can be used to measure CO diffusing capacity. The most commonly used standardized method is the single-breath DLCO, or DLCO$_{sb}$.

Indications

Measurement of DLCO is indicated to:
- Differentiate between interstitial and chest wall/neuromuscular causes of restrictive ventilatory impairments
- Evaluate, follow the progress of, and assess the degree of impairment caused by **interstitial lung disease (IDL)**
- Differentiate between emphysema and other obstructive pulmonary disorders (e.g., chronic bronchitis and asthma)
- Evaluate, follow the progress of, and assess the degree of impairment associated with chronic obstructive pulmonary disorders
- Evaluate pulmonary involvement in systemic diseases (e.g., rheumatoid arthritis, systemic lupus erythematosus)

- Evaluate the effects of chemotherapy, radiation and selected drugs (e.g., bleomycin, amiodarone) on lung function
- Assess postoperative risk in patients undergoing lung resection or transplantation
- Predict arterial desaturation during exercise in patients with lung disease
- Evaluate the causes of dyspnea in patients with normal spirometry

Equipment and Quality Assurance

Figure 9-13 depicts the basic apparatus used to measure DLCO$_{sb}$. The typical test gas contains 0.3% CO mixed with a tracer gas, most commonly helium, with the balance being O$_2$ and N$_2$. The test gas is delivered to the patient through a computer-controlled valve from either a reservoir bag or demand valve. The initial portion of exhaled gas (apparatus and anatomic dead space) is collected by a spirometer, with the remaining end-tidal portion diverted into a sampling system for CO and He measurement.

Volume measurements made by the DLCO apparatus should be accurate within ±3.5% over an 8-L range and checked daily. Both the He and CO analyzers should exhibit linearity, with the maximal error across the range of measurement being no more than ±0.5%. The computer timing mechanism should be accurate to ±1% over 10 seconds. The dead space of the breathing circuit should be less than 350 mL.

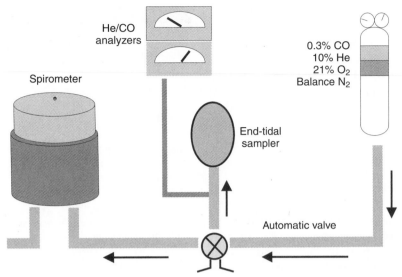

FIGURE 9-13 Apparatus used to measure the diffusing capacity of the lung using the single breath method. See text for details. (From Mottram C: *Ruppel's manual of pulmonary function testing,* ed 10, St. Louis, 2013, Mosby.)

Quality assurance testing should be done weekly by performing a DLCO measurement using a 3-L calibrated syringe, with the resulting DLCO near zero and the measured volume within 3.5% of the syringe volume. This should be supplemented by weekly testing of healthy, non-smoking biologic controls with known DLCO values.

Test Procedure and Calculations

Because transfer of CO from the lungs into the blood is affected by existing COHb levels, patients should not smoke on the day of the test. It also is important that there have been no exercise or exertional activities just before the test (which increases blood flow and DLCO). To ensure a resting state, the patient should be seated for at least 5 minutes before the test is conducted, during which time instruction can be provided and the procedure demonstrated.

In the single-breath technique, the patient first fully exhales to RV, then quickly inhales the test gas to TLC (an inspiratory VC). Then the patient performs a relaxed breath-hold with the breathing valve closed. After 10 seconds, the breathing valve opens, allowing the patient to exhale. The initial 0.5 to 0.75 L of the patient's expired gas (dead space) is discarded, with the remainder diverted by the valve to the sampling system for He and CO analysis.

Because least two acceptable tests are required, a 4- to 5-minute wait between tests is required to wash out any residual CO. Assuming proper equipment function and calibration, a DLCO test is acceptable if:
- The inspiratory vital capacity exceeds 85% of the patient's largest VC and is inspired in less than 4 seconds
- A stable, *relaxed* breath-hold is maintained for 10 ± 2 seconds, with no evidence of either active expiratory effort (Valsalva maneuver) or inspiratory effort (Mueller maneuver) against the closed breathing valve

- A smooth, unforced expiration occurs in less than 4 seconds with complete clearance of dead space and proper sampling and analysis of alveolar gas

On completion of an acceptable maneuver, the sample CO concentration (F_ACO_T) is analyzed, and the "alveolar" CO concentration at the beginning of the breath-hold is computed (F_ACO_0). The DLCO is then calculated as the log ratio of the initial alveolar CO level to that in the end-tidal sample and adjusted for alveolar volume (V_A) and breath-hold time (T) using the following equation:

$$DLCOs_b = \frac{V_A \times 60}{(P_B - 47) \times (T)} \times Ln \frac{F_ACO_0}{F_ACO_T}$$

Computation of both the "alveolar" CO concentration at the beginning of the breath-hold (F_ACO_0) and the alveolar volume (V_A) is performed using the breath's starting and ending He concentrations (or other tracer gas if used).

Results are reported in milliliters per minute per mm Hg (STPD) based on an average of at least two acceptable tests that are repeatable. Tests are repeatable if the results fall within ±3 mL/min/mm Hg of each other, or within 10% of the largest observed value. Additional measures in the report typically include the alveolar volume (V_A), the ratio of DLCO to V_A, and the average inspiratory vital capacity. In addition, both Hb content and the carboxyhemoglobin levels affect DLCO. The relationship between Hb content and DLCO is direct; that is, increases in Hb content increase the diffusing capacity. In regard to carboxyhemoglobin, the DLCO decreases about 1% for each 1% increase in COHb. For these reasons, the DLCO report should include the Hb-corrected and carboxyhemoglobin-corrected values.

Interpretation

The most commonly cited normal range for DLCO is 25 to 30 mL/min/mm Hg. However, as with other pulmonary function tests, interpretation involves comparing the patient's DLCO measurement with a reference range and its LLN and ULN. Thus, an abnormally low DLCO is one below its LLN, or below the 5th percentile of its predicted value. A reduction in DLCO below the LLN but above 60% of normal represents a mild impairment. If the patient's DLCO is less than LLN and between 40% and 60% of predicted, the impairment is considered moderate. A severe impairment exists if the DLCO is less than LLN and less than 40% of predicted.

Unfortunately, as with lung volume determinations, there are no specific prediction equations for DLCO that are generally recommended, and variation among different equations is as high as 40%. Moreover, a patient's DLCO on follow-up may need to fall by 20% to 25% before any clinical impact becomes apparent. Compounding the lack of standard reference values is the fact that DLCO is affected by so many factors, including the surface area and diffusion characteristics of the alveolar-capillary membrane, blood hemoglobin levels, pulmonary capillary blood flow and volume, and the distribution of ventilation and perfusion.

Some clinicians use the $DLCO/V_A$ ratio to help overcome some of the problems with DLCO interpreting. However, use of this ratio to support interpretation no longer is recommended. Instead, the DLCO is interpreted in combination with spirometry and lung volume measures. For example, a low DLCO in a patient with normal spirometry and lung volumes may indicate anemia, a pulmonary vascular disorder, early ILD, or early emphysema. If the FEV_1/FVC ratio exceeds the LLN, but lung volumes are reduced (a restrictive ventilatory impairment), a normal DLCO suggests a chest wall or neuromuscular disorder, whereas a reduced DLCO is consistent with an ILD. If spirometry indicates an obstructive airflow impairment that does not respond to bronchodilation, a low DLCO points to emphysema. Typical DLCO findings associated with these and other common disorders are summarized in Table 9-5.

SIMPLY STATED

In patients with restrictive ventilatory impairments, a low DLCO is consistent with an interstitial lung disease. In patients with obstructive ventilatory impairments, a low DLCO helps identify emphysema.

Specialized Tests

Specialized assessments conducted in some pulmonary laboratories include measurement of airway resistance and lung compliance, evaluation of airway hyperresponsiveness and inflammation, and selected exercise test protocols. Although normally performed by specially trained personnel, these tests can provide essential information relevant to patient management.

TABLE 9-5

Typical DLCO Results by Disease Category/Disorder

Disease Category/Disorder	Typical DLCO Findings
Airways Diseases	
Asthma	Normal*
Chronic bronchitis	Normal
Emphysema	Low
Bronchiectasis	Low
Interstitial Lung Diseases	
Idiopathic pulmonary fibrosis	Low
Collagen vascular diseases	Low
Sarcoidosis	Low
Drug-induced lung disease	Low
Diseases of Pulmonary Vasculature	
Pulmonary embolic disease	Low
Pulmonary hypertension	Low
Pulmonary vasculitis	Low
Pulmonary hemorrhage	High
Extrapulmonary Diseases	
Respiratory muscle weakness	Low
Kyphoscoliosis	Low
Obesity	Normal*
Polycythemia	High
Anemia	Low
Other	
Pneumonectomy/lobectomy	Low
Congestive heart failure	Low

*High values have also been reported.

Airway Resistance

Airway resistance is a measure of the ratio of alveolar pressure (P_{alv}) to airflow ($\dot{V}$). There are three methods used to measure airway resistance: plethysmography, the interrupter method, and the forced oscillation technique.

The standard and best validated method for measuring airway resistance is similar to that described for determining TGV by body plethysmograph, with the resulting parameter abbreviated as R_{aw}. In this case, the patient first pants with the shutter open as the system plots flow on the Y-axis against box pressure on the X-axis. Then the shutter is closed, and as the patient continues panting, the slope of box pressure–mouth pressure curve is obtained, as previously described for computing TGV. The ratio of the slopes of the closed-shutter to open-shutter curves is the R_{aw}.

The commonly cited reference range for normal R_{aw} in healthy adults is 0.5 to 2.5 cm H_2O/L/sec. However, R_{aw} varies *inversely* with lung volume, meaning that as lung volume increases, R_{aw} falls. Unfortunately, this relationship is not linear. However, the reciprocal of R_{aw} is linearly related to lung volume. The reciprocal of R_{aw} is called *conductance* and abbreviated as G_{aw}. G_{aw} computed as follows:

$$G_{aw} = \frac{1}{R_{aw}}$$

G_{aw} normally is adjusted for the volume at which it is measured, which by plethysmography is the TGV. The ratio of G_{aw} to TGV is called **specific conductance (G_{aw}/ TGV)**, which is useful in measuring the response to interventions affecting airway resistance and lung volumes, such as bronchodilator therapy.

SIMPLY STATED

Airway resistance (R_{aw}) varies inversely with lung volume; as lung volume increases, R_{aw} falls, and as lung volume decreases, R_{aw} rises.

Although R_{aw} determined by plethysmography is the gold standard, it requires a cooperative patient able to perform the required maneuvers in a laboratory setting. The interrupted method requires only quiet breathing and can be conducted at the bedside or in the clinic. This method measures tidal airflow and mouth pressure before and after closure of a shutter incorporated into a pneumotachograph. To differentiate it from R_{aw} determined by plethysmography, this measure is called the *interrupter resistance* (R_{int}). Reference ranges are available, but current evidence suggests that R_{int} may underestimate R_{aw} as determined by plethysmography, especially if the obstruction is severe.

Like the interrupter method, the forced oscillation technique (FOT) requires only tidal breathing and can be conducted at the bedside or in the clinic. FOT measures resistance by superimposing flow oscillations generated by a loudspeaker on the airways during spontaneous breathing. As the flow changes, so too does the airway pressure. The ratio of pressure to flow of each of the oscillation frequencies is computed as the respiratory system impedance (Z_{rs}). The $P/\dot{V}$ relationship that occurs in phase with these oscillations is the respiratory system resistance (R_{rs}). As with the interrupter technique, reference ranges are available for R_{rs}. One major advantage of the FOT method over plethysmography and the interrupted techniques is that it can "partition" a patient's airflow resistance by location. In large airway obstruction, R_{rs} is elevated independent of oscillation frequency. On the other hand, in small airway obstruction, R_{rs} is highest at low frequencies and decreases with increasing frequencies.

Lung and Chest Wall Compliance

Compliance is defined as the ease of inflation and is measured as volume change per unit pressure change. The total compliance of the respiratory system (C_{L+T}) measures the overall distensibility of the lung and thorax together. C_{L+T} can be partitioned into two components: lung compliance (C_L) and thorax/chest wall compliance (C_T). These two components work in parallel, with the relationship expressed in the following equation:

$$\frac{1}{C_{L+T}} = \frac{1}{C_L} + \frac{1}{C_T}$$

Lung compliance (C_L) is measured using a spirometer or other volumetric device to measure volume change and a pressure transducer to measure pressure change. To measure C_L, the applicable pressure is the transpulmonary pressure gradient (P_L), which equals alveolar pressure (P_{alv}) minus the pleural pressure (P_{pl}). Pleural pressure is estimated from the pressure within a balloon placed in the esophagus. The subject inhales to TLC and begins a slow exhalation. During exhalation, the volume and pressure are recorded as flow at the airway opening (P_{ao}) is interrupted at several descending steps. At times of zero flow, P_{ao} equals P_{alv}. Thus, P_L is calculated as $P_{ao} - P_{pl}$. The lung volumes and corresponding transpulmonary pressures are plotted to provide a lung compliance curve. The slope of the curve ($\Delta V/\Delta P$) at any given volume represents the lung compliance, or C_L. Typically, the slope between 500 and 1000 mL above the FRC is chosen for the measurement. Because this parameter is based on measurements made at zero flow, it is referred to as the *static* lung compliance. The commonly cited normal static lung compliance for a healthy adult is 0.2 L/cm H_2O or 200 mL/cm H_2O.

SIMPLY STATED

Lung compliance is computed as the lung volume divided by the transpulmonary pressure gradient (alveolar-pleural pressure). Typically, multiple measurements are made and plotted on a curve, with slope of the curve between 500 to 1000 mL above the FRC taken as the patient's measurement.

Example lung compliance curves are shown in Figure 9-14. For reference, the middle curve represents normal static compliance. The lower, flatter curve reflects a stiff lung, as may be observed in pulmonary fibrosis. The upper curve with the greater slope is consistent with greater than normal lung compliance, as can occur in emphysema, owing to loss of elastic recoil.

During the measurement of static lung compliance, the transthoracic pressure gradient (P_W) also may be recorded. P_W equals the difference between the alveolar pressure and atmospheric pressure ($P_{alv} - P_B$). Dividing the lung volume by P_W yields the *total compliance* of the respiratory system (C_{L+T}). The commonly cited normal total compliance for a healthy adult is 0.1 L/cm H_2O or 100 mL/cm H_2O.

Given a patient's lung and total compliance measures, one can then compute thorax/chest wall compliance (C_T) using the previously provided compliance equation. The commonly cited normal thorax/chest wall compliance for a healthy adult is 0.2 L/cm H_2O or 200 mL/cm H_2O.

Airway Hyperresponsiveness and Inflammation

Airway hyperresponsiveness (AHR) represents an abnormally exaggerated airway response to a provoking stimulus. The provoking stimulus most often is an

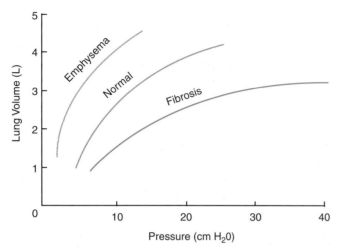

FIGURE 9-14 Example lung compliance curve plotting lung volume vs. transpulmonary pressure. The slope of the curve ($\Delta V/\Delta P$) at any given volume represents the lung compliance, or C_L. (Modified from Martin L: *Pulmonary physiology in clinical practice: the essentials for patient care and evaluation,* St. Louis, 1987, Mosby.)

inflammatory immune response causing bronchoconstriction, as in asthma.

Two different approaches can be used to assess for AHR. The first is to actually challenge the airways with a provoking agent, a method called **bronchoprovocation testing**. A newer alternative approach is to assess the actual level of airway inflammation through analysis of an inflammatory marker, exhaled nitric oxide (NO).

Bronchoprovocation Testing

Bronchoprovocation testing involves exposing a subject to increasing concentrations of a drug agent that can provoke bronchospasm in order to determine the level at which airway response occurs. The most common drug used is methacholine, a potent cholinergic agent.

Methacholine bronchoprovocation testing is indicated to:
- Rule out a diagnosis of asthma
- Assess the severity of AHR
- Evaluate for occupational asthma
- Assess response to AHR treatment

This test is contraindicated if the patient has severe airflow limitation (FEV_1 < 50% predicted or < 1.0 L), has had a heart attack or stroke in last 90 days, or has uncontrolled hypertension or a known aortic aneurysm.

Patients scheduled for provocation testing should avoid taking any short-acting inhaled bronchodilator medication for 8 hours before testing, with those receiving long-acting bronchodilators ceasing administration 48 hours in advance.

Two different methods are used for methacholine bronchoprovocation testing: the 2-minute tidal breathing method and the dosimeter method. Laboratories using the tidal breathing method have the patient inhale aerosol from a calibrated jet nebulizer, outputting at a rate of 0.13 mL/minute. With the dosimeter method, the device delivers 9 µL of aerosolized solution at the beginning of each of five IC maneuvers that end in a 5-second breath-hold. Regardless of method, a rescue protocol and advanced cardiac life support (ACLS) equipment must be in place to deal with any untoward patient response to the provoking agent.

In both methods, the patient receives an initial normal saline solution (0.9%) aerosol, followed by an FEV_1 measurement (the baseline or control). Thereafter, increasing concentrations of methacholine solution are administered every 5 minutes, typically ranging from an initial dose of 0.03 mg/mL up to 16 mg/mL. At each incremental dosage, two repeat FEV_1 measurements are made, 30 and 90 seconds after inhalation. At each step, the percentage decrease in FEV_1 compared with baseline is computed and plotted on a dose-response curve. The test ends when either the maximal dose of methacholine has been given or the FEV_1 has fallen by 20% or more from baseline. In the latter case, the provocative concentration of methacholine resulting in the 20% or greater fall in FEV_1 (termed the **PC_{20}**) is computed from the log concentration versus dose-response curve. After the test, the patient normally receives bronchodilator treatment to restore normal airway function, which is confirmed by repeat spirometry.

SIMPLY STATED

The PC_{20} is the concentration of methacholine that causes a 20% or greater fall in FEV_1 during bronchoprovocation testing. Moderate to severe airway hyperresponsiveness is present if the PC_{20} occurs at a methacholine concentration of 1 mg/mL or less.

Table 9-6 outlines the recommended interpretation of the PC_{20}, which assumes a normal FEV_1 at baseline. If the FEV_1 does not fall by at least 20% with the highest concentration of methacholine, the test is interpreted as negative, and a diagnosis of AHR or asthma can be ruled out. If the PC_{20} occurs at less than 1 mg/mL methacholine concentration, moderate to severe AHR is present, which is consistent with a diagnosis of asthma. PC_{20} values between 1 and 16 mg/mL suggest but do not confirm a diagnosis of asthma.

Exhaled Nitric Oxide ($F_E NO$) Analysis

NO is a chemical mediator produced by endothelial and epithelial cells, macrophages, and eosinophils. Because it is a gas, NO appears in the exhaled breath, with its concentration increasing in the presence of airway inflammation. For this reason, measurement of the exhaled fraction of NO (**$F_E NO$**) has been found useful in both diagnosis and management of asthma. Specifically, $F_E NO$ testing is used to:
- Help assess respiratory symptoms (cough, wheeze, dyspnea)
- Help identify the eosinophilic asthma phenotype

TABLE 9-6

Interpretation of Methacholine Test Results

PC_{20} (mg/mL)	Interpretation
>16	Normal airway responsiveness
4-16	Borderline AHR
1-4	Mild AHR
<1	Moderate to severe AHR

AHR, airway hyperresponsiveness.
Adapted from American Thoracic Society: Guidelines for methacholine and exercise challenge testing-1999. *Am J Respir Crit Care Med* 161(1):309-329, 2000.

- Monitor chronic persistent asthma
- Assess response to and compliance with inhaled steroids
- Guide changes in dosing and discontinuation of inhaled steroids
- Assess whether other factors are contributing to poor asthma control (e.g., sinusitis, anxiety, gastroesophageal reflux disease [GERD], continued allergen exposure)

F_ENO typically is measured using chemiluminescence or electrochemical methods. Both provide rapid, real-time sampling during exhalation, with graphic display of F_ENO (similar in concept to capnography). Because NO concentrations are so low, they are measured in parts per billion (ppb). For this reason, NO analyzers used to sample expired gas must have a sensitivity and accuracy of 1 ppb or better and a rapid response time (<500 msec). In addition, NO analyzers should undergo daily two-point calibrations according to the manufacturer's specifications, ideally using a zero NO gas and one at the high end of the measurement range.

Because many nondisease factors can influence F_ENO levels, it is important to instruct patients before testing to refrain from exercise, alcohol consumption, smoking, and eating for at least 1 hour before testing. In addition, since both steroids and beta-agonists alter F_ENO levels, all medications being taken and time of administration should be recorded. Last, because forced expiratory efforts decrease F_ENO levels, NO analysis should be conducted *before* any spirometry testing.

The basic procedure is simple. The patient inhales NO-free air through the analyzer to TLC, then exhales slowly while the measurement takes place. Key quality considerations in conducting the procedure are outlined in Box 9-4.

F_ENO levels are flow dependent, and measurements must be made at a constant low expiratory flow. The recommended standard flow is 0.05 L/second or 50 mL/second. Typically, this is achieved by having the patient exhale against a fixed resistance, with the monitored flow proportional to the generated back-pressure.

Because NO levels in air can be higher than those coming from the lungs, the inhaled gas should contain as little NO as possible. Typically, NO is removed from the inhaled air by exposing it to a filter containing a chemical NO scavenger.

Box 9-4   Quality Considerations in Measuring Exhaled Nitric Oxide (F_ENO)

- Patient should be seated comfortably in the upright position.
- Use nose clips only if the patient cannot avoid nasal breathing.
- Avoid any breath holding preceding the test maneuver.
- Have the patient:
  - Exhale normally without the mouthpiece.
  - Inhale NO-free air through the mouthpiece for 2 to 3 seconds to total lung capacity.
  - Maintain a steady low expiratory flow for at least 6 seconds (>4 seconds for children).
- Terminate maneuver once the test is deemed acceptability.
- Repeat until acceptability and repeatability criteria are met.
- Allow at least a 30-second interval between maneuvers.

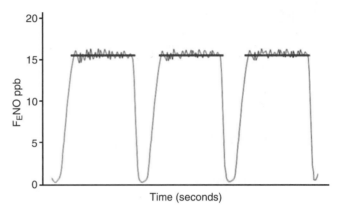

FIGURE 9-15 Graph of exhaled nitric oxide fraction (F_ENO) measured over three breaths in a normal subject. Note the consistent plateau levels of about 16 ppb occurring toward the end of each breath, indicating both acceptability and repeatability of the maneuvers. (Courtesy of Strategic Learning Associates, LLC, Little Silver, NJ)

NO contamination also can result from gas coming from the nose, which typically has higher NO concentrations than that coming from the lungs. This problem is averted because the back-pressure created by the analyzer's expiratory flow resistance closes off the soft palate.

To assure quality in F_ENO testing, at least three acceptable maneuvers should be obtained. Figure 9-15 provides an example graphic display of three such maneuvers provided by a rapidly responding F_ENO analyzer on a patient with normal F_ENO levels. Box 9-5 provides the basic acceptability and repeatability criteria for this measurement. The reported F_ENO is the mean value of at least two plateau measurements, the concentrations of which fall within 10% of each other.

Recently, the ATS has recommended using cut-off points rather than reference values when interpreting F_ENO, in part because F_ENO values are not normally distributed in the population, and there is large overlap between mean F_ENO levels in healthy subjects and those diagnosed with asthma. Table 9-7 provides interpretive guidelines based on these recommended cut-off points, which differ for adults and children. Of course, as with all pulmonary function tests, reliance solely on the F_ENO for diagnosis or disease management is inappropriate. F_ENO values should always be interpreted in light of the patient's history, physical examination, and related diagnostic procedures, including pulmonary function tests.

SIMPLY STATED

An adult patient who reports recurrent episodes of coughing, wheezing, and shortness of breath and who has a measured F_ENO greater than 50 ppb likely has eosinophilic asthma.

Box 9-5	Acceptability and Repeatability Criteria for F_ENO Maneuvers

- Acceptability criteria for F_ENO maneuvers
  - Free from any leaks
  - Exhalation of at least 6 seconds (at least 4 seconds in children < 12 years old)
  - F_ENO plateau at standard flow of 50 mL/sec (± 10%) held constant for ≥ 3 seconds
  - Variation in F_ENO during the plateau phase is no more than 10%
- Repeatability
  - Three maneuvers with F_ENO plateau values within 10% or two maneuvers within 5% of each other

Exercise Tests

Many different protocols involve assessment of a patient's exercise capacity or its effect on body functions. These tests range from simple evaluation of exercise tolerance to complex protocols requiring concurrent assessment of cardiovascular, pulmonary, and metabolism measures. Here, we review the basics involved in the two most common exercise tests, the 6-Minute Walk Test and the treadmill-based cardiopulmonary exercise test.

6-Minute Walk Test

The 6-Minute Walk Test measures how far a patient can walk in the specified time, with the resulting distance termed the **6MWD**, measured in meters. The test evaluates tolerance for mild exertion and is commonly used to assess a patient's overall functional capacity. Preassessment and postassessment of the 6MWD also can help determine the effect of medical or surgical treatments such as volume reduction surgery or pulmonary rehabilitation. The test is contraindicated in patients with recent myocardial infarction or unstable angina, and caution should be taken with those who are severely hypertensive or have high resting heart rates.

The test should follow the standard protocol published by the ATS. An oxygen source, automated defibrillator, and telephone should be available to handle potential emergencies. The walking course should be 30 meters long with a clear start line and turnaround point, marked off every 3 meters. Box 9-6 summarizes the key points in the ATS recommended test protocol.

If the patient complains of chest pain or severe dyspnea, becomes diaphoretic, or develops a pale or ashen

TABLE 9-7			
F_ENO Cut-Offs and Related Clinical Considerations for Adults and Children			
	Low Cut-Off	Intermediate Values	High Cut-Off
Adult	<25 ppb	25-50 ppb	>50 ppb
Child	<20 ppb	20-35 ppb	>35 ppb
Eosinophilic inflammation	Unlikely	Interpret based on clinical context	Likely
Response to steroids	Unlikely	Interpret based on clinical context	Likely
Diagnostic considerations	Consider other causes of symptoms, e.g., CF, sinusitis, COPD, GERD, anxiety	Be cautious; monitor F_ENO trends	In symptomatic patients (not taking steroids), generally confirms diagnosis of asthma
Management considerations for asthmatic patients	• If symptoms persist consider other diagnoses • In asymptomatic patients on inhaled steroids, indicates good compliance with treatment—consider decreasing dose	• In symptomatic patients may indicate persistent allergen exposure, inadequate inhaled steroid dose, poor adherence • In asymptomatic patients indicates adequate inhaled steroid dosing, good adherence	• May indicate poor treatment compliance, poor inhaler technique, inadequate inhaled steroid dose or steroid resistance • Increased risk for exacerbation; inhaled steroid withdrawal may lead to relapse

Adapted from Dweik RA, Boggs PB, Erzurum SC: An official ATS clinical practice guideline: interpretation of exhaled nitric oxide levels (F_ENO) for clinical applications. *Am J Respir Crit Care Med* 184(5):602-615, 2011.
CF, cystic fibrosis; COPD, chronic obstructive pulmonary disease; GERD, gastroesophageal reflux disease.

appearance, the test should be discontinued, the patient seated and administered O_2, and the physician immediately contacted.

Based on existing prediction equations for normal subjects, a 6MWD of less than 350 meters for women or 450 meters for men provides a useful cut-off point for identifying those with abnormal functional capacities. When assessing the effect of a medical or surgical intervention, one should look for at least a 10% to 20% increase in the 6MWD as an indicator of treatment effectiveness.

Although useful as a global assessment of functional capacity, the 6-Minute Walk Test is not diagnostic of any specific condition. It does not measure maximal oxygen uptake nor help identify the factors limiting a patient's exercise tolerance. To obtain such information requires a comprehensive cardiopulmonary exercise test.

Cardiopulmonary Exercise Testing

Cardiopulmonary exercise testing involves analysis of heart and lung function during incremental levels of work, typically performed on a treadmill. The standard workload measure for exercise testing is the **metabolic equivalent of task (MET)**; 1 MET = 3.5 mL O_2 consumption per kilogram of body weight, roughly equal to the average resting O_2

Box 9-6	American Thoracic Society 6-Minute Walk Protocol

1. Have the patient sit at rest for at least 10 minutes before the test starts.
2. Assemble all equipment, e.g., stopwatch, Borg Scale, recording worksheet.
3. With the patient resting, gather the needed demographic data and record the vital signs.
4. If SpO_2 is to be monitored, be sure to record the baseline value.
5. Have the patient stand, and rate his/her baseline dyspnea and exertion levels using the Borg scale.
6. Position the patient at the start line and review the procedure.
7. As soon as the patient starts to walk, begin timing.
8. Remain at the start line while you record completed laps (1 lap = down and back).
9. Each minute, provide encouragement to the patient and specify the time remaining.
10. At exactly 6 minutes, firmly say "Stop!" and place a marker at the stop point.
11. If using a pulse oximeter, record the end-of-walk SpO_2 and pulse rate.
12. Have the patient sit in a chair while you repeat the dyspnea and exertion assessment.
13. Record the number of laps and additional distance covered in the final partial lap, if any.
14. Calculate and record the total distance walked, rounding to the nearest meter.

Adapted from American Thoracic Society: ATS statement: guidelines for the six-minute walk test. *Am J Respir Crit Care Med* 166:111-117, 2002.

---

consumption per minute. Treadmill protocols are designed such that specific speeds and inclinations correspond to specific MET levels. Most exercise protocols increase exercise intensity by 1 to 2 METs at each workload increment.

Exercise testing normally is performed under direct physician supervision in a cardiac, pulmonary, or exercise physiology laboratory. A fully stocked crash cart with defibrillator, oxygen, suction, and airway equipment must be immediately available, with all staff involved in testing proficient in advanced life support.

The classic cardiac electrocardiogram (ECG) stress test measures the patient's 12-lead ECG, heart rate, and blood pressure and is indicated to:

- Diagnose obstructive coronary artery disease (CAD)
- Assess risk and prognosis in patients with a prior history of CAD
- Assess prognosis after myocardial infarction (MI)
- Provide the basis for heart patients' activity or rehabilitation prescriptions
- Help evaluate the impact of medical therapies for CAD and congestive heart failure

Measured parameters are carefully monitored at each workload increment, as well as patient symptoms, such as chest pain. ST depression or elevation (≥ 1 mm for at least 60 to 80 msec following the QRS) indicates myocardial ischemia and constitutes a positive test result.

When combined with measurement of tidal volume, respiratory rate, O_2 consumption, and CO_2 production, exercise testing also can be used to:

- Differentiate between factors limiting exercise capacity (cardiac vs. pulmonary)
- Evaluate responses to therapy intended to increased exercise tolerance
- Determine the intensity for exercise training in rehabilitation programs
- Evaluate exercise capacity in heart transplantation candidates
- Assess cardiopulmonary fitness in disability evaluations

The measurements made during exercise capacity testing, their definitions, and their typical values at peak capacity are described in Table 9-8.

The primary criterion for evaluating overall exercise capacity is the $\dot{V}O_2max$. Test results are considered normal if patients can attain their predicted $\dot{V}O_2max$ and a heart rate at or near their predicted maximum (**HRmax**) at peak exercise capacity. Normal patients also can readily increase their ventilation in proportion to metabolic demands and maintain normal SpO_2 levels during exercise.

SIMPLY STATED

To estimate the maximal heart rate of a patient at peak exercise capacity, subtract the patient's age from 220.

As a rule of thumb, poor exercise capacity is present if either the $\dot{V}O_2max$ is less than 15 mL/kg or the patient

TABLE 9-8

Measurements Made During Testing for Exercise Capacity and Its Limitations

Measurement	Definition	Typical Values at Peak Exercise Capacity
$\dot{V}O_2$max	Maximal uptake of O_2 per minute at peak exercise capacity	Men: 35-90 mL/kg/min Women: 25-75 mL/kg/min
Anaerobic threshold	Exercise intensity beyond which progressive increases in blood lactate occur	>40% $\dot{V}O_2$max
HRmax	Maximal heart rate at peak exercise capacity	220 – age
Breathing reserve	Proportion of MVV that is unused after reaching maximal minute ventilation at peak exercise	>30%
SpO_2	O_2 saturation (pulse oximetry)	>88%
O_2 pulse	Oxygen consumption per heart beat at peak exercise capacity	Men: >12 mL/beat Women: >8 mL/beat

HR, heart rate; MVV, maximal voluntary ventilation; $\dot{V}O_2$, oxygen consumption.

cannot achieve a peak exercise level of at least 5 METs. Poor exercise capacity can be due to poor physical conditioning or the presence of a cardiovascular or pulmonary disorder.

Low exercise capacity due to *poor conditioning* is associated with a low $\dot{V}O_2$max but a normal **anaerobic threshold** (>40% of the $\dot{V}O_2$max). Poorly conditioned patients also tend to exhibit abnormally high heart rates at peak exercise capacity.

Patients in whom a cardiovascular disorder is the primary factor limiting exercise have a reduced anaerobic threshold, low O_2 pulse, and higher than predicted heart rate at peak exercise capacity. The reduced O_2 pulse occurs because the diseased heart cannot increase stroke volume sufficiently to meet increased exercise demands.

Patients in whom a pulmonary disorder is the primary factor limiting exercise may have adequate stroke volumes but cannot increase their ventilation sufficiently to meet exercise demands. This limitation is evident as a reduction in breathing reserve. Normal individuals have a breathing reserve of at least 30%, meaning that at peak exercise, they are only using about 70% or less of their MVV to meet their metabolic demands. Patients with pulmonary disorders typically exhibit breathing reserves below 30%. In addition, these patients also may exhibit a reduced SpO_2 during exercise. This occurs most often in those with advanced COPD and interstitial lung diseases who have marginal arterial oxygen saturation at rest.

Simple exercise testing also may be conducted in the pulmonary function laboratory or outpatient clinic to:
- Assess for exercise-induced bronchospasm and it response to therapy
- Determine whether arterial desaturation occurs with exercise and titrate needed supplemental O_2

The test is used to detect exercise-induced bronchospasm, before and after spirometry is conducted, with a drop of 20% or more in the patient's FEV_1 after exercise constituting a positive test.

General contraindications against exercise testing include acute myocardial infarction, uncontrolled heart failure, unstable angina, significant cardiac dysrhythmias, acute pulmonary disorders, and severe hypertension. An exercise test should be terminated if a wide swing in blood pressure occurs, angina or dyspnea becomes severe, a serious dysrhythmia occurs, or the patient becomes dizzy, confused, or cyanotic.

Infection Control

With the increasing use of bacterial filters and disposable breathing circuits and flow sensors, cross-contamination has become less of an issue in pulmonary function testing. Of course, any reusable components such as breathing valves and manifolds should be disinfected or sterilized regularly. The ideal frequency for disinfection or sterilization of reusable components has not been established. However, any reusable components that show visible breath condensation should undergo high-level disinfection or sterilization between patients.

In terms of the methods used to disinfect or sterilize reusable components, it is essential to adhere to the manufacturer's recommendations for processing. This is because some processing methods can cause damage to critical components, such as flow sensors or valve seals. It is important to note that after disassembly, cleaning, and disinfection, nondisposable sensors usually requires recalibration before use.

If closed-circuit methods using a volumetric spirometer are employed in testing, the bell or bellows should be flushed with room air at least five times between tests. This is necessary to eliminate the possibility of cross-contamination due to the persistence of droplet nuclei in these systems. In addition, the full breathing circuit, including the mouthpiece, should be decontaminated or changed between patients. When using open-circuit methods in which the patient only exhales into the device, only those elements through which rebreathing occurs need to be decontaminated or changed.

Placement of a disposable bacterial filter between the patient and circuit eliminates the need to regularly decontaminate or change system components. Systems using such filters must still meet the minimal quality assurance standards, as previously discussed. In addition, pulmonary function testing filters must exhibit minimum flow resistance and create little or no back-pressure. Specifications proving that their filters have no effect on measurements should be provided by the manufacturer.

To protect oneself from infection, pulmonary function testing should be conducted using standard precautions. Airborne precautions should be employed when there is potential exposure to infectious agents transmitted by that route, such as tuberculosis. Hands should always be washed between patients and immediately after direct handling of used circuit components, whether reusable or disposable.

KEY POINTS

- ▶ The vital capacity is the maximal volume of air that can be exhaled after a maximal inhalation, typically 4 to 5 L in normal adults and varying primarily with an individual's height.
- ▶ Total lung capacity equals the sum of all four lung volumes: $RV + V_T + ERV + IRV$.
- ▶ Basic spirometry is indicated primarily to detect abnormal lung function, quantify the severity of disease, and assess a patient's response to treatment.
- ▶ Slow vital capacity measured at the bedside using a simple respirometer is used to assess for postoperative risk and need for mechanical ventilation.
- ▶ The ratio of FEV_1 to FVC (FEV_1/FVC) is the proportion of the FVC expired during the first second of the maneuver and is the key spirometry measure used to identify obstructive ventilatory impairments.
- ▶ Although effort dependent, the peak expiratory flow (PEF) can be used by patients with asthma to monitor for bronchospasm and help make self-management decisions. Values below 80% of the patient's personal best indicate the need for action.
- ▶ The width of a maximal inspiratory-expiratory flow-volume curve is the forced vital capacity or FVC (X-axis); the maximal positive deflection on the flow axis (Y-axis) is the PEF, with the maximal negative deflection on this axis being the peak inspiratory flow (PIF).
- ▶ A patient's estimated MVV = measured $FEV_1 \times 40$.
- ▶ Spirometer volume measurements should be should be checked daily and be accurate to ±3.5% of the true value (includes 0.5% syringe inaccuracy); flow measurements should be accurate to ±5% of the true value over a range of −14 to +14 L/sec
- ▶ A valid FVC maneuver requires that the subject exhale for at least 6 seconds.
- ▶ An acceptable FVC should be free from artifacts; exhibit a rapid, forceful start; and achieve complete exhalation. The results of the test are repeatable if after three acceptable maneuvers the two largest FVC and FEV_1 values are within 0.150 L of each other.

KEY POINTS—cont'd

- ▶ A spirometry value is considered abnormally low if it is below the 5th percentile of the predicted normal, a boundary called the lower limit of normal, or LLN.
- ▶ If a patient's FVC, FEV_1, and FEV_1/FVC all exceed the LLN, results are normal; an obstructive ventilatory impairment exists if the FEV_1 is low and the FEV_1/FVC ratio is less than the LLN; the combination of a reduced FVC, normal or reduced FEV_1, and FEV_1/FVC above the LLN suggests either a restrictive ventilatory impairment or poor effort.
- ▶ An obstructive ventilatory defect is considered reversible if, after bronchodilator administration, the FEV_1 or FVC increase by more than 12% and 200 mL.
- ▶ Static lung volume determinations are used to confirm a restrictive disease pattern, assess the response to medical or surgical interventions, and measure the extent of gas trapping.
- ▶ The helium dilution and N_2 washout methods for FRC determination only measure lung volume in communication with the airways. The volume of air trapped in the lungs is not measured. Trapped air can only be measured by body plethysmography.
- ▶ The classic pattern of a restrictive ventilatory impairment is a reduced TLC due to a reduction in inspiratory capacity and a decrease in FRC or RV, or both.
- ▶ The primary indication for measuring D_{LCO} is to help differentiate between interstitial and chest wall or neuromuscular causes of restrictive ventilatory impairments; D_{LCO} measurement also is indicated to evaluate pulmonary involvement in systemic diseases and the effects of chemotherapy, radiation, and selected drugs on lung function.
- ▶ A valid single-breath D_{LCO} maneuver requires that the patient inspire quickly to at least 85% of vital capacity, properly hold the breath for at least 10 seconds, and provide a smooth, unforced expiration in less than 4 seconds.
- ▶ In patients with restrictive ventilatory impairments, a normal D_{LCO} suggests a chest wall or neuromuscular disorder, whereas a reduced D_{LCO} is consistent with interstitial lung disease.
- ▶ The commonly cited reference range for normal airway resistance in healthy adults is 0.5 to 2.5 cm H_2O/L per second.
- ▶ The slope of the lung volume–versus–transpulmonary pressure curve at any given volume represents the lung compliance.
- ▶ The methacholine bronchoprovocation test ends when either the maximal dose of methacholine has been given or the FEV_1 has fallen by 20% or more from baseline.
- ▶ Moderate to severe airway hyperresponsiveness is indicated when the provocative concentration of methacholine resulting in the 20% or greater fall in FEV_1 (PC_{20}) is less than 1 mg/mL.
- ▶ Measurement of the exhaled fraction of NO is useful in both the diagnosis and management of asthma, including assessing the response to inhaled steroids
- ▶ An F_ENO greater than 50 ppb in symptomatic adults not taking steroids generally confirms the diagnosis of asthma; for patients with asthma, this measure may indicate poor treatment compliance, poor inhaler technique, or inadequate inhaled steroid dosing.

CASE STUDY

A 70-year-old man has a chief complaint of severe dyspnea on exertion. The dyspnea has increased gradually over the past several years. He has had severe kyphoscoliosis from his teenage years. He denies a history of cough, sputum production, smoking, working in a polluted environment, or respiratory disease. Physical examination reveals tachypnea, tachycardia, jugular venous distention, ankle edema, and kyphoscoliosis.

Personal Data
Age: 70 years
Height: 66 inches
Weight: 155 lb
Sex: male

Spirometry Report	Predicted	Observed	Predicted %
FVC (L)	3.78	1.46	39
FEV_1 (L)	2.57	1.40	54
FEV_1/FVC	75%	96%	—
$FEF_{25-75\%}$ (L/sec)	2.46	2.01	82

Lung Volume Studies (body box)	Predicted	Observed	Predicted %
VC (L)	3.78	1.79	47.4
FRC (L)	2.42	2.01	83.0
RV (L)	1.75	1.86	106
TLC (L)	5.78	3.65	63.2
RV/TLC	30%	51%	—

Interpretation
Spirometry reveals a small FVC and FEV_1 with a normal FEV_1/FVC ratio and $FEF_{25-75\%}$. This suggests that the small FEV_1 is caused by restrictive lung disease and small

lung volumes rather than by an obstructive impairment with low flows. The lung volume studies demonstrate a small VC and TLC. These findings confirm restrictive lung disease.

The lung function studies are typical for a patient with kyphoscoliosis. Kyphoscoliosis causes a reduction in the size of the thoracic cage and can severely compromise lung expansion and eventually result in pulmonary hypertension (cor pulmonale), which can cause right heart failure, resulting in elevated jugular venous distention and pedal edema.

CASE STUDY

A 38-year-old man complains of long-standing dyspnea on exertion. His dyspnea has increased over the past year and now occurs with minimal exertion. He denies cough, chest pain, and sputum production. He has a 40-pack-year smoking history. There is no history of exposure to environmental pollutants. Physical examination shows large anteroposterior chest diameter and diminished breath sounds bilaterally.

Personal Data
Age: 38 years
Height: 76 inches
Weight: 188 lb
Sex: male

Spirometry Report	Predicted	Observed	Predicted %
FVC (L)	6.06	5.10	79
FEV_1 (L)	4.52	1.53	34
FEV_1/FVC	75%	28%	—

Interpretation
Spirometry reveals a markedly low FEV_1 and FEV_1/FVC, indicating a severe obstructive ventilatory impairment.

Discussion
FVC measurement pre- and post-bronchodilator and static lung volume, and D_{LCO} measurements would help further evaluate this patient's status. There should be a high index of suspicion for α_1-antitrypsin deficiency in this patient given the severity of his lung disease at such a young age.

CASE STUDY

A 72-year-old woman was admitted to the medical service complaining of weakness and shortness of breath. She recently had been diagnosed with asthma but previously was in good health. Physical examination of the chest revealed markedly diminished breath sounds. There was no wheezing, but crackles were noted at both bases. The admitting chest radiograph revealed the presence of bi-basilar atelectasis but was otherwise clear. Her admitting laboratory work was normal. Her blood gas results indicated that her pH was normal, but the $Paco_2$ was 54 mm Hg, with a Pao_2 of 58 mm Hg while breathing room air.

After 3 days of standard therapy for asthma that included inhaled bronchodilators and steroids, her respiratory symptoms did not improve. Her $Paco_2$ had increased to 62 mm Hg, and her chest radiograph was unchanged. Her weakness was a little better. Pulmonary consultation was requested.

The consultant requested bedside spirometry. More blood testing was also ordered, including a sedimentation rate and anti-acetylcholine receptor (AChR) antibody.

Personal Data
Age: 72 years
Height: 63.5 inches
Weight: 166 lb
Sex: female

Spirometry Report	Predicted	Observed	Predicted %
FVC (L)	2.80	1.45	52
FEV_1 (L)	2.13	1.19	56
FEV_1/FVC	75%	82%	—

Interpretation
Results indicate low lung volumes with a normal FEV_1/FVC. This indicates restrictive lung disease rather than obstructive lung disease such as asthma.

Discussion
Restrictive lung disease may be caused by diseases that decrease lung compliance, such as pulmonary fibrosis; by diseases that "stiffen" the chest wall, such as kyphoscoliosis; by diseases associated with muscle weakness, such as muscular dystrophy; or by neurologic disorders affecting nerve transmission, such as amyotrophic lateral sclerosis or myasthenia gravis. Results in this case confirm a restrictive impairment. Blood testing for antibodies against the neurotransmitter acetylcholine makes the specific diagnosis of myasthenia gravis. As myasthenia gravis worsens, respiratory muscles weaken, and the patient develops hypercapnic respiratory failure ("myasthenia crisis"). This is the reason for the patient's rising $Paco_2$. The patient's chest radiograph findings of small volumes and bi-basilar atelectasis are also explained by weakening respiratory muscles, causing an inability to take a deep breath.

ASSESSMENT QUESTIONS

See Appendix for answers.

1. What is the term used to describe the volume of gas that can be exhaled maximally after a full inspiration?
   a. Total lung capacity
   b. Vital capacity
   c. Functional residual capacity
   d. Expiratory reserve volume
2. What volume is obtained by subtracting the VC from the TLC?
   a. Residual volume
   b. Tidal volume
   c. Inspiratory reserve volume
   d. Expiratory reserve volume
3. Which of the following tests would you recommend to quantify the disease severity of a patient diagnosed with asthma?
   a. Basic spirometry
   b. Diffusing capacity
   c. Static lung volumes
   d. Exercise capacity
4. Which of the following slow vital capacity measurements indicates inadequate ventilatory reserve?
   a. 10 mL/kg
   b. 30 mL/kg
   c. 50 mL/kg
   d. 70 mL/kg
5. What percentage of the FVC is normally exhaled in the first second?
   a. 50%
   b. 65%
   c. 75%
   d. 85%
6. What spirometry parameter would you recommend to assist a patient with asthma in monitoring her day-to-day status and need for treatment?
   a. FEV_1
   b. PEF
   c. FEV_3
   d. FVC
7. Which parameter is represented as the maximal positive deflection on the Y-axis of a standard inspiratory-expiratory flow-volume curve?
   a. PIF
   b. FVC
   c. PEF
   d. FEV_1
8. Spirometry results for a patient indicate a FVC of 3.5 L and an FEV_1 of 2.5 L. What is this patient's estimated MVV?
   a. 100 L/min
   b. 140 L/min
   c. 80 L/min
   d. 60 L/min
9. In addition to calibration with a 3-L syringe, which of the following methods should be used to validate spirometer performance and accuracy of software computations?
   a. Leak testing of the system
   b. Testing with biologic controls
   c. Random testing of patients
   d. Checking the program code

10. A valid FVC maneuver requires that the subject exhale for at least:
    a. 1 second
    b. 3 seconds
    c. 6 seconds
    d. 10 seconds

11. When performing bedside spirometry, you observe an S-shaped plotted FVC-versus-time curve on the display. Which of the following is the likely problem with this maneuver?
    a. Failure to achieve complete exhalation
    b. Early termination/cut-off of exhalation
    c. Coughing/breathing during the maneuver
    d. Failure to achieve a rapid start to exhalation

12. The upper and lower limits of normal spirometry data are calculated as being how many standard deviations (SD) from the mean?
    a. ±1 SD
    b. ±2 SD
    c. ±3 SD
    d. ±4 SD

13. Bedside spirometry results for a patient indicate an FVC lower than the LLN, with the FEV_1 and FEV_1/FVC both being higher than the LLN. Which of the following are possible interpretations?
    1. The patient has a restrictive impairment
    2. The results are inconsistent and therefore invalid
    3. The patient is not providing maximal effort
    4. The patient has an obstructive impairment
        a. 1 only
        b. 4 only
        c. 1 and 3
        d. 2 only

14. Which of the following pre- and post-bronchodilator spirometry results is most indicative of a reversible obstructive disorder?
    a. PEF increases 1 L/sec
    b. FVC increases 100 mL
    c. FEV_1 increases by 15%
    d. FRC increases by 15%

15. Based on their basic spirometry results, which of the following patients would you recommend for static lung volume determination (FRC/TLC measurement)?
    a. Patient A: FVC < LLN, FEV_1/FVC > LLN
    b. Patient B: FVC > LLN, FEV_1/FVC > LLN
    c. Patient C: FVC < LLN, FEV_1/FVC < LLN
    d. Patient D: FVC > LLN, FEV_1/FVC < LLN

16. Which of the following tests would you recommend to measure the extent of gas trapping in a patient with emphysema?
    a. Closed-circuit He dilution FRC measurement
    b. Single-breath diffusing capacity of the lung
    c. Open circuit N_2 washout FRC measurement
    d. Body plethysmography measurement of TGV

17. Which of the following are consistent with obstructive lung disease?
    a. Decreased lung volumes and decreased flows
    b. Increased lung volumes and decreased flows
    c. Decreased lung volumes and increased flows
    d. Increased lung volumes and increased flows

18. Which of the following tests would you recommend to help differentiate between interstitial and chest wall/neuromuscular causes of a restrictive ventilatory impairment?
    a. Closed-circuit He dilution FRC measurement
    b. Single-breath diffusing capacity of the lung
    c. Body plethysmography measurement of TGV
    d. Exercise capacity testing with O_2 consumption

19. Which of the following would invalidate the results of a single-breath D_{LCO} maneuver?
    a. Patient holding the breath for more than 5 seconds
    b. Patient exhaling smoothly in less than 4 seconds
    c. Patient performing a Valsalva maneuver during breath hold
    d. Patient inspiring to 90% of best vital capacity

20. After comprehensive pulmonary laboratory assessment, a patient has the following results: FVC < LLN, FEV_1/FVC > LLN, TLC < LLN, IC < LLN, D_{LCO} > LLN. Which of the following is the most likely cause?
    a. Pulmonary emphysema
    b. A neuromuscular disorder
    c. An interstitial lung disease
    d. A pulmonary vascular disorder

21. Static lung compliance is computed using which of the following formulas?
    a. Lung volume ÷ transpulmonary pressure gradient
    b. Lung volume ÷ transthoracic pressure gradient
    c. Lung volume ÷ transrespiratory pressure gradient
    d. Transpulmonary pressure gradient ÷ airflow

22. Which of the following patient(s) would you recommend for methacholine bronchoprovocation testing?
    1. A patient who experiences unexplained wheezing at his job site
    2. A patient with a history of nighttime shortness of breath and coughing
    3. A patient with spirometry data indicating severe obstruction (FEV_1 < 1 L)
        a. 1 only
        b. 1 and 2
        c. 2 and 3
        d. 1, 2, and 3

23. After progressive step-up to 16 mg/mL methacholine, a patient exhibits a 15% decrease in FEV_1 compared with baseline. You would interpret this result as indicating:
    a. Normal airway responsiveness
    b. Borderline hyperresponsiveness
    c. Mild hyperresponsiveness
    d. Severe hyperresponsiveness

24. Which of the following would invalidate the results of an expired nitric oxide (F_ENO) maneuver?
   a. Performance after spirometry
   b. Exhalation > 6 sec
   c. F_ENO plateau > 3 sec
   d. ±5% variation in plateau F_ENO

25. An adult patient with recurrent episodes of shortness of breath, wheezing, and coughing has an expired nitric oxide (F_ENO) level of 15 ppb. Which of the following diagnosis is *least* likely?
   a. Cystic fibrosis
   b. Eosinophilic asthma
   c. Sinusitis
   d. Gastroesophageal reflux

26. Which of the following patients' 6-Minute Walk Test results indicate an abnormally low functional capacity?
   a. Male patient, 6MWD 500 meters
   b. Female patient, 6MWD 400 meters
   c. Male patient, 6MWD 400 meters
   d. Female patient, 6MWD 500 meters

27. Which of the following are indications for cardiopulmonary exercise testing?
   1. To diagnose obstructive coronary artery disease (CAD)
   2. To differentiate between cardiac and pulmonary limitations to exercise
   3. To determine whether arterial desaturation occurs with exercise
      a. 1 only
      b. 1 and 2
      c. 2 and 3
      d. 1, 2, and 3

28. What would be the estimated maximal heart rate at peak exercise capacity for a 60-year-old man?
   a. 120 beats/min
   b. 140 beats/min
   c. 160 beats/min
   d. 180 beats/min

29. Exercise capacity test results for a 55-year-old woman are as follows:
   • $\dot{V}O_2$max decreased
   • Anaerobic threshold normal
   • O_2 pulse normal
   • Breathing reserve decreased
   Which of the following is the most likely cause of the decreased $\dot{V}O_2$max?
   a. Cardiovascular limitation to exercise
   b. Pulmonary limitation to exercise
   c. Poor physical conditioning
   d. Cannot determine from these data

30. Proper methods to minimize cross-contamination between patients performing tests that only require exhalation into the apparatus include which of the following?
   1. Change only those elements through which rebreathing occurs
   2. Change the entire breathing circuit, including mouthpiece and valves
   3. Place a disposable bacterial filter between the patient and breathing circuit
      a. 1 only
      b. 1 and 3
      c. 1 and 2
      d. 2 and 3

Bibliography

American Association for Respiratory Care. Clinical practice guideline. Single-breath carbon monoxide diffusing capacity, 1999 update. *Respir Care* 1999;**44**(5):539–46.

American Association for Respiratory Care. Clinical practice guideline. Methacholine challenge testing: 2001 revision and update. *Respir Care* 2001;**46**(5):523–30.

American Association for Respiratory Care. Clinical practice guideline. Static lung volumes: 2001 revision and update. *Respir Care* 2001;**46**(5):531–9.

American Thoracic Society and American College of Chest Physicians. ATS/ACCP Statement on cardiopulmonary exercise testing. *Am J Respir Crit Care Med* 2003;**167**(2):211–77.

American Thoracic Society and European Respiratory Society. ATS/ERS recommendations for standardized procedures for the online and offline measurement of exhaled lower respiratory nitric oxide and nasal nitric oxide. *Am J Respir Crit Care Med* 2005;**171**(8):912–30.

American Thoracic Society. Guidelines for methacholine and exercise challenge testing—1999. *Am J Respir Crit Care Med* 2000;**161**(1):309–29.

American Thoracic Society. ATS statement: guidelines for the six-minute walk test. *Am J Respir Crit Care Med* 2002;**166**(1):111–7.

Brazzale DJ, Upward AL, Pretto JJ. Effects of changing reference values and definition of the normal range on interpretation of spirometry. *Respirology* 2010;**15**(7):1098–103.

Busse WW. What is the best pulmonary diagnostic approach for wheezing patients with normal spirometry?. *Respir Care* 2012;**57**(1):39–46.

Chipps BE. Spirometry versus flow volume inspiratory and expiratory loop. *Ann Allergy Asthma Immunol* 2011;**107**(2):183.

Cooper B. Spirometry standards and FEV1/FVC repeatability. *Prim Care Respir J* 2010;**19**(3):292–4.

Cockcroft DW. Airway hyperresponsiveness in asthma: its measurement and clinical significance. *Chest* 2010;**138** (Suppl. 2):18S–24S.

D'Urzo AD, Tamari I, Bouchard J, et al. New spirometry interpretation algorithm: Primary Care Respiratory Alliance of Canada approach. *Can Fam Physician* 2011;**57**(10):1148–52.

Dweik RA, Boggs PB, Erzurum SC. An official ATS clinical practice guideline: interpretation of exhaled nitric oxide levels (F_ENO) for clinical applications. *Am J Respir Crit Care Med* 2011;**184**(5):602–15.

Enright P. FEV1 and FVC repeatability goals when performing spirometry. *Prim Care Respir J* 2010;**19**(2):194.

Enright P. The new all-age spirometry reference equations are the best available for Caucasians, regardless of where they live. *Respirology* 2011;**16**(6):871–2.

European Respiratory Society Task Force on Respiratory Impedance Measurements. The forced oscillation technique in clinical practice: methodology, recommendations and future developments. *Eur Respir J* 2003;**22**(6):1026–41.

Fletcher M, Loveridge C. Recommendations on repeatability of spirometry. *Prim Care Respir J* 2010;**19**(2):192.

Hankinson JL, Odencratz JR, Fedan KB. Spirometric reference values from a sample of the general US population. *Am J Respir Crit Care Med* 1999;**159**(1):179-87.

Hayes Jr D, Kraman SS. The physiologic basis of spirometry. *Respir Care* 2009;**54**(12):1717-26.

Haynes JM. Comprehensive quality control for pulmonary function testing: it's time to face the music. *Respir Care* 2010;**55**(3):355-7.

Hnatiuk OW. What is the role of PFTs in monitoring adverse effects of surgery, drug treatments, radiation therapy, and during hospitalization? *Respir Care* 2012;**57**(1):75-82.

Kaminsky DA. What does airway resistance tell us about lung function?. *Respir Care* 2012;**57**(1):85-96.

Kreider ME, Grippi MA. Impact of the new ATS/ERS pulmonary function test interpretation guidelines. *Respir Med* 2007;**101**(11):2336-42.

Laszlo G. Standardisation of lung function testing: helpful guidance from the ATS/ERS Task Force. *Thorax* 2006;**61**(9):744-6.

Lim KG, Mottram C. The use of fraction of exhaled nitric oxide. *Chest* 2008;**133**(5):1232-42.

Macintyre N, Crapo RO, Viegi G, et al. Standardisation of the single-breath determination of carbon monoxide uptake in the lung. *Eur Respir J* 2005;**26**(4):720-35.

Macintyre NR. Spirometry for the diagnosis and management of chronic obstructive pulmonary disease. *Respir Care* 2009;**54**(8):1050-7.

Miller A, Enright PL. PFT interpretive strategies: American Thoracic Society/European Respiratory Society 2005 guideline gaps. *Respir Care* 2012;**57**(1):127-33.

Miller MR, Crapo R, Hankinson J, et al. General considerations for lung function testing. *Eur Respir J* 2005;**26**(1):153-61.

Miller MR, Hankinson J, Brusasco V, et al. Standardisation of spirometry. *Eur Respir J* 2005;**26**(2):319-38.

Moore AJ. Spirometer calibration check procedures. *Respir Care* 2007;**52**(3):341-2.

Pellegrino R, Viegi G, Brusasco V, et al. Interpretative strategies for lung function tests. *Eur Respir J* 2005;**26**(5):948-68.

Perez-Padilla R, Vazquez-Garcia JC, Marquez MN, et al. Spirometry quality-control strategies in a multinational study of the prevalence of chronic obstructive pulmonary disease. *Respir Care* 2008;**53**(8):1019-26.

Pichurko BM. Exercising your patient: which test(s) and when? *Respir Care* 2012;**57**(1):100-10.

Powell CA, Caplan CE. Pulmonary function tests in preoperative pulmonary evaluation. *Clin Chest Med* 2001;**22**(4):703-14.

Quanjer PH, Ruppel GL, Diagnosing COPD. high time for a paradigm shift. *Respir Care* 2011;**56**(11):1861-3.

Ruppel GL. What is the clinical value of lung volumes? *Respir Care* 2012;**57**(1):26-35.

Ruppel GL, Enright PL. Pulmonary function testing. *Respir Care* 2012;**57**(1):165-75.

Stocks J, Quanjer PH. Reference values for residual volume, functional residual capacity and total lung capacity. *Eur Respir J* 1995;**8**(3):492-506.

Stoller JK. Quality control for spirometry in large epidemiologic studies: "breathing quality" into our work. *Respir Care* 2008;**53**(8):1008-9.

Wang JS. Pulmonary function tests in preoperative pulmonary evaluation. *Respir Med* 2004;**98**(7):598-605.

Wang X, Dockery DW, Wypij D, et al. Pulmonary function between 6 and 18 years of age. *Pediatr Pulmonol* 1993;**15**(2):75-88.

Wanger J, Clausen JL, Coates A, et al. Standardisation of the measurement of lung volumes. *Eur Respir J* 2005;**26**(3):511-22.

Chest Imaging

ZAZA COHEN*

CHAPTER OUTLINE

LEARNING OBJECTIVES

After reading this chapter, you will be able to:
1. Describe how the chest radiograph is produced.
2. Define the terms radiolucent and radiopaque.
3. Discuss how the appearance of a certain organ or tissue on a radiograph depends on its density.
4. Explain how the spatial relationship between the x-ray source, the patient, and the x-ray film affects the magnification of images on the radiograph. Identify the clinical indications for the use of a chest radiograph.
5. Discuss different types of radiograph orientations.
6. Recognize the proper technique for performing a systematic descriptive evaluation (interpretation) of the chest radiograph.
7. Explain the significance of the following special radiographic evaluation signs:
 a. Silhouette sign
 b. Air bronchogram
 c. Deep sulcus sign
 d. Kerley B lines
 e. Coin lesions

*James Dexter MD, FACP, FCCP contributed some of the content for this chapter as the coeditor of prior editions.

LEARNING OBJECTIVES—cont'd

8. Discuss the limitations of the chest radiograph.
9. Appraise the typical clinical and chest radiographic findings for the following lung disorders:
   a. Atelectasis
   b. Pneumothorax
   c. Hyperinflation
   d. Interstitial lung disease
   e. Congestive heart failure
   f. Pleural effusion
   g. Consolidation
   h. Pneumonia
10. Describe the correct position for endotracheal tube placement as seen on a chest radiograph.
11. Identify the value and limitations of using radiographs to determine a position of tubes and catheters
12. List situations that require obtaining a postprocedure chest radiograph.
13. Explain the technique, indications, and advantages and disadvantages for computed tomography scanning.
14. Discuss the relative use and indications for magnetic resonance imaging in lung disease.
15. Explain the technique and indications for performing nuclear medicine lung scans.
16. Explain the technique and indications for the use of pulmonary angiography.
17. Discuss the utility of ultrasound, fluoroscopy, and interventional radiology in diagnosis and treatment of lung diseases.
18. Give a brief overview of radiation safety.

KEY TERMS

air bronchogram
anteroposterior (AP) view
apical lordotic view
atelectasis
bronchoscopy
chest radiograph
chest ultrasound
computed tomography (CT)
deep sulcus sign
expiratory view

exudate
fluoroscopy
interventional radiology
Kerley B lines
lateral decubitus view
magnetic resonance imaging (MRI)
oblique view
pneumothorax
positron emission tomography (PET)

posteroanterior (PA) view
pulmonary angiography
radiolucent
radionuclide lung scanning
radiopaque
silhouette sign
target
thoracentesis
transudate

The introduction of x-ray technology in the early part of the last century gave medical workers a chance to see a silhouette of the structures inside the human for the first time. The result of this advance was revolutionary. A physician's ability to detect disease expanded beyond what could be identified with the history and physical examination. The use of radiographic examination expanded rapidly because of the simplicity of the technique and the information provided by radiographs. Within a decade or two, radiology became a hospital-based department, and soon thereafter, it became a special discipline within the field of medicine.

This chapter begins with a short description of the physics related to radiographs. The use of standard and special views in assessment of the patient with pulmonary disease is presented next. This is followed by a discussion of techniques for interpreting the chest image. Finally, some of the more common pathologic abnormalities seen on chest radiographs and their related clinical findings are presented. Other imaging modalities, such as **computed tomography (CT)** and **positron emission tomography (PET)** scanning, **chest ultrasound**, and **magnetic resonance imaging (MRI)**, as well as radiation safety issues, are discussed at the end of the chapter.

Production of the Radiograph

X-rays are electromagnetic waves that radiate from a tube through which an electric current has been passed. The tube is made of a cathode that is attached to a low-voltage electron source (transformer). The end of the cathode wire is inside the vacuum-sealed tube, and as electrons flow through the wire, they are "boiled off," accelerate across a short gap, and strike a positively charged tungsten plate called the *anode*. The electrons coming off the cathode wire are focused to hit a small area on the anode. This area is called the **target**.

On striking the target, the electrons undergo physical changes that result in the emission of x-rays. The origins of

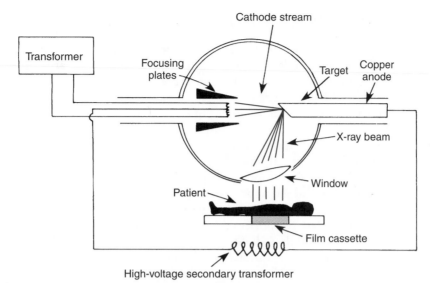

FIGURE 10-1 Electric current is generated by the transformer, passes through focusing plates, and arrives at the cathode. Electrons are "boiled off," making a cathode stream. The cathode stream then strikes the anode target and is transformed into x-rays. X-rays leave the sealed vacuum x-ray tube through a window and strike the patient, pass through the patient, and cast a shadow on the image cassette, making an image on the image. (From Scanlan CL, Spearman CB, Sheldon RL: *Egan's fundamentals of respiratory therapy,* ed 5. St. Louis, 1996, Mosby.)

the name *x-rays* are rather remarkable. Wilhelm Roentgen, a physicist from the 19th century, who is unanimously credited for the discovery of x-rays, was experimenting with various types of electromagnetic radiation. He called a particular type of radiation that he was studying x-rays, "x" for the unknown. Since then, the electromagnetic radiation in general and x-rays in particular have been extensively studied, but the name x-rays still persists, although in some countries they are referred to as *Roentgen radiation*. These x-rays are emitted in all directions, but because of the construction of the tube, only the few that escape through the window are actually used; the rest are absorbed harmlessly into the wall of the x-ray machine (Fig. 10-1). X-rays are not reflected like light rays but penetrate most matter. Their ability to penetrate matter depends on the density of the matter. Dense objects, such as bone, absorb more x-rays (allow less penetration) than air-filled objects, such as lung tissue.

A **chest radiograph** is generated by placing a sheet of film next to the patient's thorax opposite the x-ray tube. The x-ray machine emits x-rays, which pass through the patient and are absorbed by the film inversely proportional to the density of the tissue through which they pass. X-rays that pass through low-density (air-filled) tissue strike the film in great numbers and turn it black (**radiolucent**). Radiolucent areas on the chest radiograph are seen as dark shadows. X-rays that strike bone are partially absorbed; therefore, fewer x-rays strike the film, and there is less darkening of the corresponding area on the radiograph (**radiopaque**). Radiopaque areas are seen as white shadows on the film. The whole concept of "film" has recently changed with the advent of digital image processing.

In the past, a sheet of film that had the image of the x-rays would have to be "developed" (much like the old film photography) and then viewed by placing it on a box that would provide a background light in a dark room. Instead, we now use cassettes that acquire the images digitally and then transfer that digital image of the x-ray onto a computer database to be viewed electronically or placed in the patient's electronic medical record. After transfer, the cassette that was just used in the last x-ray production is ready to record a new image, much like a modern memory card can store new images after the old ones have been erased or transferred. Just as with digital still photography, digital x-ray imaging provides many tools for the interpreter (magnification, change of contrast, inversion, to name a few) that were not available in the old-fashioned films. One might argue that the use of the term film is now outdated because the actual film is not used in either production or viewing of the x-ray images. Despite this conceptual change, many clinicians will continue to use the term film to describe digital x-ray images. We will perpetuate this misnomer throughout the chapter and will call *the film* the cassette that acquires the x-ray images as well as the computer that produces the images.

One major flaw of all radiographs that a clinician needs to remember is that they present a two-dimensional view of a three-dimensional object. Structures on the same horizontal level produce the same shadow on the image whether they are inside or outside of the body. For example, a coin taped to the outside of the patient's chest (either in the front or back) will produce the same shadow as a round lung mass—hence, many round-shaped lung masses (or nodules) are called *coin lesions*. Similarly, nipple shadows often cause concern because they cannot be easily distinguished from lesions originating from lung parenchyma.

Four distinct densities recognized on radiographs are that of bone, which is very dense; water, which is less dense; fat, which is mildly radiolucent; and air, which is very radiolucent. Most tissues in the body have a characteristic density based on the mixture of these materials. The anatomy of the chest makes radiographs extremely useful for studying diseases of the chest. The contrast between the bony structures of the chest, the heart, the vascular structures of the mediastinum, and the diaphragm, which appear radiopaque on radiographs, and the lungs, which appear radiolucent, allows for easy recognition of these structures on the image and various diseases that affect them. For a comparison, muscles in the thigh are uniformly radiolucent, and there is not much contrast between the various parts of the thigh when radiographs are taken. This makes radiographs of the thigh not helpful, unless one is looking for bony fractures or air that has been introduced from infection or a penetrating wound.

X-rays leave the x-ray tube from a single point and scatter so that they cover the whole x-ray film. This leads to more magnification of shadows on the film if the patient is close to the x-ray tube and less magnification if the patient is not close to the x-ray source. This concept can be demonstrated easily by placing your hand below a lamp and observing the shadow created on the surface below. The shadow becomes smaller and sharper as your hand is moved away from the light source and closer to the surface. The concept of magnification of shadows farther away from the film will become important later in this chapter when we discuss various x-ray techniques. The radiation scatter is important because individuals within the 6 feet radius from the x-ray source are exposed to significant radiation. Radiation safety will be discussed in more detail at the end of the chapter.

SIMPLY STATED

X-rays passing through low-density tissue (e.g., lung parenchyma) create a dark area on the image, and dense tissues (e.g., bone) create a white area on the image.

Indications for the Chest Radiograph Examination

The ability to "see inside" the body with the use of radiographs has proved to be of great benefit, especially when assessing the contents of the chest. Production of the chest radiograph has become one of the most popular and important procedures performed in the hospital. It can be used in the following ways:

- Detecting alterations of the lung caused by pathologic processes
- Determining the appropriate therapy
- Evaluating the effectiveness of treatment
- Determining the position of tubes and catheters

- Observing the progression of lung disease
- Assessing the patient after an invasive procedure

Although the chest radiograph provides important information about the status of the lungs, obtaining and interpreting the image must never delay fundamental treatment of the patient with obvious signs of hypoxia. In most situations, when the members of the health care team are well trained and work together, a chest image can be obtained without interrupting assessment and treatment.

Although only the physician can order a chest radiograph, the respiratory therapist (RT) may want to suggest to the attending physician that a chest image may be needed in certain circumstances. For example, an undiagnosed **pneumothorax** may suddenly cause deterioration of a mechanically ventilated patient. In the setting of a tension pneumothorax (discussed in detail later in this chapter), there may not be time even for an urgent radiograph, and treatment may have to be started solely on clinical grounds. However, in a less urgent situation, a portable chest film may be very helpful in confirming the suspected pneumothorax. The RT is often at the bedside of the mechanically ventilated patient and may be the first person to see the signs consistent with a pneumothorax, or another potentially serious complication, and would be the first to recognize the need for an urgent chest radiograph. For this reason, all RTs should be familiar with the clinical indications for a chest radiograph (Box 10-1).

Radiographic Views
Standard and Special Views

The standard chest radiographs are taken in two directions: posteroanterior and lateral views. First, with the patient standing upright with the back to the x-ray tube, the anterior thorax is pressed against a metal cassette containing the film, and the patient's arms are positioned out of the way. The patient is instructed to take a deep breath and hold it just before the radiograph is taken. The x-ray beam leaves the source, strikes the patient's posterior chest, moves through the chest, exits through the front (anterior), and then strikes the film. This is called a **posteroanterior (PA) view** because the beam moves from posterior to anterior. The heart is in the anterior half of the thorax, so there is less cardiac magnification with a PA view. The patient is then turned sideways, and a lateral or side view is obtained. Generally, a left lateral view (left side against the cassette) is preferred. The left lateral view provides less cardiac magnification (as explained earlier, the proximity of the heart is the cause of lesser magnification) than the right lateral view. On a lateral image, the shadows of the left and right lung are often superimposed and cannot be distinguished. For this reason, the lateral image is often obtained with the patient slightly oblique (about 5 degrees) to the image (an **oblique view**), to allow easier identification of the individual lung shadows.

Other views are sometimes obtained to elucidate special problems. A lateral decubitus view is taken with the

Box 10-1   Clinical Indications for the Chest Radiograph

SYMPTOMS
New or unexplained dyspnea
Cough, sputum, and fever
Chest pain
Hemoptysis

MEDICAL HISTORY
Recent history of chest trauma
History of aspiration of foreign body
History of tuberculosis
History of chronic obstructive pulmonary disease
Significant smoking history
History of pulmonary fibrosis
Employment history consistent with inhalation of certain dusts

PHYSICAL EXAMINATION
Crackles or wheezes on auscultation
Sudden drop in blood pressure during mechanical ventilation
Unilateral decrease in breath sounds
Extensive use of accessory muscles
Respiratory rate >30 breaths/min at rest
Loud P_2 sound
Pedal edema
Cardiac murmurs
Signs of trauma

ARTERIAL BLOOD GAS LEVELS
Severe hypoxemia
Acute hypercapnia

PULMONARY FUNCTION TESTS
Evidence of air trapping (e.g., increase in residual volume or functional residual capacity)
Reduction in expiratory flows or lung volumes
Reduced diffusing capacity of lung for carbon monoxide

POSTPROCEDURE
Intubation
Central venous pressure line or pulmonary artery catheter placement
Nasogastric tube placement
Chest tube placement
Thoracentesis
Pericardiocentesis
Bronchoscopy with transbronchial biopsy
Percutaneous needle biopsy of the lung
Abdominal or thoracic surgery

OTHER
Sudden increase in peak airway pressure (with volume-targeted ventilation) during mechanical ventilation
After cardiopulmonary resuscitation
Routinely for mechanically ventilated patients
Routine screening for infectious disease

---

patient lying on the right or left side to see whether free fluid (pleural fluid) is present in the chest. As little as 50 to 100 mL of pleural fluid can be detected with the lateral decubitus view. This view is also helpful in the identification of pneumothorax. Air tends to rise and water tends to fall; therefore, patients with a suspected pneumothorax should be placed on the opposite side for radiologic examination, and patients with suspected pleural fluid should be placed on the same side as the suspected disease.

Projections made at approximately a 45-degree tube angulation from below, referred to as an **apical lordotic view**, are sometimes required for a closer look at the right middle lobe or the top (apical region) of the lung. When the tube is angled upward, the shadows of the clavicles are projected above the thorax, and the tops of the lungs are much more easily visible.

Oblique views are helpful in delineating a pulmonary or mediastinal lesion from the structures that become superimposed on those lesions on the PA and lateral views (review the limitations of radiographs as two-dimensional views of a three-dimensional objects discussed earlier). Oblique views are often obtained to help localize an abnormality. In this view, the patient is turned 45 degrees to either the right or left, with the anterolateral portion of the chest against the film.

Although chest radiographs are usually taken with the patient at full inspiration, an **expiratory view** can be helpful in certain situations. For example, a small pneumothorax can be difficult or impossible to detect in a routine inspiratory image. As the patient exhales, however, the lung volume is reduced, whereas the pleural air volume remains the same. The pneumothorax now occupies a greater percentage of the thoracic volume and therefore stands out more. In addition, the lung is denser in the expiratory position, and the contrast allows for the air density within the pleural space to be more easily visualized.

With the advance of the technology, CT scans are now readily available, easy to obtain, and able to provide information about thoracic structures that is above and beyond what can be obtained by a variety of special radiographic views. In many instances, these special views have become obsolete and have retained only teaching and historical value.

Portable Chest Image (Anteroposterior View)

Patients in intensive care units are too sick to be transported to the radiology department for a standard PA view. In this instance, a portable radiograph machine is brought to the patient's bedside and positioned in front of the patient. The film cassette is placed carefully behind the patient's back. Thus, the x-ray beam moves from front to back (anterior to posterior), generating an **anteroposterior (AP) view** instead of the usual PA view. The distance from the patient to the beam's origin is typically 4 feet in these conditions, so there is more magnification artifact than with a regular PA view.

Interpreting an AP chest radiograph presents a special challenge because often it is not centered, is rotated, is either overexposed or underexposed, or is not taken when the patient is in full inspiration. There may be many extrathoracic shadows superimposed on the film. These extra shadows include bedding, gowns, electrocardiogram (ECG) leads, and tubing. The clinician has to be able to read the film accurately despite these confounding factors.

SIMPLY STATED

The standard chest radiograph is taken with the patient's chest pressed against the film cassette. The x-ray passes from back (posterior) to front (anterior), and the resulting chest radiograph is called a PA film. The portable chest radiograph is obtained with the x-ray passing from front (anterior) to back (posterior), producing an AP film.

AP portable films are obtained to evaluate lung status, to gain information on how well lines and tubing are positioned, and to see the results of invasive therapeutic maneuvers. Some of the lines and tubes needing evaluation are discussed later in the chapter under Postprocedure Chest Radiograph Evaluation.

Evaluation of the Chest Radiograph

This section introduces the basic principles of chest radiograph evaluation. Interpreting chest images is a skill obtained only through hours of dedicated practice. The beginner is encouraged to view chest images initially with the help of qualified experts.

Familiarity with the anatomic landmarks seen on normal chest images is extremely helpful in learning to recognize abnormalities. Figure 10-2 identifies the important landmarks on a normal PA chest radiograph.

Review of Clinical Findings

The clinician will benefit from reviewing the patient's history and physical examination findings before viewing the chest image. This information can provide insight into the abnormalities to be looked for on the chest image.

Systematic Approach to the Chest Radiograph

The first step in evaluating the chest radiograph is to determine the technical quality of the image. The adequacy of exposure can be judged by looking at the vertebral bodies. The clinician should be able to just about visualize the vertebral bodies through the cardiac shadow. If the vertebral bodies are easily seen, the image is probably overexposed, and the lungs will appear black. Underexposure makes identification of the vertebral bodies more difficult, and the lung fields appear whiter than on a properly exposed image. The pulmonary vascularity and some pulmonary abnormalities may be misinterpreted with overexposure or underexposure.

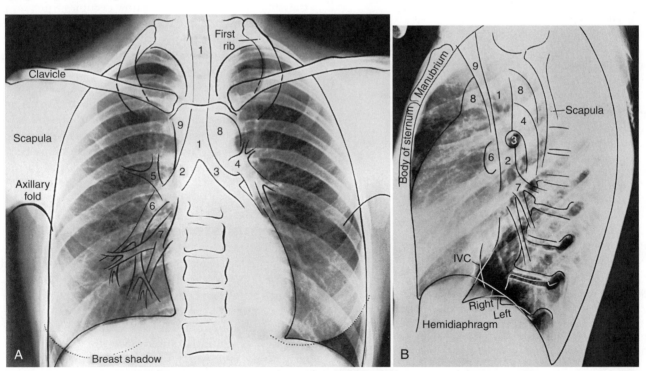

FIGURE 10-2 A, Posteroanterior projection of normal chest image showing the trachea (1), right main bronchus (2), left main bronchus (3), left pulmonary artery (4), right upper lobe pulmonary artery (5), right interlobar artery (6), right lower and middle lobe vein (7), aortic knob (8), and superior vena cava (9). **B,** Lateral projection of normal chest image showing trachea (1), right main bronchus (2), left main bronchus (3), left interlobar artery (4)—not visible in this view (5), right main pulmonary artery (6), confluence of pulmonary veins (7), aortic arch (8), and brachiocephalic vessels (9). IVC, inferior vena cava. (From Fraser RS, Pare RD: *Diagnosis of diseases of the chest.* Philadelphia, 1970, WB Saunders.)

The chest radiograph should be evaluated to make sure that the patient was not rotated when the chest image was obtained. If the patient is rotated, uniform exposure of both lungs will not be obtained, and one side of the image will be darker than the other. The shadows of the heart and other mediastinal structures may also appear enlarged if the patient is rotated. Patient rotation is assessed by identifying the relationship of the spinous processes of the vertebral column to the medial ends of the clavicles (Fig. 10-3). The spinous processes should be centered between the ends of the clavicles and directly behind the tracheal air shadow. If the medial end of one clavicle appears closer to the spine, the patient probably was rotated.

Finally, the degree of the patient's inspiratory effort is evaluated by counting the posterior ribs visible above the diaphragm. On a PA image, 10 ribs indicate a good inspiratory effort. A poor inspiratory effort may cause the heart to appear abnormally enlarged and increase the density of the lung fields so that they appear too white to allow detection of certain lung abnormalities.

SIMPLY STATED

A good inspiratory effort results in 10 posterior ribs visible above the diaphragm. The depth of the patient's inspiration is assessed to help determine the quality of the chest image.

Interpretation

Interpretation of the chest image requires a complete understanding of the x-ray principles introduced at the beginning of this chapter. The clinician must remember that x-ray penetration of structures is inversely proportional to the density of the structure, and thus the greater the density, the less the penetration. X-rays that do not penetrate fully are absorbed, resulting in less exposure of the film and the casting of a white shadow on the image.

Normal lung tissue has a low density (air density) so that few x-rays are absorbed, and normal lung fields appear as dark shadows on the chest radiograph. If an area of the lung consolidates (increases in density) because of pneumonia, tumor, or collapse, that area will absorb more x-rays and appear as a white patch on the film. Abnormalities that decrease lung tissue density, such as cavities and blebs, absorb fewer x-rays and result in darker areas on the film.

The heart, diaphragm, and major blood vessels are considered to have the density of water. Water is denser than air, and water densities result in less exposure and therefore whitish-gray shadows on the chest radiograph. The heart, diaphragm, and major blood vessels rarely alter in density but may change in size, shape, and position. Evaluation of the shadows produced on the chest radiograph by these structures allows a clear view of any deviation from normal in position or size.

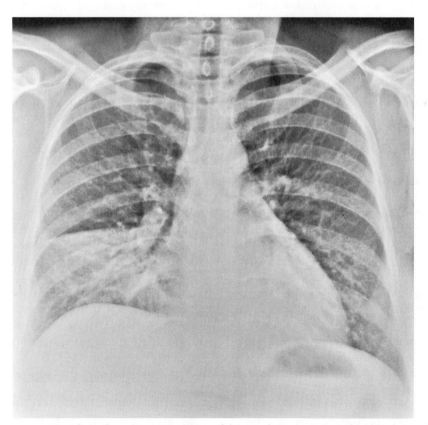

FIGURE 10-3 Note how the spinous processes of the vertebrae are centered within the tracheal air shadow, indicating that the patient was not rotated when the chest image was obtained. Also note the consolidation in the patient's right lung. The infiltrate must be in the right middle lobe because the right heart border is blurred (see description of silhouette sign in text).

It is important to note that the lung shadow on a normal chest radiograph is not uniformly black. The pulmonary vessels that are perpendicular to the x-ray plane give round shadows, and the vessels that are parallel to the plane give tubular shadows. So the normal lung will appear "peppered" with dots and lines that represent pulmonary vasculature. This appearance is sometimes called *normal lung architecture*. As a result of the absence of the lung vasculature, blebs and the air contained in pneumothorax do not have this particular lung architecture appearance, which makes it easier to distinguish them from the normal lung tissue.

The structures in the chest with the greatest density are the bones, including the ribs, clavicles, scapulae, and vertebrae. They are seen on the radiograph as white shadows. Fractures and changes in position and density of bones may be evaluated with a chest radiograph. It should be obtained to evaluate the bony structures of the chest when the patient's history or physical examination suggests chest trauma.

Identification of the abnormalities visible on the chest radiograph requires a systematic review of all the structures shown on it. The sequence in which the structures are evaluated is not important as long as all are included. Many experts encourage beginners to develop a habit of evaluating the bony structures and peripheral areas of the radiograph first. This helps prevent overlooking subtle but important abnormalities in the less conspicuous areas of the radiograph. Once the peripheral soft tissues and bony structures have been viewed, the lung, mediastinum, heart, and diaphragms are inspected carefully. A system using the alphabet—A to Z—has been recommended to remind the examiner which parts of the chest image to study. This system, starting with A for airway, B for bones, C for cardiac shadow, and so forth, may prove useful in organizing the approach to reading the chest radiograph. An alternative approach is to follow a comfortable pathway around the chest radiograph. The major goal is to use the same method of complete review in every individual case.

The ability to localize abnormalities within the thorax is aided by special radiographic signs. Two of the most important radiographic signs are the silhouette sign and the air bronchogram.

Silhouette Sign

The **silhouette sign** is useful primarily in determining whether a pulmonary infiltrate is in anatomic contact with another thoracic structure. Normally, the significant difference in density between two adjoining structures will sharply delineate their borders. This allows a person viewing the chest radiograph to see the heart border, the aortic knob, and the diaphragm shadows on the background of radiolucent lung—a natural contrast between the thoracic tissues that makes the chest radiograph a great diagnostic tool (see comparison to thigh radiograph earlier in this chapter). If the lung tissue in contact with either heart border or sections of diaphragm becomes consolidated, the contrast in densities is lost, and the corresponding heart or diaphragm border is blurred (Fig. 10-4; see Fig. 10-3). This phenomenon is called the silhouette sign.

The heart is located in the anterior thorax, and any infiltrate that obliterates the heart border must also be located in the anterior segments of the lungs (lingula or the right middle lobe). Infiltrates that appear to overlap the heart border on the image but do not affect its sharpness are located in posterior segments and are not in anatomic contact with the heart. An infiltrate in the mid-lung zone on a chest radiograph may be located anteriorly or posteriorly, and the silhouette sign often allows a better localization (a lobe, rather than more vague "zone") of the infiltrate. Infiltrates that create a silhouette sign by blurring the diaphragm border are thought to be in the lower lobes.

> ### SIMPLY STATED
>
> Infiltrates in the lung that blur the edges of the heart, the diaphragm, or other thoracic structures are thought to be adjacent to those structures and allow better localization of the infiltrate.

Air Bronchogram

The presence of **air bronchograms** is useful in determining whether an abnormality seen on the radiograph is located within lung tissue. Intrapulmonary bronchi are not normally visible on chest images because they contain air and are surrounded by air-filled alveoli. Bronchi surrounded by consolidated alveoli are visible because the air within their lumina will stand out in contrast to the surrounding consolidation and fluid. In this situation, the bronchi are seen as linear branching air shadows, signifying that the lesion is within lung tissue. Diseases that both consolidate lung tissue and fill the airways will not produce air bronchograms. Therefore, the presence of an air bronchogram confirms intrapulmonary disease, whereas the absence of an air bronchogram does not rule it out.

Limitations

Although the chest radiograph provides important information about the pathologic changes within the thorax, it does have certain limitations. Small lesions and those located in "blind" areas may not be seen. In addition, the chest image is often normal in patients experiencing significant respiratory symptoms. In the setting of asthma with acute bronchospasm, or acute pulmonary embolism (PE), even though the patient may be severely symptomatic, the chest radiograph often appears normal.

Clinical and Radiographic Findings in Lung Diseases

This section reviews the radiographic findings typical of the more common respiratory disorders. Familiarity with this information is helpful in the interpretation of the chest radiograph. In addition, this section presents the

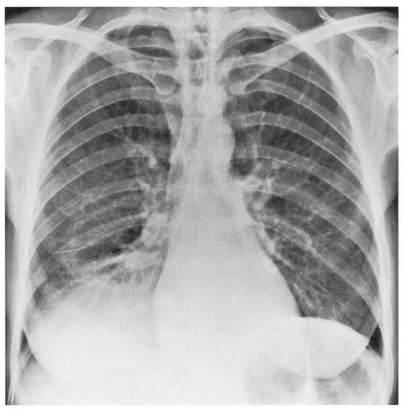

FIGURE 10-4 Right lower lobe pneumonia. Note how the right heart border is clearly seen, indicating that the infiltrate must be in the lower lobe, which is posterior to the heart. Also note that the right hemidiaphragm is obscured. This provides further evidence that the consolidation is in the right lower lobe.

clinical findings typically associated with the different pathologic abnormalities described. In most cases, the most efficient and accurate assessment is achieved when clinical and radiographic findings are used together. The following categories of chest disorders are presented:

- Atelectasis
- Hyperinflation
- Interstitial lung disease
- Congestive heart failure (CHF)
- Pleural effusion
- Consolidation

Atelectasis

Loss of air in a portion of lung tissue results in a condition called **atelectasis** (Fig. 10-5), a word formed from the Greek *ateles* (incomplete) and *ektasis* (extension). Atelectasis may occur as a result of changes in the transpulmonary distending pressure and in such cases is called *compression atelectasis*. It may also be caused by obstruction of one or more airways, which allows distal gas to be absorbed. The latter type of atelectasis may be called *obstructive* or *absorption atelectasis*.

Compression Atelectasis

Compression atelectasis is seen in patients with pleural effusion, pneumothorax, hemothorax, and any space-occupying lesion. The degree of pulmonary compromise

with compression atelectasis depends on the extent of the problem. Severe atelectasis may shift the mediastinum enough to compromise cardiac output and overall hemodynamic status.

Obstructive Atelectasis

Obstructive atelectasis is caused by blockage of an airway so that ventilation of the affected region is absent. Many clinical situations can obstruct an airway, leading to partial or complete lung collapse (atelectasis). Tumor, aspirated foreign body, and mucous plugs are some of the more common causes of obstructive atelectasis.

As long as the airway obstruction remains incomplete, the distal lung will remain inflated. In fact, partial obstruction of a bronchus can lead to hyperinflation of the lung if the obstruction causes a one-way valve effect, allowing air to enter the lung but not escape. Complete obstruction of a larger airway usually leads to atelectasis of the distal lung.

A related form of atelectasis occurs in patients after surgery. It is not uncommon for atelectasis to develop in the postoperative period, especially if the patient has had upper abdominal or thoracic surgery or if the patient is obese or has a history of chronic lung disease. After surgery, lung secretions tend to be retained in the lung because of mucociliary stasis and suppression of coughing and deep breathing. Retained secretions can obstruct multiple small

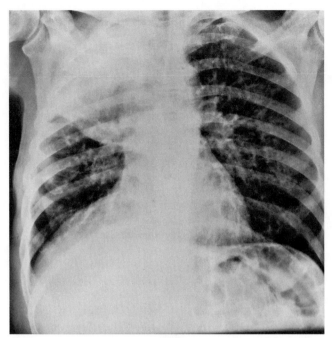

FIGURE 10-5 This patient's right upper lobe has become consolidated because of a tumor obstructing the right upper lobe bronchus. As a result, pneumonia has developed distal to the obstruction. Note the well-outlined horizontal fissure, slightly rotated up and delineating the inferior boundary of the right upper lobe. The upward displacement of the horizontal fissure suggests atelectasis in the right upper lobe.

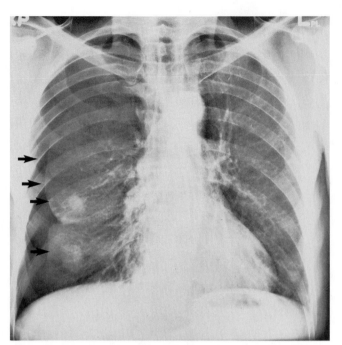

FIGURE 10-6 Good example of pneumothorax involving the right lung. Note the pleural line along the right lateral chest wall where the lung has pulled away from the chest wall as it collapsed toward the hilum.

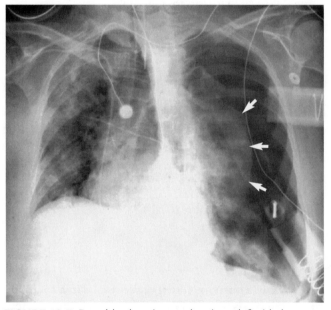

FIGURE 10-7 Portable chest image showing a left-sided tension pneumothorax. Note that the pressure in the left hemithorax has depressed the diaphragm on that side and forced the heart into the right side of the chest. A chest tube must be inserted immediately into the left chest.

airways, leading to underventilation and microatelectasis in the affected regions.

The physical examination findings of atelectasis vary with the amount of lung involved. With significant loss of lung volume, as occurs with lobar collapse, the findings are striking and usually include the following:

- Rapid shallow breathing
- Decreased to absent breath sounds
- Decreased to absent vocal fremitus
- Decreased resonance to percussion
- Cyanosis
- Shift of the mediastinum toward the affected side

The chest radiograph in most cases demonstrates the loss of lung volume caused by the atelectasis. Collapse of entire segments or lobes produces characteristic densities that show on the chest radiograph. Shift of the trachea, heart, and major thoracic vessels toward the affected side may be seen with lobar atelectasis. The radiographic findings seen with postoperative microatelectasis often are much more subtle or may be absent altogether.

Pneumothorax

Pneumothorax often causes atelectasis (Fig. 10-6). Pneumothorax is a condition in which air enters the pleural space either externally from a hole in the chest wall or internally from a hole in the lung. This leads to loss of the negative pressure normally found in the pleural space. As a result, the lung's normal elasticity causes it to contract, and the lung collapses.

This is serious enough, but the lung can develop a potentially more serious problem called *tension pneumothorax* (Fig. 10-7). With a tension pneumothorax, the air cannot get out of the pleural space, and pressure builds up. This pressure eventually shifts the heart away from the involved lung and puts pressure on the mediastinum and the other lung, altering blood and airflow. The good lung's ability to oxygenate is severely compromised, and venous return of blood to the heart may be compromised. Not all pneumothoraces develop "tension."

Physical findings with a small pneumothorax may be absent or minimal. With a tension pneumothorax, physical findings are as follows:

- Chest wall: reduction in movement in the chest wall on the side where the pneumothorax has occurred
- Auscultation of the lung: loss of breath sounds or distant breath sounds on the affected side
- Percussion: increased resonance to percussion on the affected side
- Heart: usually a rapid heart rate (tachycardia) and low blood pressure
- Other: cyanosis, an external wound, or bruising on the affected side
- Absent whispered voice sounds and tactile fremitus

Radiographic changes seen with a tension pneumothorax include shift of the mediastinal structures (the trachea and heart) away from the involved side and deviation of the trachea away from the affected side. Another sign suggestive of pneumothorax is **deep sulcus sign** (see Sabar and Nilles, 2012, in Bibliography). A pleural line represents the outer margin of the lung (see Fig. 10-6). It is expected that an experienced clinician (physician, nurse, RT) should be able to diagnose tension pneumothorax on clinical examination and not waste time on obtaining and evaluating radiographs to confirm the diagnosis. The treatment should be started emergently and consists of immediate chest tube placement or needle decompression followed by chest tube placement.

> **SIMPLY STATED**
>
> Tension pneumothorax is a life-threatening condition that is seen on the chest image as extreme hyperlucency on the affected side, with a shift of the mediastinal structures away from the air-filled pleural space.

Hyperinflation

Lung hyperinflation is seen commonly in patients with emphysema. This is seen on chest radiograph as small heart size (Fig. 10-8A), increased AP diameter, a large retrosternal air space (Fig. 10-8B), and flattening of the diaphragm (see Fig. 10-8A and B). The chest radiograph is neither very sensitive nor specific for the diagnosis of chronic obstructive pulmonary disease (COPD) but often provides supporting evidence for the diagnosis. Pulmonary function testing is much more sensitive and specific in diagnosis of COPD.

The physical examination findings that correlate with the radiographic examination include the following:

- Large barrel chest, with increased AP diameter of the chest wall

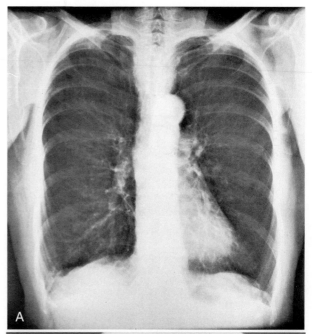

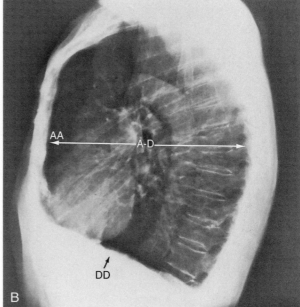

FIGURE 10-8 **A,** Posteroanterior chest image. Note marked hyperinflation with large lung volumes; low-set diaphragm; small, narrow heart; and enlarged intercostal spaces. **B,** Lateral view. Hyperinflation is manifested by increased anterior air space, depressed diaphragm, and increased anteroposterior chest dimensions (barrel chest). AA, anterior air space; DD, depressed diaphragm; A-D, anteroposterior dimension.

- Increased resonance to percussion
- Decreased breath sounds
- Limited motion of low-set diaphragms
- Wheezing (may not be present with emphysema)
- Prolonged expiratory phase
- Rapid respiratory rate
- Use of accessory muscles to breathe

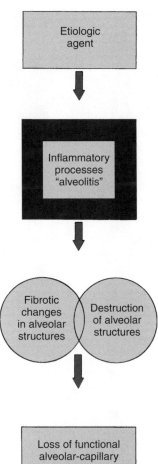

FIGURE 10-9 Theoretical explanation for development of pulmonary fibrosis. Patients who develop interstitial fibrosis are prone to develop other complications such as pneumothorax, cancer, and pneumonia. (Modified from Simmons DH: *Current pulmonology*. New York, 1981, Elsevier.)

SIMPLY STATED

The severity of the emphysema and pulmonary hyperexpansion in the patient with COPD is often predicted by the size of the retrosternal air space. The larger it is, the more severe the emphysema.

Interstitial Lung Disease

About 200 different diseases and syndromes can cause interstitial lung disease (Figs. 10-9 to 10-11, Box 10-2). The term *interstitial lung diseases* implies that most of the disease activity is contained within the interstitium (a microscopic anatomic space between the structural elements) of the lung; however, this implication is incorrect. Many interstitial lung diseases affect various parts of the lung, including airways, lung parenchyma, the interstitium, and the pleura. A more inclusive name of *diffuse parenchymal lung disease* has been suggested as a replacement for interstitial lung diseases; however, the latter is still commonly used. A simplified classification with a few representative diseases

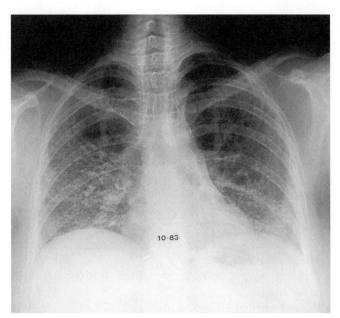

FIGURE 10-10 Severe interstitial fibrosis in the chest. (From Kacmarek RM, Stoller JK, Heuer AJ: *Egan's fundamentals of respiratory care,* ed 10. St. Louis, 2013, Mosby-Elsevier).

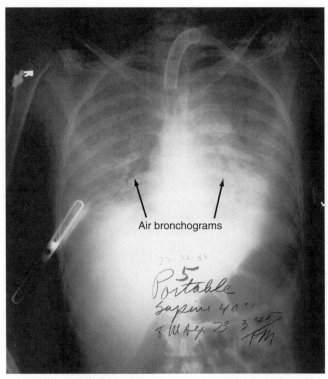

FIGURE 10-11 Typical alveolar filling pattern.

or syndromes causing interstitial lung disease is included to acquaint the reader with the terms (see Box 10-2). A more detailed review of the classification and clinical features of these diseases is available in the Bibliography.

The basic pathologic process associated with pulmonary fibrosis is shown in Figure 10-9. Some substance (etiologic

Box 10-2	Interstitial Lung Diseases

INFECTIONS
Influenza
Chickenpox
Pneumocystis

EXPOSURES
Asbestosis
Silicosis
Bleomycin
Radiation
Various organic and inorganic dusts

NEOPLASTIC CAUSES
Bronchoalveolar carcinoma
Lymphangitic or hematologic spread of metastases

CONGENITAL OR FAMILIAL CAUSES
Niemann-Pick disease
Hermansky-Pudlak syndrome

SYSTEMIC DISEASES
Rheumatoid arthritis
Systemic lupus erythematosus

IDIOPATHIC (UNKNOWN CAUSES)
Sarcoidosis
Pulmonary fibrosis

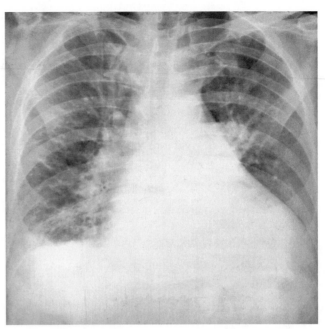

FIGURE 10-12 Congestive heart failure with upper lobe redistribution of vasculature markings, especially on the right, increased cardiothoracic ratio, and increased interstitial markings. Cardiac shadow should not be over half of the entire width of the thoracic cage; here it is well over half.

agent) activates the patient's immune system, causing the lung to scar or become fibrotic. The fibrotic process usually is progressive over a period of months to years. The end result for most of these patients is combined cardiac and respiratory failure. In a few instances, the disease is self-limited, and spontaneous resolution has been seen.

Initially, the patient with pulmonary fibrosis may notice a dry, nonproductive cough and dyspnea on exertion (DOE). This usually brings the patient in for medical care. The history is probably the most important element in helping to determine what has incited the immune response, causing the lung damage. A history of industrial exposure to silica or asbestos is crucial. A history of systemic symptoms, such as swallowing disorders or joint or muscle pain, may suggest a collagen vascular disease causing the fibrosis.

The pattern seen on the chest radiograph may give a clue to the cause of the abnormality. Examples include large hilar and paratracheal lymph nodes, suggesting sarcoidosis; calcified pleural or diaphragmatic nodules, suggesting asbestosis injury; honeycomb-sized cavities in the lungs, suggesting end-stage pulmonary fibrosis; and large air bronchograms with thick walls, suggesting bronchiectasis.

Physical examination of the patient with interstitial lung disease typically identifies a rapid and shallow breathing pattern. The interstitial fibrosis causes a decrease in lung compliance that results in the patient breathing with a smaller tidal volume (V_T). As the V_T decreases, the respiratory rate must increase to maintain adequate ventilation. Auscultation usually identifies fine inspiratory crackles that do not clear with deep breaths or changes in position.

The crackles often are more noticeable over the lower lobes. If the interstitial lung disease is severe, hypoxemia and cyanosis may be present.

In the evaluation of a patient with interstitial lung disease, **bronchoscopy** is commonly done to exclude a few diseases, like infections, malignancy, and sarcoidosis. In most cases, bronchoscopy does not lead to a final diagnosis, necessitating a surgical lung biopsy.

Congestive Heart Failure

Early CHF causes the following changes on the chest radiograph (Fig. 10-12):

- Redistribution of pulmonary vasculature with engorgement (cephalization) of the upper lobe vessels. The normal chest image shows the pulmonary blood vessels most prominent in the lower lobes. Left heart failure increases venous pressure, and the increased pressure distends upper lobe vessels that would otherwise carry very little blood.
- Fluid collection in the dependent portions of the lung.
- Increase width of the heart in relation to that of the thorax. Normally, the base of the heart occupies about half of the width of the thorax. In CHF, that ratio increases, and the heart appears larger (see Fig. 10-12). Increase in the width of the shadows of the mediastinal structures is another sign of fluid overload.
- Development of **Kerley B lines.** These lines, usually seen in the right base, are less than 1 mm thick and approximately 1 to 2 cm in length. They are horizontal and start at the periphery, extending into the lung approximately 1 to 2 cm. They are pleural lymphatic vessels filled with

fluid. Kerley B lines are very subtle, often difficult to find on an actual image, and nearly impossible to reproduce in print. An interested reader is instructed to view the article by Koga and Fujimoto (see Bibliography) on a high-resolution monitor to appreciate them.

- Miscellaneous signs:
  - Increased interstitial markings caused by fluid collecting around the lymph channels
  - Pleural effusion greater in the right hemithorax than the left hemithorax
  - Enlarged pulmonary artery segments caused by increased pulmonary artery pressure
  - Fluid collection around the vessels causing the margins to appear blurred
  - Increased size of the azygos vein caused by increased venous pressure
  - Fluffy perihilar opacities caused by fluid collection in lung tissue

CHF in patients with severe hyperinflation (especially emphysema) may not result in some of these previously mentioned signs. The development of an enlarged heart may be delayed in patients with emphysema because of the pathologic changes already present in the thoracic cage. With tissue destruction, common in emphysema, redistribution to the upper lobes already may have occurred before CHF develops. Physical examination findings include the following:

- Fine inspiratory crackles
- Rapid heart rate, either regular or irregular in rhythm. Third heart sound (S_3), a consistent finding in CHF
- Jugular venous distention
- Enlarged liver (hepatomegaly)
- Hepatojugular reflex
- Ankle edema (swelling)

SIMPLY STATED

Heart size is increased with congestive heart failure. An enlarged heart is present if the width of the heart exceeds 50% of the width of the thorax on a PA chest radiograph.

Pleural Effusion

The pleural space usually contains approximately 30 mL of viscous fluid on each side. The major function of this fluid is to lubricate the pleural surfaces and decrease friction between them as the lung moves. Pleural fluid is in constant flux; it is secreted and reabsorbed to maintain its volume and composition. During various pathologic conditions, the amount of fluid in the pleural space may increase, leading to formation of pleural effusion (Figs. 10-13 and 10-14). Usually, 100 mL must be present before the fluid can be seen on the chest radiograph. The fluid can be a clear watery material, caused by the imbalance in hydrostatic pressures (more fluid being secreted under higher pressure or less fluid being reabsorbed under lower pressure). This type of pleural fluid is low in protein content (<3 g/dL) and called a **transudate**. Alternatively, infection,

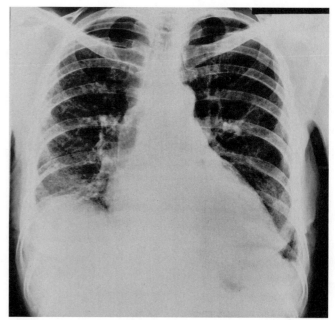

FIGURE 10-13 A small pleural effusion has developed in the right chest, resulting in a blunted right costophrenic angle and partially obscured right hemidiaphragm.

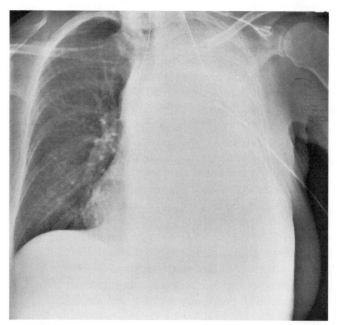

FIGURE 10-14 Large massive pleural effusion involving the left hemithorax. This has caused the x-ray image to appear as a whiteout of the involved side, completely obscuring all structures in the left chest.

inflammation, or blockage of the lymphatic flow by tumor can lead to production of fluid with a high protein content (>3 g/dL), called an **exudate**. Although transudates are almost always free flowing, exudates are often loculated, or compartmentalized. Loculated pleural effusions are more difficult to manage because different pockets of fluid do not communicate with each other, making them difficult

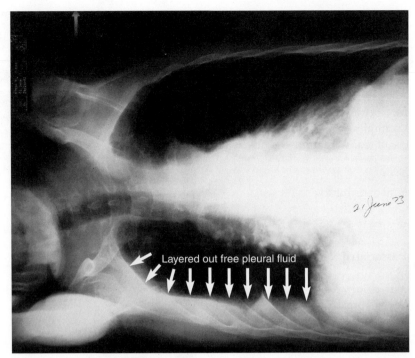

FIGURE 10-15 Patient lying on his side so that pleural effusion fluid has moved to the dependent area of the chest cavity (line indicated by *arrows*). This is called a *lateral decubitus view*. Important information is available from this view: confirmation of the effusion's presence and the fact that the effusion is free and not loculated, or trapped, by adhesions in one area of the chest cavity.

to drain. Open thoracotomy with decortication (stripping of the pleural surfaces) may be necessary.

The causes of transudative pleural effusion include CHF, hepatic failure, and atelectasis. Each of these causes either low protein in the blood or high pressure within the pleural veins favoring fluid movement into pleural space. The possible causes of exudative pleural effusions are more numerous and include bacterial pneumonia, PE, malignancy, viral disease, tuberculosis, and fungal infections.

Other fluids that collect in the pleural space include blood (hemothorax), a fatty fluid called *chyle* (chylothorax), and pus (empyema or pyothorax). Sometimes, there will be a mixture of air, fluid, and blood or pus in the pleural space (hydropneumothorax or pyopneumothorax).

The radiographic findings of pleural effusion depend on the volume of fluid collected in the pleural space. Small volume findings (see Fig. 10-13) are as follows:

- Blunting of the otherwise sharp angle between the chest wall and the point at which the diaphragm touches the chest wall laterally (the costophrenic [CP] angle).
- Small meniscus sign, which is seen when fluid starts to fill the space between the lung and chest wall, forming an opaque white crescent (meniscus) next to the chest wall; partially obscured diaphragm with elevation of the diaphragm from its normal position.

Large (massive) volume findings (see Fig. 10-14) are as follows:

- Complete or nearly complete whiteout of the involved side

- Complete obscuring of the hemidiaphragm
- Shift of the thoracic organs away from the effusion

It is illustrative to compare the findings of a massive pleural effusion and the mediastinal shift to the contralateral (opposite) side (see Fig. 10-14) to the complete lung collapse and the mediastinal shift to the ipsilateral (same) side (see Fig. 10-17, later).

If there is a question as to whether an effusion is present or if the fluid is free to move about, a lateral decubitus image is obtained. This study requires only that the patient lie on the side suspected of having the pleural effusion while the radiograph is taken. This is called the **lateral decubitus view** (Fig. 10-15). Free fluid will layer along the new horizontal plane on the lateral decubitus view, and loculated fluid, pneumonia, or tumor will be unchanged from the upright view.

The physical findings with pleural effusion are related to the volume of free fluid in the chest. The patient may complain of pain on inspiration; a dull, heavy feeling in the involved area; coughing; or shortness of breath. Small volumes of fluid are symptom free and undetectable on physical examination. However, when the size of the pleural effusion is significant, the findings may include the following:

- Dullness to percussion in the involved area
- Egophony just above the area of dullness
- Decreased or absent breath sounds on the affected side
- Tachypnea

Lung Consolidation

Bacterial pneumonia is the most common cause of lung consolidation. The infection causes copious mucus production that fills lung tissue so that it becomes airless but does not collapse. Less common causes of consolidation include obstruction of the airway by aspirated foreign bodies (e.g., peanuts or very small toys) or tumorous growths. Figures 10-3 and 10-4 show good examples of lung consolidation.

The radiographic signs of consolidation include the following:

* Minimal loss of volume
* Usually lobar or segmental distribution
* Homogeneous density
* Air bronchogram if the airway leading to the consolidated area is open

The physical findings associated with a consolidated lung include the following:

* Reduced resonance to percussion over the involved area
* Bronchophony and bronchial breath sounds
* Fine crackles often heard over the involved area
* Whispered voice sounds increased, and egophony present (if airway is patent)
* Tachypnea and fever

Postprocedural Chest Radiograph Evaluation

Tracheal Intubation

The AP chest image often is used to evaluate the position of the endotracheal (ET) tube to be sure that the inferior tip rests appropriately 3 to 5 cm above the carina after intubation (Fig. 10-16). Although the carina may be difficult to see on some chest images, it is often located at the space between the T-4 and T-5 vertebrae in many adults. It is also important to note that the position of the ET tube can vary by neck position and can move as much as a total of 4 cm as the neck moves from full extension (high position) to full flexion (low position). Therefore, whenever possible, the chest radiograph should be taken while the patient's neck is in a neutral position.

Accidental placement of the ET tube in the right or left mainstem bronchus or esophagus must be recognized immediately to minimize potential harm to the patient. All manufacturers include a thin radiopaque strip in the wall of the entire length of the ET tube to allow visualization of the tube's precise position in the chest on the radiograph. It must be remembered that the AP chest image helps determine position of the ET tube only on a two-dimensional (front-to-back) basis. Therefore, an ET tube placed in the esophagus 3 cm above the carina might very well produce a similar (if not the same) shadow on an AP chest image as one placed in the trachea. Therefore, it is imperative that other clinical findings, such as capnometry, rise of the chest wall, bilateral breath sounds, absence of gastric sounds, and esophageal detector devices, be used in addition to chest radiographs to ensure proper placement of the ET tube.

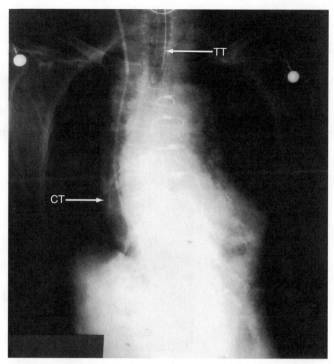

FIGURE 10-16 Pulmonary artery catheter (Swan-Ganz catheter) in its usual position in the right lower lung field. This view does not indicate whether the catheter is anterior or posterior within the chest. CT, catheter tip; TT, tracheal tube.

Figure 10-17 shows a common incorrect ET tube placement. Note that the tip of the ET tube has come to rest in the right mainstem bronchus and the mediastinal structures are shifted to the left (ipsilateral or same) side of the lung collapse (see Fig. 10-14 for comparison). Such improper tube placement may cause severe hypoxia due to $\dot{V}/\dot{Q}$ mismatch (left lung being perfused, but not ventilated), overdistention (large tidal volume being delivered to the right lung), or pneumothorax (with additional risk of shock, hypoxia, and even death). After the tube is repositioned, the number of centimeters seen on the tube at the position of the patient's teeth should be noted in the patient record (ventilator-patient flowsheet), the tube carefully taped, and a repeat radiograph obtained for documentation that the tube's malposition has been corrected.

Central Venous Pressure Line

Evaluation of the CVP line is necessary to be sure that the catheter tip is in the proper position. The catheter is placed into the right or left subclavian or jugular vein and should come to rest just above where the superior vena cava and the right atrium of the heart join together. During placement of central catheters, it is possible to enter the lung accidentally by passing through the wall of the vein, entering the pleural space, and thus causing the lung to collapse. If fluids are being delivered (e.g., blood replacement or total parenteral nutrition), the fluid will end up in the chest cavity instead of the bloodstream. An AP portable chest image is required immediately after the line is

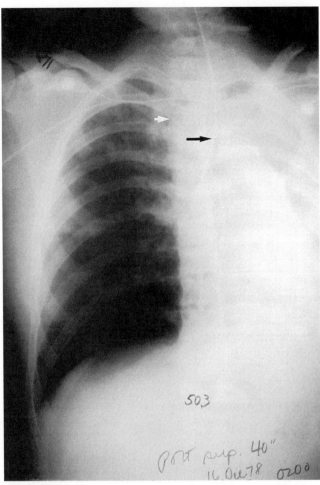

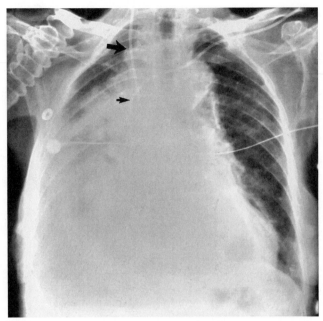

FIGURE 10-18 Anteroposterior chest image demonstrating a central venous pressure line in the right jugular vein (*large arrow*). The line has punctured the vein and entered the right lung. Fluids have been infused into the right pleural space. Note that a left subclavian central venous pressure line is in good position (*small arrow*).

FIGURE 10-17 Anteroposterior chest image demonstrating placement of the endotracheal tube in the right mainstem bronchus (*black arrow*). The left lung has collapsed because of atelectasis. The central venous pressure line is in good position (*white arrow*).

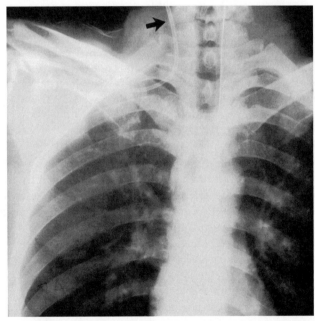

FIGURE 10-19 Anteroposterior chest image showing a central venous pressure line in the right subclavian vein. The tip of the line has moved retrograde up the internal jugular vein (*arrow*) and must be repositioned.

thought to be in position and before fluid is given through the central line.

In Figure 10-18 the post-placement radiograph shows two CVP lines. Although both appear to be in proper position on the chest radiograph, the catheter "placed" in the right jugular vein missed the vein, entered the pleural space, nicked the lung, and caused a pneumothorax. To make matters worse, fluid delivery was started before the error was discovered. The fluid is seen in the pleural space. A second invasive procedure (chest tube) is now required to relieve the pneumothorax and drain off the fluid. The line placed in the left subclavian vein just above where the superior vena cava and the right atrium join together seems to be in the proper position, but clinical confirmation is necessary before its use.

Radiographs obtained for verification of CVP line placement are at risk for the same limitations as the ones for the placement of ET tube. Therefore it is imperative that physicians, nurses, or other members of the patient care team confirm the intravascular position of the line by aspirating

blood from it. Sometimes, when it is unclear whether the line has been placed in the vein or the artery, blood gases are obtained, or pressure tracings are reviewed to ensure proper positioning.

Figure 10-19 shows another common malpositioning of a subclavian CVP line. It has gone up the neck on the

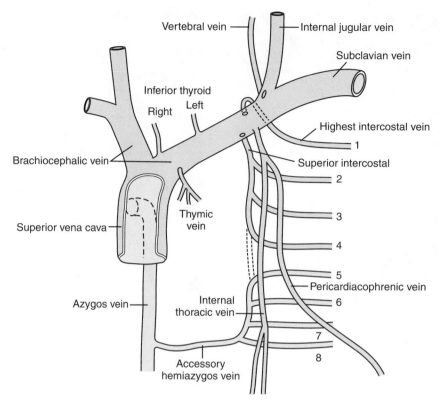

FIGURE 10-20 Venous anatomy of the neck. The central venous pressure line is intended to be located in the lower part of the superior vena cava.

right. Figure 10-20 shows the venous anatomy in the area of the neck and upper thorax. Every vein shown has the potential to receive a misdirected CVP line.

Pulmonary Artery Catheter Placement

After the pulmonary artery (Swan-Ganz catheter) is inserted, an AP portable chest radiograph is obtained to identify the position of the catheter tip. This catheter usually stays in the patient for several days, and daily radiographs are used to monitor its position and effect on the pulmonary circulation. Figure 10-21 shows a pulmonary artery catheter in good position: the right midlung near the hilum.

Nasogastric Feeding Tubes

The AP chest radiograph is useful to evaluate the position of the nasogastric (NG) feeding tube to ensure that it is located appropriately in the stomach or small bowel. Occasionally, the NG tube can be inserted accidentally into the trachea. In the alert patient, the accidental placement of an NG tube into the trachea causes severe coughing and dyspnea. The patient complains and alerts caregivers to the problem. However, these tubes are often placed in heavily sedated or comatose patients who cannot complain. NG tubes have been placed accidentally into the trachea, down the mainstem bronchus, and deep into the lung. This can lead to numerous problems such as pneumonia and pneumothorax.

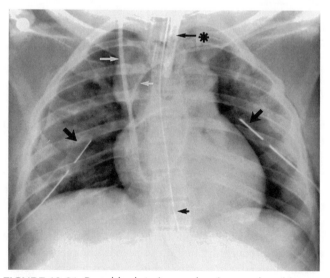

FIGURE 10-21 Portable chest image showing good position of the pulmonary artery catheter as it passes through the right side of the heart and into the right pulmonary artery (*long white arrow*). Note the position of the right and left chest tubes (*large black arrows*), endotracheal tube (*black arrow with asterisk*), and nasogastric tube (*small black arrow*). A *short white arrow* points to the left subclavian central venous pressure line in good position.

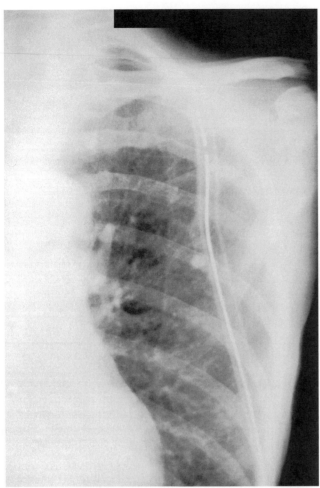

FIGURE 10-22 Close-up view of a chest image showing a left chest tube in good position. Note that three distinct lines are seen along the tube. The thicker line in the middle is a radiopaque stripe that allows visualization of the entire length of the tube. The other two lines are the edges of the tube itself; they would not be visible if the tube were accidentally placed in the soft tissues of the chest wall.

Chest Tubes

Chest tubes are large drainage tubes placed into the left or right thorax and attached to a suction device at approximately 20 cm H_2O pressure. The purpose is to drain excess air, blood, pus, or pleural fluid from the pleural cavity.

Placing the chest tube can be very painful for the patient and may require conscious sedation. Pain medication is usually needed as long as the tube remains in the chest. With proper precautions (monitoring the ECG and oxygen saturation [Sp_{O_2}]), the tube can be placed at the bedside and not in an operating room.

A portable chest radiograph is commonly obtained after the chest tube has been inserted. Figure 10-22 shows good placement of the tube for the purposes of draining pneumothorax (superior and anterior, as air collects in the gravity nondependent areas). The proper position of the tube is often dependent on the indication for its placement. For example, chest tubes placed for the drainage of

pleural fluid would have their tips directed inferiorly and posteriorly (fluid collects in gravity-dependent areas). For loculated fluid collections, the tube may have to be placed by an interventional radiologist (see Interventional Radiology later in this chapter) and properly directed under the ultrasound guidance. Once placed, the tube is sutured in place and heavily bandaged to reduce pain if the patient inadvertently rolls onto the insertion wound. Periodic portable chest radiographs may be needed to ensure that the tube remains in the correct position.

For additional procedures requiring evaluation with an AP portable chest radiograph, see Box 10-3.

SIMPLY STATED

The chest radiograph is used not only to diagnose lung disease but also to confirm the correct placement of tubes and catheters and the effect of procedures on the lung.

Computed Tomography

CT scanning is based on mathematical modeling of the tissues through which many small electron beams have passed. Standard CT scan presentation shows a slice of the body equivalent in thickness and orientation to a slice of bread. High-resolution CT scanning shows the slices in 1- to 2-mm thicknesses so that very fine detail can be seen. Newer mathematical modeling techniques allow presentation of either standard resolution or high-resolution slices in any dimension or even three-dimensional portrayal of any specific organ or part of the body. Injection of contrast material during the CT scan allows additional information about thoracic vessels. The very accurate three-dimensional information provided by CT scanning

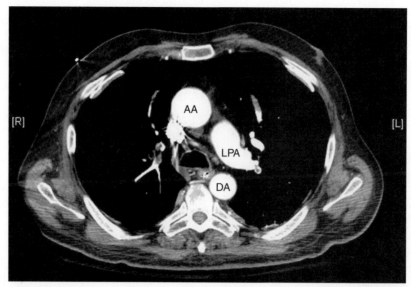

FIGURE 10-23 Computed tomographic scan of the chest with intravenous contrast demonstrates multiple filling defects (*arrows*) within pulmonary arteries, indicative of pulmonary embolism. Note that the ascending aorta (AA), descending aorta (DA), and left pulmonary artery (LPA) are all completely opacified with contrast.

allows the equipment to guide needle aspirations of tissue masses or catheter placement into tissue cavities.

The clarity of the image produced has made CT scanning indispensable in the medical management of pulmonary disease. As we discuss the utility of chest CT below, it must be remembered that CT scanning exposes the patient to a significant amount of radiation and repeated testing (often indicated for follow-up or screening) can lead to increased risks from radiation exposure.

Lung Tumors

CT scans easily show tissue masses that are hidden by dense tissues on plain radiographs. CT contrast scans help differentiate lymph nodes or tumor masses from blood vessels. High-resolution CT scans can show tissue nodules as small as 2 to 3 mm. CT scans can also provide information regarding the density of pulmonary nodules. Very dense nodules are likely to contain calcium and are less likely to be cancer.

Screening for Lung Cancer

Lung cancer remains the second most common type of cancer and the leading cause of cancer death in the United States as well as worldwide. Over the past decades, many types of screening modalities have been tried, but have been proved not helpful in prevention of the morbidity and mortality associated with lung cancer. A recent landmark study showed that using screening with low-dose chest CT may increase the survival in selected patients at risk for lung cancer. Unfortunately, for every patient diagnosed with cancer, many more have to undergo unnecessary additional testing (CT scanning as well as biopsies) for what eventually is proved to be a benign disease. This type of screening has not yet become a standard of care because many such screening studies are subject to certain biases, when the result of the study (positive, negative, or neutral) depends on the statistical inaccuracies, inherent to the study methods, rather than true biologic effects of the screening. Additional issues to be considered with this new screening tool are cost (financial as well as emotional, stemming from unnecessary follow-up tests and biopsies) as well as the potential for repeated radiation exposure causing complications many years later.

Pulmonary Embolism

Over the past few decades, CT scanning after administration of intravenous contrast has become the test of choice for the diagnosis of suspected PE. A rapid bolus of contrast is typically given, immediately followed by acquisition of CT images. When done properly, this technique leads to near-complete opacification of pulmonary vasculature by the contrast. Many well-done studies allow examination of small segmental and subsegmental branches of the pulmonary artery, so the procedure is often called *CT angiography*. In the presence of a PE, the lumen of the pulmonary vessel with the thrombus will be incompletely opacified, leading to a "filling defect" (Fig. 10-23). In addition to providing vivid images of the pulmonary vasculature, CT scan with contrast also allows examination of the pulmonary parenchyma, leading a physician toward a potential alternative diagnosis, even when there is no evidence of PE. A great deal of emphasis is placed in proper (rapid) administration of the contrast, so many radiology centers will request a dedicated large-bore intravenous line. Patient participation is also important because breath holding during the acquisition of images enhances the overall quality and accuracy of the test. This becomes important in patients with severe dyspnea, who cannot hold their breath even for a few seconds, as well as in patients on mechanical ventilator.

Chronic Interstitial Lung Disease

High-resolution CT scanning is superior to conventional radiographs in the evaluation of diffuse interstitial lung disease. The CT scan can demonstrate characteristic changes in patients with mild pulmonary fibrosis even when the conventional radiograph appears to be normal. In a few cases, the pattern of abnormality is so specific that a diagnosis can be made without biopsy. However, in most cases, the CT scan shows the nature and extent of the abnormality and suggests the best location for a lung biopsy.

Acquired Immunodeficiency Syndrome

CT scanning can be useful in the early detection of pneumonias that occur as a result of acquired immunodeficiency syndrome (AIDS). The technique is also useful in detecting abscesses and cavities. The mediastinum also can be evaluated for enlarged lymph nodes caused by infection or the lymphomas seen in AIDS.

Occupational Lung Disease

The lung diseases resulting from the inhalation of dusts, fumes, irritant gases, organisms, and smoke are called pneumoconioses, or extrinsic alveolitis. Inhaling dusts and fumes can cause pulmonary fibrosis. CT scanning is very helpful in identifying the changes seen in the pleura and the lung tissue associated with these occupational lung diseases. They initially cause nodules and subsequently fibrosis, both of which are seen clearly on CT scan. Pleural plaques seen with asbestosis are also readily demonstrated with CT scan.

Pneumonia

The cost of CT and the risks associated with high radiation exposure have restricted its use in the evaluation of most pneumonias. CT scans of the lung are superior to conventional chest radiographs in the visualization of pneumonias and related pathologic changes in the hila and pleura. CT scan is often ordered when radiographic findings do not resolve after clinical improvement, suggesting an alternative etiology (most commonly, malignancy). In general, radiographic resolution tends to lag behind clinical resolution by 6 to 8 weeks, so it is advised that a clinician should wait at least 8 weeks until the chest radiograph is repeated or a CT scan is ordered in a clinically stable patient.

Bronchiectasis

Bronchiectasis is caused by infection around the airways. As the infection clears and the concurrent scarring retracts, the airways are pulled widely open. Airways are always adjacent to blood vessels and are usually about the same size as

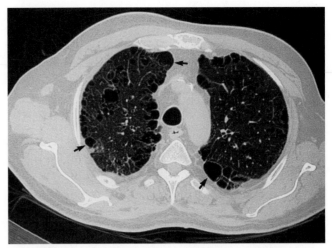

FIGURE 10-24 Computed tomography slice through the upper lungs in a patient with pulmonary emphysema. Numerous cystic lucencies are present in both lungs. Note the absence of bronchovascular markings within the lucencies. Most of the emphysematous areas are located in a peripheral distribution (*arrows*) along the pleural surface (paraseptal). (From Kacmarek RM, Stoller JK, Heuer AJ: *Egan's fundamentals of respiratory care,* ed 10. St. Louis, 2013, Mosby-Elsevier).

the adjacent blood vessel. Bronchiectasis thus shows up on CT scan as a very characteristic signet-ring pattern with the blood vessel appearing to be a small stone set against the much larger ring of bronchial tissue.

Chronic Obstructive Pulmonary Disease

CT scans of the emphysematous chest are remarkable in their clarity and detail. The diagnosis of emphysema or COPD using conventional radiography based on pulmonary hyperexpansion and bullae formation is 65% to 80% accurate. With CT scanning, emphysematous changes of even mild to moderate degree are seen with such ease as to make diagnosis consistently in the high 90% range (Fig. 10-24). It is important to note that radiographic appearance of COPD often does not correlate with clinical or physiologic measures, such as degree of dyspnea or airflow limitation on pulmonary function tests.

Magnetic Resonance Imaging

The role of MRI in the diagnosis of lung disease has been limited by breathing artifacts caused by slow cameras. Although there may be certain clinical scenarios in which MRI is superior to CT scan in the diagnosis of lung pathology, such scenarios are rare, especially when CT scans are enhanced with intravenous contrast or with simultaneous CT-PET scanning (see later). This leads to few MRIs being ordered for the diagnosis of lung diseases, which leads to even fewer radiologists being experienced in reading them. Overall, MRIs of the lung are not commonly done, except in rare instances. In contrast, cardiac MRI has become a new and exciting assessment tool to diagnose heart diseases.

Although MRI is not as common as other imagining studies, it is important for the RT to remember that special precautions need to be followed when accompanying a respiratory patient to the MRI, such as one who is mechanically ventilated. Even when the MRI is not fully operational, it emits a powerful magnetic force that can intensely draw to it equipment and devices containing ferrous (iron-containing) metals. In addition, data stored on magnetic strips on computer storage devices and identification cards can be wiped out. Therefore, in such settings, special tanks, regulators, ventilators, and other equipment need to be used, patients should be prescreened for implanted devices, and precautions must be taken to protect data storage devices and identification cards.

Radionuclide Lung Scanning

Radionuclide lung scans are obtained by measuring radiation emitted from the chest after radiopharmaceuticals are injected into the bloodstream or inhaled into the lung, or both. The two most commonly used lung scans are the $\dot{V}/\dot{Q}$ scan and gallium scan. The $\dot{V}/\dot{Q}$ scan is useful for studying the comparative distribution of ventilation and perfusion and the effects disease may have on these two important functions. The major clinical application of $\dot{V}/\dot{Q}$ lung scanning is in the evaluation of patients suspected of having a PE.

Distribution of perfusion is measured by attaching radioactive particles to albumin molecules that are so large they cannot get through the lung capillaries. These radioactive particles are injected into a peripheral vein through a standard intravenous catheter. They follow the bloodstream to the lung where they are trapped by the capillary system. An image will then be produced that will mimic the distribution of the radioactive particles within the lung. Areas of high blood flow will have high levels of radioactive particles and appear "hot" or very black on film. Areas of low flow will have few radioactive particles and appear "cold" or clear on film (Fig. 10-25). A reduction in blood flow occurs with PE or any respiratory disease that causes a localized area of vasoconstriction.

Distribution of ventilation is measured by having the patient breathe a radioactive gas. Well-ventilated areas will absorb a lot of radioactivity and appear hot or black on film. Poorly ventilated regions will absorb little radioactivity and will appear cold or clear on film. The ventilation scan can be compared with the perfusion scan to identify correlation between ventilation and perfusion (Fig. 10-26). When a PE is present, the ventilation scan usually is normal, and

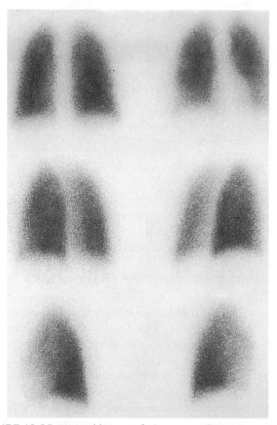

FIGURE 10-25 Normal lung perfusion scan. There is no evidence of perfusion defects in the anterior, posterior, oblique, or lateral views of the lungs.

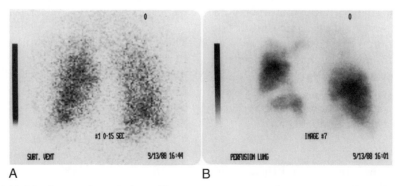

A   B

FIGURE 10-26 Abnormal ventilation-perfusion scan. The ventilation study (**A**) demonstrates bilateral lung filling without gross defects; however, the perfusion scan (**B**) shows multiple subsegmental perfusion defects of both lungs. These findings are highly suggestive of pulmonary emboli.

the perfusion scan shows a defect in the affected region. In patients with pneumonia, atelectasis, COPD, and many other lung diseases, the relationship between the ventilation and perfusion in a given area is not as straightforward, which leads to $\dot{V}/\dot{Q}$ scans that are often difficult to interpret. The accuracy of such interpretation is poor and may lead to more clinical uncertainty. In addition, image interpretation is often subject to interobserver variability (meaning two different radiologists might give conflicting reading of the same study). When studied systematically, it appeared that $\dot{V}/\dot{Q}$ scanning gave meaningful clinical information (ruled in or ruled out PE) in a minority of cases. However, widespread use of the helical CT with intravenous contrast has essentially replaced $\dot{V}/\dot{Q}$ scanning as the diagnostic test of choice for PE owing to superior image quality and additional information for PE diagnosis.

Gallium scanning is another **radionuclide lung scanning** method that is being used less commonly today. The idea of gallium scan is based on the fact that inflamed tissues excessively take up gallium, making certain areas of lung (or the rest of the body) involved in inflammation appear hot. This may be useful in directing the surgeon to the location of the biopsy specimen to be taken in patients with pulmonary fibrosis or other interstitial diseases. Alternatively, gallium uptake in lung hila, mediastinal lymph nodes, and most important, lacrimal glands could be very helpful in the diagnosis of sarcoidosis.

Positron Emission Tomography

PET scanning (Fig. 10-27) uses a glucose analog (fluorine-18-fluorodeoxyglucose) attached to a positron emitter. The patient fasts for several hours, is injected with the radiopharmaceutical labeled "sugar water," and is then allowed to remain supine and perfectly quiet for about an hour. Metabolically active tissue will take up the sugar water and thus show hot or black on film. Metabolically inactive tissues will not use much sugar water as fuel and will be cold or clear on film. Tumors and areas of infection increase the local rate of metabolic activity and cause hot spots. This allows the clinician to determine whether a lung mass is metabolically active. Especially helpful are combined CT-PET scans, when both CT and PET images are obtained simultaneously and then superimposed one on another. This allows better correlation between the two imaging studies and determination of whether a lesion seen on CT scan appears malignant or not.

For instance, in the diagnosis of coin lesions of 1 cm or greater, PET scans have shown the ability to identify tumor with sensitivities of 95% and specificities of 78%. PET scanning can also demonstrate tumor spread to local and distant tissues, such as lymph nodes in the hilar and mediastinal area, and distant spread to bone and adrenal glands. Brain usually uses glucose exclusively for energy and often appears hot on PET scans. For this reason, PET scanning is not helpful for the diagnosis of brain metastases in most cases.

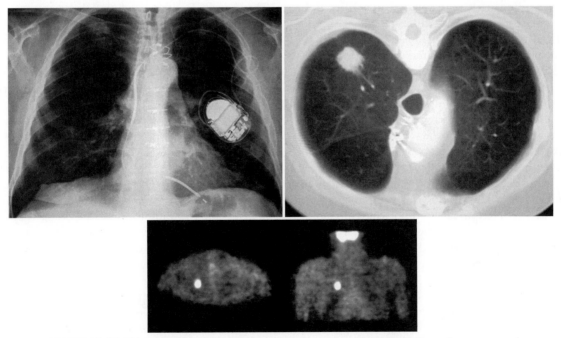

FIGURE 10-27 This series of images shows a coin lesion on routine chest radiograph, a computed tomography (CT) scan of the lesion, and a positron emission tomography (PET) scan. Only the PET scan is able to indicate, with a high sensitivity and specificity, that this lesion is actually cancerous. The routine chest radiograph shows a faint density on the right, behind the right clavicle. The presence of the pacemaker overlying the left chest tends to direct the examiner's eye away from the right upper lobe lesion. The CT scan shows this lesion to be ominous. Is it a cancer or an old scar, and thus benign? Two views from the PET scan show this lesion "lights up." It is a cancer.

Pulmonary Angiography

Angiography of the pulmonary circulation is rarely used today. In the past, it was generally done only if $\dot{V}/\dot{Q}$ lung scanning and CT angiogram were nondiagnostic and the patient was considered to be at risk for PE. Pulmonary angiography is performed by threading an intravascular catheter up a vein to the right heart, past the tricuspid valve and the pulmonary valves, and into the pulmonary artery, and then injecting contrast medium into the pulmonary artery or one of its branches. Angiographic proof of PE is considered to be identification of one or more filling defects. Nowadays, CT angiography, when done properly, can obtain equal, if not better, imaging of the pulmonary vasculature. In addition, it does not require placement of a catheter into the pulmonary artery and therefore has essentially replaced **pulmonary angiography** and $\dot{V}/\dot{Q}$ scanning as the diagnostic test of choice in patients with suspected PE.

> **SIMPLY STATED**
>
> Widespread availability and the ease of use of helical CT for the diagnosis of suspected PE has essentially made $\dot{V}/\dot{Q}$ scanning and pulmonary angiography obsolete.

Chest Ultrasound

Ultrasound waves are sound waves with the frequency above the upper limit of human hearing. These sound waves, much like electromagnetic waves (x-rays), are reflected differently by various tissues and structures and give additional methods of imaging the human body. One major quality that distinguishes ultrasound waves from the electromagnetic waves is that the former is considered harmless to humans, including fetuses, allowing much greater use of ultrasound in certain clinical scenarios. Another feature of the ultrasound is its portability, allowing complete bedside examinations—an important feature for critically ill patients. Portable ultrasound has become nearly as important as the stethoscope in the hands of an experienced emergency department or intensive care unit physician. It allows rapid and bedside evaluation of many internal organs' structure as well as function. The common chest ultrasound applications in the diagnosis of lung diseases are as follows:

- Visualization of pleural effusion
- Guidance of needle placement during thoracentesis
- Guidance of catheter placement during chest tube insertion
- Guidance of needle placement during central vein line placement
- Further assessment of a consolidation seen on chest radiograph
- Sniff test for unilateral diaphragm paralysis
- Visualization of pneumothorax
- Visualization of ET tube placement
- Assessment of the heart function (echocardiography)

Fluoroscopy

During **fluoroscopy**, real-time continuous radiographs are obtained and displayed, much like a movie of "still" x-rays. This technique is especially important when the needle or a catheter is guided into an internal structure to ensure its proper placement. Fluoroscopy is commonly used during cardiac catheterization, bronchoscopy, and many other invasive procedures. During bronchoscopy, it is typically used to establish the position of the bronchoscope or that of the biopsy forceps in relation to the lesion that is not directly seen through the bronchoscope. Although immensely helpful in diagnosing coin lesions, they are still subject to sampling error. As discussed earlier, x-rays provide two-dimensional images of three-dimensional objects, so a biopsy forceps placed on the outside of the patient's chest, directly above the coin lesion, would appear to be piercing that lesion on fluoroscopy.

One important feature of fluoroscopy is that it uses and emits much greater radiation that is used during conventional radiographs. For this reason, all health care personnel, whether performing, assisting, or observing the fluoroscopy procedure, must wear protective equipment (see Radiation Safety). Similarly, pregnant individuals are instructed to leave the room to avoid exposing the fetus to damaging radiation.

Interventional Radiology

The use of CT, ultrasound, and fluoroscopy allows visualization of and image-guided access to nearly every part of the human body. With such precise guidance, needle drainage of a deep tissue abscess is more desirable, rather than invasive surgery. This simple concept has led to the development of a whole new subspecialty, called **interventional radiology**. Today's interventional radiologists offer first-line diagnosis and treatment modalities for a wide variety of diseases. In many instances, interventional radiology procedures have replaced costly and complex surgical interventions with simpler alternatives and provided novel approaches in situations in which no other diagnostic or therapeutic options were available. Commonly performed interventional radiology procedures, as they pertain to lung diseases, are transcutaneous lung biopsy, bronchial artery embolization, ultrasound-guided **thoracentesis**, and small-bore chest tube placement.

Radiation Safety

As stated earlier, x-rays are a type of ionizing electromagnetic radiation and in large doses are harmful to the human body. A routine chest radiograph (PA and lateral) delivers 0.06 to 0.1 mSv (millisievert) or 6 to 10 mrem (millirem) of radiation. For a comparison, an individual residing in the United States will annually absorb approximately 3 mSv (300 mrem) of background radiation. So, having a chest radiograph exposes the patient to an equivalent of 2% to 3% of the annual background radiation. The amount of radiation increases with more sophisticated studies, such as CT or PET scanning. An annual exposure to more than 100 mSv is considered dangerous to human health.

Health care workers are often exposed to scatter radiation. For example, a nurse or an RT standing outside of the patient's room while radiographs are being taken receives a small part of the radiation used to produce the x-ray. Even that small amount of radiation can become dangerous when multiplied by many such instances of scatter radiation, occurring over the decades of a clinical career. The exposure can be much greater if one is performing or assisting during fluoroscopy. Typically, the real-time images require more radiation to obtain, and there are often more than 20 images obtained during a single procedure like bronchoscopy. It is mandatory that everyone (performing, assisting, or observing) present during fluoroscopy wear protective clothing made from lead that absorbs all x-rays. Such clothing must cover the neck (thyroid gland area) as well as the chest, abdomen, and pelvis to shield the internal organs from radiation.

Many health care workers who are frequently exposed to scatter radiation must wear small chips (about the size of a modern-day memory card) that record the amount of radiation absorbed by that individual. These chips are periodically exchanged for new ones, with the old ones sent to the local radiation safety office for review and measurements. Fortunately, the amount of radiation tapers off dramatically as one moves away from the source. The best way to avoid exposure to the scatter radiation is to stay as far away as possible. It is accepted that there is no additional radiation exposure 6 feet away from the x-ray source.

A different aspect of radiation safety is performing radiographs or other imaging studies using radiation on pregnant women. Even with abdominal shielding, the radiographs directed to the chest scatter and reach the fetus. Although MRI and ultrasound are generally considered safe, pros and cons of using any test that uses ionizing radiation (e.g., x-rays, CT scan, radionuclide scans) have to be carefully considered. The urgency of the test and the information obtained from it often outweigh the risks of radiation exposure, but each case must be considered by members of the patient care team on an individual basis.

KEY POINTS

- Dense body tissue appears white (radiopaque), and air-filled body tissue appears black (radiolucent) on x-rays.
- The magnification of organs by x-rays is reduced by reducing the distance between the organ and the film.
- Increasing ventilator pressures may indicate development of a pneumothorax and should prompt an order for a chest radiograph.

KEY POINTS—cont'd

- The right mainstem bronchus is straighter, wider, and shorter than the left mainstem bronchus, making it the usual site for an ET tube placed too deeply, which will usually result in atelectasis of the left lung and overdistention of the right lung.
- CT scans show structural information using x-rays but use digital enhancement to provide much clearer detail and more specific information about density than chest radiographs provide.
- MRI uses a strong magnetic field rather than x-rays to provide images of the body.
- $\dot{V}/\dot{Q}$ lung scans are helpful only if they are completely normal or if they are highly suggestive for the presence of pulmonary emboli.
- CT scan of the chest with intravenous contrast has become the diagnostic study of choice in patients suspected for pulmonary embolism.
- PET scan uses a radioactively tagged sugar water injection to demonstrate metabolically active tissue, such as cancer or infection.
- Chest radiograph interpretation requires evaluation of the following:
  - Proper patient name
  - Image exposure
  - Patient placement in relation to the film (rotation)
  - Bony structures and other extrapulmonary tissues
  - Trachea and mediastinum
  - Heart and lungs
  - Pulmonary arteries and lung hilum
- The presence of the silhouette sign allows more precise location of the infiltrate.
- Air bronchograms suggest fluid in the lung tissue surrounding patent airways.

ASSESSMENT QUESTIONS

See Appendix for answers.

1. Which of the following tissues is normally the most radiolucent?
   a. Blood
   b. Lungs
   c. Muscle
   d. Fat

2. Which of the following is true regarding the distance between the x-ray source, image, and patient when taking a chest radiograph?
   a. Distance has no effect on the image on the film.
   b. As the distance between the source and the patient decreases, magnification increases.
   c. As distance between the source and patient decreases, the image becomes more sharply focused.
   d. The distance between the patient and the x-ray machine varies with the size of the patient.

3. Which of the following is the standard distance between the x-ray source and the image for a posteroanterior x-ray?
   a. 3 feet
   b. 4 feet
   c. 5 feet
   d. 6 feet

4. A chest radiograph would be indicated to:
   a. Assess the progression of a patient's pneumonia
   b. Confirm ET tube placement during cardiopulmonary resuscitation
   c. Confirm tension pneumothorax in an unstable patient
   d. Screen for lung cancer in a patient with risk factors for cancer

5. Which of the following is/are true regarding a posteroanterior chest radiograph?
   a. Patient rotation usually is present and makes interpretation difficult.
   b. Heart size is subject to less magnification.
   c. It is the standard for bedridden hospitalized patients.
   d. Lateral image provides little additional information

6. Which of the following views helps to evaluate for the presence of small amounts of free pleural fluid?
   a. Apical lordotic
   b. Expiratory
   c. Anteroposterior
   d. Lateral decubitus

7. Which of the following is a true statement about a portable (anteroposterior) chest radiograph?
   a. Apical areas of the lung are well visualized
   b. It provides the best view for pleural effusion diagnosis
   c. Lateral image is usually obtained in addition
   d. Patient is often not centered on the image

8. The type of chest radiographic image most helpful in identifying a pneumothorax is:
   a. Lateral
   b. Oblique
   c. Expiratory
   d. Lateral decubitus

9. In a properly intubated adult patient, an ET tube tip should be this far from the carina:
   a. 0-1 cm
   b. 2-3 cm
   c. 3-5 cm
   d. 7-9 cm

10. After insertion of a CVP line, a chest radiograph is obtained to:
   a. Confirm that the line was placed in the vein, rather than artery
   b. Help with the estimation of central venous pressure
   c. Ensure that the line was not placed in the pleural cavity
   d. Evaluate the position of the line in relation to other thoracic structures

11. In which of the following clinical scenarios is CT scanning most useful?
   a. Interstitial lung disease
   b. Pneumonia
   c. Emphysema
   d. Screening for lung cancer

12. An MRI of the chest is most useful for the detection of:
   a. Interstitial lung diseases
   b. Pneumonia
   c. Cardiac diseases
   d. Emphysema

13. In which of the following clinical scenarios is gallium lung most useful?
   a. Lung cancer
   b. Emphysema
   c. Pulmonary embolism
   d. Sarcoidosis

14. Which of the following is the best method to evaluate for the presence of pulmonary embolism?
   a. $\dot{V}/\dot{Q}$ lung scan
   b. CT angiography
   c. Standard angiography
   d. MRI

15. The depth of inspiration on an x-ray is considered adequate if the lung shadows span the posterior shadows of this many ribs
   a. 5
   b. 7
   c. 8
   d. 10

16. The significance of the silhouette sign is that:
   a. It allows differentiation between alveolar and interstitial infiltrates.
   b. It can aid in detecting pleural effusion.
   c. It helps determine the location of a pulmonary opacity.
   d. It confirms proper positioning of the ET tube.

17. The chest radiograph finding most consistent with tension pneumothorax is:
   a. Increased radiolucency on the affected side
   b. Mediastinal shift toward the affected side
   c. Engorgement of the blood vessels on the affected side
   d. Air bronchograms and silhouette sign of the affected side

18. Which of the following is a radiographic sign of atelectasis?
   a. Enlarged heart
   b. Hilar shift away from atelectasis
   c. Vascular engorgement
   d. Hemidiaphragm elevation

19. The chest radiograph finding most suggestive of heart failure is:
   a. Low and flat diaphragm
   b. Increased cardiothoracic ratio
   c. Tracheal deviation
   d. Increased retrosternal air space on a lateral image

20. The chest radiograph finding most suggestive of pneumonia is:
    a. Silhouette sign
    b. Deep sulcus sign
    c. Coin lesion
    d. Kerley B lines
21. Which of the following chest radiograph findings is consistent with hyperinflation?
    a. Kerley B lines
    b. Enlarged heart
    c. Peripheral pleura line
    d. Large lung volumes
22. Which of the following chest radiograph findings is consistent with a small pleural effusion?
    a. Blunted costophrenic angle
    b. Air bronchograms on the affected side
    c. Peripheral pleural line
    d. Elevated hemidiaphragm

Bibliography

American Thoracic Society website: http://www.thoracic.org/education/breathing-in-america/resources/chapter-10-interstitial-lung-disease.pdf; Accessed March 12, 2012.

Brenner DJ, Hall EJ. Computed tomography: an increasing source of radiation exposure. *N Engl J Med* 2007;**357**:2277.

Kacmarek RM, Stoller JK, Heuer AJ. *Egan's fundamentals of respiratory care*. 10th ed. St. Louis: Mosby-Elsevier; 2013.

Koga T, Fujimoto K, Kerley's A. B and C lines. *N Engl J Med* 2009;**360**:1539.

Mason RL, Broaddus VC, Murray RJ. *Murray and Nadel's textbook of respiratory medicine*. Philadelphia: WB Saunders; 2004.

Moore CL, Copel JA. Point-of-care ultrasonography. *N Engl J Med* 2011;**364**:749.

National Lung Screening Trial Research Team. Reduced lung-cancer mortality with low-dose computed tomographic screening. *N Engl J Med* 2011;**365**:395.

Patz EF, Goodman PC, Bepler G. Current concepts: screening for lung cancer. *N Engl J Med* 2000;**343**:1627.

Sabbar S, Nilles EJ. Images in clinical medicine: deep sulcus sign. *N Engl J Med* 2012;**366**:552.

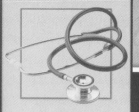

Chapter 11

Interpretation of Electrocardiogram Tracings

ALBERT J. HEUER*

CHAPTER OUTLINE

LEARNING OBJECTIVES

After reading this chapter, you will be able to:

1. Describe the clinical value of the electrocardiogram (ECG).
2. Describe the clinical findings that indicate the need for an ECG recording.
3. Identify the key components of the electrical conduction system of the heart and the role of each component.
4. Define depolarization and repolarization.
5. Describe the specific electrical activity of the heart associated with each wave and interval of the normal ECG.
6. Identify the normal values for the PR interval and the QRS complex.
7. Identify the ventricular rate and position of the mean QRS vector from an ECG recording.
8. List the steps for ECG interpretation.
9. Describe the ECG criteria for each of the following abnormalities:
   a. Sinus bradycardia
   b. Sinus tachycardia
   c. Sinus dysrhythmia
   d. Premature atrial contraction
   e. Atrial flutter
   f. Atrial fibrillation
   g. Premature ventricular contractions
   h. Ventricular tachycardia

---

*Dr. Robert Wilkins, PhD, RRT, contributed some of the content for this chapter as the coeditor of the prior edition.

LEARNING OBJECTIVES—cont'd

    i. Ventricular fibrillation
    j. Asystole
    k. First-, second-, and third-degree atrioventricular (AV) block
10. Describe the ECG abnormalities associated with chronic lung disease.
11. Identify ischemia, injury, and infarction using the 12-lead ECG tracing.
12. Explain how to assess and help treat patients with chest pain.

KEY TERMS

action potential	escape beat	QT interval
atrial kick	first-degree block	repolarization
automaticity	focus	RR interval
depolarization	heart block	ST segment
dysrhythmias	hypertrophy	ST-elevation myocardial
ectopic impulse	QRS complex	infarction (STEMI)

Given the hands-on nature of respiratory care, the likelihood of a respiratory therapist (RT) observing a patient during the acute onset of an ischemic cardiac event or lethal dysrhythmia is relatively high. Thus it is vital for RTs to have basic knowledge in electrocardiogram (ECG) interpretation. The RT may serve as the first link in the chain of survival for a patient experiencing a cardiac arrest and represent an important part of the medical team providing management of the patient once stabilized. Early recognition of a serious cardiac problem may potentially minimize cardiac damage or prevent death caused by a myocardial infarction. In addition, understanding the significance of the subtle and often progressive aspects of ECG changes enhances the RT's or other clinician's assessment of a patient's cardiopulmonary health and may help optimize interdisciplinary care planning.

This chapter describes the electrophysiology of normal and abnormal ECG tracings. Ultimately, it is intended to explain how to recognize basic and life-threatening ECG patterns that may be observed while performing respiratory care. After a review of cardiac physiology related to the production of electrical activity within the heart, numerous abnormal rhythms (dysrhythmias) are described. Criteria for recognition and possible causes are reviewed for each abnormality presented.

What Is an Electrocardiogram?

An ECG (also called an EKG) is an indirect measurement of the electrical activity within the heart. A recording of the electrical currents within the heart is obtained by placing electrodes containing a conductive media to each extremity and to numerous locations on the chest wall to create a 12-lead ECG. Each specific position of an electrode provides a tracing referred to as a *lead*. The purpose of using 12 leads is to obtain 12 different views of the electrical activity in the heart and therefore a more complete picture.

Current standard of practice in most hospitals calls for patients at risk for cardiac events or dysrhythmias to be initially placed on continuous ECG monitoring using the 3-lead or 5-lead system. These systems use only 3 or 5 leads, placed on the patient's chest, which is less cumbersome and allows for more patient mobility than a 12-lead ECG. Although 3- and 5-lead systems do not provide the level of detail that a 12-lead ECG does, they may help facilitate a rapid assessment of gross abnormalities in the electrical conduction system of the heart. Identification of a rhythm abnormality on a 3-lead or 5-lead tracing often indicates the need to obtain a more detailed 12-lead view of the heart.

What Is the Value of an Electrocardigram?

The ECG provides valuable information about the cardiac status of a patient presenting with signs and symptoms suggestive of heart disease. For example, if a patient presents with dyspnea and chest discomfort, an ECG can aid in the diagnosis of an ischemic cardiac event. In addition, the ECG may indicate an increased workload on the myocardium as a compensatory response to the chronic dysfunction of another body system such as the respiratory system. Both acute and chronic conditions may have adverse effects on the heart. The severity of such effects (e.g., myocardial infarction, ventricular hypertrophy, or abnormal heart rhythms known as *dysrhythmias*) may be assessed on interpretation of the ECG. The ECG may also be used to monitor the heart's response to treatment of an event that causes changes in the ECG. Therefore, several ECGs may be needed over the course of treatment.

It is important to note that the ECG tracing does not measure the pumping ability of the heart. It is not unusual for a patient with a low cardiac output to have a normal ECG tracing. This is because the ECG does not directly depict abnormalities in cardiac structure such as defects in the heart valves or interventricular septum. Another limitation worth noting is that the probability of any patient having an acute problem, such as myocardial infarction, generally cannot be predicted from a resting ECG tracing.

SIMPLY STATED

The resting ECG does not reflect the pumping ability of the heart or the likelihood that the patient may have a myocardial infarction in the near future.

When Should an Electrocardiogram Be Obtained?

Because an ECG is noninvasive and does not present a risk to the patient, it is reasonable to obtain an ECG when the patient has signs and symptoms suggestive of an acute or chronic cardiac disorder such as myocardial infarction or congestive heart failure (CHF) (Box 11-1). An ECG is often used as an assessment tool to help determine the patient's general health status or as a screening tool before major surgery. An ECG is especially helpful in this situation if the patient is older or has a history of heart disease. If an abnormality is identified early, treatment can be promptly started, thus potentially improving the longer term prognosis. Of course, the process of obtaining the ECG should never delay the initiation of critically needed care such as oxygen therapy, airway placement, or cardiopulmonary resuscitation (CPR).

It should also be noted that different clinical situations dictate whether a 3-, 5- or 12-lead ECG is warranted. Suffice to say that 3- or 5-lead ECG's may be adequate for more routine monitoring such as ongoing telemetry or for initial preliminary cardiac screening. However, the most diagnostic value can be gathered from a standard 12-lead ECG. In essence, a 12-lead ECG provides a more complete assessment of the electrical activity of the heart by viewing it from 12 different angles. As a result, the focus of this chapter is the 12-lead ECG.

Cardiac Anatomy and Physiology

Before discussing the interpretation of ECGs, it is important to review the cardiac anatomy and physiology related to electrical activity within the heart. The heart is made up of four chambers: two upper chambers called *atria* and two lower chambers called *ventricles* (Fig. 11-1). The heart typically is described as having two sides, the right and the left. The right atrium receives deoxygenated blood from the venae cavae and directs the blood into the right ventricle. Right ventricular contraction ejects blood into the pulmonary artery, which carries blood to the lungs for

Box 11-1	Clinical Findings Suggestive of the Need for an ECG

MEDICAL HISTORY

CHIEF COMPLAINTS

Chest pain (centrally located and may radiate to the shoulder or back)

Dyspnea on exertion in a patient older than 40 years

Orthopnea

Paroxysmal nocturnal dyspnea

Pedal edema

Fainting spells

Palpitations

Unexplained and persistent nausea and indigestion in a high-risk patient

PAST MEDICAL HISTORY

History of heart disease

History of cardiac surgery

PHYSICAL EXAMINATION

Unexplained tachycardia at rest

Hypotension

Decreased capillary refill

Abnormal heart sounds or murmurs

Pedal edema

Cool, cyanotic extremities

Abnormal heaves or lifts on the precordium

Diaphoresis

Jugular venous distention

Abnormal sensorium

Hepatojugular reflex

Bilateral inspiratory crackles in the dependent lung zones

oxygenation. The oxygenated blood returns to the left atrium of the heart via the pulmonary veins, where it is directed into the left ventricle. Left ventricular contraction ejects blood into the aorta, which branches off into the systemic circulation. Since the left side of the heart pumps blood throughout the entire body, it normally has a significantly larger muscle mass than the right side.

Cardiac muscle is referred to as the *myocardium*. Myocardial contraction occurs as a response to electrical stimulation. For the heart to move blood effectively, stimulation of the myocardium must be coordinated. Initiating and coordinating the electrical stimulation of the myocardium is the responsibility of the electrical conduction system, which is made up of special pacemaker and conducting cells (Table 11-1).

Normally, the electrical activity of the heart is initiated in the sinus node, also known as the sinoatrial (SA) node located in the right atrium (Fig. 11-2). The SA node is a collection of specialized cells capable of spontaneously generating electrical signals. Cells that have the ability to generate electrical activity spontaneously are said to have **automaticity**. Because the SA node normally has the greatest degree of automaticity of all the cardiac cells, it usually controls the rate at which the heart beats. In this way, the

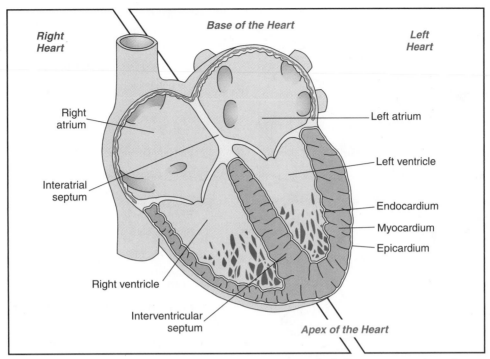

FIGURE 11-1 Anatomy of the heart. (From Huszar RH: *Basic dysrhythmias: interpretation and management*, ed 3. St Louis, 2007, Mosby.)

TABLE 11-1	
Types of Heart Cells	
Pacemaker cells	Specialized cells that have an extensive ability to generate their own electrical activity (automaticity) and provide the electrical power for the heart
Conducting cells	Cells that conduct the electrical impulse throughout the heart
Myocardial cells	Cells that contract in response to electrical stimuli and pump the blood

SA node serves as the primary pacemaker of the heart, discharging at about 60 to 100 beats/min at rest.

The SA node is strongly influenced by the autonomic nervous system. For this reason, the rate at which the SA node fires can vary significantly. Increased activity of the sympathetic system increases the heart rate. Stimulation of the sympathetic system occurs with stress, anxiety, exercise, hypoxemia, and the administration of certain medications. On the other hand, slowing of the heart rate occurs as a result of vagal stimulation, which is a parasympathetic response.

Once the SA node initiates the electrical signal, the impulse spreads across the atria in a wavelike fashion. The electrical impulse travels through the atria by way of the internodal also known as *interatrial pathways*, causing depolarization and then contraction. Contraction of the atria just before ventricular contraction (systole) aids in filling the ventricles with blood and accounts for about 10% to 30% of subsequent stroke volume. This atrial contraction is often referred to as the **atrial kick**.

After the electrical impulse passes through the atria, it reaches the atrioventricular (AV) junction. This junction acts as an electrical bridge between the atria and the ventricles. The AV junction contains the AV node and the bundle of His (see Fig. 11-2). Once the electrical impulse reaches the AV node, it is delayed for approximately 0.1 second before passing on into the bundle of His. The delay is believed to serve the purpose of allowing more complete filling of the ventricles before ventricular contraction, further adding to the atrial kick. In addition, the AV node can protect the ventricles from excessively rapid atrial rates that the ventricles could not tolerate. Damage to the AV junction, as may occur with a myocardial infarction, usually leads to excessive delays of the electrical impulse passing into the ventricles. This causes a condition known as **heart block**.

The AV junction normally guides only the electrical impulse from the atria into the ventricles. Under certain circumstances, however, it can also serve as the backup pacemaker. The AV junction has automaticity qualities similar to those of the SA node. If the SA node fails to function properly and does not pace the heart, the AV junction can serve as the pacemaker for the ventricles. When this occurs, the ventricular rate is usually between 40 and 60 beats/min and the ECG reveals a distinct pattern, described later in this chapter (Fig. 11-3).

After the electrical impulse leaves the AV node, it travels rapidly through the bundle of His and then into the left and right bundle branches (see Fig. 11-2). The stimulus travels simultaneously through the bundle branches into the myocardium. At the end of the bundle branches are

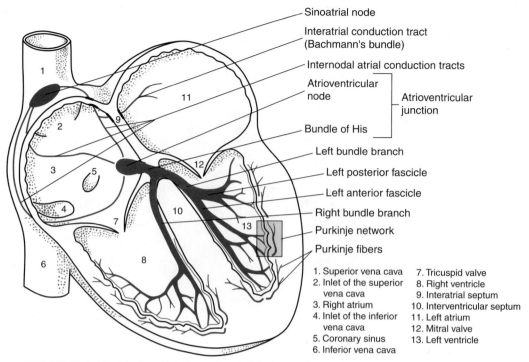

FIGURE 11-2 Electrical conduction system of the heart. (From Huszar RH: *Basic dysrhythmias: interpretation and management*, ed 3. St Louis, 2007, Mosby.)

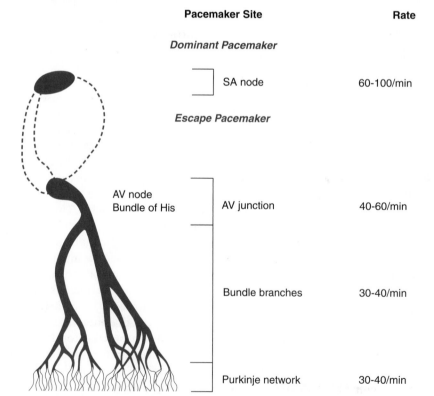

FIGURE 11-3 Dominant and escape pacemakers. AV, atrioventricular; SA, sinoatrial. (From Huszar RH: *Basic dysrhythmias: interpretation and management*, ed 3. St Louis, 2007, Mosby.)

countless fingerlike projections called *Purkinje fibers*. The Purkinje fibers pass the electrical impulse rapidly throughout the myocardium to create a coordinated contraction of the left and right ventricles.

SIMPLY STATED

The SA node normally has the greatest degree of automaticity and therefore normally controls the pace of the heart at a normal rate of 60 to 100 beats/minute. The AV junction acts as the backup pacemaker, with an inherent rate of 40 to 60 beats/minute.

Because most of the cardiac cells have automaticity characteristics, the heartbeat may be paced by heart tissue other than the SA node. When this occurs, it often indicates that the SA node is not functioning normally or that myocardial tissue is irritated. Any impulse that originates outside the SA node is called an **ectopic impulse**, and the site from which the ectopic impulse originates is called the **focus**. Ectopic impulses can originate from foci in either the atria or the ventricles. When the ectopic impulse results from depression of the normal impulse origin, it is called an **escape beat**.

The myocardium must receive a constant supply of oxygen and nutrients to pump blood effectively. Oxygen and nutrients are supplied to the myocardium via the left and right coronary arteries and their branches. The main coronary arteries arise from the ascending aorta and direct arterial blood into branches that feed various regions of the heart. Blockage of one or more of the coronary vessels leads to regionalized ischemia and tissue death (infarction). The size and location of the region affected by the coronary vessel blockage determines the resulting physiologic and clinical impact. Infarction of a major portion of the left ventricle is likely to cause significant arterial hypotension, abnormal sensorium, and a backup of blood into the pulmonary circulation. Infarction of the tissues associated with pacing the heart (e.g., the SA or AV junction) can lead to significant dysrhythmias and diminished blood flow to all regions of the body.

SIMPLY STATED

Blockage of one of the coronary arteries leads to ischemia and infarction of a portion of the myocardium. This leads to dysrhythmias and reduced cardiac output in most cases.

Causes and Manifestations of Dysrhythmias

Disturbances in cardiac conduction are called **dysrhythmias**. Dysrhythmias can occur even in healthy hearts. Often, minor dysrhythmias produce no symptoms and resolve without any treatment. More serious dysrhythmias indicate significant acute or chronic heart disease. When serious dysrhythmias occur, medication or electrical therapy often is required to increase or decrease the ventricular rate or to suppress an irritable area within the myocardium. Occasionally, surgical intervention or thrombolytic therapy is needed to prevent the progression of injury or infarct, thereby salvaging viable tissue. The application and improved delivery of oxygen often is a key factor in reducing or eliminating cardiac irritability. Causes of dysrhythmias include the following:

- **Hypoxia:** Hypoxia results from inadequate delivery of oxygen to the heart muscle or myocardium, and may be caused by hypoxemia or low blood flow known as *ischemia*. Inadequate delivery may be caused by reduced arterial oxygen levels, reduced hemoglobin levels, reduced perfusion (blood flow), or a combination of such factors.
- **Ischemia:** Ischemia is low blood flow, which can lead to cardiac tissue hypoxia further resulting in myocardial injury and infarction. Myocardial cells deprived of oxygen do not conduct nor contract well.
- **Sympathetic stimulation:** Physical or emotional stress from fear or anxiety and conditions, such as hyperthyroidism and CHF, can elicit dysrhythmias. Sympathetic stimulation can also result in cardiac ischemia caused by an increased workload on the myocardium without concurrent increase in blood flow such as in the case of diseased coronary arteries.
- **Drugs:** Many prescribed medications taken in nontherapeutic ranges or in the presence of inadequate biotransformation or clearance may produce dysrhythmias. Illegal use of sympathomimetic agents, such as cocaine or methylphenidate (Ritalin), may cause myocardial irritability and even infarction.
- **Electrolyte imbalances:** Electrical activity in the heart results from the exchange of electrolytes within cardiac tissue, known as the **action potential.** As a result, abnormal serum concentrations of electrolytes, such as potassium, magnesium, and calcium, can cause dysrhythmias.
- **Hypertrophy:** Overdevelopment of the heart muscle due to a genetic disorder or a consequence of increased workload on the myocardium (e.g., pulmonary and/or systemic vaso-constriction), resulting in smaller heart chambers and/or abnormal pumping action.
- **Rate:** Rhythms that are too slow or too fast result in inadequate cardiac output. Cardiac output is a product of stroke volume and cardiac rate. Stroke volume is the volume of blood pumped by one ventricle during one beat. Therefore, if the heart rate is too slow and the stroke volume is not increased proportionally, the cardiac output will be reduced. On the other hand, if the heart rate is too fast, the ventricles do not have enough time to fill with blood and stroke volume may be significantly reduced, resulting in poor cardiac output.
- **Stretch:** How much the atrium or ventricle stretches open so it can fill and then contract. With all else equal, greater stretch is associated with more stroke volume according to Frank Starling's Law.

Important Abbreviations and Acronyms

Before coming in contact with a patient, the RT will receive a verbal report from the RT from the preceding shift regarding the patient's clinical status and notable aspects of their medical record (see Chapter 21). It is important to understand the meaning of descriptive terms, abbreviations, and acronyms related to cardiology and ECG interpretation that may be presented while receiving a report or reviewing the medical record. Table 11-2 provides a list of some of the most common cardiology abbreviations and acronyms that may assist in the assessment of the patient's underlying disease process or cardiac conduction abnormalities.

Basic Electrocardiogram Waves

The spread of electrical stimuli throughout the heart by way of the action potential initially causes depolarization of the myocardial cells. Depolarization occurs when a polarized cell is stimulated. Polarized cells carry an electrical charge on their surface; the inside of the cell is more negatively charged than the outside of the cell. The sudden loss of the negative charge within the cell is called **depolarization**, which is a result of potassium moving out of the cell and sodium moving into the cell. The return of the negative electrical charge is called **repolarization** (Fig. 11-4) and is a result of potassium moving back into the cell and sodium moving out of the cell. This process of depolarization and repolarization produces waves of electrical activity that travel back and forth across the heart. These waves of electrical activity are represented by waves detected by the ECG electrodes. The magnitude or amplitude of each wave is determined by voltage generated by depolarization of a particular portion of the heart.

Depolarization of the atria corresponds with atrial contraction and creates the initial wave of electrical activity detected on the ECG tracing, known as the *P wave* (Fig. 11-5). Because the atria usually are small, the atria generate less voltage than the ventricles and the resulting P wave is small. Repolarization of the atria is not seen on the ECG because it usually is obscured by the simultaneous depolarization of the ventricles.

Depolarization of the ventricles corresponds with the ventricular contraction and is represented by the *QRS complex*. Because the ventricular muscle mass is larger than the atria and produces more voltage during depolarization, the QRS complex is normally taller than the P wave in most cases (see Fig. 11-5). Ventricular repolarization corresponds to ventricular relaxation between contractions and is seen as the *T wave*. The T wave is normally upright and rounded.

Just after the T wave but before the next P wave, a small deflection known as the *U wave* is sometimes seen. The U wave is thought to represent the final phase of ventricular

TABLE 11-2

Common Cardiology Abbreviations

AIJR	Accelerated idiojunctional rhythm
AIVR	Accelerated idioventricular rhythm
ARP	Absolute refractory period
A-tach	Atrial tachycardia
AV	Atrioventricular
BBB	Bundle branch block
bpm	Beats per minute
BVH	Biventricular hypertrophy
CABG	Coronary artery bypass graft
CAD	Coronary artery disease
CK-MB	Creatine kinase-myocardial band
CO	Cardiac output
CV	Cardiovascular
ECG	Electrocardiogram
EF	Ejection fraction
EKG	Electrocardiogram (German abbreviation)
EMD	Electromechanical dissociation (see *PEA*)
EP	Electrophysiologic
f wave	Fibrillatory wave
F wave	Flutter wave
HR	Heart rate
ICD	Implantable cardioverter/defibrillator
IVR	Idioventricular rhythm
LA	Left atrial
LAE	Left atrial enlargement
LAP	Left atrial pressure
LBBB	Left bundle branch block
LVH	Left ventricular hypertrophy
mA	Milliamperes
MAT	Multifocal (or multiformed) atrial tachycardia
MCL	Modified chest lead
msec	Milliseconds
mV	Millivolt
NSR	Normal sinus rhythm (see *RSR*)
PAC	Premature atrial contraction
PEA	Pulseless electrical activity
PJC	Premature junctional contraction
PJT	Paroxysmal junctional tachycardia
PMI	Point of maximal impulse
PSVT	Paroxysmal supraventricular tachycardia
PTCA	Percutaneous transluminal coronary angioplasty
PVC	Premature ventricular contractions
PVR	Pulmonary vascular resistance
QTc	QT interval corrected for heart rate
RAE	Right atrial enlargement
RBBB	Right bundle branch block
RVH	Right ventricular hypertrophy
SA	Sinoatrial
SVR	Systemic vascular resistance
SVT	Supraventricular tachycardia
SSS	Sick sinus syndrome
TdP	Torsades de pointes
VF	Ventricular fibrillation
VSD	Ventral septal defect
VT	Ventricular tachycardia
WAP	Wandering atrial pacemaker (multifocal atrial rhythm)
WPW	Wolff-Parkinson-White syndrome
1° AVBL	First-degree AV block
2° AVBL	Second-degree AV block types I or II
3° AVBL	Third-degree AV block

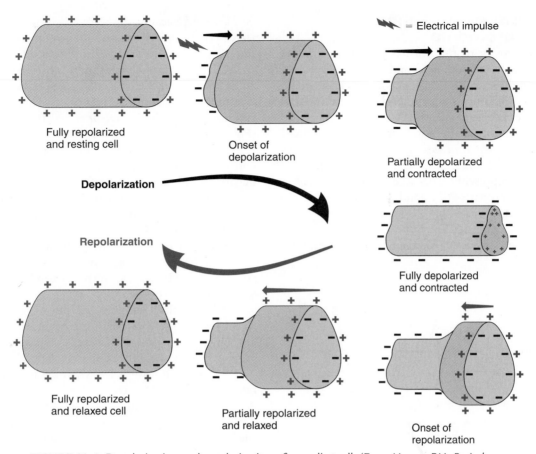

FIGURE 11-4 Depolarization and repolarization of a cardiac cell. (From Huszar RH: *Basic dysrhythmias: interpretation and management*, ed 3. St Louis, 2007, Mosby.)

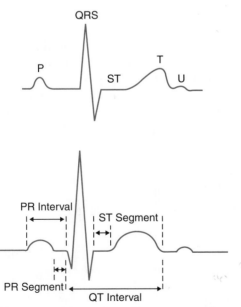

FIGURE 11-5 Normal configuration of electrocardiogram waves, segments, and intervals.

repolarization. In most cases the U wave is not seen. The clinical significance of its presence or absence is not known.

QRS complexes usually consist of several distinct waves, each of which has a letter assigned to it as a label. This labeling system is needed because the precise configuration of the QRS complex can vary from one lead to the next and from one patient to the next. To establish a standardized labeling system, several guidelines have been developed. If the first deflection of the QRS complex is downward (negative in lead II), it is labeled a *Q wave*. The initial upward (positive) deflection is called an *R wave*. The first negative deflection following an R wave is called an *S wave* (Fig. 11-6). If the QRS complex has a second positive deflection, it is labeled *R′* (R prime), and if a second S wave is also present it is called *S′* (S prime). A negative deflection can be called a Q wave only if it is the first wave of the complex. In clinical practice, each ventricular depolarization complex is called a **QRS complex** whether it has all three waves or not.

SIMPLY STATED

The QRS complex is important in evaluating the ECG because it reflects the electrical activity of the ventricles.

Electrocardiogram Paper and Measurements

The electrical activity of the heart is recorded on paper that has gridlike boxes with light and dark lines running horizontally and vertically (Fig. 11-7). The light lines circumscribe small boxes (1 × 1 mm) and the dark lines circumscribe larger boxes (5 × 5 mm).

Time is measured on the horizontal axis of the ECG paper. The ECG paper moves through the electrocardiograph at a speed of 25 mm/sec. Therefore each small square (1 mm) represents 0.04 second and each larger square (5 mm) represents 0.2 second. Five large boxes represent 1.0 second.

On the vertical axis, voltage, or amplitude, of the ECG waves is measured. The exact voltage of any ECG wave can be measured because the electrocardiograph is standardized so that 1 mV produces a deflection 10 mm in amplitude. Therefore, the standard for most ECG recordings is 1 mV = 10 mm. Each small square represents 1 mm.

To measure the amplitude of a specific wave, the isoelectric baseline must be identified. This is the flat line seen just before the P wave or right after the T or U wave (Fig. 11-8). Any movement of the ECG stylus above this line is considered positive; any downward movement is considered negative. To measure the degree of positive or negative amplitude of a specific wave, the isoelectric line is used as a reference point marking zero voltage.

R waves are measured from the isoelectric line to the top of the R wave. Q and S waves are measured from the isoelectric line to the bottom of the wave (see Fig. 11-6). P waves can be either positive or negative and are also measured from the isoelectric line to the top (if positive) or bottom (if negative) of the wave.

In addition to the amplitude of any wave, the duration of waves, intervals, and segments can be measured. A *segment* is a straight line between two waves. An *interval* encompasses at least one wave plus the connecting straight line.

The normal P wave is less than 2.5 mm in height and not more than 0.11 second in length. The *PR interval* is an important measurement that provides information regarding conduction time. This interval is measured from the beginning of the P wave, where the P wave lifts off the isoelectric line, to the beginning of the QRS complex (see Fig. 11-5). The PR interval represents the time it takes for the electrical stimulus to spread through the atria and to pass through the AV junction to the ventricles. The normal PR interval is between 0.12 and 0.20 second (3 to 5 small boxes). If conduction of the impulse through the AV junction is abnormally delayed, the PR interval will exceed 0.2 second. A prolonged PR interval is called **first-degree AV block** and is discussed later in this chapter.

The duration of ventricular depolarization is determined by measuring the *QRS interval*. This interval is measured from the first wave of the QRS complex to the end of the last wave of the QRS complex. Normally the QRS interval does

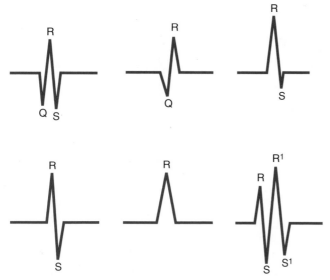

FIGURE 11-6 QRS nomenclature. See text for explanation.

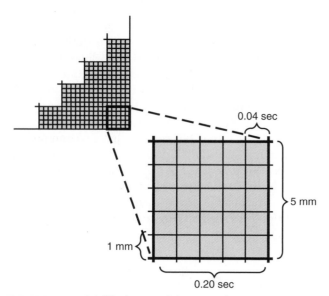

FIGURE 11-7 Gridlike boxes of electrocardiogram paper illustrating the 1-mm and 5-mm boxes.

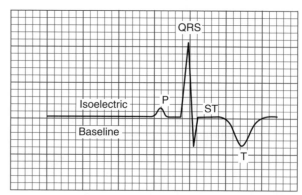

FIGURE 11-8 Isoelectric baseline used for measuring voltage of electrocardiogram waves. (From Goldberger AL: *Clinical electrocardiography: a simplified approach*, ed 7. St Louis, 2006, Mosby.)

not exceed 0.10 seconds (2 1/2 small boxes). The amplitude of the QRS complex may range from 2 to 15 mm, depending on the lead and the size of the ventricular mass.

A very important segment to evaluate is the **ST segment.** This segment is the portion of the ECG cycle from the end of the QRS complex (even if no S wave is present) to the beginning of the T wave (see Fig. 11-5). It measures the time from the end of ventricular depolarization to the start of ventricular repolarization. The normal ST segment is isoelectric (no positive or negative voltage) or at least does not move more than 1 mm above or below baseline. Certain pathologic abnormalities, such as myocardial ischemia or injury, cause the ST segment to be elevated or depressed (Fig. 11-9). The duration of the ST segment is not as important as its configuration.

The **RR interval** is useful in identifying the rate and regularity of ventricular contraction. The distance in millimeters is determined from one R wave to the next in successive QRS complexes. This is done for several different RR intervals. ECG calipers can be helpful in making this measurement. The average of the measurements is determined and converted to time. Remember that each large box is equal to 0.2 second and 5 large boxes equal 1.0 second. If the RR interval is 1.5 seconds, the heart rate is 40 beats/min (60 seconds divided by 1.5 = 40). If the RR interval is 1.0 second, the heart rate is 60 beats/min. If the RR interval is 0.5 second, the heart rate is 120 beats/min. This method for determining the heart rate is easy to apply if the RR interval falls conveniently on one of the numbers just described. Unfortunately, this is not usually the case. Other methods for calculating the heart rate are described later. Marked variation in the RR interval from one interval to the next indicates that the heartbeat is irregular and may be a sign of sinus dysrhythmia, which is described in more detail in the section on dysrhythmia identification.

The **QT interval** is measured from the beginning of the QRS complex to the end of the T wave (see Fig. 11-5). This interval represents the time from the beginning of ventricular depolarization to the end of ventricular repolarization. The normal values for the QT interval depend on the heart rate. As the heart rate increases, the QT interval normally shortens; as the heart rate decreases, the QT interval increases. As a general rule, the QT interval that exceeds one half of the RR interval is prolonged if the heart rate is 80 beats/min or less. Common causes of an abnormally prolonged QT interval include hypokalemia (low potassium), hypocalcemia (low calcium), and the side effects of certain medications such as quinidine.

Evaluating Heart Rate

If the heart rate is regular, one of the easiest ways of determining the heart rate is to count the number of large (0.2 second) boxes between 2 successive QRS complexes and divide this number into 300. For example, if there is one large box between successive R waves, then each R wave is separated by 0.2 second. Over the course of 1.0 second there will be 5 QRS complexes and 300 QRS complexes in 60 seconds. Therefore the heart rate is 300 beats/min. Following this logic:

2 large boxes = rate of 150 beats/min (300/2=150)
3 large boxes = rate of 100 beats/min (300/3=100)
4 large boxes = rate of 75 beats/min (300/4=75)
5 large boxes = rate of 60 beats/min (300/5=60)
6 large boxes = rate of 50 beats/min (300/6=50)

If the heart rate is irregular, this method will not be accurate because the spacing between QRS complexes will vary from beat to beat. In such cases, the average rate can be determined by counting the number of QRS complexes in a 6-second interval (30 large boxes) and multiplying the number by 10. Because the top of the ECG paper is marked with small vertical dashes every 3 seconds, 6-second intervals are easy to identify.

An increase or decrease in heart rate by more than 20% of the baseline value is generally regarded as a significant change and should be evaluated further. An abnormally slow heart rate may reduce cardiac performance to the point of compromised perfusion. Recall that cardiac output is a product of stroke volume and heart rate. A heart rate below 60 beats/min is referred to as an *absolute bradycardia*. However, bradycardia that may require intervention is relative to the individual patient. For example, a well-conditioned runner may present with a heart rate of 50 beats/min with no signs of inadequate cardiac output. On the other hand, a person with poor myocardial contractility that presents with a heart rate of 50 beats/min is likely to show signs of compromised perfusion or even cardiogenic shock in severe cases. At the other extreme, an adult heart rate greater than 100 beats/min is known as *tachycardia*. An increase in heart

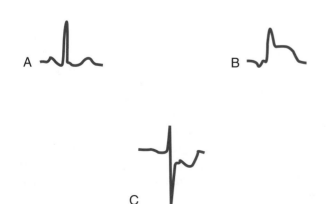

FIGURE 11-9 ST segments. **A,** Normal. **B,** Abnormal elevation. **C,** Abnormal depression.

rate above 130-140 beats/min may compromise cardiac performance. This is because an abnormally rapid heart rate will increase myocardial oxygen demand, possibly to the point of inducing ischemia if the demand exceeds the supply. Additionally, significant tachycardia may further induce ischemia because it shortens the diastolic period, which is the period when most coronary perfusion occurs. In instances of extreme tachycardia where the heart rate exceeds 160 beats/minute, the ventricular filling time may be too short to permit adequate refilling, thus reducing cardiac output. In severe tachycardia, the combined effects of increased oxygen demand and decreased cardiac output is potentially dangerous, especially for those patients with pre-existing cardiac conditions. Such patients should be monitored carefully and the attending physician notified immediately.

Electrocardiogram Leads

Because the heart is a three-dimensional organ, a more complete picture of the electrical activity in the heart will be obtained if it is viewed from several different angles. The standard ECG uses 12 different leads to provide 12 different views from different angles of the heart. Interpretation of the 12 leads is a little more difficult, but the information obtained is more complete and abnormalities are not likely to be missed.

The 12 leads can be subdivided into two groups: 6 extremity (limb) leads and 6 chest leads. To obtain the six limb leads, two electrodes are placed on the patient's wrists and two on the patient's ankles. The ECG machine can vary the orientation of these four electrodes to one another to create the six limb leads. The chest leads are created by attaching six electrodes across the patient's chest. The chest leads are discussed after the limb leads are reviewed.

Limb Leads

The six limb leads are called *leads I, II, III, aV_R, aV_L, and aV_F*. Leads I, II, and III are bipolar. Each lead is created by comparing the difference in electrical voltage between two electrodes. For lead I, the ECG machine temporarily designates the electrode on the left arm as a positive lead and the electrode on the right arm as negative. The measured difference in voltage between these two leads results in lead I. For lead II, the right arm electrode remains negative and the left leg electrode is positive. Lead III is created by making the left arm negative and the left leg positive.

The other three limb leads (aV_R, aV_L, and aV_F) are called *augmented leads* because the ECG machine must amplify the tracings to get an adequate recording. The augmented leads are created by measuring the electrical voltage at one limb lead, with all other limb leads made negative. For the augmented leads, the ECG machine must augment the recorded voltages by about 50% to get an adequate recording. Lead aV_R is created by making the right arm positive

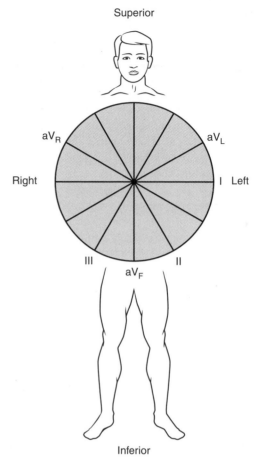

FIGURE 11-10 Frontal plane showing spatial relationships of six extremity leads. (Modified from Goldberger AL: *Clinical electrocardiography: a simplified approach*, ed 7. St. Louis, 2006, Mosby.)

and all the others negative. Lead aV_L calls for the left arm to be positive, and lead aV_F is created by making the left leg positive.

The six limb leads view the heart in a vertical plane called a *frontal plane*. Any electrical activity that is directed up, down, left, or right is recorded by the limb leads (Fig. 11-10). The frontal plane can be envisioned as a giant circle that surrounds the patient and lies in the same plane as the patient. This circle can be marked off in 360 degrees, as shown in Figure 11-10.

The angle of orientation for each of the bipolar limb leads can be determined by drawing a line from the designated negative lead to the designated positive lead. For lead I, the angle of orientation is 0 degrees; for lead II, +60 degrees; and for lead III, +120 degrees. For the augmented leads, the angle of orientation can be determined by drawing a line from the average of the other three limb leads to the one that is designated as the positive lead. The angle of orientation is −150 degrees for lead aV_R, −30 degrees for lead aV_L, and 90 degrees for lead aV_F.

In review, the limb leads consist of three bipolar leads and three unipolar leads. The three bipolar leads are called

The 12 Leads of an Electrocardiogram and the Myocardial Wall that Each Set Views

Lead	View
I, aV$_L$, V$_5$, V$_6$	Lateral
II, III, aV$_F$	Inferior
V$_1$, V$_2$	Septal
V$_3$, V$_4$	Anterior
Cells and Function	
Pacemaker cells	Specialized cells that have a high degree of automaticity and provide the electrical power for the heart
Conducting cells	Cells that conduct the electrical impulse throughout the heart
Myocardial cells	Cells that contract in response to electrical stimuli and pump the blood

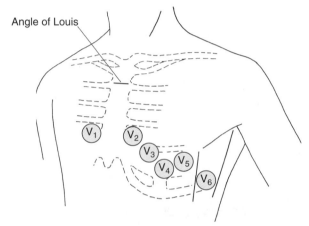

FIGURE 11-11 Position of the six chest leads. V$_1$ is located in the fourth intercostal space right of the sternum. V$_2$ is located in the fourth intercostal space left of the sternum. V$_3$ is placed between V$_2$ and V$_4$. V$_4$ is placed in the fifth intercostal space in the midclavicular line. V$_5$ is placed between V$_4$ and V$_6$. V$_6$ is placed in the fifth intercostal space in the midaxillary line. (Modified from Goldberger AL: *Clinical electrocardiography: a simplified approach*, ed 7. St. Louis, 2006, Mosby.)

leads I, II, and III. The three unipolar leads are called aV$_R$, aV$_L$, and aV$_F$. The abbreviation *a* refers to augmented, *V* to voltage, and *R, L,* and *F* to right arm, left arm, and left leg (foot), respectively. The limb leads measure the electrical activity in the heart that occurs in the frontal plane, and each lead has its own specific view or angle of orientation to the heart (Table 11-3).

Chest Leads

The six chest leads, or precordial leads, are called *leads V$_1$, V$_2$, V$_3$, V$_4$, V$_5$, and V$_6$.* The chest leads are unipolar leads that are placed across the chest in a horizontal plane. Figure 11-11 shows the correct placment of the six chest leads. The chest leads define a horizontal or transverse plane and view electrical voltages that move anteriorly and posteriorly. Like the

limb leads, each chest lead has its own view or angle of orientation. Leads V$_1$ through V$_4$ often are called the *anterior leads* because they view the anterior portion of the heart. Leads V$_5$ and V$_6$ view the left lateral portion of the heart and are therefore called the *left lateral leads* (see Table 11-3). More specifically, leads V$_1$ and V$_2$ are positioned next to the sternum and normally view the interventricular septum, leads V$_3$ and V$_4$ are placed on the left anterior chest to view the anterior wall of the left ventricle, and V$_5$ and V$_6$ are positioned on the axillary area of the left chest and therefore view the lateral wall of the left ventricle.

SIMPLY STATED

The normal ECG has six limb leads that examine the heart in the vertical plane and six chest leads that examine the heart in the horizontal plane.

Evaluating the Mean QRS Axis

The QRS axis represents the general direction of current flow during ventricular depolarization. Although depolarization spreads through the ventricles in different directions, an average or mean direction can be determined. Normally, the mean QRS axis (vector) points leftward (patient's left) and downward, somewhere between 0 and 90 degrees in the frontal plane previously described (Fig. 11-12).

The ECG records a positive (upward) QRS complex when the mean QRS axis is moving toward a positive electrode. When the mean QRS axis is moving toward a negative lead, the QRS complex is negative (downward). Because each of the six limb leads has its own angle of orientation as defined in the hexaxial reference system, a review of the recorded limb leads should identify the mean QRS axis in the frontal plane.

To identify the mean QRS axis, begin by sketching the hexaxial reference system, including labels for the points where the limb leads are located on the circle. Next, identify which limb lead has the QRS complex with the most voltage (positive or negative). This is accomplished by identifying the QRS complex with the largest deflection from baseline. If the largest deflection is positive (R wave), the mean QRS axis points toward the lead with the tallest QRS. If the most voltage is negative (Q or S wave), the mean axis points away from that lead. For example, if the most voltage is found to be in lead II and it is positive, then the mean QRS axis must be about +60 degrees because this is where lead II is located on the hexaxial reference system (see Fig. 11-12). This would be considered a normal axis because it falls between 0 and +90 degrees. If the most voltage is found in lead I and is negative, then the QRS axis is approximately 180 degrees because lead I is located at 0 degrees. This would be consistent with right-axis deviation.

In some situations, the most voltage may be equally present in two leads. If two leads exhibit equal positive voltage,

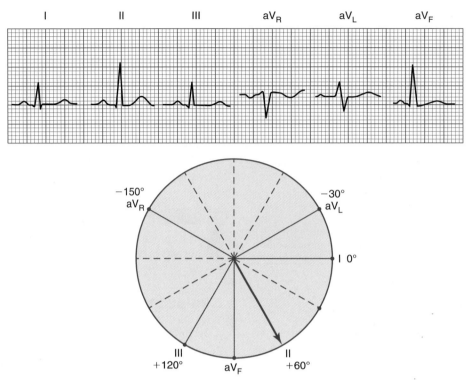

FIGURE 11-12 Normal mean QRS axis of 60 degrees. (From Goldberger AL: *Clinical electrocardiography: a simplified approach*, ed 8. St. Louis, 2013, Mosby.)

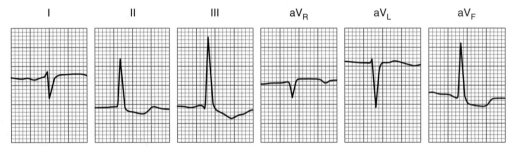

FIGURE 11-13 Sample electrocardiogram showing right-axis deviation. Note the positive QRS complex (R wave) in leads II and III and the negative QRS complex (S wave) in lead I. (From Goldberger AL: *Clinical electrocardiography: a simplified approach*, ed 8. St. Louis, 2013, Mosby.)

the mean axis must fall midway between the two leads. If the most voltage is equally negative in two leads, the mean axis is opposite the midpoint between the two leads.

As mentioned, a normal QRS axis is approximately −35 to +90 degrees. If the axis is found to be between +90 and 180 degrees, right-axis deviation is present. Right-axis deviation is common in patients with cor pulmonale (right ventricular enlargement due to chronic lung disease). In such cases, the QRS complex will be negative in lead I but positive in lead aV$_F$. Leads II and III are both positive in most cases of right-axis deviation; however, lead III will be taller than lead II (Fig. 11-13 and Table 11-4). Right-axis deviation is important to recognize early in the care of the patient since it often indicates significant chronic pulmonary

TABLE 11-4

Quick Axis Determination

Lead	Axis
I is positive II is positive	Normal
I is positive II is negative	Left deviation
I is negative II is positive	Right deviation
I is negative II is negative	Extreme right deviation

hypertension. This is most often related to chronic hypoxemia from chronic obstructive pulmonary disease (COPD).

Left-axis deviation is present when the mean axis is found to be between -35 and -90 degrees. Left-axis deviation can occur in several different conditions, including left ventricular hypertrophy and blocks of the left bundle branch. In such cases, the QRS complex is positive in lead I and negative in lead aV_F. In addition, the QRS complex in lead III will demonstrate negative voltage with left-axis deviation.

If the mean QRS axis is found to be between −90 and −180 degrees, extreme left or right-axis deviation is present. This condition is not common. When the ECG recording indicates that it may be present, the extremity leads should be checked to make sure they are attached properly.

The same principles of axis evaluation can be applied to the P wave as to the QRS complex. When normal sinus rhythm is present and the atria are normal in size, the P wave is positive in lead II and negative in lead aV_R. Therefore the normal P wave is directed toward lead II and away from lead aV_R, making the normal mean P wave axis about +60 degrees. In cor pulmonale, right atrial enlargement is common. The ECG will show tall, narrow P waves in leads II, III, and aV_F in such cases.

SIMPLY STATED

The normal mean axis is somewhere between −35 and +90 degrees. Right-axis deviation indicates that the right ventricle is enlarged; left-axis deviation suggests that the left ventricle is enlarged.

Steps of Electrocardiogram Interpretation

First and most importantly, the patient's condition must be evaluated. All dysrhythmias should be interpreted and evaluated in accordance with the patient's clinical presentation and medical history. Important signs and symptoms that may be associated with dysrhythmias may include the following:
- Chest pain
- Dyspnea
- Fine, inspiratory crackles in the lower lobes
- Palpitations
- Nausea
- Pale, cool, clammy skin
- Dizziness or syncope
- Sense of impending doom
- Hypotension
- Altered level of consciousness

Interpretation of dysrhythmias can be accomplished on three levels. The first level is simply identifying ventricular response. The contraction of the ventricles determines the majority of the cardiac output and perfusion of blood to the tissues. The ventricular response is determined by evaluating the QRS complexes and subsequent pulse strength.

Second, dysrhythmias can be placed into categories based on the origin of the impulse formation, which may include the following:
- Atrial
- Junctional
- Ventricular

Third, dysrhythmias can be evaluated based on the electrophysiology (or pathway) of the conduction disturbance. These can be categorized as follows:
- Ectopic beats or rhythms
- Escape beats or rhythms
- AV blocks
- Bundle branch blocks

To make sure that all components of the ECG tracing are reviewed by the RT or other member of the patient care team, a systematic method should be used. It is important to avoid assumptions resulting from quickly glancing at an ECG strip, because they may lead to misinterpretation. Every strip should be read from left to right and the step-by-step process described here should be followed, generally in the order they are listed. The steps are as follows:

1. *Identify the heart rate.* Most modern ECG monitors provide a display of the heart rate. Always take the patient's pulse to verify that the monitor is calculating the heart rate correctly. Note that the monitor may not provide an accurate rate if the rhythm is irregular. If this is the case, a strip should be printed and calculation should be done as mentioned in the section on Evaluating Heart Rate. Rhythms are called *bradycardia* if the rate is below 60 beats/min and *tachycardia* if the heart rate is over 100 beats/min (see Table 11-4).

2. *Evaluate the rhythm.* Note whether the spacing between the QRS complexes is equal. Small variations of 0.04 second (40 msec) are considered normal. If the spaces are greater than 0.04 second, the rhythm is irregular. Irregularity may occur randomly or in patterns (e.g., occur every other beat or change with respirations). Irregular rhythms are present with the following dysrhythmias:
   - Ectopic beats
   - Escape beats
   - Second-degree AV blocks
   - Atrial fibrillation
   - Sinus dysrhythmia

3. *Note the presence of P waves.* A normal P wave generally is positive, depending on the lead, and has a rounded shape. Normal P waves are less than 0.11 second (110 msec) wide and less than 2.5 mm (21/2 small boxes) tall. Oddly shaped P waves may indicate atrial enlargement. Normal rhythms will only have one P wave preceding each QRS complex, and each P wave should have the same configuration as the others. If there

appears to be more than one P wave preceding a QRS complex, the rhythm may be the following:
- Atrial flutter
- Atrial fibrillation (no distinguishable P-waves with a fibrillatory baseline waveform)
- Second-degree AV block
- Third-degree AV block

4. *Measure the PR interval.* The normal PR interval is 0.12 to 0.20 second (120 to 200 msec) wide. A PR interval that is wider than 0.20 second indicates a delay in conduction through the AV node, indicating the possibility of a block (Table 11-5).

5. *Measure the width of the QRS complex.* The normal QRS complex is less than 0.10 second (120 msec) wide. Wide QRS complexes can occur with the following:
- Bundle branch blocks
- Ectopic beats originating in the ventricles (premature ventricular contractions)
- Ventricular dysrhythmias such as ventricular tachycardia, idioventricular rhythm, or premature ventricular complexes
- Third-degree AV block

6. *Inspect the ST segment in all leads.* ST segment elevation may indicate myocardial injury whereas ST segment depression may indicate myocardial ischemia. The portion or wall of the heart that is ischemic can be determined by identifying the leads looking at that portion of the heart (see Table 11-3). The ST segment is measured from the J point: the junction between the QRS complex and the ST segment (see Fig. 11-8).

7. *Identify the mean QRS axis.* Most 12-lead ECG tracings indicate the QRS axis. Normal axis is 0 to +90 degrees. Left-axis deviation is −35 to −90 degrees, and right-axis deviation is +90 to +180 degrees (see Fig. 11-12 and Table 11-4). Box 11-2 lists causes of axis deviation.

8. *Assess the waveform morphology.* Some QRS complexes may have additional deflections. If there is a second deflection, the second portion is called *prime* (see Fig. 11-6). For example, a second R wave would be labeled R′.

R′

9. *Evaluate the Q wave.* A Q wave is considered normal (or physiologic) if it is less than 0.04 second (40 msec) wide and less than one-third the amplitude of the R wave. Q waves that exceed either of these values are considered pathologic and indicate a new or possibly old infarction.

10. *Look for signs of chamber enlargement.* High-voltage R waves in the precordial leads indicate ventricular hypertrophy. Large or abnormally shaped P waves indicate atrial enlargement (see review later in this chapter).

SIMPLY STATED

A systematic step-by-step evaluation of the ECG is needed to find all abnormalities.

Normal Sinus Rhythm

Recognizing abnormal rhythms from an electrocardiographic strip is easier if you have an appreciation for the normal tracing (see Fig. 11-5). The normal sinus rhythm begins with an upright P wave that is identical from one complex to the next. As summarized in Table 11-5, the PR interval is consistent throughout the rhythm strip and is 0.12 to 0.20 second. The QRS complexes are identical and no longer than 0.10 second. The ST segment is flat. The R-R interval is regular and does not vary more than 0.12 second between QRS complexes. The heart rate is between 60 and 100 beats/min.

Identification of Common Dysrhythmias

This section discusses the characteristics of some of the most commonly seen dysrhythmias. It is always important to treat a symptomatic dysrhythmia, but it is just as important to determine the underlying cause. Some of the most common causes of each dysrhythmia are also discussed.

Box 11-2	Causes of Axis Deviation

RIGHT AXIS
Left ventricular infarction
Right ventricular hypertrophy
Chronic obstructive lung disease
Acute pulmonary embolism
Infants up to 1 year of age (normal)
Biventricular hypertrophy
Left posterior fascicular

LEFT AXIS
Right ventricular infarction
Left ventricular hypertrophy
Abdominal obesity
Ascites or large abdominal tumors
Third-trimester pregnancy
Left anterior fascicular block

TABLE 11-5

Summary of Normal Values for the Electrocardiogram Interpretation and Common Alterations

Variable	Normal Range	Common Alterations
Rate	60-100/min	Rates > 100= tachycardia
		Rates < 60 =bradycardia
PR interval	0.12-0.20/sec	>0.20 = First-degree AV block
QRS interval	<0.10/sec	>0.10 = Ectopic foci
ST segment	Isoelectric	Elevated or depressed = myocardial ischemia
T wave	Upright, round and asymmetrical	Inverted with ischemia, tall and peaked with electrolyte imbalances

Sinus Bradycardia

Sinus bradycardia meets all the criteria for a normal sinus rhythm except for the heart rate, which is less than 60 beats/min. It is important at this point to understand the difference between an absolute bradycardia and a relative bradycardia. Absolute sinus bradycardia is simply a heart rate less than 60 beats/min and may be normal for a particular patient or tolerated well by the patient. For example, a conditioned runner may present with a heart rate of 55 beats/min with no negative cardiopulmonary signs and symptoms. By definition, this is an absolute bradycardia, but it is probably the patient's normal heart rate. On the other hand, a relative sinus bradycardia or a heart rate that is significantly below a patient's baseline is generally not tolerated well because it often compromises cardiac performance. Marked relative sinus bradycardia may result in hypotension, syncope, diminished cardiac output and shock.

Transient bradycardia may be caused by an increase in vagal tone as a result of direct carotid massage, manipulation of tracheostomy ties or tube, tracheal suctioning, or the Valsalva maneuver. Damage to the SA node, as may occur with a myocardial infarction, can cause a long-term bradycardia. Hypothyroidism, hypothermia, and hyperkalemia, and certain drugs may also result in bradycardia (Fig. 11-14).

Sinus Tachycardia

Sinus tachycardia is present when the heart rate is 100 to 150 beats/min, the SA node is the pacemaker, and all the normal conduction pathways in the heart are followed. Sinus tachycardia may be well-tolerated by the patient; however, it increases myocardial oxygen demand and decreases the diastolic period, both of which can lead to myocardial ischemia. Sinus tachycardia results from sympathetic nervous system stimulation and may indicate a significant physiologic problem or be self-limiting and cease once the underlying cause is addressed. Fever, pain, hypoxemia, hypovolemia, hypotension, sepsis, and heart failure are causes of sinus tachycardia. It is especially important for the RT to note that tracheal suctioning, especially if it is performed without adequate oxygenation, can cause sinus tachycardia as a compensatory mechanism to hypoxemia. In addition, many beta-agonist bronchodilators and excessive intake of caffeine often increase heart rate (Fig. 11-15).

Sinus Dysrhythmia

Sinus dysrhythmia is a benign dysrhythmia that meets all the criteria for normal sinus rhythm except that the rhythm is irregular. It usually does not produce symptoms in the patient and requires no treatment. In most cases of sinus dysrhythmia, no abnormality of the heart is present. Often the irregularities are related to the patient's breathing pattern. This suggests that the changes in intrathoracic pressure associated with breathing in and out are causing changes in the tone of the vagus nerve, which may produce mild alterations in regularity of the heart rate.

Systematic Evaluation

Rate	60 to 100 beats/min, may also present as a bradydysrhythmia (<60)
Rhythm	Irregular
P waves	Normal configuration. Each P wave is followed by a QRS complex
PR interval	Less than or equal to 0.2 second in length
QRS complex	Less than 0.10 second in width

Paroxysmal Atrial Tachycardia

Paroxysmal atrial tachycardia (PAT) occurs when an ectopic focus in the atrium usurps the pacemaking function of the SA node and paces the heart, usually at an abnormally rapid rate of 160 to 240 beats/min. It appears on the monitor as a series of normal-looking QRS complexes, each associated with a P wave. Because of the rapid rate, the P wave may be obscured by the preceding T wave.

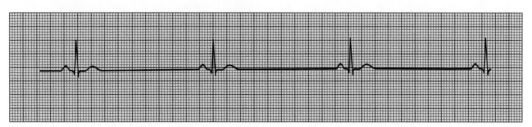

FIGURE 11-14 Electrocardiogram tracing of sinus bradycardia.

Systematic Evaluation

Rate	Less than 60 beats/min
Rhythm	Regular
P waves	Normal configuration; each P wave is followed by a QRS complex
PR interval	Less than or equal to 0.2 sec in length
QRS complex	Less than 0.10 sec in width

Onset of this dysrhythmia is sudden and spontaneous; termination is similarly abrupt. PAT is seen in patients with normal hearts and in those with organic heart disease. The hazard of PAT is that it increases myocardial oxygen demand while decreasing pump effectiveness as a result of the diminished "filling time." PAT may precipitate hypotension or an ischemic episode. PAT is especially dangerous for patients with compromised cardiovascular function, myocardial ischemia, preexisting heart failure, and recent myocardial infarction. Patients with PAT often complain of lightheadedness or palpitation. Occasionally, PAT will cause the patient to faint. Some possible causes of PAT may include emotional stress, mitral valve disease, rheumatic heart disease, digitalis toxicity, or the use of alcohol, caffeine, or nicotine (Fig. 11-16).

Atrial Flutter

Atrial flutter is a dysrhythmia that produces a very distinctive ECG pattern, usually caused by a rapidly firing ectopic site in the atria that presents as a characteristic sawtooth pattern between normal-appearing QRS complexes. The sawtooth pattern of flutter waves (often referred to as *F waves*) represents the rapid flutter or contraction of the atria on stimulation by a reentry circuit or accelerated automaticity. Atrial flutter results in diminished atrial "filling time," which results in minimal atrial assistance in filling the ventricles. Recall that the term atrial kick refers to the contraction of the atria forcing out blood at the latter part of systole and results in about 10% to 30% of cardiac output in a healthy person but is diminished in atrial flutter. A secondary problem with atrial flutter is that the pattern of blood flow in the atria causes areas of diminished blood movement near the atrial walls. This stagnation of blood promotes the formation of thrombi, often referred to as *mural thrombi*, along the wall of the atria. Hence, RTs and other members of the patient care team should be mindful that patients with untreated atrial flutter are at higher risk for pulmonary emboli and stroke caused by the migration of a mural thrombus.

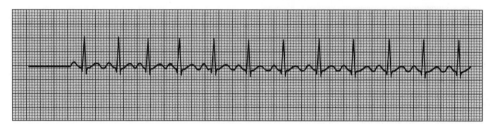

FIGURE 11-15 Electrocardiogram tracing of sinus tachycardia.

Systematic Evaluation

Rate	100 to 150 beats/min
Rhythm	Regular
P waves	Normal configuration; each P wave is followed by a QRS complex
PR interval	Less than or equal to 0.2 sec in length
QRS complex	Less than 0.10 sec in width

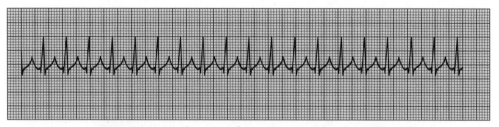

FIGURE 11-16 Short run of paroxysmal atrial tachycardia.

Systematic Evaluation

Rate	160 to 240 beats/min
Rhythm	Regular
P waves	Abnormal configuration. May precede the QRS complex or may be hidden within the QRS complex. Usually appear pointed because of combined amplitude with the previous T wave. If observable, each P wave is followed by a QRS complex
PR interval	Usually not measurable
QRS complex	Less than 0.10 sec in width

Atrial flutter usually is a short-lived dysrhythmia; it usually deteriorates to atrial fibrillation or the patient's previous rhythm returns spontaneously. Some possible causes of atrial flutter may include valvular heart disease, myocardial infarction, hypertensive heart disease, cardiomyopathy, myocarditis, and pericarditis (Fig. 11-17).

Atrial Fibrillation

In atrial fibrillation, the electrical activity of the atria is completely chaotic and without coordination because it is arising from multiple ectopic sites within the atria. This results in a quivering of the atrial myocardium and complete loss of atrial pumping ability. Because the atria provide useful assistance in filling the ventricles from the atrial kick, there is a decrease in ventricular filling during atrial fibrillation. In most cases, the reduction in cardiac output is not serious enough to produce symptoms, although it reduces cardiac reserve and may limit the normal activities of daily living. Similar to atrial flutter, patients with atrial fibrillation are at greater risk for mural thrombi formation and embolization due to blood stagnation in the atria. As a result, RTs and other clinicians should be on the alert for pulmonary emboli and stroke in such patients. Some possible causes of atrial fibrillation include all of those mentioned under atrial flutter but may also include hyperthyroidism, pulmonary disease, and congenital heart disease.

The ECG tracing shows a chaotic baseline between QRS complexes, with no regular pattern or organization. This irregular baseline is composed of what are called *fibrillatory waves* (f waves) that all have a different configuration because of their origin from different ectopic sites in the atria (Fig. 11-18).

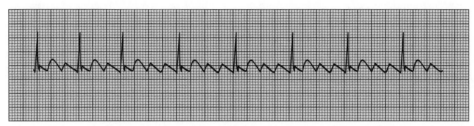

FIGURE 11-17 Electrocardiogram tracing of atrial flutter.

Systematic Evaluation

Atrial rate	180 to 400 beats/min
Ventricular rate	Varies but always less than the atrial rate
Rhythm	Regular
P waves	A uniform sawtooth baseline configuration. The relationship between the flutter waves and the QRS complexes may be regular (e.g., four flutter waves to each QRS complex) or variable
PR interval	Not measurable
QRS complex	Less than 0.10 sec in width

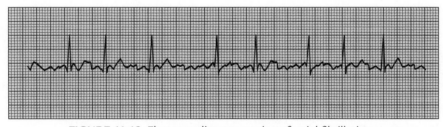

FIGURE 11-18 Electrocardiogram tracing of atrial fibrillation.

Systematic Evaluation

Atrial rate	Difficult to determine
Ventricular rate	Varies but always less than the atrial rate
Rhythm	Irregularly irregular
P waves	All f waves have a different configuration. The relationship between the f waves and the QRS complexes is irregular
PR interval	Not measurable
QRS complex	Less than 0.10 sec in width

Premature Ventricular Contractions

Premature ventricular contractions (PVCs) represent ecto-pic beats originating in one of the ventricles as a result of irritable foci. QRS intervals of PVCs are generally wider than normal (>0.10 sec) PVCs occur in both the normal and the diseased heart. PVCs commonly occur with anxi-ety or excessive use of caffeine, alcohol, or tobacco. Cer-tain medications, such as epinephrine and theophylline,

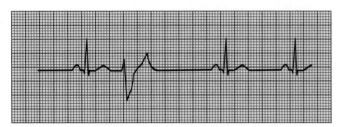

FIGURE 11-19 Electrocardiogram tracing of a single premature ventricular contraction.

Systematic Evaluation

Rate	That of the underlying rhythm
Rhythm	Underlying rhythm is usually regular but irregular with a PVC
P waves	None associated with the PVC
PR interval	Not measurable
QRS complex	Generally more than 0.10 sec in width, abnormal configuration, and premature. T wave after the PVC is deflected in a direction opposite to that of the QRS complex. There is a full compensatory pause after the PVC confirmed by measuring the interval between the normal QRS complex immediately before the PVC and the normal QRS complex immediately after the PVC; it will be double the normal RR interval for that patient

may also provoke PVCs in patients with normal hearts. Myocardial ischemia is a common cause of PVCs in patients with heart disease. Other causes may include aci-dosis, electrolyte imbalance, CHF, myocardial infarction, and hypoxia.

A single PVC poses no threat to the patient (Fig. 11-19), but certain configurations of PVCs may signal a serious cardiac problem that may need immediate treatment. Although the idea that PVCs are "warning" dysrhythmias has not been proved by clinical research, the following con-ditions warrant further investigation and indicate the need for close monitoring of the patient:

- *Increased frequency*: Multiple PVCs occur in 1 minute (Fig. 11-20).
- *Multifocal PVCs*: The QRS complexes of the PVCs have more than one configuration (Fig. 11-21); this indicates that more than one area of the ventricles is irritated.
- *Couplets*: Two PVCs occur in a row.
- *Salvos*: Three or more PVCs occur in a row (sometimes called a *short run of ventricular tachycardia*).
- *R-on-T phenomenon*: The PVC occurs during the downslope of the T wave of the preceding beat; this poses a real dan-ger because it can precipitate ventricular tachycardia (Fig. 11-22).

Ventricular Tachycardia

Ventricular tachycardia appears on the monitor as a series of broad QRS complexes, occurring at a rapid rate, each without an identifiable P wave. This condition originates from an ectopic focus in the ventricles that may also be associated with enhanced automaticity or reentry. By defi-nition, ventricular tachycardia is a run of three or more consecutive PVCs. It may be classified as *sustained ven-tricular tachycardia*, which lasts more than 30 seconds and requires immediate medical attention, or *nonsustained ven-tricular tachycardia*, which terminates spontaneously after

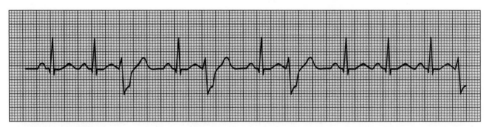

FIGURE 11-20 Electrocardiogram tracing of frequent premature ventricular contractions.

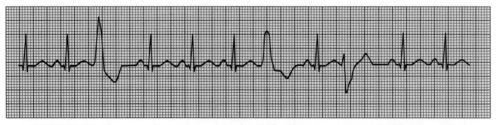

FIGURE 11-21 Electrocardiogram tracing of multifocal premature ventricular contractions.

a short burst. The rhythm is regular, and the rate is usually in the range of 140 to 300 beats/min. The majority of patients deteriorate rapidly with this dysrhythmia; therefore it must be treated as an emergency. Without appropriate treatment, sustained ventricular tachycardia may lead to ventricular fibrillation (described later). When ventricular tachycardia occurs, the patient may become hypotensive and be slow to respond. If cardiac output deteriorates significantly, the patient usually becomes unresponsive. In addition, such patients in ventricular tachycardia may not have a detectable carotid pulse, in which case the American Heart Association (AHA) Basic Life Support (BLS) and Advanced Cardiac Life Support (ACLS) rescue protocols should be immediately initiated. Ventricular tachycardia is often caused by problems similar to those that cause PVCs. When the heart is hypoxic, as occurs with severe myocardial ischemia, ventricular tachycardia is common and is a sign that the patient needs immediate care (Fig. 11-23).

Ventricular Fibrillation

Ventricular fibrillation is the presence of chaotic, completely unorganized electrical activity in the ventricular myocardial fibers. It produces a characteristic wavy, irregular pattern on the ECG monitor. Depending on the amplitude of the electrical impulses, it can be mistaken for asystole or ventricular tachycardia. Because the heart cannot pump blood when fibrillation is occurring, the cardiac output drops to zero and the patient becomes unconscious immediately. This dysrhythmia is life threatening and must be treated immediately in accordance with the BLS and ACLS resuscitation protocols, including chest compressions between each defibrillation attempt. Ventricular fibrillation often is caused by the same factors that precipitate ventricular tachycardia (Fig. 11-24).

Asystole

Asystole is cardiac standstill and is invariably fatal unless an acceptable rhythm is rapidly restored. In fact, asystole is one of the criteria used for the determination of clinical death. Asystole is recognized on the ECG monitor as a straight or almost straight line. In accordance with AHA resuscitation protocols, the RT or other clinician should quickly assess for a pulse and patient responsiveness early in any rescue effort because what may initially appears to be asystole on an ECG monitor, may simply be a disconnection of the ECG leads, which can resemble asystole. In addition, the AHA guidelines call for the confirmation of asystole in more than one lead during resuscitation efforts to ensure it is not fine ventricular fibrillation. Clinically, asystole is characterized by immediate pulselessness and loss of consciousness. The ECG tracing shows a line that is flat or almost flat, without discernible electrical activity (Fig. 11-25).

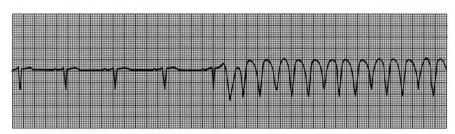

FIGURE 11-22 Electrocardiogram tracing of R-on-T phenomenon.

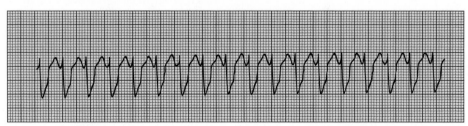

FIGURE 11-23 Electrocardiogram tracing of ventricular tachycardia.

Systematic Evaluation

Rate	140 to 300 beats/min
Rhythm	Regular
P waves	None associated with the QRS complex. They may occasionally occur because the sinoatrial node is still functioning
PR interval	Not measurable
QRS complex	Abnormal and greater than 0.10 sec in width

Pulseless Electrical Activity

Pulseless electrical activity (PEA) is not a discrete dysrhythmia but rather an electromechanical condition that can be diagnosed clinically. As the name implies, there is a dissociation of the electrical and the mechanical activity of the heart. In other words, the pattern that appears on the ECG monitor does not generate a pulse. Fortunately, PEA is rare and does not occur without a precipitating event. Tension pneumothorax, cardiac trauma, hypothermia, and severe electrolyte or acid-base disturbances are among the most common causes of PEA. PEA sometimes is seen as a terminal event in an unsuccessful cardiac resuscitation effort.

There is no relationship between the electrical pattern appearing on the ECG monitor or tracing and the mechanical activity of the heart. PEA therefore is any rhythm that

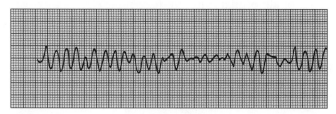

FIGURE 11-24 Electrocardiogram tracing of ventricular fibrillation.

Systematic Evaluation

Rate	None
Rhythm	Irregular, chaotic waves
P waves	None
PR interval	None
QRS complex	No waves appear with any regularity on the tracing. There may be occasional low-amplitude waves that appear somewhat like ventricular-origin complexes, but they are sporadic in occurrence and totally irregular

does not produce a pulse with the exception of ventricular tachycardia, ventricular fibrillation, and asystole.

Atrioventricular Heart Block

AV heart block is a general term that refers to a disturbance in the conduction of impulses from the atria to the ventricles through the AV node. However, the block may be at the level of the AV node or the bundle of His or in the bundle branches. Classification of the AV blocks is based on the site of the block and the severity of the conduction disturbance.

Disturbances in AV conduction can occur as an adverse effect of medications, such as digitalis, or when damage to the conduction system occurs with myocardial infarction. In some cases of complete heart block, the patient may develop symptoms associated with hypotension (fainting and weakness) if the ventricles are beating too slowly. In milder forms of heart block, the patient often is asymptomatic.

First-Degree AV Block

The mildest form of heart block is first-degree block, which is present when the PR interval is prolonged more than 0.2 second. In first-degree block, all the atrial impulses pass through to the ventricles but are delayed at the AV node. First-degree AV block may or may not compromise cardiac output. It is important to assess the patient as discussed earlier in the section on Steps of ECG Interpretation. Some potential causes of first-degree AV block include adverse effects of medications such as digitalis, increased vagal tone, hyperkalemia, myocarditis, and degenerative disease (Fig. 11-26).

Second-Degree AV Block Type I (Mobitz I)

Second-degree AV block type I, also known as *Wenckebach*, is an intermediate form of heart block that presents with a PR interval that becomes progressively longer (changes in length) until the stimulus from the atria is blocked completely for a single cycle (dropped QRS complex). After the blocked beat, relative recovery of the AV junction occurs, and the progressive increasing of the PR interval starts all over again. The ventricular rhythm is almost always irregular. As with first-degree AV block, second-degree AV block type I may or may not compromise cardiac output; thus it is important to assess the patient in conjunction with rhythm interpretation. Causes of second-degree AV block type I are similar to those of first-degree AV block (Fig. 11-27A).

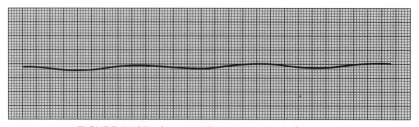

FIGURE 11-25 Electrocardiogram tracing of asystole.

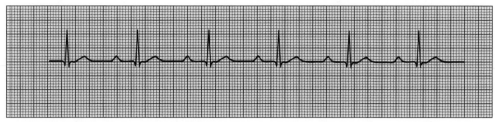

FIGURE 11-26 First-degree atrioventricular block with a PR interval of 0.30.

Systematic Evaluation

Rate	Underlying rhythm rate
Rhythm	Regular
P waves	Normal sinus configuration, each preceding a QRS complex
PR interval	Greater than 0.20 sec in length and constant
QRS complex	Less than 0.10 sec in width

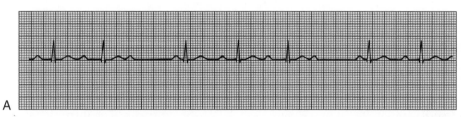

A

FIGURE 11-27 A, Second-degree atrioventricular block type I. Wenckebach

Systematic Evaluation

Rate	Varies, but ventricular rate is always less than the atrial rate
Rhythm	Regular
Ventricular rhythm	Irregular
P waves	Normal sinus configuration, not always followed by QRS complex
PR interval	Varies, lengthens, and then drops a QRS complex
QRS complex	Less than 0.10 sec in width

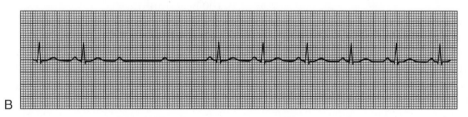

B

B, Second-degree atrioventricular block type II.

Systematic Evaluation

Rate	Varies, but ventricular rate is always less than the atrial rate
Atrial rhythm	Regular
Ventricular rhythm	May be regular if there is a constant conduction ratio or irregular if conduction is not constant
P waves	Normal sinus configuration, not always followed by QRS complex
PR interval	Normal or prolonged but always constant
QRS complex	Less than 0.10 sec in width

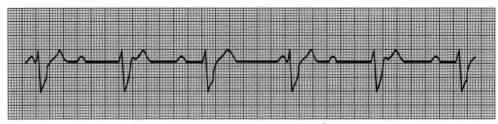

FIGURE 11-28 Third-degree heart block characterized by independent atrial (P wave) and ventricular activity. The atrial rate is always faster than the ventricular rate.

Systematic Evaluation

Rate	Usually less than 60 beats/min but may vary; ventricular rate is always less than the atrial rate
Rhythm	Both atrial and ventricular rates are regular
P waves	Normal sinus configuration, not always followed by QRS complex
PR interval	Varies, no relationship
QRS complex	Usually greater than 0.10 sec but may also be less than 0.10 sec in width

Second-Degree AV Block Type II (Mobitz II)

Second-degree AV block type II is a rarer but more serious form of second-degree AV block and is characterized by a series of nonconducted P waves followed by a P wave that is conducted to the ventricles. It is important to note that each time the P wave is followed by a QRS complex, the PR interval is always fixed (not changing in length). This will help differentiate between the two types of second-degree AV block. Sometimes the ratio of nonconducted to conducted P waves is fixed (at 3:1 or 4:1, for example). This block should be considered serious and treated promptly. Common causes of second-degree AV block type II include extensive damage to the bundle branches after an acute anteroseptal myocardial infarction or degenerative disease (Fig. 11-27B).

Third-Degree AV Block

The most extreme form of heart block is third-degree AV block, which is caused by conduction disturbances below the AV node in the bundle of His (producing a narrow QRS complex) or bundle branches (producing a wide QRS complex). This block does not allow any conduction of stimuli from the atrium to the ventricles. In this situation, the ventricles and atria beat independently of one another. Thus there is no distinguishable pattern between the atria and ventricles. Third-degree AV block may be transient or permanent but is always considered serious and should prompt immediate intervention. Possible causes of transient third-degree AV block may include inferior myocardial infarction, increased vagal tone, myocarditis, and digitalis toxicity. Permanent causes may include degenerative disease or acute anteroseptal myocardial infarction (Fig. 11-28).

Idioventricular Rhythm

Idioventricular rhythm occurs when the normal pacemaker does not set the pace for the ventricles. In this case, an ectopic focus in one of the ventricles becomes the pacemaker for the ventricles. The intrinsic rate of the ventricular tissue is usually less than 40 beats/min, so the ventricular rate is very slow (Fig. 11-29). In idioventricular rhythm, the ECG pattern appears as a slow series of wide and bizarre QRS complexes. The slower ventricular rate and the loss of assistance in ventricular filling provided by the atria decrease cardiac output significantly and can lead rapidly to heart failure and more severe dysrhythmias.

There is a variation of idioventricular rhythm called *accelerated idioventricular rhythm*. In accelerated idioventricular rhythm, the rate is in the normal range (40 to 100 beats/min).

Junctional Rhythm

In a junctional rhythm, an area in the AV junction assumes the pacemaking role and sends impulses down the normal conduction pathways in the ventricles. Because the normal conduction pathways in the ventricles are being used, the QRS complexes appear normal. The P wave may be present or absent. If present, it may appear immediately after the QRS, plainly demonstrating retrograde conduction. In this case, the P wave is typically inverted, indicating that depolarization of the atria followed a retrograde path. The P wave may appear before the QRS, but when it does, the PR interval is less than normal duration (0.10 second). This indicates that there was not sufficient time for the P wave to be responsible for initiating the associated QRS complex. Some potential causes of a junctional rhythm may include AV node damage, electrolyte disturbances, digitalis toxicity, heart failure, valvular disease, rheumatic fever, and myocarditis (Fig. 11-30).

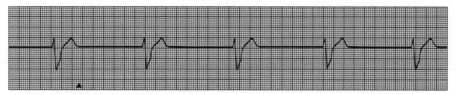

FIGURE 11-29 Electrocardiogram tracing of idioventricular rhythm.

Systematic Evaluation

Rate	30 to 40 beats/min or slower, unless accelerated, then it may be between 40 and 100 beats/min
Rhythm	Regular
P waves	Absent
PR interval	None
QRS complex	Greater than 0.10 sec

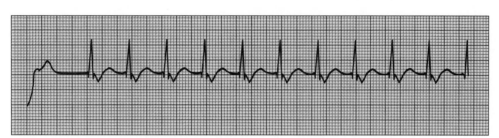

FIGURE 11-30 Electrocardiogram tracing showing junctional tachycardia.

Systematic Evaluation

Rate	Normal intrinsic junctional rate, 40 to 60 beats/min Accelerated junctional rate, 60 to 100 beats/min Junctional tachycardia, >100 beats/min
Rhythm	Regular
P waves	Absent or inverted
PR interval	Short if present
QRS complex	Less than 0.10 sec

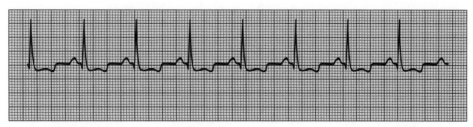

FIGURE 11-31 Electrocardiogram tracing showing ST-segment depression.

Evidence of Cardiac Ischemia, Injury, or Infarction

Normally, the ST segment is isoelectric, which means that it is in the same horizontal position as the baseline, or isoelectric line. Significant deviations (1 mm) of the ST segment from baseline, either up or down, suggest an abnormality in myocardial perfusion and oxygenation.

Cardiac ischemia is often seen on the ECG as depression of the ST segment (Fig. 11-31) or inversion of the T waves. At this point, there is no permanent damage to the heart, and proper therapy usually reverses any ECG

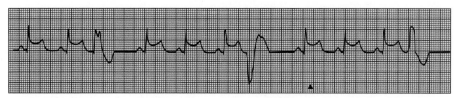

FIGURE 11-32 Electrocardiogram tracing showing ST-segment elevation with a PVC.

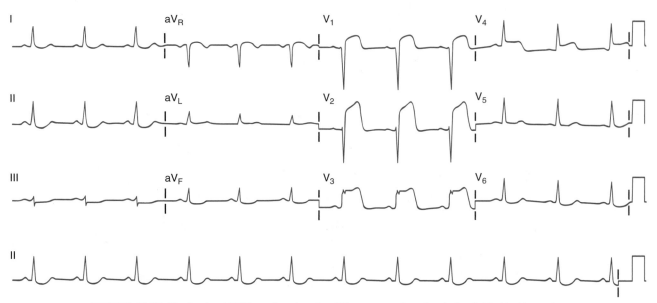

FIGURE 11-33 Twelve-lead ECG tracing showing ST-segment elevation in leads V_1, V_2, V_3, and V_4. This pattern is indicative of acute anteroseptal myocardial injury.

abnormalities. In many cases of myocardial infarction, however, this pattern of ischemia may not be seen because the event has already progressed to the injury phase.

When ischemia persists, the heart muscle can become permanently injured due to inadequate oxygen delivery for a sustained time period. This is known as **ST-elevation myocardial infarction (STEMI).** In cases involving a STEMI, the typical manifestation on an ECG tracing is an ST elevation in the leads monitoring the electrical activity of the corresponding injured heart tissue (Fig. 11-32). For example, an acute myocardial injury to the anteroseptal part of the heart will cause ST segment elevation in the leads that examine the anteroseptal portion of the heart (Fig. 11-33; see Table 11-3). In general, the degree of damage to the heart caused by the ischemia determines the degree of ST segment elevation. In addition, other symptoms

It can be helpful to identify ST segment abnormalities by drawing a straight line over the imaginary isoelectric line. This will reveal whether ST segment elevation or depression is present and to what degree. If the deviation from the isoelectric line is greater than 1 mm, significant changes have occurred and further investigation is appropriate. The patient should be monitored closely when this abnormality is identified.

It should be noted that rapid identification and treatment of STEMI is critical in achieving favorable clinical outcomes. As a result, the AHA has issued specific guidelines for identifying patients with suspected STEMI. In addition to ECG changes, these include chest discomfort, shortness of breath, weakness, diaphoresis, nausea and lightheadedness, particularly in the presence of a prior cardiac history or other risk factors such as smoking and obesity.

In patients with STEMI, the ST segment abnormality often resolves when perfusion is restored. However, it should be noted that at some point after myocardial infarction, significant Q waves (0.04 second in length) will be seen on the ECG in the corresponding leads. Q waves may develop within hours of an infarction but may not evolve for several days in some patients. They persist for the remainder of the patient's life.

SIMPLY STATED

T-wave inversion and ST-segment depression indicate myocardial ischemia. ST-segment elevation indicates that an acute myocardial injury has occurred and indicates the presence of an ST-elevation myocardial infarction, or STEMI.

Assessing Chest Pain

The significance of pain as a general clinical finding is discussed in Chapter 3. Pain and distress are subjective to the patient's perception of his or her condition and may be difficult to assess. However, it is essential that signs and symptoms associated with cardiac events be accurately reported both verbally and on the patient's chart. The following sequence will provide you with a reference for assessing these signs and symptoms. Ask the patient the following:

O   When and how abrupt was the *o*nset of the symptoms?

P   What *p*rovoked the symptoms? (e.g., exercise, sleep, emotional upset)

Q   How would you describe the *q*uality of the pain? (e.g., sharp, dull)

R   Does the pain *r*adiate anywhere?
       Does anything provide *r*elief from the pain?
       In what *r*egion is the pain located?
       Does the pain change with deep *r*espiration?

S   Placing severity on a *s*cale of 0 to 10, how would you rate your pain?

T   What is the *t*ime frame of your symptoms? Is this chronic or acute?

U   What do *y*ou think is wrong? Is this different from any previous episodes?

The AHA recommends that for chest pain or associated symptoms not relieved by nitroglycerin, a myocardial infarction should be suspected until proven otherwise. Remember that "time is muscle," and treatment interventions, such as thrombolytic therapy or surgical intervention, should be implemented quickly to minimize damage to the myocardium.

The role of an RT in such cardiac events is to notify the patient's physician, evaluate and optimize oxygen delivery, obtain a 12-lead ECG, and stand by to participate as a member of the cardiac arrest team if needed.

SIMPLY STATED

For a patient with severe cardiac symptoms, the role of the RT is to quickly notify the physician, optimize oxygen delivery, obtain an ECG, and assist in resuscitation if the patient worsens.

Electrocardiogram Patterns with Chronic Lung Disease

The majority of patients with COPD have ECG abnormalities. Hyperinflation of the lungs and flattening of the diaphragm are associated with a more vertical position of the heart. This causes a clockwise rotation and contributes to the right-axis deviation associated with COPD. (For quick axis determination, see Table 11-4.) Additionally, chronic pulmonary hypertension is common in patients with COPD and causes an enlargement of the right side of the heart. Enlargement of the right atrium causes the following:

- Rightward deviation of the P-wave axis
- Enlarged positive P waves greater than 2.5 mm in leads II, III, and aV_F
- A prominent and negative P wave in lead I
- This syndrome is called *cor pulmonale.* Right ventricular enlargement may be associated with this syndrome and is recognized certain characteristics, including:
- Right-axis deviation of the QRS complex
- Increased R-wave voltage in leads V_1, V_2, and V_3
- Reduced voltage in the limb leads (I, II, and III) is seen when severe pulmonary hyperinflation (emphysema) is present. This is seen as QRS complexes that are less than 5 mm tall in leads I, II, and III. Reduced voltage in precordial leads V_5 and V_6 may also be present. The reduced measured voltage appears to be caused by the following two factors:
- Reduced transmission of electrical activity through hyperinflated lungs
- A mean QRS axis directed posteriorly and perpendicular to the frontal plane of the limb leads, causing decreased voltage on the ECG

Dysrhythmias often are seen in patients with COPD and acute lung disease. Tachycardia, multifocal atrial tachycardia, and ventricular ectopic beats are some of the more common ECG abnormalities seen in COPD. Such dysrhythmias occur as the result of hypoxemia from lung disease and from adverse effects of medications (e.g., bronchodilators) used to treat the obstructed airways. Hypoxemia often worsens during sleep in patients with COPD and increases the prevalence of nighttime dysrhythmias.

SIMPLY STATED

Patients with chronic hypoxemic lung disease often have evidence of right-axis deviation on the ECG. This is seen as a negative QRS in lead I.

KEY POINTS

- An ECG is an indirect measurement of the electrical activity of the heart.
- The normal electrical conducting pathway of the heart starts with the SA node, then travels through the AV junction, bundle of His, bundle branches, and Purkinje fibers and finally through the heart muscle known as the *myocardium.*
- The RT should recommend that an ECG be obtained whenever the patient has signs and symptoms (e.g., chest pain) of an acute cardiac disorder such as a myocardial infarction.
- Disturbances in the cardiac conduction system are called *dysrhythmias,* which can be detected with an ECG.

KEY POINTS—cont'd

▶ The RT should remember that dysrhythmias can occur for many reasons, including hypoxemia, myocardial ischemia, sympathetic nerve stimulation, and certain drugs.

▶ On an ECG, the initial wave of electrical activity or P wave signals atrial depolarization, the QRS complex represents ventricular depolarization, and the T wave occurs with ventricular repolarization.

▶ On ECG paper, time is measured on the horizontal axis, and voltage or amplitude is measured on the vertical axis.

▶ On ECG paper, each small square represents 0.04 second, and each large square is 0.2 second. Therefore, if the interval between R waves (RR interval) is five large boxes (1 second) and the rhythm is regular, then the rate is 60 beats/minute.

▶ An ECG involves the placement of six leads on the extremities and another six chest leads across the chest to measure cardiac electrical activity from several different angles.

▶ There are several steps involved in ECG interpretation, including identifying the heart rate, evaluating the rhythm and presence of P waves, and measuring both the PR interval and the QRS complex.

▶ Sinus tachycardia in an adult is a common dysrhythmia characterized by a heart rate of 100 to 150 beats/minute, a regular rhythm, and normal P waves, PR interval, and QRS complex. It may be caused by hypoxemia and selected respiratory medications such as certain β-agonist bronchodilators.

▶ Sinus bradycardia in an adult is characterized by a regular rhythm and heart rate less than 60 beats/minute as well as normal P waves, PR interval, and QRS complex. This dysrhythmia can be caused by vagal stimulation associated with suctioning or tracheostomy tube manipulation.

▶ PVCs can occur in a normal heart as a result of causes such as hypoxemia, or they can signal a diseased heart. PVCs can occur several times per minute, two or more in a row, as different shapes tend to be considered more serious.

▶ Dysrhythmias, such as ventricular fibrillation characterized by chaotic electrical activity or asystole (cardiac standstill), should be considered by the RT as medical emergencies that require immediate and aggressive intervention according to resuscitation protocols.

▶ In an apparent case of asystole, the RT should quickly assess for a pulse and patient responsiveness early in any rescue effort because what may initially appear to be asystole on an ECG monitor may simply be a disconnection of the ECG leads.

▶ The AHA guidelines indicate that during resuscitation efforts, asystole should be confirmed in more than one ECG lead to rule out fine ventricular fibrillation.

▶ Rapid identification and treatment of ST-elevation myocardial infarction (STEMI) is critical in achieving favorable clinical outcomes. As a result, the AHA has issued specific guidelines for identifying patients with suspected STEMI. In addition to ECG changes, these include chest discomfort, shortness of breath, weakness, diaphoresis, nausea, and lightheadedness.

▶ The role of the RT for a patient experiencing severe chest pain is to notify the physician, evaluate and optimize oxygen delivery, help ensure that a 12-lead ECG is quickly obtained, and be ready to participate as part of the cardiac resuscitation team.

ASSESSMENT QUESTIONS

See Appendix for answers.

1. ECGs are useful to evaluate all of the following, except:
   a. Impact of lung disease on the heart
   b. Pumping ability of the heart
   c. Severity of the myocardial infarction
   d. Heart rhythm

2. What clinical findings are most suggestive of the need for an ECG?
   a. Headache and flulike symptoms
   b. Orthopnea and chest pain
   c. Fever and cough
   d. Joint pain and swelling

3. For an adult, what is the normal intrinsic rate of the heart's primary pacemaker?
   a. 90 to 110 beats/min
   b. 60 to 100 beats/min
   c. 40 to 80 beats/min
   d. 40 to 60 beats/min

4. What is the normal intrinsic rate of the heart's secondary pacemaker?
   a. 80 to 100 beats/min
   b. 60 to 100 beats/min
   c. 40 to 60 beats/min
   d. 30 to 40 beats/min

5. What does the P wave on the ECG recording represent?
   a. Atrial depolarization
   b. Atrial repolarization
   c. Ventricular depolarization
   d. Ventricular repolarization

6. What does the QRS wave on the ECG recording represent?
   a. Atrial depolarization
   b. Atrial repolarization
   c. Ventricular depolarization
   d. Ventricular repolarization

7. What does the T wave on the ECG recording represent?
   a. Atrial depolarization
   b. Atrial repolarization
   c. Ventricular depolarization
   d. Ventricular repolarization

8. Which of the following is within the normal range for a PR interval?
   a. 0.10 second
   b. 0.20 second
   c. 0.30 second
   d. 0.40 second

9. What is the upper limit of a normal QRS complex?
   a. <0.04 second
   b. <0.08 second
   c. <0.10 second
   d. <0.16 second

10. The QRS complexes are equally spaced with three large boxes between each complex. What is the heart rate?
    a. 150 beats/min
    b. 100 beats/min
    c. 75 beats/min
    d. 60 beats/min
11. A prolonged PR interval is indicative of which of the following?
    a. Sinus dysrhythmia
    b. Sinus bradycardia
    c. Sinus block
    d. AV block
12. An early, widened QRS complex with an inverted T wave and no associated P wave is consistent with which of the following?
    a. PVC
    b. Ventricular tachycardia
    c. Ventricular fibrillation
    d. Ventricular asystole
13. What ECG finding is suggestive of an acute myocardial infarction?
    a. Prolonged PR intervals
    b. Elevated ST segments
    c. Tall, peaked T waves
    d. Narrow QRS complexes
14. What ECG finding is suggestive of cor pulmonale?
    a. Inverted T waves
    b. Elevated ST segments
    c. Right-axis deviation
    d. Small QRS complexes
15. Which of the following statements is true regarding sinus tachycardia?
    a. It is caused by parasympathetic stimulation
    b. It may be caused by a vasovagal response
    c. It is a meaningless clinical finding
    d. It may be caused by fever, fear, or pain
16. For a patient experiencing severe chest pain and other acute cardiac symptoms, the immediate role of the RT is to do which of the following?
    a. Call the respiratory care supervisor
    b. Help ensure that a stat ECG is quickly obtained
    c. Administer a bronchodilator
    d. Notify the nurse and doctor and be ready to assist the cardiac arrest team

For Questions 17 thru 26, please list the Rate, Rhythm, P Wave, PR Interval, QRS and Interpretation for the following tracings.

17.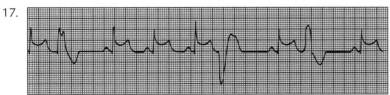

Rate:_____
Rhythm:_____
P wave:_____
PR interval:_____
QRS:_____
Interpretation:_____

18.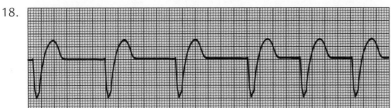

Rate:_____
Rhythm:_____
P wave:_____
PR interval:_____
QRS:_____
Interpretation:_____

19.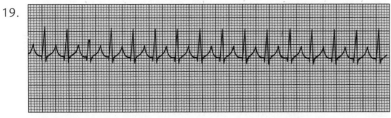

Rate:_____
Rhythm:_____
P wave:_____
PR interval:_____
QRS:_____
Interpretation:_____

20.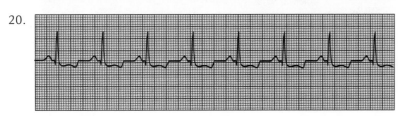

Rate:_____
Rhythm:_____
P wave:_____
PR interval:_____
QRS:_____
Interpretation:_____

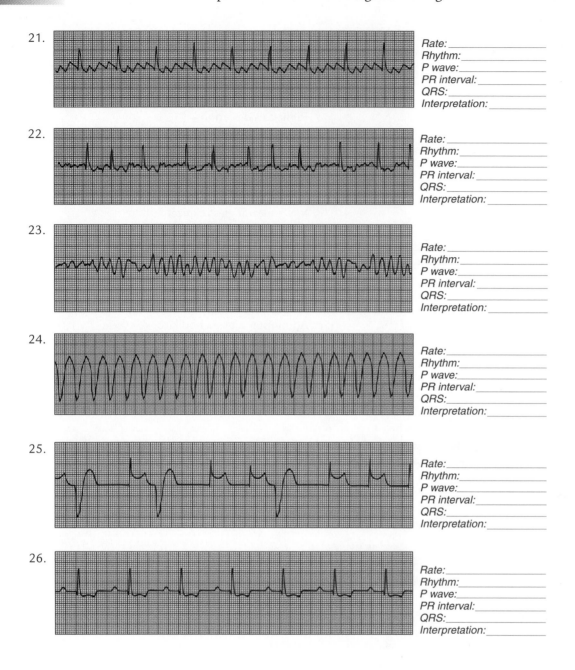

21.

Rate: _____
Rhythm: _____
P wave: _____
PR interval: _____
QRS: _____
Interpretation: _____

22.

Rate: _____
Rhythm: _____
P wave: _____
PR interval: _____
QRS: _____
Interpretation: _____

23.

Rate: _____
Rhythm: _____
P wave: _____
PR interval: _____
QRS: _____
Interpretation: _____

24.

Rate: _____
Rhythm: _____
P wave: _____
PR interval: _____
QRS: _____
Interpretation: _____

25.

Rate: _____
Rhythm: _____
P wave: _____
PR interval: _____
QRS: _____
Interpretation: _____

26.

Rate: _____
Rhythm: _____
P wave: _____
PR interval: _____
QRS: _____
Interpretation: _____

Bibliography

Aehlert BJ: *ECGs made easy.* 4th ed. St. Louis: Mosby-Elsevier; 2009.

Barrett D, Gretton M, Quinn T. *Cardiac care: an introduction for healthcare professionals.* Indianapolis: Wiley; 2006.

Darovic GO. *Hemodynamic monitoring: invasive and noninvasive clinical application.* 3rd ed. Philadelphia: WB Saunders; 2003.

Goldberger AL. *Clinical electrocardiography: a simplified approach.* 7th ed. St Louis: Mosby-Elsevier; 2006.

Hazinski MF, Samson R, Schexnayder S, editors. *Handbook of emergency cardiovascular care for healthcare providers.* Dallas: American Heart Association; 2010.

Huff J. *ECG workout: exercises in arrhythmia interpretation.* 6th ed. Philadelphia: Lippincott Williams & Wilkins; 2011.

Huszar R. *Basic arrhythmias: interpretation and management.* 3rd ed. St Louis: Mosby-Elsevier; 2007.

Phalen T, Aehlert B. *The 12-lead ECG in acute coronary syndromes.* 2nd ed. St Louis: Mosby-Elsevier; 2006.

Thaler MS. *The only ECG book you'll ever need.* 6th ed. Philadelphia: Lippincott Williams & Wilkins; 2009.

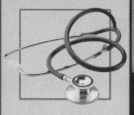

Chapter 12

Neonatal and Pediatric Assessment

NARCISO RODRIGUEZ*

CHAPTER OUTLINE

LEARNING OBJECTIVES

After reading this chapter, you will be able to:

1. Describe the type of information found in the pregnancy, labor, and delivery history and the clinical significance of common findings.
2. Explain the value of the Apgar scoring system and its interpretation.
3. Identify normal values for the vital signs in newborns and older children and the clinical implications of abnormalities.
4. Describe the clinical implications of retractions, nasal flaring, and grunting in neonates and infants.
5. Summarize the proper technique for auscultation of the infant.
6. Describe the clinical implications of abnormal breath sounds in the infant.
7. List potential causes of murmurs heard during auscultation of the infant precordium.
8. Identify the presence of a pneumothorax using a transilluminator.
9. Identify normal values for the white and red blood cell counts and partial differential for the infant at birth, 7 days of age, and 14 days of age.
10. List the possible causes of abnormalities in the white and red blood cell counts in the infant.
11. Describe the clinical implications of abnormalities in blood glucose, total protein and albumin, serum enzymes, and electrolytes.
12. Describe the limitations for sputum analysis in the infant and the child.
13. Identify normal values for arterial pH, Pao_2, $Paco_2$, HCO_3^-, and base excess at birth, 24 hours after birth, 2 days to 1 month, and 1 month to 2 years after birth.
14. Identify differences in blood gas parameters for capillary blood and arterial blood.
15. Describe the factors that can lead to misleading results from the transcutaneous oxygen monitor.
16. Describe the role of pulse oximetry assessment in the newborn for the detection of critical congenital heart disease.
17. Describe the lung volumes that can be measured in the newborn and the clinical value of such measurements.
18. Describe the lung mechanics that can be measured in the newborn and the clinical value of such measurements.
19. Describe the clinical findings that suggest the need for a chest radiograph in the infant.
20. Identify signs and symptoms of a compromised airway in infants and children with a tracheostomy.
21. List the indications and advantages of flexible bronchoscopy in infants and children.

---

*Douglas D. Deming MD contributed some of the content for this chapter as the contributor of the prior edition of this chapter.

KEY TERMS

abortion
acrocyanosis
anasarca
anterior fontanel
Apgar score
apnea
ascites
bradycardia
bradypnea
bronchopulmonary dysplasia
   (BPD)
bruit
chronologic age
coarctation of the aorta
cholestasis
cranial sutures
critical congenital heart
   disease (CCHD)
croup
crying vital capacity (CVC)
epiglottitis
estimated date of confinement
   (EDC)
extremely low birthweight
   (ELBW)
fetal hemoglobin (HbF)
gestational age

gravida
grunting
hepatomegaly
hyperbilirubinemia
hyperdynamic precordium
hyperglycemia
hyperthermia
hypoglycemia
hypothermia
hypotonia
impulse oscillometry (IOS)
interrupted aortic arch
   syndrome
intraventricular hemorrhage
   (IVH)
intrauterine growth
   retardation (IGR)
last menstrual period (LMP)
leukocytosis
leukopenia
low birthweight (LBW)
meconium
meconium aspiration
   syndrome (MAS)
nasal flaring
neutral thermal environment
   (NTE)

neutropenia
osteopenia of the premature
para
patent ductus arteriosus
   (PDA)
periodic breathing
pneumoperitoneum
polycythemia
postterm infants
preterm infants
pulmonary interstitial
   emphysema (PIE)
respiratory distress syndrome
   (RDS)
retractions
sinus bradycardia
splenomegaly
sudden infant death syndrome
   (SIDS)
tachycardia
tachypnea
term infants
thrombocytopenia
thrombocytosis
transient tachypnea of the
   newborn (TTN)
very low birthweight (VLBW)

The fundamentals for assessing the newborn and pediatric patient are a good history, thorough physical examination, and careful attention to selected laboratory and radiographic information. Although most of the basic principles that apply to adult patients also apply to newborn and pediatric patients, certain characteristics make assessment of the newborn and pediatric patient unique for the respiratory therapist (RT). These characteristics include lack of verbal communication skills, tendency to be afraid of strangers (particularly people in white coats), and inability or reluctance to follow directions, to mention just a few. This chapter reviews the assessment of the newborn and pediatric patient with respiratory disease.

For the purposes of this chapter, a neonate is a newborn baby up to 28 days old, an infant is less than 1 year old, and a child is between 12 months of age and adolescence. An infant's age can be defined as either chronologic or gestational. **Chronologic age** is the age of the infant computed from the date of birth. **Gestational age** is the age of the infant computed from the date of conception. Gestational age usually is assigned based on the history and physical examination. **Term infants** are born between 37 and 42 weeks of gestational age, **preterm infants** (premature or "preemies") are born at fewer than 37 weeks of gestational age, and **postterm infants** are born at 43 or more weeks of gestational age.

Assessment of the Newborn

History

It is essential that RTs obtain a clear picture of the prenatal environment and use this information to anticipate the mother's and newborn's immediate needs and make appropriate preparations for resuscitation and initial nursery care.

The prenatal history is obtained from several sources and covers more than just the medical history of the infant. Sources include the parents, the mother's labor and delivery chart, and the infant's own chart.

Maternal History

The newborn's history begins with the mother's history obtained during her prenatal care. Was the mother healthy before she was pregnant? Does she have chronic diseases? Is she taking medications or illicit drugs? If no prenatal care is noted, the RT should be on the alert for the potential of a high-risk delivery and possible postnatal complications.

The mother's previous pregnancy history can give the RT or other clinician valuable information. Obstetricians note this information in the mother's medical record using the terms gravida, para, and abortion. **Gravida** is a pregnant woman, **para** is a woman who delivers a live infant, and **abortion** is the delivery of a dead infant or embryo. These terms will most likely be abbreviated and followed by numbers (e.g., G2, P1, Ab0, which means this woman is in her second pregnancy, has delivered a living infant, and has not had any abortions). Abortions can be further subdivided into therapeutic and spontaneous; these are frequently abbreviated as TAb and SAb, respectively.

Other maternal factors that may indicate a high-risk pregnancy are listed in Table 12-1. Some of these factors will be discussed in the sections that follow.

Family History

It is important to inquire about family history as well as maternal history. Is there a history of spontaneous abortion during pregnancy? Is there a history of multiple early neonatal deaths? Multiple deaths during pregnancy or the early neonatal period may be clues for genetic diseases or the presence of other risks factors such as alcohol or drug abuse. Is there a history of prematurity? Have there been other infants with respiratory problems? It should be noted that the incidence and severity of diseases, such as **respiratory distress syndrome (RDS)**, are similar among siblings. RDS is discussed later in the chapter. There may also be an increased tendency for the recurrence of pneumonias caused by group B β-hemolytic streptococcus in siblings.

Pregnancy History

In evaluating the infant with respiratory disease, valuable information can be found in the pregnancy, labor, and delivery histories. In the pregnancy history, the interviewer records information about the mother and the fetus. Did the mother have any illnesses during gestation? Congenital viral infections that profoundly affect the infant may have produced only mild or even no symptoms in the mother. Did the mother have any vaginal bleeding? The mother usually is the source of bleeding, but occasionally the baby is bleeding, and these infants must be evaluated at birth for hypovolemia or low hematocrit. Did the mother note any evidence of amniotic infection or urinary tract infection? An infant delivered in the presence of infection has an increased risk for respiratory difficulty and other complications. Did the mother have a traumatic injury? A traumatic injury may compromise the uteroplacental interface and thus decrease transfer of oxygen and other nutrients to the baby. Traumatic injuries can also lead to hemorrhage and low hemoglobin and hematocrit in the newborn infant. Did the mother's uterus grow appropriately during pregnancy? If not, the infant may not have grown properly and could have pulmonary hypoplasia, severe malformations, a congenital infection, or **intrauterine growth retardation (IGR)**, a conditioned explained later on this chapter. Any of these conditions may cause significant respiratory distress in the newborn.

The incidence of respiratory disease varies with different gestational ages, and determining when the infant was actually due is important. The interviewer should attempt to identify the date of the mother's **last menstrual period (LMP)**, her estimated date of delivery (this appears as the **estimated date of confinement [EDC]** on the mother's chart), her obstetric record of uterine growth, and any reports from ultrasound examinations that she may have had.

Infants born prematurely are more susceptible to develop RDS, **pulmonary interstitial emphysema (PIE)**, **intraventricular hemorrhage (IVH)**, and **bronchopulmonary dysplasia (BPD)**. Postterm infants are more susceptible to severe perinatal asphyxia, meconium aspiration, and the development of persistent pulmonary hypertension of the newborn (PPHN).

Labor and Delivery History

The labor and delivery (L&D) history is obtained to evaluate the well-being of the newborn during the transition from intrauterine to extrauterine life. The newborn must successfully deal with cyclic decreases in uterine blood flow caused by contraction and possible umbilical cord compression as well as compression of his or her body. The clinician should consider fetal heart rate tracings, fetal activity, biophysical profile, and fetal ultrasound as well as neonatal age in order to anticipate possible complications. Information that suggests perinatal asphyxia might include variable or late heart rate decelerations, low biophysical profile score, decrease in fetal movement, presence of **meconium** (first feces of an infant) in the amniotic fluid, long labor, and abnormal vaginal bleeding. The clinician should also look for information that might suggest

TABLE 12-1	
Common Maternal High-Risk Factors	
Classification	**Factors**
Medical history	History of hypertension and preeclampsia
	Pulmonary disease
	Cardiovascular disorders
	Seizure disorder
	Pregestational diabetes
	Smoking and drug use
	Infectious and venereal diseases
Obstetric history	Cervical insufficiency
	Absence of prenatal care
	Maternal anemia
	History of ectopic pregnancy
	Previous cesarean delivery
	History of miscarriage or ectopic pregnancy
Others	Low socioeconomic status
	Minority
	Malnutrition
	Maternal age < 18 years

an infection in the infant or the mother. This information might include maternal fever, high maternal white blood cell (WBC) count, tender uterus, rupture of the amniotic membranes for more than 24 hours, foul-smelling or colored amniotic fluid, and fetal tachycardia.

A healthy fetus is capable of withstanding the challenges of labor. However, when the fetus is compromised or the labor is dysfunctional, the fetus can be taxed beyond capacity. This stress can place the fetus at risk for further compromise, including but not limited to asphyxia and intrauterine death. Box 12-1 lists some of the more significant clinical manifestations signaling abnormal transition to extrauterine life.

The delivery history should include the method of delivery for the infant: vaginal or cesarean; spontaneous, forceps, or vacuum extraction; or low, middle, or high forceps. Newborns who successfully withstand the labor process are usually born by spontaneous or low forceps vaginal deliveries. Those who have trouble during labor and delivery are more likely to be delivered by vacuum extraction,

middle or high forceps, or cesarean delivery. Some cesarean deliveries are performed because the infant is positioned in such a manner that vaginal delivery would be high risk, not because the infant is in trouble. These infants are at greater risk for respiratory diseases, such as **transient tachypnea of the newborn (TTN)**, caused by a failure to reabsorb fetal lung fluid after birth. It is also helpful to know what type of anesthetic the mother had for delivery (e.g., narcotics, local, epidural, spinal, or general). Narcotics and general anesthetics may enter the fetus's bloodstream and produce respiratory depression in the newborn. Spinal anesthetics may lower the mother's blood pressure, thus compromising the oxygen supply to the fetus.

The most standard objective measurement of the newborn's well-being during the perinatal period is the Apgar score.[1,2] The **Apgar score** is a simple, quick, and reliable means to assess and document the newborn's status immediately after birth. It assigns the infant points for the presence of five specific physical criteria (Table 12-2). Most infants are evaluated and assigned Apgar scores at 1 and 5 minutes. However, if the infant is having difficulty during the transition to extrauterine life, Apgar scores can be assigned more often and over a longer time span. For example, a sick infant may have 1-, 2-, 5-, 10-, 15-, and 20-minute Apgar scores. The process of assigning an Apgar score must not delay the initiation of resuscitative measures.

The Apgar score is useful in identifying neonates who may need further resuscitation and assistance. Those who are adjusting well to extrauterine life usually have 1-minute scores of 7 to 10 but may still show **acrocyanosis** (bluish coloration of hands and feet), irregular respirations, or **hypotonia** (decreased muscle tone). Such neonates usually require only routine newborn care such as drying, temperature maintenance, and clearing of the airway. These neonates may occasionally require supplemental oxygen or bag-mask ventilation (BVM) for a brief period. Moderately depressed infants with 1-minute scores of 4 to 6 may need more than routine care and often require an increased fraction of inspired oxygen (F_IO_2) with BVM ventilation. Most infants respond well to this therapy and improve in a few minutes. Infants who have 1-minute scores of 0 to 3 are severely depressed and need extensive medical resuscitation that may include intubation and mechanical ventilation.

Box 12-1	Manifestations Indicating Abnormal Transition to Extrauterine Life

- Persistent tachypnea, nasal flaring, grunting, and retractions
- Fixed bradycardia
- Diffuse and persistent fine crackles on auscultation
- Persistent cyanosis ($Spo_2 < 90\%$) in room air and prolonged requirements for supplemental oxygen (after 2 to 3 hours of age)
- Episodes of prolonged apnea (>20 sec) and bradycardia (<80 beats/min)
- Marked pallor or ruddiness
- Persistent temperature instability after 2 to 3 hours of age
- Poor capillary refill (>3 sec) and blood pressure instability
- Unusual neurologic behavior (lethargy, hypotonia, jitteriness)
- Excessive oral secretions, drooling, and chocking or coughing spells accompanied by cyanosis

Modified from Hernandez JA, Thilo E: Routine care of the full-term newborn. In Osbon LC, DeWitt TG, First LR, et al, editors: *Pediatrics*, St. Louis, 2005, Mosby.

TABLE 12-2

Apgar Scores

Sign	Score 0	Score 1	Score 2
Heart rate	Absent	<100 beats/min	>100 beats/min
Respiratory effort	Absent	Gasping, irregular	Good
Muscle tone	Limp	Some flexion	Active motion
Reflex irritability	No response	Grimace	Cry
Color*	Body pale or blue, extremities blue	Body pink, extremities blue	Completely pink

*Skin pigmentation and race may affect this evaluation. In this case, assess oral mucosa and nail beds for a more accurate assessment. Beware of acrocyanosis in hands and feet, as explained later in this section.

Although the 1-minute Apgar score is a useful tool in screening infants who might require resuscitation, the 5-minute Apgar score is a better predictor of the infant's neurologic outcome. For preterm and term infants, neonatal survival increases with increasing Apgar scores; low 5-minute scores (e.g., 0 to 3) are associated with the highest risk for neonatal morbidity and mortality.[3]

SIMPLY STATED

Newborns are evaluated at 1- and 5-minute intervals after birth with the Apgar score. This score calls for evaluation of the infant's color, heart rate, respiratory rate, muscle tone, and reflex irritability (normal score is 7 to 10, moderate depression is 4 to 6, and severe depression is 0 to 3).

Postnatal History

After the delivery, the clinician should document the magnitude of the infant's resuscitation, presence of disease, treatment of disease, length of the hospital stay, condition at discharge, and problems that have developed since the infant was last seen. For most infants, all of this information is normal, and the postnatal history is brief. All newborns require some form of resuscitation. The simplest resuscitation required is clearing the airway and drying the skin. It is important to document whether the infant required only this simple intervention; a more significant intervention with oxygen, manual ventilation with bag and mask, or intubation; or chemical resuscitation with the administration of drugs to support cardiac output. How did the infant respond to resuscitation? Was the response immediate or slow?

If the infant is still hospitalized, the only further information needed for an adequate assessment is what diseases the infant has, what treatment has been initiated, and what the response to treatment has been. If the infant has been discharged and is now being readmitted, seen again in a practice office, or seen at home, the clinician must inquire about the infant's condition since discharge. Was the infant still sick at the time of discharge? Did the infant require continuing treatment at home? How is the infant doing with the current treatment? What kind of problem does the infant have now?

Fetal Assessment

Useful information about the future well-being of the infant can be determined from the prenatal assessment of the fetus. This information could include but it is not limited to the following:

- Fetal movement monitoring
- Genetic karyotyping during amniocentesis and biophysical profile to assess fetal growth and development
- Lecithin-to-sphingomyelin (L/S) ratio
- Presence of phosphatidylinositol (PI) and phosphatidylglycerol (PG) to assess lung maturity
- Fetal monitoring tracings and nonstress tests (NSTs) to assess for proper neurologic development

Fetal movement monitoring is easily accomplished using three widely available tools: maternal observation, fetal ultrasound, and fetal Doppler ultrasound. The simplest of these tools is having the mother keep a log of the timing, strength, and duration of the fetal movements for a period of time. Fetal ultrasound and Doppler ultrasound provide more quantifiable data but for shorter periods. Having a history of decreased fetal movement should alert the clinician of the possibility of the fetus being in trouble. This could indicate prenatal asphyxia and impending death or the possibility of severe neuromuscular disease, in which the newborn will be unable to support spontaneous independent respiration after birth. See Figure 12-1 for a representation of the events leading to neonatal death.

The biophysical profile is an ultrasound evaluation of fetal breathing, body movement, tone, reactive heart rate, and amniotic fluid volume that predicts the presence or absence of fetal asphyxia and, ultimately, the risk for fetal death. Like the Apgar score, each of these parameters has a maximal score of 2 and a minimal score of 0. The score for a normal fetus is 8 to 10. With lower biophysical profile scores, the chance of significant fetal and newborn problems increases (Table 12-3). These potential problems include IGR, significant fetal acidosis, stillbirth, and neonatal death (see Fig-12-1).

Amniocentesis also allows for the evaluation of the L/S ratio to assess pulmonary lung maturity. The L/S ratio is the ratio of two surfactant phospholipids: lecithin and sphingomyelin. Increasing levels of lecithin indicate improving maturation of the lung's surfactant system. Like lecithin, the presence of PI and PG is usually indicative of advancing lung maturation. In general, L/S ratios of less than 2:1 and the absence of PG are associated with high risks for RDS.[4]

Fetal monitoring is a continuous graphic method of recording the fetal heart rate and uterine contractions. Various patterns (fetal tachycardia, variable decelerations, and late decelerations) are signs that a fetus may be in trouble

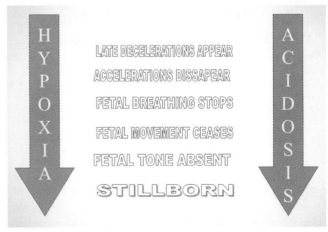

FIGURE 12-1 Events leading to neonatal death. (Courtesy of Narciso Rodriguez.)

in the uterine environment. Knowing that a fetus has any of these heart rate patterns should alert the health care team that this infant may need a more extensive resuscitation and more careful evaluation after birth.

The fetal NST is a method of evaluating the stability of the fetus's physiology within the uterine environment. The NST monitors the acceleration of the fetal heart rate in response to fetal movement. A healthy fetus has a minimum of an increase in heart rate of at least 15 beats/minute in response to fetal movement. To be considered reactive, the fetus needs to have a minimum of two accelerations exceeding 15 beats/minute in 20 minutes for term pregnancies. A fetus is considered nonreactive when it fails to have heart rate response in two consecutive 20-minute periods. Nonreactivity may be associated with prolonged fetal sleep states, immaturity, maternal ingestion of sedatives, and fetal cardiac or neurologic anomalies.[5] A fetus that is nonreactive is at greater risk for serious complications and fetal death. This will prompt the obstetrician to consider the possibility of an accelerated or operative delivery (cesarean). Knowing that a fetus has a nonreactive NST should alert the health care team that this infant may need a more extensive resuscitation and more careful evaluation after birth.

Physical Examination of the Newborn and Infant

Unlike the adult patient, the nonverbal neonate communicates primarily by behavior. Through objective physical observations and evaluations, the clinician can interpret this behavior into information about the individual neonate's condition during the postnatal period.

Examination of a newborn is based on three of the four classic principles of physical examination as described in Chapter 5: inspection, palpation, and auscultation. Percussion is rarely used in examining newborns because of their small cavity and organ sizes and the possibility of injury.

Therefore, percussion is not described in this chapter. Careful inspection reveals clues about the type and severity of respiratory disease. It is important to inspect the overall appearance of the infant carefully because respiratory pathology in the newborn is often manifested by extrapulmonary signs. Palpation is useful in assessing growth and gestational age and in determining the cause of respiratory distress and the severity of side effects from the lung disease and its treatment. As in the adult, auscultation is used to define characteristics of the disease process occurring in the lung. However, statements about the internal location of the pathologic process must be made with greater caution in newborns because localization by auscultation is difficult in the small chest cavity.

Growth and Gestational Age Assessment

Preterm infants are also classified based on their birthweight, as follows:
- **Low birthweight (LBW):** less than 2500 g
- **Very low birthweight (VLBW):** less than 1500 g
- **Extremely low birthweight (ELBW):** less than 1000 g

Newborn classification based on birthweight and gestational age is a valuable tool in predicting possible complications in the postnatal period and neonatal diseases. In any gestation, the poorest outcome is seen in infants born with marked IGR.

Based on their weight and gestational age, newborn infants are further classified as:
- Appropriate for gestational age (AGA): weight is appropriate for the gestational age
- Small for gestational age (SGA): smaller than expected, the weight falls below the 10th percentile for the gestational age
- Large for gestational age (LGA): heavier than expected, the birthweight is above the 90th percentile for the gestational age

TABLE 12-3		
Biophysical Profile		
Biophysical Variable	**Normal (Score 2)**	**Abnormal (Score 0)**
Breathing	At least 30 sec of sustained FBMs observed over a 30-min period	Fewer than 30 sec of sustained FBMs observed over a 30-min period
Movements	At least three discrete body/limb movements in a 30-min period	Absent or less than three movements in a 30-min period
Tone	At least one movement of a limb from a position of flexion to one of extension, with a rapid return to flexion	Fetal limb in extension with no return to flexion with movement
FHR	Two or more episodes of acceleration of ≥15 beats/min and of >15 beats/min associated with fetal movement within 20 min	One or more episodes of acceleration of fetal heart rate or acceleration of <15 beats/min within 20 min
AFV	At least a single amniotic fluid pocket measuring 2 × 2 cm in two perpendicular planes	No amniotic fluid pocket that measures at least 2 × 2 cm in two perpendicular planes

AFV, amniotic fluid volume; FBM, fetal breathing movements; FHR, fetal heart rate.
Adapted from Oyelese Y, Vintzileos AM: Uses and limitations of the fetal biophysical profile. *Clin Perinatol* 38(1):47-64, 2011.

Gestational age is assigned by the maternal dates, fetal ultrasound, and gestational assessment examination. Assessment of gestational age should be done to assign a newborn classification, determine neonatal mortality risk, assess for possible morbidities, and quickly initiate the proper interventions to address the identified risk factors.

Most women know approximately when they conceive. This is frequently confirmed by an early fetal ultrasound examination. Sometimes, the mother does not know the date of conception, or there is significant disagreement between the maternal dates and the fetal ultrasound. In those situations, the gestational age assessment can be performed with a gestational assessment tool.

The original assessment tools were developed by Dubowitz and Dubowitz. These tools have been modified and validated over many years. Most nurseries currently use a Ballard examination (Fig. 12-2), which is a modification of the Dubowitz examination. Gestational age assessment should be performed for all newborns.

The Ballard examination is divided into two sections: neuromuscular maturity and physical maturity. The infant's neuromuscular and physical characteristics are scored by matching the infant's characteristics to the table's descriptions and then marking the table. Each column of the table has a numerical value ranging from −1 to +5. The numerical values for all of the marked cells are added together. It is important that a cell is marked in each

NEWBORN MATURITY RATING & CLASSIFICATION

ESTIMATION OF GESTATIONAL AGE BY MATURITY RATING
Symbols: X - 1st Exam O - 2nd Exam

Gestation by Dates ____________ wks

Birth Date ________ Hour ________ am pm

APGAR ________ 1 min ________ 5 min

NEUROMUSCULAR MATURITY

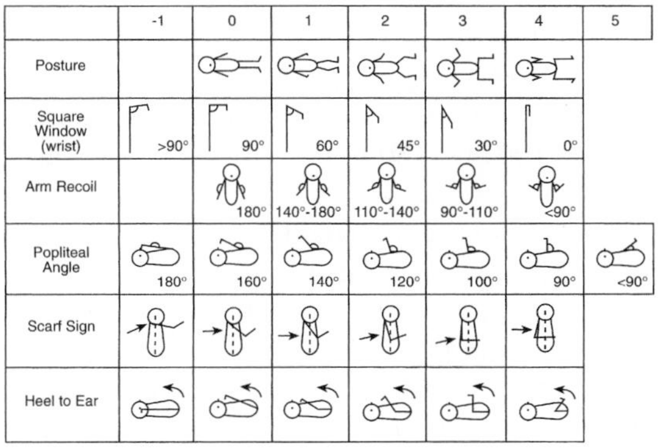

PHYSICAL MATURITY

	-1	0	1	2	3	4	5
Skin	sticky; friable; transparent	gelatinous; red; translucent	smooth; pink; visible veins	superficial peeling &/or rash; few veins	cracking; pale areas; rare veins	parchment; deep cracking; no vessels	leathery; cracked; wrinkled
Lanugo	none	sparse	abundant	thinning	bald areas	mostly bald	
Plantar Surface	heel-toe 40-50 mm: -1 <40 mm: -2	>50 mm; no crease	faint red marks	anterior transverse crease only	creases ant. 2/3	creases over entire sole	
Breast	imperceptible	barely perceptible	flat areola; no bud	stippled areola; 1-2 mm bud	raised areola; 3-4 mm bud	full areola; 5-10 mm bud	
Eye/Ear	lids fused loosely: -1 tightly: -2	lids open; pinna flat; stays folded	sl. curved pinna; soft; slow recoil	well-curved pinna; soft but ready recoil	formed & firm; instant recoil	thick cartilage; ear stiff	
Genitals male	scrotum flat; smooth	scrotum empty; faint rugae	testes in upper canal; rare rugae	testes descending; few rugae	testes down; good rugae	testes pendulous; deep rugae	
Genitals female	clitoris prominent; labia flat	prominent clitoris; small labia minora	prominent clitoris; enlarging minora	majora & minora equally prominent	majora large; minora small	majora cover clitoris & minora	

Scoring system: Ballard JL, Khoury JC, Wedig K, Wang L, Eilers-Walsman BL, Lipp R. New Ballard Score, expanded to include extremely premature infants. *J Pediatr.* 1991;119:417-423.

MATURITY RATING

score	weeks
-10	20
-5	22
0	24
5	26
10	28
15	30
20	32
25	34
30	36
35	38
40	40
45	42
50	44

SCORING SECTION

	1st Exam=X	2nd Exam=O
Estimating Gest Age by Maturity Rating	______ Weeks	______ Weeks
Time of Exam	Date ______ am Hour ______ pm	Date ______ am Hour ______ pm
Age at Exam	______ Hours	______ Hours
Signature of Examiner	______ M.D./R.N.	______ M.D./R.N.

FIGURE 12-2 Ballard gestational age scoring system. (From Ballard JL, Khoury JC, Wedig K, et al: New Ballard Score, expanded to include extremely premature infants. *J Pediatr* 119:417-423, 1991.)

row. The sum is then compared with the maturity scale, and a gestational age is assigned. The Ballard examination is accurate to within 2 weeks of the gestational age.[3]

Vital Signs Assessment

Body Temperature. The range of normal body temperature in the newborn does not differ from that in the adult. Humans maintain body temperature by balancing heat production with heat loss. The newborn loses much more heat to the environment than the older child or adult, largely because heat loss is determined by the ratio of the surface area of the body to the total body mass (Table 12-4). The neonatal surface area-to-mass ratio is more than three times the surface area-to-mass ratio of an adult male. For premature neonates, the problem becomes even more significant owing to the lack of brown fat tissue and a very low surface area-to-mass ratio. Brown fat tissue, which is present in a full term neonate, is a major source of heat production for the newborn and helps to maintain internal body temperature. A 28-week gestational age neonate has a body surface area of approximately 0.15 m^2 and a body mass of 1 kg. This results in a surface area to mass ratio of 0.15 m^2/kg, which is more than six times greater than that of an adult male. Therefore, newborn term and preterm infants lose heat easily and are extremely dependent on the environment to help them maintain a **neutral thermal environment (NTE)**. An NTE is the environmental temperature at which the infant's metabolic demands and therefore oxygen consumption are the least (Fig. 12-3).

Neonates, like all physical objects, lose heat to the environment by one of four mechanisms: conduction (touching a cold or wet object), convection (gas blowing over the skin surface), evaporation (liquid evaporating from the skin surface), and radiation (attempting to warm a cold surface not in contact with the skin). All these mechanisms must be considered when helping newborns deal with their environment.

SIMPLY STATED

Newborns are very prone to heat loss because of their high ratio of surface area to body mass. Maintaining an NTE is essential to avoid stressing the infant and causing "cold stress."

TABLE 12-4

Ratio of Surface Area to Body Mass

	Surface Area (m^2)	Mass (kg)	Area/Mass (m^2/kg)
Adult male	1.7	80	0.02
Term infant	0.25	3.5	0.07
28-week-old infant	0.15	1.0	0.15

Hyperthermia is a core body temperature of more than 37.5° C or 99.5° F. Hyperthermia in the newborn usually is caused by environmental factors. The infant may be wrapped in too many clothes, placed too close to a heater, or placed in an isolette or radiant warmer that is too warm. It is uncommon, although not rare, for an infant with hyperthermia to have an infection.

Hypothermia is a core body temperature of less than 36.5° C or 97.7° F. Hypothermia is a more common and significantly more serious sign of infection in the newborn than in the older child or adult. Hypothermia probably occurs because the newborn is unable to maintain normal heat production or there is an increase in heat loss caused by environmental factors around the neonate. The newborn, in contrast to the adult, does not shiver when hypothermic.

Assessment of Body Temperature. The most common methods to measure temperature are axillary and rectal temperatures. In addition to noting body temperature, the RT or other clinician should also note the temperature of the infant's environment. Most sick infants are placed in an NTE (see Fig. 12-3). If the environmental temperature leaves the neutral thermal range, the infant usually can maintain a stable body temperature, but at the cost of a significant increase in oxygen consumption. NTEs are defined for an infant based on weight and gestational and chronologic age.

Pulse. The normal pulse rate for newborns is between 100 and 160 beats/minute. Their heart rate is age and size dependent and is usually a function of the developmental age of the neonate. The normal resting heart rate is higher in premature infants than in a full-term newborn. The resting heart rate also decreases with increasing chronologic age. Newborns and infants cannot significantly change their cardiac output by increasing stroke volume (volume of blood ejected from the heart with ventricular contraction) because their stroke volume at rest is normally more than

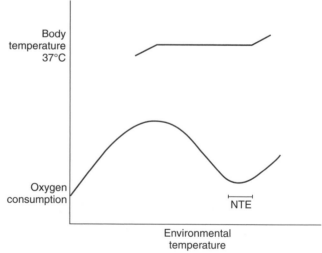

FIGURE 12-3 Effect of environmental temperature on oxygen consumption and body temperature. NTE, neutral thermal environment.

90% of maximal stroke volume. Neonates and infants increase their cardiac output by increasing their heart rate. However, too high a rate (>180 beats/minute) may impede ventricular refill and lead to cardiovascular collapse and shock in the small infant or child.

Tachycardia in the newborn is a heart rate greater than 160 beats/minute, and **bradycardia** is a heart rate of less than 100 beats/minute. Tachycardia in the newborn can be caused by crying, pain, decrease in the circulating blood volume, drugs, hyperthermia, and heart disease. Bradycardia can be caused by hypoxia, Valsalva maneuver (often occurs during crying), heart disease, hypothermia, vagal stimulation (e.g., passing a nasogastric tube), **critical congenital heart disease (CCHD)**, and certain drugs. In addition, there are a few infants with **sinus bradycardia** (a normal variant) and resting heart rates between 70 and 100 beats/minutes.

Assessment of Pulse Rate. The pulse usually is evaluated at the brachial or femoral artery because of the small size of the radial arteries. To evaluate the brachial pulse, the clinician places his or her index finger pad over the brachial artery just above the elbow, with the baby in a supine position. The femoral artery pulse can be assessed at the groin, about halfway across the thigh (Fig. 12-4). On a newborn, the pulse can also be felt at the base of the umbilical cord. This is the preferred site in the L&D room during resuscitation of the neonate.

Respiratory Rate. The normal respiratory rate for neonates and infants is between 30 and 60 breaths/minute and is a function of the developmental age of the infant. The normal respiratory rate decreases as gestational age increases. Infants' respiratory rates are higher than those of older children and adults because of mechanical properties of their chest walls and airways. Infants' chest walls are more compliant, leaving them more prone to excessive inward movement of the chest (retractions) on inhalation. As a result, infants normally breathe rapidly and shallowly to help avoid retractions and chest wall collapse.

Tachypnea is a respiratory rate greater than 60 breaths/ minute, and **bradypnea** is a respiratory rate of less than 30 breaths/minute in an infant (<40 breaths/minute in

a newborn). In newborns and infants, tachypnea can be caused by hypoxemia, metabolic and respiratory acidosis, CCHD, anxiety, pain, hyperthermia, and crying. Bradypnea is not a normal physiologic response in newborns. Bradypnea can be caused by certain medications (e.g., narcotics), hypothermia, and central nervous system diseases, and it may be an important clinical sign of the imminent decompensation from fatigue of the newborn with significant lung disease. Nonintubated infants with lung disease usually are tachypneic. As the disease progresses and the infant or child tires from the increasing work of breathing, bradypnea occurs just before ventilator respiratory failure.

All newborns display an irregular breathing pattern. Respiratory rates that exceed 60 breaths/minute but normalize over the next several hours may indicate TTN.

Another common respiratory pattern of infants is **apnea**, or the cessation of respiratory effort. Apnea is a pathologic condition in which breathing ceases for longer than 15 to 20 seconds. Apnea may be accompanied by cyanosis, bradycardia, pallor, and hypotonia. More than six events of apnea accompanied by bradycardia in an hour (A&Bs) should be further investigated and their cause properly treated or addressed. A phenomenon known as **periodic breathing** also exists in newborns. During periodic breathing, the infant has multiple episodes of respiratory pauses or short apnea interspersed with normal-appearing ventilation. This pattern of breathing may continue for several minutes to several hours. All episodes of apnea must be investigated to establish the cause.

Assessment of Respiratory Rate. The respiratory rate can be obtained by visually observing chest motion or counting respirations while listening with a stethoscope. Visual observation provides a respiratory rate closer to the infant's resting rate. However, because the normal infant breathes rapidly with a small tidal volume, visualization of all of the true breaths may be difficult. If the RT or other member of the patient care team thinks this is a possibility, the respiratory rate should be assessed by listening with a stethoscope. The infant is likely to respond to the touch of the stethoscope with a temporary increase in respiratory rate.

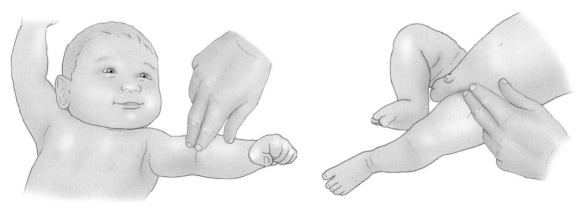

FIGURE 12-4 Position of brachial and femoral pulses in the newborn.

TABLE 12-5		
Normal Newborn Blood Pressures in the First Hours of Life		
Birthweight (g)	Systolic (mm Hg)	Diastolic (mm Hg)
501-750	50-62	26-36
751-1000	48-59	23-36
1001-1250	49-61	26-35
1251-1500	46-56	23-33
1501-1750	46-58	23-33
1751-2000	48-61	24-35
2001-3000	59	35
>3000	66	41

Adapted from Hegyi T, Carbone MT, Anwar M, et al: Blood pressure changes in premature infants. I. The first hours of life. *J Pediatr* 124:627-633, 1994.

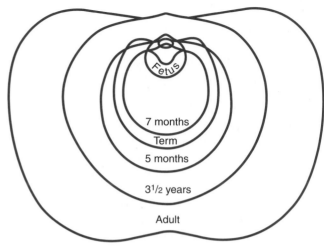

FIGURE 12-5 Changes in anteroposterior chest configuration with age.

The infant's respirations are assessed for rate as well as for regularity and depth. Many premature infants have normal rates but very irregular breathing patterns, which may include brief periods of apnea as described before. In addition, infants with significant lung disease may have normal respiratory rates but tidal volumes so small that they have minimal effective ventilation. Gasping respiratory efforts are never to be considered normal respiratory patterns in newborns.

Blood Pressure. The normal values for blood pressure depend on the size of the infant or neonate, with pressures decreasing with lower weights (Table 12-5). Usually, a term neonate's systolic blood pressure should be no higher than 70 mm Hg, with diastolic pressure no higher than 50 mm Hg. Normal pulse pressure (the difference between systolic and diastolic blood pressure) in a term infant is between 15 and 25 mm Hg.

Assessment of Blood Pressure. There are two common methods of determining blood pressure in newborns: use of a blood pressure cuff (sphygmomanometer) and direct arterial pressure monitoring. The more common method is to use a blood pressure cuff. The other common method for obtaining blood pressure in newborns is the direct measurement of pressure through an arterial cannula, also known as an arterial pressure catheter (see Chapter 15). In the newborn, it is important to measure the blood pressure in all four extremities after birth. Difference in blood pressure between upper and lower extremities can be an indication of a CCHD such as **coarctation of the aorta** (a narrowing of the ascending or descending aorta in a newborn).

Morphometric Measurements

In newborns, there are three important measurements, two of which are not usually thought of in the physical examination of adults: weight, length, and head circumference. There are standard tables of normal growth for all gestational and developmental ages for these measurements. These measurements provide important clues to assessing

the infant's past nutritional environment and current state and predicting the infant's long-term growth. They are also essential to determine whether IGR has occurred during fetal development.

Lung Topography

The infant's lungs are situated in the chest much as in the adult, but the infant's chest has a greater anteroposterior (AP) diameter than the adult's chest. The AP diameter of the infant's chest decreases proportionally and becomes more like the adult configuration with growth (Fig. 12-5). The imaginary lines and thoracic cage landmarks are the same in infants as in adults (see Chapter 5).

Techniques of Examination
Inspection

Inspection is probably the most important and often the most neglected portion of the physical examination of a newborn. The infant should be unclothed and in a supine position initially in a quiet environment. The RT or other clinician should look first at the infant's overall appearance to identify level of illness, presence of malformations, and whether the infant's body position is appropriate for the gestational age (Fig. 12-6). The full-term neonate at rest flexes the arms and legs into a fetal position. Premature infants at earlier gestational ages have less muscle tone, and their extremities are less flexed at rest.

The RT should also look at the infant's skin to see whether the infant is cyanotic. Some caution must be used in interpreting these findings. Infants with hypothermia or infants with **polycythemia** (hematocrit level > 65%) may have bluish extremities, yet they are not really hypoxemic. The mucosal color of infants who are preterm and immature with thin skin can look quite pink when they are really hypoxemic. The color of the mucous membranes in the mouth and tongue and the nail beds in the extremities

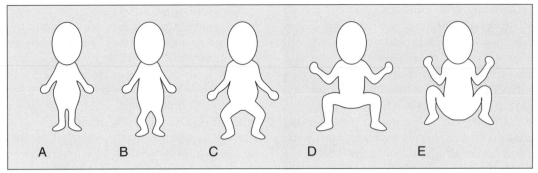

FIGURE 12-6 Progression in body position with gestational age. **A,** A 26-week infant. **B,** A 28-week infant. **C,** A 32-week infant. **D,** A 36-week infant. **E,** A 40-week term infant.

give a more reliable indication of the infant's true level of oxygenation. Acrocyanosis, which is peripheral cyanosis of the hands and feet during the first 24 to 72 hours of life, is normal and is due to immature development of peripheral capillary beds.

The effort involved in breathing and the breathing pattern should be noted, especially the regularity of respirations. An infant with respiratory distress characteristically exhibits tachypnea (discussed earlier), retractions, nasal flaring, and sometimes grunting.

Retractions. Sinking inward of the skin around the chest wall during inspiration (**retractions**) occurs when the lung's compliance is less than the compliance of the chest wall or when there is a significant airway obstruction. Thus, retractions are a sign of an increase in the work of breathing. The diaphragm contracts during inspiration, lowering the negative pressure in the intrapleural space. In the normal respiratory system, the lung is the most compliant structure and will inflate to relieve this negative pressure. Furthermore, in a healthy infant, the chest wall is as compliant as the lungs. Any lung disease that causes a decrease in compliance can cause the lung to become less compliant than the chest wall. The chest wall then represents the most compliant structure in the respiratory system and collapses inward in response to the increasing negative intrathoracic pressure generated by diaphragmatic contraction.

Retractions tend to be in different locations, depending on the cause of the respiratory distress. Three common points of collapse are the intercostal area (between the ribs), the subcostal area (below the lower rib margin), and the substernal area (below the bottom of the sternum). A fourth point of collapse is the supraclavicular area (above the clavicles) (Fig. 12-7).

Infants with lung disease tend to have retractions toward the center of the body (substernal and subcostal). Infants with heart disease tend to have intercostal retractions on the sides of their bodies because their large hearts prevent backward motion of the sternum. Finally, infants with obstructed airways tend to have large suprasternal retractions due to the pronounced use of accessory respiratory muscles.

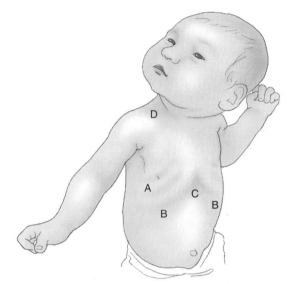

FIGURE 12-7 Retractions commonly occur in these areas: intercostal (A), subcostal (B), substernal (C), and supraclavicular (D).

SIMPLY STATED

Retractions in the infant generally indicate a decrease in lung compliance, and a serious increase in the work of breathing or airway resistance, or both. Further assessment and monitoring of the infant are necessary.

Nasal Flaring. The dilation of the alae nasi during inspiration is called **nasal flaring**. Infants are obligatory nose breathers, and the minute ventilation they require must be achieved through their nose. Nasal flaring is an attempt by the infant to achieve airway dilation to decrease airway resistance, increase gas flow, and achieve a larger tidal volume. It is generally an attempt to compensate for increased work of breathing.

SIMPLY STATED

Nasal flaring is a cardinal sign of respiratory distress and increased work of breathing in the infant.

Grunting. **Grunting** is a sound heard at the end of expiration just before rapid inspiration. Grunting is caused by closure of the glottis during expiration in an attempt to provide increased positive end-expiratory pressure and to maintain lung volume and functional residual capacity (FRC). The infant accomplishes this by occluding the airway with glottic closure and actively exhaling against the closed glottis after the end of inspiration. The grunting sound is produced when the infant suddenly opens the glottis and quickly exhales, inhales, and again closes the glottis (Fig. 12-8). Grunting is typically heard in infants with diseases that decrease lung volume (e.g., RDS).

Precordium. While observing the respiratory pattern and effort, the RT or clinician should look at the precordium (area over the heart) for any increase in motion. Increased motion is present if the chest wall is visibly lifting or moving as the heart contracts. This increase in motion, or **hyperdynamic precordium**, is an indication of increased volume load on the heart, usually secondary to a left-to-right shunt of blood through the ductus arteriosus or any other shunt.[6] If a preterm newborn has a **patent ductus arteriosus (PDA)**, the anatomic connection between the aorta and pulmonary artery remains open and blood from the aorta flows into the pulmonary artery, which can cause congestive heart failure and pulmonary edema. The presence of a hyperdynamic precordium is a clue that the infant's respiratory distress may not be completely of pulmonary origin and requires further evaluation.

Palpation

In infants, palpation is an important tool for physical assessment. However, the use of palpation in the physical examination of infants is directed less at the lungs than at other organ systems that may influence pulmonary function.

The easiest organ to palpate is the skin. Palpation of the skin can give the RT or other clinician valuable information about the infant's cardiac output and fluid volume status, both of which are clinically important in the evaluation of the infant's pulmonary status.

The three aspects of the skin that are useful in evaluating cardiac output are the skin perfusion, skin temperature, and peripheral pulses. To check the skin perfusion, or capillary refill, the RT or other clinician should gently blanch the infant's skin at the palm of the hands and feet and note how long it takes for the blanched area to recover its color. Capillary refill is checked on the trunk and extremities. Capillary refill should be less than 3 seconds and will be greater than 3 seconds if the infant has a low cardiac output or decreased peripheral perfusion. The clinician should keep in mind that other pathologic states, such as acidosis, hypoxemia, **hypoglycemia** (low blood glucose), and hypothermia, can decrease blood flow to the skin and prolong capillary refill.

An approximation of the infant's skin temperature can be determined by feeling the skin. The dorsum, or back side, of the examiner's hand and fingers is more sensitive to temperature than the front side or palmar surface. Infants with hypothermia, low cardiac output, shock, or any abnormality that decreases skin blood flow have skin that feels cool.

Comparing the central and peripheral arterial pulses gives the clinician valuable clues about the infant's cardiac output. A careful RT or other clinician should be able to palpate the pulses of the radial, brachial, posterior tibial, and dorsalis pedis arteries. The infant should be examined closely for a decrease in cardiac output if these pulses are not easily palpable or if there is a big discrepancy between them and the central arterial pulses of the femoral or axillary arteries. The clinician should also look for any discrepancies between the intensity of the pulses in the upper and lower extremities. As previously mentioned, if pulses in the lower extremities are weaker than those in the upper extremities, the infant may have an aortic obstruction such as coarctation of the aorta or **interrupted aortic arch syndrome**.

> **SIMPLY STATED**
>
> Palpation of the infant for skin temperature, capillary refill, and quality of peripheral pulses is helpful in determining the general quality of cardiac output and perfusion.

Finally, the RT or other clinician can achieve a rough idea about the fluid volume of the infant by feeling the turgor or fullness of the infant's skin. Infants with low fluid volume have a loss of skin turgor. This is manifested by "tenting," or gathering of the skin when it is lightly pinched together.

Palpation of the abdomen may be helpful in assessing an infant's pulmonary status. An infant's abdomen and abdominal organs move significantly with respiration because the diaphragm is the major source of power for respiration and an infant's abdominal wall musculature is relatively weak. Anything that impedes the motion of the abdomen or its organs hinders the infant's respiration.

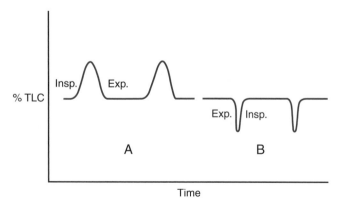

FIGURE 12-8 Comparison of lung volumes during tidal breathing: **A,** Adult. **B,** Grunting infant. exp., Expiratory; insp., inspiratory; TLC, total lung capacity.

Liver or spleen enlargement (**hepatomegaly** or **spleno-megaly**, respectively); enlargement of other organs, such as kidneys, bladder, or bowel; or intra-abdominal tumors can impede abdominal motion and affect respiration. Distention of the abdomen by fluid (ascites) or air (gaseous bowel distention) or **pneumoperitoneum** (free air in the abdomen) also impedes abdominal motion.

Gentleness is important when palpating an infant's abdomen. The liver should be soft and mobile and palpable on the right side of the abdomen parallel to and 1 to 2 cm below the costal margin. The spleen may be palpable as a soft tip below the left costal margin at the anterior axillary line. The kidney can be palpated in the immediate newborn period by compressing it between one hand placed under the posterior flank and the other hand firmly pressing in from the anterior abdominal wall. In infants with significant chronic **cholestasis** (internal obstruction to bile flow), the liver and spleen may be so large that their lower edge may be close to the pelvis and would be missed if the RT or other clinician started palpation in the midabdomen.

Major central nervous system diseases, such as IVH and hydrocephalus, are causes of respiratory problems in preterm infants. The clinician should evaluate the tension of the **anterior fontanel** (the soft spot on top of the infant's head). Infants who have had a major IVH or hydrocephalus may have a full, tense fontanel. In addition, the **cranial sutures** (junctions between two skull bones) may be widely separated in these conditions. The anterior fontanel would be depressed in a newborn with mild to severe hypovolemia.

Auscultation

The last of the classic techniques routinely used in newborn examination is auscultation. Auscultation is the least definitive of the three examination techniques discussed, but this does not mean it is unimportant. Auscultation yields the best information if the infant is quiet; therefore, auscultation is the first examination performed after inspection. Auscultation should be performed with a warm chest piece that has a small (1.0 to 1.5 cm diameter) diaphragm and bell. This allows for maximal localization of the findings. For auscultatory examination of the lungs, the infant is ideally in the prone position. However, because most neonates are in a supine position or on one side, the RT or other member of the patient care team should try to complete most of the examination before moving the infant. If the infant's position does not allow an adequate examination, the clinician should gently move the infant to a more desirable position. Normal infant breath sounds are bronchovesicular in character and harsher than in the adult. The techniques for use of the stethoscope and the types of adventitious lung sounds heard are the same as in the adult (see Chapter 5).

The clinical significance of breath sounds in the infant and small child is similar to that in the adult. The mechanisms and significance of breath sounds are explained in detail in Chapter 5. The infant's thoracic cage is small, and sound is transmitted easily; therefore, breath sounds usually are not entirely absent. A decrease in breath sounds implies a decrease in gas flow through the airways, as it may occur in RDS, atelectasis, pneumothorax, or in a pleural effusion. Wheezing implies gas flow through constricted airways; infants with BPD may have wheezing. Crackles usually imply excess fluid or secretions in the lung (pulmonary edema) or the presence of pneumonia. Crackles may also be heard in neonates with RDS. A loud ripping sound like the separation of Velcro often is associated with the presence of pulmonary interstitial emphysema.

In addition to listening for the breath sounds, the clinician should listen for the presence of cardiac murmurs. The presence of a murmur does not mean that the infant has heart disease, but it may mean that the infant requires further diagnostic evaluation. Almost all infants have physiologic murmurs such as physiologic pulmonary stenosis or a venous hum. The pathologic murmurs that are characteristic of the newborn period are often caused by a PDA, ventricular septal defect, tricuspid insufficiency, or a major CCHD.

The abdomen is another area of the body where auscultation may help in pulmonary assessment. The abdomen should be auscultated when there is a question about whether an infant is properly intubated. Loud sounds of air movement are heard over the stomach during inspiration if the endotracheal tube is in the esophagus. The presence of a **bruit** (a murmur-like sound) in the liver or neck should raise the question of whether the infant has an arteriovenous malformation in the liver or in the head. This type of malformation can cause respiratory distress because of high-output heart failure.

Transillumination

Transillumination is a technique often used in examining the chest of neonates and small infants, but not an older child or adult. It can be used in small infants because their chest wall is thin enough to shine a light through. The source is usually a bright fiberoptic light, which is placed against the chest wall in a dark room. Normally, this produces a lighted halo around the point of contact with the skin. In the presence of a pneumothorax or pneumomediastinum, the entire hemithorax lights up, dispersing the light in an irregular shape (Fig. 12-9). This technique is quick and allows rapid treatment of a serious condition. The procedure should be performed by a clinician who is familiar with the technique because some fiberoptic lights can cause cutaneous burns and it is possible to be misled by the area of transilluminance.

Clinical Laboratory Data

Two crucial issues face anyone who wants to use the clinical laboratory in pulmonary assessment of newborns. The first and most obvious issue is that the normal values for

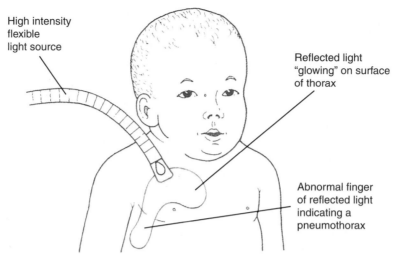

High intensity
flexible
light source

Reflected light
"glowing" on surface
of thorax

Abnormal finger
of reflected light
indicating a
pneumothorax

FIGURE 12-9 Transillumination of a pneumothorax.

TABLE 12-6

White Blood Cell, Neutrophil, and Platelet Counts of Very-Low-Birthweight Infants During the First 6 Weeks of Life

		PERCENTILES				
Day of Life	n^*	10	25	50	75	90
WBCs (10^9/L)						
3	376	4.8	7.1	9.5	14.4	24.5
12-14	180	8.1	9.7	12.3	15.2	19.8
24-26	233	7.2	8.5	10.4	12.4	14.6
40-42	212	6.8	7.7	9.1	11.0	13.0
Neutrophils (10^9/L)						
3	334	1.5	2.7	4.7	8.2	14.8
12-14	161	2.2	3.1	4.6	6.8	10.6
24-26	205	1.3	1.9	2.9	4.0	5.3
40-42	175	1.0	1.4	2.2	3.1	4.6
Platelets (10^9/L)						
3	558	95	140	204	285	355
12-14	372	142	216	318	414	499
24-26	394	171	242	338	443	555
40-42	370	189	275	357	456	550

*n = Number of infants involved in calculating values.
WBCs, white blood cells.
From Martin RJ, Fanaroff AA, Walsh MC, editors: *Behrman's neonatal-perinatal medicine: diseases of the fetus and infant,* ed 8, St. Louis, 2006, Mosby.

clinical laboratory tests may be different between newborns and adults. The magnitude of these differences depends on the laboratory test in question. However, to complicate this issue further, the normal values may depend on the gestational or chronologic age of the newborn. The second, less obvious issue is the relationship between the test sample volume and the infant's blood volume.

An infant's blood volume is approximately 80 to 110 mL/kg of body weight, with premature infants tending to have higher volume per weight. Depending on the severity of the illness, most infants can tolerate an acute blood loss of no more than 10% of their blood volume at any given time. This means that for a 0.5-kg infant, all of the laboratory tests should require no more than 5.5 mL of blood.

The infant will need replacement volume if the laboratory tests require more than this amount. A corollary of this issue is that even if the infant can tolerate the volume loss, it may not be practical or technically feasible to withdraw the sample volume. Infants have small vessels that tend to be fragile, and often it is not possible to draw large volumes by venipuncture or arterial puncture.

Hematology

The WBC count in infants tends to be higher than in older child or adult. Normal values vary with the chronologic age of the infant. Table 12-6 indicates typical values for WBCs, neutrophils, and platelets for VLBW infants at selected intervals during the first 6 weeks of life. In general, infants

TABLE 12-7

Red Blood Cell Parameters of Very-Low-Birthweight Infants During the First 6 Weeks of Life

Day of Life	n*	PERCENTILES				
		10	25	50	75	90
Hemoglobin (g/dL)						
3	559	12.5	14.0	15.6	17.1	18.5
12-14	203	11.1	12.5	14.4	15.7	17.4
24-26	192	9.7	10.9	12.4	14.2	15.6
40-42	150	8.4	9.3	10.6	12.4	13.8
Hematocrit (%)						
3	561	39	43	47	52	56
12-14	205	34	39	44	48	53
24-26	196	29	32	39	44	48
40-42	152	26	28	33	38	44
Corrected Reticulocytes (%)						
3	283	1.9	4.2	7.1	12.0	20
12-14	139	0.5	0.8	1.7	2.7	5.7
24-26	140	0.5	0.8	1.5	2.6	4.7
40-42	114	0.6	1.0	1.8	3.4	5.6

*n = Number of infants involved in calculating values.
From Martin RJ, Fanaroff AA, Walsh MC, editors: *Behrman's neonatal-perinatal medicine: diseases of the fetus and infant,* ed 8, St. Louis, 2006, Mosby.

closer to delivery have higher WBC counts. Over the first week of life, total WBCs tend to fall to a plateau that is just slightly higher than the normal values for adults.

Leukocytosis, or a WBC count greater than 15,000/mm³, usually is a reflection of the infant's environment rather than of infection, as in the older child or adult. When evaluating an infant with a high WBC count, the clinician should consider infection as well as crying, hyperthermia from excess wrapping or high environmental temperature, and other environmental stresses. **Leukopenia**, particularly **neutropenia** (absolute neutrophil count < 2000/mm³), is a more ominous sign. Usually, neutropenia indicates an infection and implies that the infant may be developing an overwhelming infection. The neutropenia from infection can be caused by one of two mechanisms: peripheral consumption of neutrophils or failure to produce and release neutrophils from the bone marrow.

There is still a great deal of debate about whether the newborn's leukocytes function as well as those of an older person. It is fair to say that even a term newborn's response to infection is not optimum, but why this is and what cellular or immunologic function is involved are still being investigated.

SIMPLY STATED

In the infant, significant leukocytosis (WBC > 15,000/mm³) is more often the result of environmental stress (e.g., hyperthermia) than infection, as it is in the older child or adult. Neutropenia (absolute neutrophil count < 2000 neutrophils/mm³) is a serious condition and needs to be evaluated immediately.

The normal values for the red blood cell (RBC) count, hematocrit, and hemoglobin depend on chronologic age. In utero, the fetus is stimulated to produce a large number of RBCs by the low partial pressure of arterial oxygen (PaO_2). This stimulus is withdrawn at the time of birth. The normal newborn severely limits or ceases the production of RBCs until a new stimulus is received. Anemia is the normal physiologic stimulus for this. In healthy term infants, this "physiologic" anemia occurs between 6 and 8 weeks of age. In healthy preterm infants, the lowest decrease in hemoglobin occurs between 8 and 12 weeks. Infants who have received transfusions have a 4- to 6-week delay in onset of RBC production. After an infant begins RBC production, hematocrit and hemoglobin levels rise slightly above the level of an adult and remain there throughout childhood. Table 12-7 indicates typical values for hemoglobin, hematocrit, and corrected reticulocytes (%) for VLBW infants at selected intervals during the first 6 weeks of life.

Platelet counts often are obtained in newborns and infants when they are being evaluated for thrombocytopenia, disseminated intravascular coagulation, or other bleeding disorders (see Table 12-7). Normal values are between 100,000 and 350,000/mm³; however, most clinicians will not transfuse infants with platelets unless the count is less than 25,000/mm³ and the infant is bleeding. **Thrombocytopenia** (platelet count < 100,000/mm³) may be a sign of disseminated intravascular coagulation from severe infection or one of many other causes. **Thrombocytosis** (platelet count > 350,000/mm³) usually is not a clinical problem in the newborn. Thrombocytosis can be seen in infants with iron deficiency anemia or hemolytic anemia, during recovery from thrombocytopenia, and in

TABLE 12-8

TABLE 12-8

Normal Coagulation Test Values

Category	Partial Thromboplastin Time (sec)	Prothrombin Time (sec)
Preterm infant (1500-2500 g)	21.7-51.2	10.0-16.2
Term infant, 1 day	37.1-48.7	11.6-14.4
Term infant, 5 days	34-51.2	10.9-15.3

From Martin RJ, Fanaroff AA, Walsh MC, editors: *Behrman's neonatal-perinatal medicine: diseases of the fetus and infant,* ed 8, St. Louis, 2006, Mosby.

TABLE 12-9

Normal Values for Blood Chemistries

Determination	Value
Sodium (mmol/L)	133-149
Potassium (mmol/L)	5.3-6.4
Chloride (mmol/L)	87-114
Total carbon dioxide (mmol/L)	19-22
Total protein (g/dL)	4.8-8.5
Albumin (g/dL)	2.9-5.5
Bilirubin (mg/dL)	
24 hr	1.0-6.0
48 hr	6.0-8.0
3-5 days	4.0-15.0

From Martin RJ, Fanaroff AA, Walsh MC, editors: *Behrman's neonatal-perinatal medicine: diseases of the fetus and infant,* ed 8, St. Louis, 2006, Mosby; and Meites S, editor: *Pediatric clinical chemistry: a survey of normals and instrumentation, with commentary.* Washington, DC, 1992, American Association for Clinical Chemistry.

infants whose mothers have inflammatory collagen vascular disease. Thrombocytosis can also be seen in infants after cardiac transplantation. A high normal value in infants is not well established, but clinical symptoms are not usually seen until the platelet count exceeds 1 million.

The normal values for coagulation tests, such as partial thromboplastin time, prothrombin time, and fibrinogen, are listed in Table 12-8. Values for mean corpuscular volume, mean corpuscular hemoglobin, mean corpuscular hemoglobin concentration, and reticulocyte count (see Table 12-7) in infants are close to the normal values for adults. Mean corpuscular volume and reticulocyte counts are higher in the immediate newborn period but decrease over the first few months of life to normal adult levels.

Blood Chemistry

Blood glucose probably is the most frequent blood chemistry determination made in newborns. This simple test is of tremendous importance because hypoglycemia is as detrimental to the developing newborn's brain as hypoxia. The exact levels and length of time necessary to cause damage to the central nervous system have not been determined, so most physicians treat an infant with a glucose level of less than 40 mg/dL (<20 mg/dL in preterm infants). There are easy methods for approximating serum glucose at the bedside by point-of-care testing. These methods are used as screening tests, and any abnormalities found are confirmed with serum glucose levels obtained in the clinical laboratory.

Hypoglycemia can be caused by a variety of metabolic disturbances, including infection, hyperinsulinemia secondary to maternal diabetes mellitus, and inadequate glycogen stores secondary to SGA. Although only symptomatic treatment is usually needed, an extensive evaluation of the infant's glucose control mechanisms is often necessary. **Hyperglycemia**, or blood glucose greater than 125 mg/dL in a term infant (>150 mg/dL in a preterm infant), is most often iatrogenic. However, hyperglycemia is also one of the early signs of septicemia in infants. The problems with hyperglycemia from diabetes mellitus are rare in this age group.

Total protein and albumin are useful tools in evaluating the nutritional status of the ill newborn. They may also give helpful clues for evaluating the cause of pulmonary edema (Table 12-9). Colloid osmotic pressure usually is not measured in infants because the sample volume required is large.

The serum enzymes that are so useful in adults are much less useful in newborns and the pediatric age group. For many of the enzymes, normal values have not yet been established, and the clinical significance of abnormal values often is unknown. Lactate dehydrogenase (LDH), aspartate transaminase (AST), and alanine transaminase (ALT) are used when evaluating liver function. Creatine phosphokinase (CPK), also known as creatine kinase (CK), and its isoenzymes are useful in determining myocardial injury. Alkaline phosphatase is useful in evaluating bone growth and the adequacy of an infant's nutrition.

Serum drug level determinations are becoming increasingly useful during the newborn period. As a result of their small size, there is a narrow difference between therapeutic and toxic doses of most medications for infants. The need to obtain drug levels has always been present, but it has been practical only as improving technology has permitted smaller sample volumes. Drug levels for antibiotics (vancomycin, gentamicin, and other aminoglycosides), anticonvulsants (phenobarbital and phenytoin), antiarrhythmics, caffeine, and theophylline are often used. Digitalis and cyclosporine levels are used less often.

Serum bilirubin determination is often used in evaluating newborns. Probably more than 70% of infants have a bilirubin determination during the first week of life. There are many causes for **hyperbilirubinemia** during the newborn period. Some abnormalities in bilirubin metabolism are likely to affect pulmonary function. First is hyperbilirubinemia from any cause that requires treatment by phototherapy. Second is hyperbilirubinemia caused by hemolytic disease that requires an exchange transfusion. An exchange transfusion is a procedure in which the infant's blood is replaced with donor blood by cyclically withdrawing the infant's blood and gradually transfusing donor blood. Finally, the most severe and most rare is hyperbilirubinemia associated with severe hemolytic disease and hydrops fetalis. In this disorder, the hyperbilirubinemia is not the fundamental problem. The infant has **anasarca** (massive total body edema) with pleural effusions and abdominal **ascites** that may cause profound respiratory failure.

Electrolytes, blood urea nitrogen (BUN), and serum creatinine determinations are all useful laboratory tests for newborns. The normal values depend on the infant's chronologic age, nutritional status, and fluid status. They are generally similar to adult values, with serum potassium being slightly higher and BUN and creatinine levels lower. These values are useful in a variety of clinical situations, from assessing the infant's fluid status to evaluating renal function (see Table 12-9).

Calcium and phosphorus levels are indirectly important in the evaluation of a newborn with chronic lung disease. Infants with BPD or other chronic lung diseases have increased work of breathing and increased metabolic and nutritional needs. The metabolism of calcium and phosphorus is a valuable clue to the nutritional status of the chronically ill infant. A chronically ill infant with poor nutrition has low levels of calcium and phosphorus and an increased risk for developing rickets. **Osteopenia of the premature** (a rickets-like disease caused by chronically low phosphorus intake) may worsen the infant's pulmonary status by increasing the chest wall compliance secondary to a decrease in the mineralization of the ribs and decreasing the infant's depth of respiration secondary to pain from rib fractures.

Microbiology

The sputum analysis that is useful in adults is not possible in newborns. Until a child is about 6 years old, sputum is swallowed and not expectorated. However, if the infant is intubated, samples can be obtained with sterile suction catheters through the endotracheal tube. In an older infant or young child, samples may be obtained from the stomach through nasogastric tubes. Samples obtained from the stomach should be interpreted with caution. Even samples obtained through the endotracheal tube may reflect bacterial colonization rather than infection. In addition to the Gram stain, culture, and sensitivity, a polymorphonuclear neutrophil (PMN) count is useful. High PMN counts in tracheal or stomach samples are strongly suggestive of infection rather than colonization.

Newborn Blood Gases

Monitoring the blood gas status of newborns is performed either by analysis of the gas in a blood sample or by transcutaneous monitoring. Analysis of blood samples is performed on blood obtained from arterial, capillary, or venous sources. The clinician must consider the limitations of the different techniques and sources of the blood

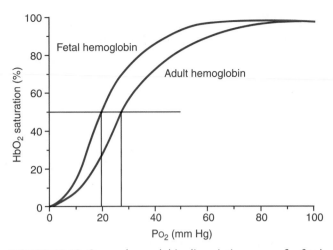

FIGURE 12-10 Oxygen hemoglobin dissociation curves for fetal and adult hemoglobins. Fetal hemoglobin P_{50} is approximately 18.6. Adult hemoglobin P_{50} is approximately 27.

when drawing clinical conclusions from blood gas results on neonates, infants, and children alike.

Fetal Hemoglobin

The newborn's oxygen-carrying mechanism is significantly different from that of the older infant, child, or adult. The presence of **fetal hemoglobin (HbF)** has significant effects on the transport of oxygen. HbF meets the needs of the fetus in the oxygen-poor environment of intrauterine life. The fetal hemoglobin curve is shifted to the left of the adult hemoglobin (HbA) curve (Fig. 12-10). Thus, HbF has a higher affinity for oxygen than HbA. This means that HbF absorbs oxygen more readily but also releases it more slowly. The half-life for RBCs with HbF is about 45 days. Thus, a newborn infant will typically have a significant portion of the RBC population with HbF until about 60 to 90 days of life.

Arterial Blood Gases

Arterial blood samples are the most reliable source for blood gas analysis in newborns. Normal values in newborns depend on the age of the infant when the blood is drawn (Table 12-10). Once infants are beyond the transitional period after delivery (usually 4 to 12 hours), their arterial oxygen (Pa_{O_2}), carbon dioxide (Pa_{CO_2}), and pH values should be similar to those of the older child or adult. During the transitional period, Pa_{O_2} is lower, Pa_{CO_2} is higher, and pH is lower compared with later in the newborn's development. Sick infants who require supplemental oxygenation or mechanical ventilation often have values for Pa_{O_2}, Pa_{CO_2}, and pH that are not quite normal for this age but are accepted because of the complications that result from oxygen therapy and mechanical ventilation.

The fact that an arterial blood sample provides the most reliable source for blood gas analysis in newborns must be weighed against the problems associated with arterial puncture in newborns and young infants. Arterial

TABLE 12-10

Normal Values for Arterial Blood Gases in Infants at Room Air

Age	pH	Pao$_2$ (mm Hg)	Paco$_2$ (mm Hg)	HCO$_3^-$ (mmol/L)	Base Excess
Newborn	7.25-7.35	50-70	26-40	17-23	−10 to −2
24 hr	7.30-7.40	60-80	26-40	18-25	−4 to +2
2 days to 1 mo	7.32-7.43	85-95	30-40	16-25	−6 to +1
1 mo to 2 yr	7.34-7.46	85-105	30-45	20-28	−4 to +2

pH, Hydrogen ion concentration in blood; Pao$_2$, partial pressure of oxygen in arterial blood; Paco$_2$, partial pressure of carbon dioxide in arterial blood; HCO$_3^-$, plasma bicarbonate concentration.
Unpublished data from author's laboratory and data from Meites S, editor: *Pediatric clinical chemistry: a survey of normals, methods and instrumentation, with commentary*, Washington, DC, 1982, American Association for Clinical Chemistry.

puncture is technically possible, but it requires good technique and often extra assistance. Newborns and young infants have small arteries and are notoriously uncooperative, moving their extremities and making the arterial puncture difficult. This also increases the risk for arterial damage. In addition, arterial blood does not always reflect the resting state for the newborn or young infant because the discomfort associated with the puncture usually causes the baby to cry. Infants who are crying change their ventilation in one of two patterns: they either hyperventilate or hold their breath and stop ventilating. Either of these changes in ventilation rapidly alters the values for oxygen, carbon dioxide, and pH in the blood.

In the newborn, the placement of an umbilical arterial catheter allows the clinician to obtain arterial blood samples without altering the infant's physiology in the immediate newborn period. This is useful in evaluating sick infants without causing them the pain and discomfort of percutaneous arterial puncture. Umbilical arterial catheters are widely used in neonatal intensive care units. The use of these catheters presents some significant risks such as embolization, thrombosis, vasospasm, and infection. Their use by experienced personnel minimizes these risks.

Capillary Blood Gases

Many nurseries and pediatric units obtain blood gas samples by capillary puncture because of the risk and the technical expertise involved in obtaining arterial blood gas (ABG) samples. Although the results require special consideration, less technical expertise and fewer people are required to do a capillary blood gas (CBG) than an arterial puncture. In general, capillary samples are obtained by puncturing the skin of the infant's warmed heel. Fingers and earlobes can also be used for obtaining capillary samples.

When the values of capillary carbon dioxide tension (Pcco$_2$) and pH are compared with those obtained by arterial sample, Pcco$_2$ is 2 to 5 mm Hg higher and pH is 0.01 to 0.03 units lower. These small differences are inconsequential in most clinical situations. However, when the values of the capillary oxygen tension (Pco$_2$) are compared

with those obtained by arterial samples, the differences are not so slight. Unfortunately, there is no fixed ratio for Pao$_2$/Pco$_2$. An infant with a Pco$_2$ of 50 mm Hg may have a Pao$_2$ of 50 to 90 mm Hg or higher. The only statement that can be made about Pao$_2$ by knowing only Pco$_2$ is that Pao$_2$ is probably higher than Pco$_2$. Pulse oximetry or transcutaneous oxygen monitoring should be used to monitor the oxygenation status if needed.

When capillary blood gas sampling is appropriate, the person drawing the sample and the person evaluating the results need to remember the underlying problems that must be overcome in obtaining the sample. A capillary sample that closely reflects arterial blood must be obtained from a warmed extremity (skin temperature should be approximately 39° C or 102° F). Caution must be used in warming the extremity so that the infant is not burned and the warming device does not cool and secondarily cool the extremity if left in place for too long. All the values will be unreliable if the extremity is edematous, acrocyanotic, or not warmed or if the infant has poor peripheral circulation. In addition, because this procedure is painful, like arterial puncture, it reflects the infant's condition during crying, which may be vastly different from rest. Finally, if there is difficulty obtaining the sample, the results may reflect air or tissue contamination rather than the infant's true status.

SIMPLY STATED

Capillary blood samples from the infant usually reflect Pco$_2$ and pH values reasonably close to those of arterial blood; however, the Po$_2$ of capillary blood is often significantly below that of arterial blood and should not be used for clinical decision making.

Venous Blood Gases

Venous blood samples can also be obtained for gas analysis. These are useful in computing the oxygen extraction or carbon dioxide production of tissues (see Chapter 14). Great care should be exercised if using venous blood samples for routine gas analysis. The values obtained by this method may be very misleading.

Noninvasive Monitors

One of the most significant advances in monitoring sick newborns has been the development of transcutaneous oxygen and carbon dioxide monitors. These monitors give caregivers up-to-date information that would otherwise be unavailable. In newborn intensive care units, these devices can be used around the clock to monitor sick infants and for trending.

Transcutaneous Oxygen Monitors. Transcutaneous oxygen pressure ($tcPO_2$) monitors measure electrical current that is directly proportional to the number of oxygen molecules present in the electrode (like the Clark electrode).[6] The $tcPO_2$ electrode measures oxygen present in the underlying capillaries and tissue of the skin and not PaO_2 directly, but $tcPO_2$ usually approximates PaO_2, with $tcPO_2$ slightly lower than PaO_2. Any condition that decreases blood flow under the electrode, such as acidosis, shock, hypovolemia, or hypoglycemia, can cause $tcPO_2$ to be falsely lower than PaO_2.

The $tcPO_2$ monitor is a good method of evaluating the physiologic changes that occur with blood gas sampling. The pain of blood gas sampling can cause changes in the infant's resting condition. The infant can produce an increase in $PaCO_2$ and a decrease in PaO_2 by becoming apneic. If the infant cries and hyperventilates, the $PaCO_2$ might decrease and the PaO_2 might increase. The person obtaining the sample should note the $tcPO_2$ value three times: before disturbing the infant, at the beginning of blood flow, and 40 to 60 seconds after completion of sampling. These three values can then be used to assess the infant's resting condition, the physiologic changes the procedure caused, and the correlation between PaO_2 and $tcPO_2$.

In a neonate with a CCHD or heart condition, the position of the $PtcO_2$ electrode will also allow for the comparison of preductal and postductal PO_2 values. The right upper chest just below the right clavicle is the recommended site for the preductal electrode position. Any other position in the body is considered postductal except the right arm.

Transcutaneous Carbon Dioxide Monitors. Transcutaneous carbon dioxide pressure ($tcPCO_2$) electrodes are used clinically. Similar to the $tcPO_2$ electrodes, they measure the gas present in the underlying skin and not gas present in the blood. The $tcPCO_2$ electrode has merit as a trend monitor for carbon dioxide.

There are still problems with both $tcPO_2$ and $tcPCO_2$. Both techniques use heated electrodes, which must be repositioned every 2 to 4 hours. The heater element in the electrode can cause burns. The tape used to secure the electrode may tear the fragile skin of a preterm infant during repositioning. The monitors have slow response times and are subject to multiple skin perfusion artifacts. Other than difficulty validating the $tcPO_2$ and $tcPCO_2$ against the patient's arterial values, the most common problem with transcutaneous monitoring is air leaks around the adhesive ring. Air leaks always cause a dramatic fall in $tcPCO_2$.

If the leak is large, the $tcPO_2$ and $tcPCO_2$ values will mimic those in room air ($PO_2 \sim 150$ mm Hg; $PCO_2 \sim 0$ mm Hg). In these cases, you should reapply the sensor using a new adhesive ring.

New available technologies in blood gas monitoring have improved some of these drawbacks and have made transcutaneous gas monitoring a more reliable source for clinical information and decision making in the neonatal intensive care unit.

Pulse Oximeters. Pulse oximetry has become a useful monitoring tool and a standard of care in neonatal and pediatric medicine. Pulse oximeters measure the changing transmission of red and infrared light through a pulsating capillary bed to identify the saturation of the hemoglobin. They overcome many of the problems of the transcutaneous monitors. The oximeter is not heated; therefore, it does not require repositioning and does not cause burns. It has a much faster response time, and it does not require tight taping to the skin. (See Chapter 14 for a further discussion of pulse oximeters.)

Pulse oximetry screening for CCHD is recommended for all newborns. Pulse oximetry screening during the first 48 hours of life can identify some infants with a CCHD before they show any signs.

A finding of oxygen saturation of less than 95% in both extremities warrants a repeat screen (after 1 hour) to reduce false-positive results. A second finding of less than 95% warrants a third screen. A positive pulse oximetry screen is defined as a greater than 3% absolute difference in oxygen saturation between the right hand and foot on three measures, each separated by 1 hour.[7] A negative screen was defined as a finding 95% or higher in either extremity with 3% or less absolute difference in oxygen saturation between the upper and lower extremities. Once identified, babies with a CCHD can receive specialized care and treatment that could prevent death or disability early in life.[8]

SIMPLE STATED

Pulse oximetry screening is a low-cost and safe procedure that when performed both preductally and postductally, can detect 100% of infants with pulmonary duct dependent circulation (e.g., PDA). When combined with routine clinical examination during the first 24 hours of life before hospital discharge, it may also detect infants with CCHD and has a higher detection rate than physical examination alone.[9]

Pulmonary Function Testing
Volumes

Pulmonary function can be tested in newborns and small infants. In the past few years, standard computerized equipment for infant pulmonary function testing has become available. This has taken pulmonary function testing in this age group out of the realm of the research laboratory and made it available to the clinician. Although nurseries that measure pulmonary function usually are still found in major teaching and research institutions, now small institutions without major research support can be involved in pulmonary function testing. A variety of technologies that compute pulmonary functions exist. These devices are capable of traditional lung mechanics, active and passive exhalation mechanics, and FRC measurements using either helium dilution or nitrogen washout techniques. New techniques are being developed to measure FRC that use ultrasonic washout methods.[9]

The fundamental difference between newborn and adult pulmonary function testing is the patient's ability to cooperate. The pulmonary function tests for adults and older children depend on the patient's ability to follow simple commands. The tests performed on infants must be reproducible without patient cooperation.

Three volumes can be measured easily in newborns independent of their cooperation: FRC, thoracic gas volume (TGV), and **crying vital capacity (CVC)**. However, a certain degree of caution must be exercised when interpreting the results of these tests. The range of normal values is great, and all three tests are subject to error. To compare the results of these tests for two babies or even for the same baby at different times, the results must be described against a standard unit. Usually, this is done with the body weight in kilograms (e.g., milliliters of gas per kilogram), body length in centimeters (e.g., milliliters of gas per centimeter), or body surface area (e.g., milliliters of gas per square meter).

FRC is measured by two methods: closed-system helium dilution and open-system nitrogen washout. Both methods are available with the computerized pulmonary function machines. TGV requires the use of a plethysmograph and measures all of the gas in the thoracic cavity whether it is communicating with the airway or not. By comparing the TGV with the FRC, the clinician can determine the presence of trapped gas in the thorax. The use of plethysmography in infants and children is very difficult and is not typically available in most centers.

CVC is the measurement of tidal volume while the infant is crying. It is useful in following infants who have lung diseases that cause changes in FRC (e.g., RDS), in whom it is difficult to measure FRC. CVC does require that the infant be able to cry vigorously, which may be difficult for sick infants.

A method of measuring distribution of ventilation is available using a nitrogen washout curve. The pulmonary clearance delay (PCD)[10] divides the lung into fast, intermediate, and slow ventilating areas based on calculations from expired nitrogen concentrations obtained during a nitrogen washout. The PCD can be used to evaluate what percentage of the lung is ventilating effectively.

The most important clinical lung volume measurement is the FRC. The lung mechanics are affected if the FRC is either too high or too low, so it is imperative that clinicians be able to regulate FRC. In either situation (high or low FRC), the compliance decreases, the resistance increases,

and $Paco_2$ is significant elevated. Low FRC can also cause the Pao_2 to drop significantly.

RDS causes the FRC to be decreased. **Meconium aspiration syndrome (MAS)** and PIE are diseases in which FRC is increased. Diseases such as pneumonia and BPD may have either decreased or increased FRCs, depending on the current stage of the disease and the respiratory support being used.

Mechanics

Compliance. Compliance is a measure of the distensibility of the lung. It is calculated by dividing change in volume by change in pressure and requires measurement of tidal volume and transpulmonary pressure. Tidal volume can be measured in newborns by either pneumotachography or plethysmography. Plethysmographs are tricky to use with infants because making an airtight seal around the face is difficult. In addition, plethysmographs for infants are all custom made. Therefore, most nurseries measure tidal volume by pneumotachography.

Transpulmonary pressure is the difference between alveolar pressure and pleural pressure. It is approximated by measuring airway and esophageal pressure in intubated infants and esophageal pressure in nonintubated infants. Either an air-filled balloon or saline-filled catheter in midesophagus can be used. Tidal volume is integrated from the pneumotachometer signal, a pressure-volume loop is constructed, and the compliance of the lung is calculated. The compliance of the chest wall can also be measured by changing the two pressure sources from airway minus esophageal to esophageal minus atmospheric pressure.

Compliance is significantly lower in infants with RDS. Compliance begins to improve dramatically with the return of surfactant function in the lung. Compliance is also lower in infants with BPD, PIE, and pneumonia.

Resistance. Resistance is a measure of the inhibition of gas flow through airways. It is calculated by dividing change in transpulmonary pressure by change in flow. These measurements are obtained with the same equipment used for compliance.

Resistance is elevated in infants with MAS and BPD. The airway resistance in infants with MAS remains elevated for several weeks until the chemical inflammatory phase of the disease is resolved. Infants with BPD will probably have increased airway resistance all of their lives.

Work of Breathing. The work of breathing (WOB) is the cumulative product of the pressure generated and the volume at each instant of the respiratory cycle. It is usually calculated by planimetry of the pressure-volume curve or by electrically integrating the pressure and volume signals.[11] Airway resistance is the major contributor to the planimetric area of a pressure-volume loop, and work of breathing is increased in the diseases that have major resistive components: MAS and BPD.

Lung Mechanics with Mechanical Ventilators. The newer, more sophisticated infant ventilators can measure the mechanical properties of the respiratory system in the newborn during mechanical ventilation. These new ventilators allow the clinician to match the settings of the ventilator with the individual needs of the infant. It is possible to diagnose overdistention (Fig. 12-11), air leak (Fig. 12-12), short inspiratory time (Fig. 12-13), and other dysfunctional ventilator-patient interactions. These ventilators are capable of synchronizing the mechanical cycle with the infant's spontaneous breaths.

Newer modes of ventilation, such as airway pressure release ventilation-assist (APRV), neurally adjusted ventilatory assist (NAVA), and closed-loop ventilation, among others, will respond to the patient's chest and lung mechanics as well as to physiology parameters as determined by the mode and the RT and other members of the patient care team. These newer modes provide lung-protective strategies, improve patient-ventilator synchrony, and optimize gas exchange and lung volumes in neonates and infants.[12,13] They also provide a plethora of clinical data regarding the infant's lung and the patient-ventilator interface, helping to fine-tune the ventilatory management of neonates and children.

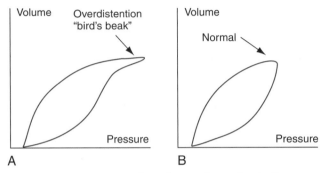

FIGURE 12-11 Pressure-volume loops of a mechanically ventilated infant showing overdistention (**A**) and normal inflation pressures (**B**).

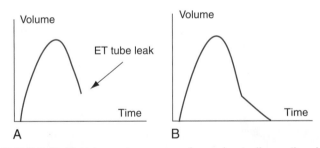

FIGURE 12-12 Volume-time curves of a mechanically ventilated infant show air leak around the endotracheal (ET) tube (**A**) and no air leak (**B**).

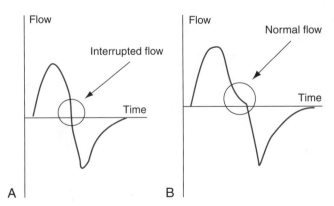

FIGURE 12-13 Flow-time curves of a mechanically ventilated infant show interrupted inspiratory flow secondary to inadequate inspiratory time (**A**) and normal inspiratory flow with adequate inspiratory time (**B**).

Chemoreceptor Response

Sudden infant death syndrome (SIDS) has stimulated a tremendous amount of research into the way infants control respiration. Some investigators have shown that newborns have a blunted response to hypercapnia and a severely diminished or paradoxical response to hypoxia. Many nurseries have the ability to look at carbon dioxide and oxygen responses. These studies are usually performed by measuring tidal volume, minute ventilation, end-tidal oxygen and carbon dioxide, and transcutaneous oxygen levels. The infant's minute ventilation is then plotted against $Paco_2$ or F_1o_2 to assess the infant's ventilatory response to increased $Paco_2$.

Radiographs

Chest radiography is discussed in detail in Chapter 10. However, radiographic views and the methods for obtaining radiographs are significantly different between infants and older children. In the older pediatric patient, the preferred position for taking x-ray films is upright. Infants cannot be placed upright easily, and they dislike being forced to lie on their stomachs; thus, most chest x-ray films are taken with the infant in the supine position, lying on the x-ray film. The x-ray beam passes from the front to the back of the infant (AP view). Most adult radiographs are taken in the posteroanterior (PA) view, which minimizes distortion and enhances the quality of the film.

The typical views used to evaluate an infant's lung are AP and lateral chest films. As in the older patient, these two views allow the RT or other clinician to see all areas of the lung in a standard presentation. It is important that the viewer approach the reading of these films systematically. The viewer should evaluate the airways, including the larynx, trachea, and major bronchi, for deviation from external masses or pressure, for filling defects from internal masses or hypoplasia, and for normal location in the chest.

Occasionally, decubitus films of the chest and abdomen are helpful in evaluating the status of the newborn. They can be useful in detecting the presence of fluid or air in the pleural space. Inspiratory and expiratory chest films are also useful in evaluating the presence of a foreign body. Most aspirated foreign bodies are radiolucent and will not show in a chest radiograph. In an expiratory film, the lung area below the mechanical obstruction will remain hyperinflated when compared with an inspiratory film on the same patient, letting the clinician know the probable position of the foreign body.

Chest radiographs should be done in infants who have unexplained tachypnea, cyanosis, abnormal breath sounds, malformations of the chest or airway, or an overall generalized sick appearance. In addition, any infant who has a significant worsening of clinical status should have a chest radiograph. This might include infants who suddenly have an increase in respiratory rate, the appearance or worsening of retractions, or a sudden increase in $Paco_2$. Less obvious, but equally important, is the need to obtain a chest radiograph in mechanically ventilated infants who suddenly improve clinically. This is especially true for infants who are being mechanically ventilated with high-frequency ventilators, which can make physical assessment much more difficult (e.g., breath sounds cannot be evaluated).

The two classic newborn lung diseases are RDS and MAS. RDS is a disease of inadequate surfactant production. The immature alveoli have increased surface tension and collapse. The chest radiograph of these infants is fairly typical. It includes a diffuse, hazy ground-glass appearance; air bronchograms extending out to the periphery of the lungs; and low lung volumes (Fig. 12-14). MAS is primarily an airway disease. The stressed mature fetus passes meconium into the amniotic fluid and then with gasping respirations inhales the meconium-laden amniotic fluid into its lungs. The disease has two phases: an early mechanical phase and a late chemical phase. The chest radiograph shows a typical pattern of mixed atelectasis and local emphysema (Fig. 12-15).

TTN is another disease that has diagnostic radiographs. In TTN, the amniotic fluid in the lung is incompletely resorbed at the time of delivery. The characteristic chest radiograph shortly after birth shows diffuse streakiness and fluid in the major and minor fissures. This is impossible to distinguish from the chest radiograph of pneumonia. The characteristic of TTN is the rapid resolution of the disease. By 24 hours of age, the newborn's chest radiograph is typically normal (Fig. 12-16). A description of radiologic findings for additional neonatal and pediatric pathologies can be found in Table 12-11.

Other imaging techniques available for the assessment of the fetus and neonate are high-resolution ultrasound, rapid-sequencing magnetic resonance imaging (MRI), and even three-dimensional computed tomography (CT). These techniques provide exquisite detail regarding the fetus and the intrauterine environment.[14]

Imaging advances in fluoroscopy, ultrasound, MRI, and CT continue to provide improved care of the neonate. Fluoroscopy can quickly identify life-threatening abnormalities of the gastrointestinal tract such as meconium ileus and atresia. Ultrasound remains essential in neonatal imaging of the brain, chest, and abdomen because of the lack of radiation, the portability, and the lack of sedation requirements. MRI-compatible incubators have improved the safety of

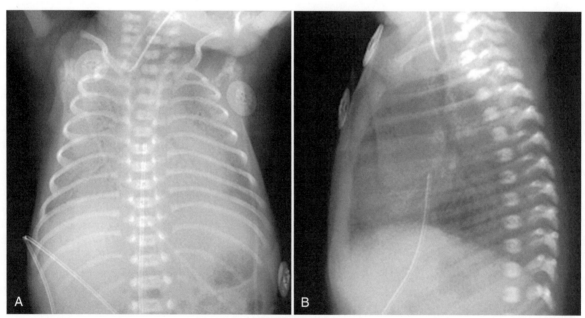

FIGURE 12-14 Anteroposterior (**A**) and lateral (**B**) chest radiographs of a preterm infant with respiratory distress syndrome. Both views show diffuse, hazy ground-glass appearance, air bronchograms, and low lung volumes.

performing the examination on unstable infants. Multi-detector CT with multiplanar reconstruction and three-dimensional volume rendering are infrequently used in neonates because of the high radiation exposure; however, they can quickly provide critical information in the unstable infant with pulmonary or vascular abnormalities.[14]

Apnea Monitoring

Apnea monitoring is designed to warn of life-threatening respiratory and cardiac events, most often in neonates. Apnea monitors use two electrodes placed on the chest wall to detect respiratory movements through changes in electrical impedance, with most units also able to detect heart rate through the electrocardiogram signal.

Apnea monitoring is indicated in neonates at risk for recurrent apnea, bradycardia, and hypoxemia. This procedure may also be considered for infants:

- Receiving drug therapy (e.g., caffeine) for a history of apnea and bradycardia
- With bronchopulmonary dysplasia, especially those requiring supplemental oxygen
- With symptomatic gastroesophageal reflux (GER)
- Born to substance-abusing mother if clinically symptomatic

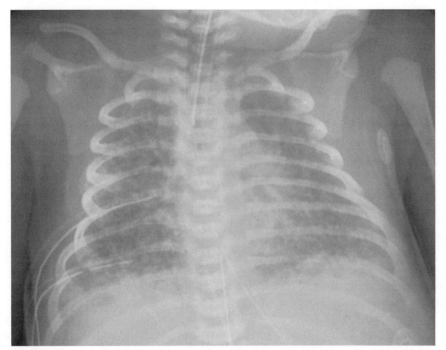

FIGURE 12-15 Anteroposterior chest radiograph of a term infant with meconium aspiration syndrome. This view shows the typical pattern of mixed atelectasis and local emphysema. An endotracheal tube is seen in good position.

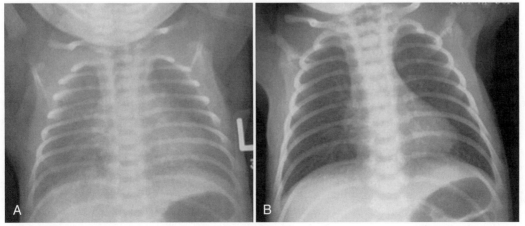

FIGURE 12-16 Two anteroposterior chest radiographs of an infant with transient tachypnea of the newborn. **A,** First day of life. **B,** Second day of life.

TABLE 12-11		
Most Common Radiologic Findings in the Neonatal and Pediatric Population		
Disease	**Pathology**	**Description**
Bronchopulmonary dysplasia (BPD)	This is a complication from a combination of respiratory distress, mechanical ventilation, and high concentration of oxygen over a prolonged period of time (>28 days)	Radiograph findings of stage 4 BPD may show multiple pneumothoraces and spongelike, "honeycomb" pattern with flattened diaphragm
Pulmonary interstitial emphysema	Occurs when air is present outside the normal airways within the interstitium of the lung; it may develop into a pneumothorax or pneumomediastinum	Chest radiograph findings show air trapping with barrel chest or increased anteroposterior diameter and irregular "bubbles" in the hilar area radiating outward
Pneumonia	Commonly caused by lower respiratory tract infections. Viruses are the most common cause in children	Chest radiograph may resemble respiratory distress syndrome or BPD and have bilateral infiltrates and diffused lung markings. Consolidation of a lobe or segment is very rare in neonates
Tetralogy of Fallot	Critical congenital heart disease consisting of four specific malformations: ventricular septal defect, malpositioned aorta, pulmonary stenosis, and right ventricular hypertrophy	Echocardiogram and chest radiograph show a boot-shaped heart. Pulmonary congestion may appear with patchy infiltrates and increased vascular markings
Transposition of the great vessels	Reversal of the origin of the aorta and the pulmonary artery such that the right ventricle leads to the aorta and the left to the pulmonary artery	Echocardiogram and chest radiograph show an egg-shaped heart as well as the transposed vessels
Congenital diaphragmatic hernia	Results from the absence or incomplete development of one of the hemidiaphragms, allowing the abdominal organs to enter the thorax	Chest radiograph shows abdominal organs in the thoracic area and atelectasis; 90% of hernias occurs on the left

- With a tracheostomy or an airway abnormality that increases the risk for obstruction
- With neurologic or metabolic disorders affecting respiratory control

Apnea monitoring is often done within a hospital or clinic but continues to be performed from the home once the patient is discharged. In the case of home monitoring (see Chapter 20), it is essential that the parents and all other caregivers receive proper training on the apnea monitoring equipment and on responding to actual episodes of apnea and bradycardia, before the patient is discharged.

Assessment of the Critically Ill Infant

Airway

Evaluation of airway patency in newborns is not as easy as it is in adults and older children. Infants with obstructed airways still have chest wall motion, and with chest auscultation, they may even make noises that could be misinterpreted as breath sounds. The RT or other clinician needs a thorough knowledge of normal newborn breath sounds and chest wall motion to be able to evaluate airway patency in infants.

Even experienced clinicians can be deceived about the adequacy of the airway in intubated infants because the signs usually used in the older patient may not be reliable in the newborn. For example, an infant whose right mainstem bronchus is intubated may still have breath sounds in the left hemithorax as well as left chest wall motion. This can occur because of the short tracheal lengths (<10 cm)

and the increased compliance of the chest wall. The RT or other clinician must be careful to compare all of the lung fields when auscultating. A misplaced endotracheal tube creates a subtle difference in breath sounds, particularly in the apices, which can be picked up by the careful clinician.

The synchrony of spontaneous ventilation rate compared with mechanical ventilation rate is more important than its frequency in the newborn. An infant who exhales during the inspiratory phase of the ventilator can generate tremendous intrathoracic pressures, potentially damaging the lung. Asynchronous breathing between the infant and the ventilator usually is seen during the hours and days immediately after intubation and the start of mechanical ventilation. The clinician must watch the infant's chest wall motion while listening to the ventilator cycle to document this asynchronous breathing. An inward motion of the chest or absence of an outward motion of the chest wall during mechanical inspiration may indicate that the infant is breathing asynchronously with the ventilator.

One major cause of neonate/infant ventilator asynchrony is the trigger setting in the ventilator, also called ventilator sensitivity. Mechanical ventilators use a variety of triggers for the infant to control the initiation of the breath. These triggers are volume (through either pneumotachography or hot-wire anemometry), abdominal wall motion, thoracic impedance, and flow triggering. The important characteristics that must be present for any of the systems to be useful are sensitivity to small changes and rapid response time.

The airway pressures monitored in infants are the peak inspiratory pressure, mean airway pressure, positive end-expiratory pressure, and occasionally, esophageal pressure. These pressures are interpreted like their counterparts in the adult intensive care unit (see Chapter 14).

Static airway pressure, intrapleural pressure, lung volume, and expired gas analysis generally are not used in the clinical management of newborns. Airway resistance and lung compliance are being used clinically more often with the advent of reproducible, easy-to-use neonatal pulmonary function equipment.

Tracheostomy

Special assessment consideration should be given to the infant or older child that has undergone a tracheotomy procedure. Congenital defects, acquired airway lesions, tracheal malacia, neuromuscular disorders, and ventilator dependency are the most common indications for this procedure in the infant population.[15] Emphasis should be put on assessment of airway patency and signs of distress to prevent short- and long-term complications. Caregiver education and monitoring of the child play an important role in preventing complications.

Factors to consider when assessing risk for complications in a child with a tracheostomy include age, size of the tracheostomy, degree of airway obstruction, behavior of the child, underlying airway pathology, presence of other medical conditions, and social environment. Common signs and symptoms that may indicate airway patency compromise include rattling or "noisy" secretions, thick and inspissated secretions, inability to cough and clear secretions, silent cough, absent or diminished breath sounds, lack of air movement felt around the tracheostomy or mouth, increased work of breathing, and pallor or cyanosis. For some high-risk tracheostomy patients who have a history of airway instability, 24-hour home nursing monitoring may be necessary.[16]

Hemodynamic Assessments

Hemodynamic monitoring in the critically ill infant is in some ways easier and in other ways more difficult than in the adult. The presence of patent umbilical vessels makes cannulation of the aorta and inferior vena cava simple. However, cannulation of the pulmonary artery is difficult and usually must be performed in a cardiac catheterization laboratory in specialized centers. In addition, the newborn may have varying degrees of right-to-left shunt, depending on the pulmonary vascular resistance, with the presence of a PDA and a patent foramen ovale (PFO). This makes calculation of cardiac output difficult if not impossible.

Cannulation of the umbilical artery and vein is a routine practice in most nurseries. The technique for such a cannulation is easy, and although there are risks to indwelling central catheters, they can be minimized by using a good technique and appropriate indications. In addition, many nurseries are now using percutaneous cannulation of radial arteries and subclavian veins

in neonates. The indications for umbilical artery catheterization include a source for frequent ABG sampling, continuous blood pressure monitoring, and large-scale blood replacement (e.g., exchange transfusion). The indications for umbilical venous catheterization include central venous pressure monitoring and large-scale blood replacement. The course of the umbilical artery and vein is shown in Figure 12-17.

These two methods of hemodynamic monitoring are susceptible to many of the same problems that exist in adults and older children. Signal damping is a major concern for several reasons: the small internal lumina of the catheters involved, softer materials used in catheter production, and development of fibrin sleeves. Infections, thrombus formation, embolization, and arteriospasm are also major concerns when using these monitoring methods. Newer and safer methods of monitoring hemodynamic parameters noninvasively (see Chapter 14) have been developed for adults but have not crossed over yet to the neonatal and infant population.

Assessment of the Older Infant and Child

History

The history of the older infant and the child combines that of the newborn and the adult. The parents remain the major source of information about the infant or child until adolescence. Until the age of 2 years, it is important to include the birth history as part of the evaluation of these patients. The RT or other clinician assessing the patient must begin to include a review of systems in the historical assessment at 3 months of age. The review of systems may not be of great benefit before this.

It is important to differentiate acute from chronic problems. When did the symptoms begin? How rapidly have the symptoms progressed? Is the child truly sick or just not feeling well?

The RT or other clinician inquiring about the pulmonary symptoms in an older infant or child is limited to signs that are visible or audible to the parent. Historical information about coughing, wheezing, cyanosis, purulent nasal discharge, frequent colds or infections, and change in behavior is easy to obtain. Dyspnea, chest pain, night sweats, and other symptoms that are not observable by the parent may be impossible to document. It should be remembered that hemoptysis and sputum expectoration do not occur in children. Most children swallow any mucus, blood, or purulent material that might be generated by the upper or lower airway.

In addition to experiencing the usual respiratory symptoms, the older infant and child often have extrapulmonary symptoms caused by pulmonary disease. The careful clinician queries parents about these symptoms. The most obvious of these signs is general activity. Infants and children who are sick act differently from well babies and children. The parents or guardians are the best judges of an infant's or a child's normal behavior. The clinician must be alert to a parent's statement that the child is acting differently, particularly not eating or not playing. The interviewer should inquire about the infant's feeding habits if the parents do not bring this up.

Gastrointestinal upset is a common complaint in infants and children and can lead to dehydration and hypovolemia. Vomiting and diarrhea are major causes for hospitalization in this age group. Many people who take care of infants and children forget that vomiting and diarrhea may be manifestations of pneumonia or other pulmonary diseases. In addition, diseases such as cystic fibrosis and gastroesophageal reflux may have gastrointestinal and pulmonary symptoms.

Finally, an infant or child who does not maintain growth appropriate for developmental age (failure to thrive) should be investigated for an underlying chronic pulmonary disease. In this age group, such diseases include asthma, cystic fibrosis, gastroesophageal reflux, foreign body aspiration, chronic infection (e.g., sinusitis, cytomegalovirus, tuberculosis, sarcoidosis, histoplasmosis, coccidioidomycosis, bronchiectasis, lung abscess, and empyema), nonasthmatic allergic pulmonary diseases, neuromuscular disease affecting the chest wall, and immotile cilia syndrome.

Physical Examination

The components of the physical examination discussed in Chapter 5 are the basis for the physical examination of an older infant or child. Observation, palpation, percussion, and auscultation should be used to localize the disease process within the patient's body. The uniqueness of the physical examination in the older infant or child is in the order in which the examination progresses. It is most important to gain the infant or child's trust and cooperation. The clinician should first examine the parts that upset or frighten the infant or child the least, saving for last the parts of the examination that are upsetting or frightening. If possible, the clinician should make a game out of the examination. Let the child hold and play with the stethoscope or other instruments that are used in the examination.

Two major respiratory diseases in the young child are croup and epiglottitis. **Croup** is usually a viral disease affecting the trachea and small airways in children. Croup tends to appear in children between 3 months and 5 years old, but it can happen at any age. Some children are prone to croup and may get it several times.[17] The child may have cold symptoms, such as a stuffy or runny nose, for a few days and may also have a fever. These symptoms progress to a loud, seal-like barking cough; rapid or difficult respiration; and grunting or wheezing while breathing. In severe cases, the child may develop

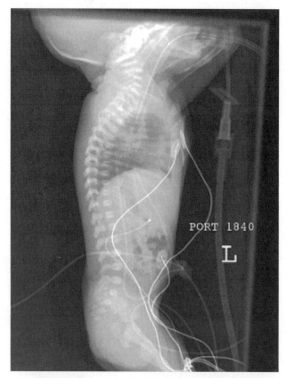
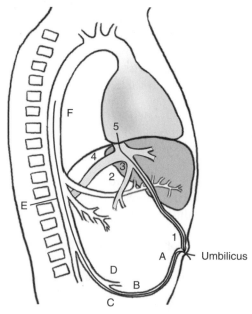

FIGURE 12-17 Lateral radiograph and diagram of the course of umbilical venous and arterial catheters. Umbilical venous catheter enters through umbilicus, passes through 1, umbilical vein; 2, portal vein; 3, ductus venosus; and 4, inferior vena cava and stops in 5, right atrium. Umbilical arterial catheter enters through umbilicus, passes through A, umbilical artery; B, hypogastric artery; C, internal iliac artery; D, common iliac artery; and E, abdominal aorta and stops in F, thoracic aorta.

stridor (high-pitched squeaking noise during inspiration) or cyanosis. An AP neck radiograph usually shows a narrowed subglottic airway (*steeple sign*). The symptoms of croup often worsen when the infant is upset or crying and at night. Scoring systems have been developed to help quantify the degree of illness with croup. These scoring systems often can be used with minimal disturbance of the sick and often anxious child. A scoring system developed by Leipzig and colleagues[18] has been widely used for children with croup (Table 12-12). It has been independently validated and has been shown to be a reliable score. A score greater than 5 is an indication of impending airway obstruction.

Epiglottitis is usually a bacterial disease that causes significant edema and inflammation of the epiglottis. Epiglottitis is now very uncommon because the *Haemophilus influenzae* type B (Hib) vaccine is a routine childhood immunization. The disease was once most often seen in children aged 2 to 6 years. Rarely, epiglottitis can occur in adults. The child with epiglottitis presents with drooling, dysphasia, and respiratory distress. All these symptoms come from the swelling and inflammation of the epiglottis. These children are usually febrile and appear sick and anxious. They often have stridor. They usually do not cough. Epiglottitis can be a life-threatening disease that should be treated as an emergency. The child with epiglottitis should not be disturbed until the airway is secured. However, if a lateral film is done, it will show a swollen epiglottis blocking the upper airway (usually called the *thumb sign*).

Asthma is an increasingly prevalent disease in children of all ages beyond infancy. Asthma is a chronic airway disease that is caused by airway inflammation and hyperresponsiveness to irritants. The typical symptoms include intermittent dry cough and expiratory wheezing. Young children may report nonfocal chest pain. Older children may report shortness of breath and chest tightness. Severe exacerbations may include airflow obstruction that can be life threatening. In 2007, the National Institutes of Health (NIH) issued their third Expert Panel Report detailing the guidelines for the diagnosis and management of asthma.[19] According to these guidelines, the functions of assessment and monitoring for asthma are closely linked to the concepts of severity, control, and responsiveness to treatment. Both severity and control include the domains of current impairment and future risk of the asthmatic patient. The ultimate goal of treatment is to enable a patient to live symptom free, and an initial assessment of the severity of the disease allows an estimate of the type and intensity of treatment needed to achieve this goal.

Clinical Laboratory Data

Older infants, children, and adolescents tend to have a narrower range of normal values on both clinical laboratory and blood gas laboratory tests. Their normal values tend to reflect the normal values seen in adults. Although some laboratory tests show a wide divergence from adult values (e.g., growth hormone and others), in most clinical situations, the normal values for adults can also be used for children.

Other special tests are occasionally used in this age group for the diagnosis of diseases that have a major pulmonary component. Sweat chloride is the most prominent of these. This test is used to diagnose cystic fibrosis. It is simple to perform, but laboratories often obtain erroneous results because of poor methods or techniques. Sweat chloride levels higher than 60 mmol/L are considered indicative

---

TABLE 12-12

Croup Assessment Scoring System

	CROUP SCORE			
	0	1	2	3
Stridor	None	Faintly audible	Easily audible	—
Sternal retraction	None	Minimal	Obvious	—
Respiratory rate (breaths/min)				
0-5 kg	<35	36-40	41-45	>45
5.1-10 kg	<30	21-24	25-30	>30
>10 kg	<20	21-24	25-30	>30
Pulse rate (beats/min)				
<3 mo	<150	151-165	166-190	>90
3-6 mo	<130	131-145	146-170	>170
7-12 mo	<120	120-135	136-150	>150
1-3 yr	<110	111-125	126-140	>140
3-5 yr	<90	91-100	101-120	>120

The respiratory rate is adjusted for body weight and the pulse rate for age.
From Jacobs S, Shortland G, Warner J, et al: Validation of a croup score and its use in triaging children with croup. *Anaesthesia* 49(10):903-906, 1994.

of cystic fibrosis. However, levels as low as 39 mmol/L have also been recommended as threshold for cystic fibrosis diagnosis.[20]

Blood Gases

The older infant and child present a unique problem in obtaining and interpreting blood gases. Their arteries are still small, and arterial puncture is not easy. Most of these patients vigorously object to having an arterial puncture performed even if they are sick. Therefore, more than one person is usually required to obtain the sample. As in the newborn, the older infant and child can quickly change ABG values by crying and hyperventilating. The clinician interpreting the ABG sample should be aware of the patient's disease as well as what conditions existed when the sample was obtained.

Pulse oximetry is more reliable in this age group than is transcutaneous monitoring. There is a greater difference between arterial and transcutaneous gas values because of the increased thickness of the skin and subcutaneous tissue. However, transcutaneous monitoring is still useful as a trending device to identify changes in the patient's status. It is also useful in estimating the true arterial gas value because the value may have changed during the sampling process.

Pulmonary Function Testing

Beyond the newborn and young infant stage, standard pulmonary function testing is not possible until the child is 5 years of age. There are two important points to remember when doing pulmonary function tests on a child. First, the validity of the results is directly related to the child's cooperativeness. Children in the 5- to 8-year age range can have remarkably short attention spans and be frustratingly uncooperative. Second, the lungs of the child are still growing, and the results of pulmonary function tests must be adjusted to body size.

Pulmonary function testing is particularly useful in children with asthma. Machines are now available for clinical use in the outpatient setting. These allow rapid diagnosis of expiratory collapse. Most of these systems use a forced exhalation, measuring peak expiratory flow. With increasing bronchospasm, the child has progressively lower peak flows and a scooped rather than linear expiratory flow pattern (Fig. 12-18).

Impulse oscillometry (IOS) is a fairly new technique being used for the diagnosis and management of respiratory and allergic diseases in children. IOS measures respiratory function during normal breathing by transmitting mixed-frequency rectangular pressure impulses down the airways and measuring the resultant pressure and flow relationships, which describe the mechanical parameters of the lungs. This technique requires little patient cooperation because only tidal volume breaths are required, and children as young as 2 years old can be readily examined.[21] Thus, measurement of pulmonary resistance in preschool-aged

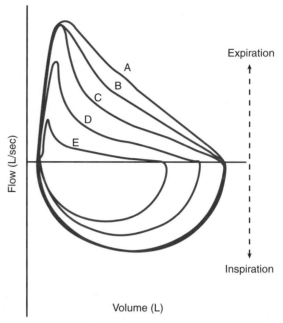

FIGURE 12-18 Forced expiratory flow-volume loops in asthmatic children showing (A) normal flow and (B to E) progressive worsening of flow with airway constriction.

children can be used to diagnose and manage respiratory diseases. Currently, this innovative technique has produced excellent results for pediatric pulmonary function assessment.

Pediatric Bronchoscopy

Traditionally, rigid bronchoscopy (see Chapter 17) has been the bronchoscopic technique of choice to use in infants and children throughout the years. However, the development of smaller, more flexible bronchoscopes has led to the widespread use of this procedure in the pediatric population.[22] Pediatric flexible bronchoscopy is now performed by many medical specialists in a variety of settings and is becoming a major tool for the evaluation of several respiratory disorders. Some of the indications of flexible bronchoscopy in children include stridor, wheeze, cough, radiographic abnormalities, foreign body aspiration, hemoptysis, and inhalation injury.

Radiographs

As the infant becomes older and progresses through childhood, radiographs become easier to obtain and interpret. After the child can sit erectly, it becomes possible to take a PA chest radiograph. Chapter 10 covers most of the chest radiograph techniques and interpretation that can also be applied to the older child.

A lateral view of the neck can help distinguish between croup and epiglottitis. Subglottic narrowing is present in laryngotracheobronchitis, and supraglottic narrowing with a large thumb-shaped epiglottis is present with epiglottitis, as mentioned in the previous section (Fig. 12-19).

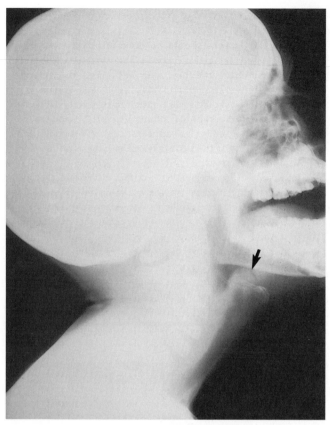

FIGURE 12-19 Lateral neck radiograph demonstrating an enlarged epiglottis (*arrow*). (Courtesy of Lionel Young, MD, Loma Linda University Children's Hospital, Loma Linda, California; from Wilkins RL, Dexter JR: *Respiratory disease: principles of patient care*, Philadelphia, 1993, FA Davis.)

KEY POINTS

- The newborn's history is obtained from several sources and covers more than just the medical history of the infant. Sources include the parents, the mother's labor and delivery chart, and the infant's chart.
- Obstetricians note the mother's previous pregnancy history in the mother's medical record using the terms gravida, para, and abortion. Gravida is a pregnant woman, para is a woman who delivers a live infant, and abortion is the delivery of a dead infant.
- In evaluating the infant with respiratory disease, valuable information can be found in the pregnancy, labor, and delivery histories. An infant delivered in the presence of infection has an increased risk for respiratory difficulty.
- The biophysical profile is an ultrasound evaluation of fetal breathing, body movement, tone, reactive heart rate, and amniotic fluid volume. Like the Apgar score, each of these parameters has a maximal score of 2 and a minimal score of 0. The score for a normal fetus is 8 to 10.
- The labor history is obtained to evaluate the well-being of the infant during the transition from intrauterine to extrauterine life.

KEY POINTS—cont'd

- The delivery history should include the method of delivery for the infant: vaginal or cesarean section; spontaneous, forceps, or vacuum extraction; or low, middle, or high forceps. Infants with uncomplicated deliveries are usually born by spontaneous or low forceps vaginal deliveries.
- The most standard objective measurement of the newborn's well-being is the Apgar score. This is a simple, quick, and reliable means of assessment. It assigns the infant points for the presence of five specific physical criteria: color, reflex irritability, muscle tone, respiratory effort, and heart rate.
- The Apgar score is useful in identifying infants who need resuscitation. Infants who are adjusting well to extrauterine life usually have 1-minute scores of 7 to 10. Infants who have 1-minute scores of 0 to 3 are severely depressed and need extensive medical care such as intubation and mechanical ventilation.
- The range of normal body temperature in the newborn does not differ from that in the adult.
- Newborn term and preterm infants lose heat easily and are extremely dependent on the environment to help them maintain body temperature.
- Hypothermia is a core body temperature of less than 36.5° C or 97.7° F. Hypothermia is a more common and significantly more serious sign of infection in the newborn than in the older child or adult.
- Most sick infants are placed in an NTE, which is the environmental temperature at which the infant's metabolic demand and therefore oxygen consumption is the least.
- The normal pulse rate for infants is age and size dependent, is usually between 100 and 160 beats/minute, and is a function of the developmental age of the infant.
- Tachycardia in the newborn can be caused by crying, pain, decrease in the circulating blood volume, drugs, hyperthermia, and heart disease.
- The normal respiratory rate for infants is between 30 and 60 breaths/minute and is a function of the developmental age of the infant.
- In newborns, tachypnea can be caused by hypoxemia, metabolic and respiratory acidosis, CCHD, anxiety, pain, hyperthermia, and crying.
- The normal values for blood pressure depend on the size of the infant, with pressures decreasing with lower weights. Usually, a term infant's systolic blood pressure should be no higher than 70 mm Hg, with diastolic pressure no higher than 50 mm Hg.
- Inspection is probably the most important and often the most neglected portion of the physical examination of a newborn.
- Retractions (sinking inward of the skin around the chest wall during inspiration) occur when the lung's compliance is less than the compliance of the chest wall or when there is a significant airway obstruction.
- Nasal flaring is the dilation of the alae nasi during inspiration. Nasal flaring is an attempt by the infant to achieve airway dilation to decrease airway resistance, increase gas flow, and achieve a larger tidal volume.

KEY POINTS—cont'd

▶ Grunting is a sound heard at the end of expiration just before rapid inspiration. Grunting is the infant's attempt to increase gas volume in the lung by holding back pressure in the airway.

▶ Capillary refill is checked on the trunk and extremities. Capillary refill should be less than 3 seconds and will be greater than 3 seconds if the infant has a low cardiac output.

▶ A decrease in breath sounds implies a decrease in gas flow through the airways, as in RDS, atelectasis, pneumothorax, or pleural effusion.

▶ Wheezing implies gas flow through constricted airways; infants with BPD may have wheezing.

▶ Crackles usually imply excess fluid or secretions in the lung (pulmonary edema) or the presence of pneumonia. A loud ripping sound like the separation of Velcro often is associated with the presence of pulmonary interstitial emphysema and atelectasis.

▶ Leukocytosis, or a WBC count greater than 15,000/mm^3, usually is a reflection of the infant's environment rather than of infection, as in the older patient.

▶ Leukopenia, particularly neutropenia (an absolute neutrophil count of <2000/mm^3), is a more ominous sign. Usually, neutropenia indicates an infection and implies that the infant is being overwhelmed.

▶ The normal values for the RBC count, hematocrit, and hemoglobin depend on the chronologic age of the infant. Blood glucose probably is the most frequent blood chemistry determination made in newborns. This simple test is of tremendous importance because hypoglycemia, or low serum glucose, is as detrimental to the developing newborn's brain as hypoxia.

▶ Monitoring the blood gas status of newborns is done by analysis of the gas in a blood sample, by transcutaneous monitoring, or by pulse oximetry.

▶ Normal ABG values in newborns depend on the age of the infant when the blood is drawn.

▶ Once infants are beyond the transitional period after delivery (usually 4 to 12 hours), their arterial oxygen (Pao$_2$), carbon dioxide (Paco$_2$), and pH values should be similar to those of the older child or adult.

▶ The tc Po$_2$ electrode measures oxygen present in the capillaries and tissue of the skin and not Pao$_2$, but tcPo$_2$ usually approximates Pao$_2$, with tcPo$_2$ slightly lower than Pao$_2$. Any condition that decreases blood flow under the electrode, such as acidosis, shock, hypovolemia, or hypoglycemia, can cause tcPo$_2$ to be falsely lower than Pao$_2$.

▶ The fundamental difference between newborn and adult pulmonary function testing is the patient's ability to cooperate.

▶ CVC is the measurement of tidal volume while the infant is crying. It is useful in following infants who have lung diseases that cause changes in FRC (e.g., RDS), in whom it is difficult to measure FRC.

▶ The most important clinical lung volume measurement in the infant is the FRC. The lung mechanics are affected if the FRC is either too high or too low, so it is imperative that clinicians be able to regulate FRC.

▶ Compliance is significantly lower in infants with RDS. This begins to improve dramatically with the return of surfactant function in the lung. Compliance is also lower in infants with BPD and pneumonia.

KEY POINTS—cont'd

▶ Chest radiographs should be done in infants who have unexplained tachypnea, cyanosis, abnormal breath sounds, malformations of the chest or airway, or a sick appearance. In addition, any infant who has a significant worsening of clinical status should have a chest radiograph.

▶ The chest radiograph of infants with RDS shows a diffuse, hazy ground-glass appearance; air bronchograms extending out to the periphery of the lungs; and low lung volumes.

▶ Impulse oscillometry (IOS) is a PFT technique that can measure oscillatory resistance in the airways and can be helpful in diagnosing allergic respiratory dysfunction in infants and children unable to fully cooperate during PFT.

▶ In a child with croup, an AP neck radiograph will show a narrowed subglottic airway, usually called the steeple sign.

▶ If a lateral film is done in a child with epiglottis, it will show a swollen epiglottis blocking the upper airway, usually called the thumb sign.

ASSESSMENT QUESTIONS

See Appendix for answers.

1. What range of gestational weeks is considered term?
   a. 32 to 36
   b. 34 to 40
   c. 37 to 42
   d. 38 to 44

2. You are looking at the chart of your patient and in the maternal history you see the following: G3, P2, Ab0. The correct interpretation of the abbreviation is that:
   a. The mother is in her third pregnancy.
   b. The mother is in her second pregnancy.
   c. The mother has delivered three healthy children.
   d. The mother has had one abortion.

3. Which of the following conditions is commonly associated with an infant born early in gestation?
   a. Meconium aspiration
   b. RDS
   c. Transient tachypnea of the newborn
   d. Perinatal asphyxia

4. All of the following are part of the biophysical evaluation of the fetus using ultrasound, *except*:
   a. Reactive heart rate
   b. Body tone
   c. Amniotic fluid volume
   d. Body temperature

5. What Apgar parameter usually deteriorates first in the hypoxic infant?
   a. Respiratory effort
   b. Heart rate
   c. Muscle tone
   d. Skin color

6. Infants needing extensive medical resuscitation at birth will have Apgar scores in the range of which of the following?
   a. 11 to 13
   b. 7 to 10
   c. 4 to 6
   d. 0 to 3

7. Which of the following is a common cause of hypothermia in the infant?
   a. Infection
   b. Heart failure
   c. Atelectasis
   d. Liver disease

8. What is the upper limit of normal range for heart rate in the newborn?
   a. 120 beats/min
   b. 140 beats/min
   c. 160 beats/min
   d. 180 beats/min

9. All of the following are a typical cause of tachypnea in the newborn, *except*:
   a. Hypothermia
   b. Hypoxemia
   c. Respiratory acidosis
   d. Pain

10. In what position should a newborn infant be placed to perform a physical examination?
    a. Prone
    b. Supine
    c. Fowler
    d. Trendelenburg

11. All of the following can account for the presence of chest retractions in a newborn, *except*:
    a. Airway obstruction
    b. Decreased lung compliance
    c. Increased work of breathing
    d. Hyperthermia

12. What is indicated by a capillary refill time longer than 3 seconds in an infant?
    a. Normal cardiopulmonary function
    b. Respiratory failure
    c. Decreased cardiac output
    d. Renal failure

13. What effect does abdominal distention have on respiration?
    a. Impedes diaphragm movement
    b. Decreases airway resistance
    c. Decreases work of breathing
    d. Produces periodic apnea

14. Transillumination of an infant's chest may be helpful in diagnosing which of the following conditions?
    a. Pneumothorax
    b. Pneumonia
    c. Meconium aspiration syndrome
    d. Transient tachypnea of the newborn

15. Leukopenia in the infant indicates what type of infection?
    a. Overwhelming infection
    b. Chronic infection
    c. Acute infection
    d. Local infection

16. What clinical problem is associated with low serum levels of calcium and phosphorus?
    a. Acute hypoxia
    b. Liver failure
    c. Poor nutrition
    d. Renal failure

17. What is the normal range for Pa_{O_2} at birth?
    a. 40 to 60 mm Hg
    b. 50 to 70 mm Hg
    c. 60 to 80 mm Hg
    d. 70 to 90 mm Hg

18. Which parameter demonstrates the largest difference when comparing capillary blood with arterial blood?
    a. P_{O_2}
    b. P_{CO_2}
    c. pH
    d. HCO_3^-

19. Which of the following conditions is least likely to cause a falsely low Pt_{CO_2} reading?
    a. Acidosis
    b. Shock
    c. Hypovolemia
    d. Hyperthermia

20. All of the lung volumes are easily measured in the newborn, *except*:
    a. Thoracic gas volume
    b. Residual volume
    c. FRC
    d. CVC

21. Which of the following findings is not an indication for a chest radiograph in an infant?
    a. Cyanosis
    b. Unexplained tachypnea
    c. Abnormal breath sounds
    d. Periodic apnea

22. What lung disease of newborns is caused by inadequate surfactant production and leads to a decrease in compliance as well as a diffuse, ground-glass appearance on the chest radiograph?
    a. RDS
    b. MAS
    c. Infant asthma
    d. TTN

23. All of the following are indications for umbilical artery catheterization in infants, *except*:
    a. A source for frequent arterial blood gas samples
    b. Continuous blood pressure monitoring
    c. Accurate cardiac output monitoring
    d. Large-scale blood replacement

24. For older infants and children, all of the following are chronic pulmonary diseases that can cause developmental delays, *except*:
    a. Cystic fibrosis
    b. MAS
    c. Bronchopulmonary dysplasia
    d. Bronchiectasis

25. Which of the following is not a recommended method for gaining the trust of a young child about to have a physical examination?
    a. Make a game out of the examination
    b. Ensure they are sedated
    c. Start by examining parts that are least likely to upset them
    d. Distract them by letting them play with the stethoscope

26. An acute viral disease affecting the trachea and small airways of young children, causing fever, barking cough, grunting, and wheezing, is known as:
    a. Epiglottitis
    b. Croup
    c. RDS
    d. Asthma

27. An acute bacterial infection causing significant edema and inflammation to the tissue around a child's glottis, often leading to dysphasia and severe respiratory distress, is known as which of the following?
    a. Croup
    b. RDS
    c. Epiglottitis
    d. Asthma

28. Which of the following is a chronic disease caused by airway inflammation and resulting in intermittent wheezing and dry cough, as well as the possible complaint of chest pain or shortness of breath by an affected child?
    a. Asthma
    b. Cystic fibrosis
    c. Croup
    d. Bronchiectasis

29. At about what age does standard pulmonary function testing become possible in children?
    a. 2 to 3 years old
    b. 3 to 4 years old
    c. 5 to 6 years old
    d. 8 to 9 years old

30. All of the following factors are considered signs of airway compromise in an infant with a tracheostomy airway, *except*:
    a. Absence of airflow
    b. Silent cough
    c. Capillary refill time of <3 seconds
    d. Copious, inspissated secretions

References

1. Wiberg N, Källén K, Herbst A, Olofsson P. Relation between umbilical cord blood pH, base deficit, lactate, 5-minute Apgar score and development of hypoxic ischemic encephalopathy. *Acta Obstet Gynecol Scand* 2010;**89**:1263.
2. Casey BM, McIntire DD, Leveno KJ. The continuing value of the Apgar score for the assessment of newborn infants. *N Engl J Med* 2001;**344**:467.
3. Sasidharan K, Dutta S, Narang A. Validity of New Ballard Score until 7th day of postnatal life in moderately preterm neonates. *Arch Dis Child Fetal Neonatal Ed* 2009;**94**:F39.
4. Tennant C, Friedman AM, Pare E, et al. Performance of lecithin-sphingomyelin ratio as a reflex test for documenting fetal lung maturity in late preterm and term fetuses. *J Matern Fetal Neonatal Med* 2012;**25**:1460–2.
5. Devoe LD. Antenatal fetal assessment: contraction stress test, nonstress test, vibroacoustic stimulation, amniotic fluid volume, biophysical profile, and modified biophysical profile-an overview. *Semin Perinatol* 2008;**32**:247.
6. Dyson A, Singer M. Tissue oxygen tension monitoring: will it fill the void? *Curr Opin Crit Care* 2011;**17**:281.
7. Middleton LJ, Ewer AK, Bhoyar A, et al. Pulse oximetry as a screening test for congenital heart defects in newborn infants: the pulse ox test accuracy study. *Arch Dis Child Fetal Neonatal* 2011;**96**(Suppl. 1).
8. Mahle WT, Newburger JW, Matherne GP, et al. Role of pulse oximetry in examining newborns for congenital heart disease: a scientific statement from the American Heart Association and American Academy of Pediatrics. *Circulation* 2009;**120**:447.
9. Fuchs SI, Sturz J, Junge S, et al. A novel sidestream ultrasonic flow sensor for multiple breath washout in children. *Pediatr Pulmonol* 2008;**432**:731.
10. Fuchs SI, Eder J, Ellemunter H, Gappa M. Lung clearance index: normal values, repeatability, and reproducibility in healthy children and adolescents. *Pediatr Pulmonol* 2009;**44**:1180.
11. Demory D, Arnal JM, Wysocki M, et al. Recruitability of the lung estimated by the pressure volume curve hysteresis in ARDS patients. *Intensive Care Med* 2008;**34**:2019.
12. Biban P, Serra A, Polese G, et al. Neurally adjusted ventilatory assist: a new approach to mechanically ventilated infants. *J Matern Fetal Neonatal Med* 2010;**23**(Suppl. 3):38.
13. Walsh MA, Merat M, La Rotta G, et al. Airway pressure release ventilation improves pulmonary blood flow in infants after cardiac surgery. *Crit Care Med* 2011;**39**:2599.
14. Bulas D. Advances in fetal and neonatal imaging: executive summary. *Pediatr Radiol* 2012;**42**(Suppl. 1):S3.
15. Corbetta HJ, Manna KS, Mitrab I, et al. Tracheostomy: a 10-year experience from a UK pediatric surgical center. *J Pediatr Surg* 2007;**42**:1251.
16. American Thoracic Society. Position statement: care of the child with a chronic tracheostomy. *Am J Respir Crit Care Med* 2000;**161**:297.
17. Everard ML. Acute bronchiolitis and croup. *Pediatr Clin North Am* 2009;**56**:119.
18. Leipzig B, Oski FA, Cummings CW, et al. A prospective randomized study to determine the efficacy of steroids in treatment of croup. *J Pediatr* 1979;**94**:194.
19. National Institutes of Health. *Expert Panel Report 3 (EPR-3): guidelines for the diagnosis and management of asthma.* Bethesda, MD: National Heart, Blood, and Lung Institute; 2007.
20. Costantinoa L, Paracchinia V, Porcaroa L, et al. Borderline sweat test: utility and limits of genetic analysis for the diagnosis of cystic fibrosis. *Clin Biochem* 2009;**42**:611.

21. Park JH, Yoon JW, Shin YH. Reference values for respiratory system impedance using impulse oscillometry in healthy preschool children. *Korean J Pediatr* 2011;**54**:64.

22. Moon CJ, Lee EJ, Chun YH, et al. Pediatric flexible bronchoscopy: clinical experience of 100 cases of bronchoscopy from a single institute. *Pediatr Allergy Respir Dis* 2011;**21**:313.

Bibliography

Gardner SL, Carter B, Enzman-Hine M, Hernandez JA. *Merenstein and Gardner's handbook of neonatal intensive care*. 7th ed. St. Louis: Mosby-Elsevier; 2011.

Kattwinkel J, Bloom RJ, editors. *American Academic of Pediatrics and American Heart Association textbook of neonatal resuscitation*. 6th ed. Elk Grove Village, IL: American Academy of Pediatrics; 2011.

Kliegman RN, Marcdante KJ, Jenson HB. *Nelson essentials of pediatrics*. 6th ed. Philadelphia: Elsevier-Saunders; 2011.

Scanlan C, Heuer AJ, Sinopoli L. *Certified respiratory therapist exam review guide*. 1st ed. Burlington, MA: Jones and Bartlett Learning; 2010.

Walsh BK, Czervinske MP, DiBlasi RM. *Perinatal and pediatric respiratory care*. 3rd ed. St. Louis: Mosby-Elsevier; 2010.

Wanger J. *Pulmonary function testing: a practical approach*. 3rd ed. Burlington, MA: Jones and Bartlett Learning; 2012.

Wilkins RL, Hodgkin JE, Lopez B. *Fundamentals of lung and heart sounds*. 3rd ed. St. Louis: Mosby-Elsevier; 2004.

Whitaker K. *Comprehensive perinatal and pediatric respiratory care*. 3rd ed. Albany, NY: Delmar-Thompson Learning; 2001.

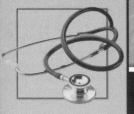

Chapter **13**

Older Patient Assessment

DAVID GOURLEY*

CHAPTER OUTLINE

Patient-Clinician Interaction
  Principles of Communication
  Reducing Communication Barriers
Age-Related Sensory Deficit
  Hearing Impairment
  Vision Impairment
Aging of the Organ Systems
  Age-Related Changes
  Pulmonary Defense Mechanisms
  Unusual Presentations of Illness

Patient Assessment
  Vital Signs
  Inspection and Palpation
  Pulmonary Auscultation
  Cardiac Auscultation
Diagnostic Tests
  Gas Exchange
  Laboratory Values
Comprehensive Geriatric Assessment
  Functional Ability

LEARNING OBJECTIVES

After reading this chapter, you will be able to:
1. Describe several techniques for reducing communication barriers with older adult patients.
2. Describe how patient loss of vision and hearing affect geriatric assessment efforts.
3. Identify techniques health care providers can use to compensate for hearing or vision loss in patients.
4. Identify age-related structural and physiologic changes in the cardiovascular and pulmonary systems.
5. Describe why older adults have a depressed immune system.
6. Describe pulmonary and cardiac assessment techniques.
7. List specific diagnostic tests that have altered, age-related normal values.
8. Describe how functional ability relates to level of health, both actual and perceived.

KEY TERMS

ageism
crepitus
fremitus
immunosenescence

isolated systolic hypertension
  (ISH)
ototoxicity
presbycusis

presbyopia
pseudohypertension
tinnitus

The purpose of this chapter is to introduce the respiratory therapist (RT) to many age-related changes in older adult patients. Gradual decline and chronic illness characterize aging. Many health care professionals are focused on treatment of acute illnesses and conditions. Clinicians may need to gain a different perspective when assessing and managing elderly patients and the chronic conditions associated with old age.

Communicating with older adults in the health care environment can be challenging owing to hearing loss, more frequent health issues, and age differences between them and members of their patient care team, including RTs. However, effective communication is a necessary component of patient care. Chapters 1 and 2 of this text describe various strategies that can be used to help optimize communication and overall outcomes with all patient populations, including older adults. Several of these strategies focus on encouraging them to participate in a dialogue about the design and implementation of their care plan. It has been shown that health

*Helen M. Sorenson, MA, RRT, FAARC, contributed some of the content for this chapter as a contributor for the prior edition of this text.

outcomes can be enhanced by having patients, including older adults, take a share of the responsibility in their plan of care.

> ### SIMPLY STATED
>
> It is important for RTs and other clinicians to understand the major age-specific physiologic changes that can occur with the aging process, including but not limited to a decline in pulmonary function.

It is also important for the RTs and other members of the patient care team to understand age-specific physiologic and structural changes in organ systems that pertain to older adults. Such changes may be apparent in general appearance, vital signs, and diagnostic tests, including pulmonary function test results (see Chapter 9). In addition, realizing that older adults have depressed immune systems and may present with unusual signs and symptoms is especially important to their disease management.

Assessment of the functional performance of an older adult patient may uncover a potential source of disability or impairment or a special need. A systematic inventory of functional abilities can lead to improved diagnostic evaluation and choice of interventions. Functional ability can be directly correlated with the index of health.

The "graying of America" will increase the number of older adults seeking medical attention. Over the next 30 years, the population of older adults will dramatically increase. In 2008, there were about 39 million adults aged 65 years and older. By 2030, this number will likely increase to over 72 million.[1] The average expenditure for consumer health care in the 64- to 74-year-old age group increased 21% from 1999 to 2006 and increased 26% in the 75 years and older age group in that same time span.[2] Additionally, the rate of visits to emergency departments by senior citizens in the United States is growing faster than in any other age group.[1] This translates to an increase in the need for clinicians, including RTs, who are knowledgeable about aging and older adults.

> ### SIMPLY STATED
>
> More than 50% of patients requiring the services of cardiopulmonary professionals are aged 65 years and older.

Patient-Clinician Interaction

The importance of patient-clinician interaction cannot be overstated. Chapter 1 discusses the stages of patient-clinician interaction. The same general techniques for establishing rapport with patients holds true for older adults, but one important difference that must not be overlooked with older patients is time. Gathering data from older patients takes more time. Wise and efficient use of time can make a difference between just recording vital signs and really

assessing the patient. Having a plan before making contact with the patient allows the clinician to gather better history and physical data, in the most efficient manner. Keep in mind that older adults who are institutionalized may be weakened by chronic or acute conditions. Asking an older patient to do unnecessary repeated maneuvers, performing unnecessary manipulations, and exposing his or her skin for long periods of time may exacerbate these conditions. Performing a structured assessment in a calm, unhurried, and respectful manner is fundamental to good geriatric patient assessment.

> ### SIMPLY STATED
>
> To maximize efficiency and conserve energy of older patients and those who are especially ill, it is important to use an organized approach to clinical assessment.

Principles of Communication

As discussed in Chapters 1 and 2, principles of communication are key factors in information gathering. Patient data that have not been gathered cannot be assessed.

Many young clinicians in their daily lives are segregated from older adults. There may be a tendency to associate aging with illness and death. The connection of aging with chronic illness and death may lead to **ageism**, or discrimination against older adults. Ageism in the health care setting can lead RTs and other members of the patient care team to listen to older patients less carefully, spend less time addressing their concerns, and treat them mechanically, without compassion. If clinicians approach their patients with an ageist attitude, communication is hindered.

Reducing Communication Barriers

Communication implies two things: the message has been delivered, and the message has been understood. When older patients know what clinicians are asking and why, they are usually more compliant.

There are many potential barriers that hinder patient-caregiver communication. Sensory deficit, such as hearing or visual impairment, are obvious barriers. Physical barriers related to poorly fitted dentures, nonfunctional hearing aids, or surgical removal of vocal chords may make it impossible for patients to talk. Aphasia, related to stroke, head trauma, or Alzheimer disease, might affect both speech and processing of language, as can the adverse effects of many medications. Emotional barriers often manifested as depression can block communication efforts. Other emotional events, such as the loss of a loved one, the death of a spouse, or even being relocated to a health care institution against the patient's wishes, may be obstacles to effective communication.

Although determining the exact cause of the communication barrier is beyond the scope of therapists, there are a few interventions that may help bridge the gap. It is always important to approach older adults in a caring

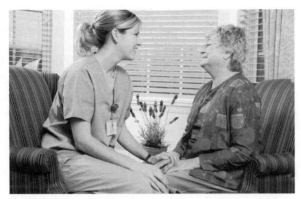

FIGURE 13-1 Patient-clinician interaction: elderly people may need very little, but they need that little so much. (From Sorrentino, SA: Mosby's textbook for long-term care nursing assistants, ed. 6, St. Louis, 2010, Mosby-Elsevier.)

manner. A smile, a pat on the hand, and a kind word while making eye contact are usually successful forms of non-verbal communication. When addressing the patient, use his or her last name preceded by the appropriate title (e.g., Ms., Mr., Dr., Father). Using the patient's last name shows respect and promotes an atmosphere of equality. Call the patient by his or her first name only if you are given permission. Calling patients "sweetie" or "dear" is too familiar, may be interpreted as condescending, and should be avoided.

Be aware of the environment. If the room is too hot, too cold, or too dark or if sunlight from a window is blinding your patient, his or her discomfort may affect your assessment efforts and thus assessment results. Introduce yourself clearly, both by name and by department. Give the patient your full attention. Let him or her know that you are performing an important job. Tell the patient you look forward to working with them and encourage them to ask questions as they arise. If the patient seems confused, a gentle reminder of your role and goal may reassure him or her. Eliminate or reduce background noise and interruptions when possible. Taking a few seconds to do this up front will save time later.

Approach the patient and position yourself at eye level (Fig. 13-1). Maintain an unhurried pace, but keep the assessment structured in a logical manner so that all subjective and objective data can be recorded. An unorganized, unstructured, and hurried approach to assessment can be counterproductive. When asking your patient a question, wait for his or her answer. Try not to put words in the patient's mouth. Older adults function better when they do not feel rushed.

Age-Related Sensory Deficit

Although research confirms the presence of age-related decremental changes in vision and hearing, it is important to remember that all older adults are neither hard of hearing nor visually impaired.

Hearing Impairment

Mild hearing loss begins in the 40s and slowly worsens as we get older. It is estimated that 40% to 50% of people over 75 years old have some level of hearing loss.

Presbycusis, an age-related, progressive, bilateral hearing loss, is the most common cause of auditory impairment in the United States. This condition affects about 23% of adults between the ages of 65 and 75 years.[3,4] In the 70- to 80-year-old group, as many as 50% of older adults have hearing impairment that actually affects their communication skills.[5] Statistics on the exact number of older adults with impaired hearing varies, depending on the source of information. A prospective patient evaluation and retrospective analysis from 576 consecutive frail elders found hearing impairment in 64% of those tested.[4] The burden of hearing loss in older adults is considerable and is often associated with diminished functional independence.

Tinnitus, defined as a symptom rather than a disease, is also more prevalent in elderly people.[5] Tinnitus is an auditory perception not caused by external sounds. It may be described as ringing, buzzing, roaring, or chirping in the ears. Depending on the severity of symptoms, tinnitus can result in mental status changes ranging from mild irritation to depression and suicidal thoughts. Tinnitus can be a result of ototoxicity, so drug-induced hearing impairment should always be considered in older adults. **Ototoxicity** is defined as a damaging effect on the eighth cranial nerve or in the organs of hearing or balance. The diminished hearing capacity that clinicians observe in institutionalized patients may be inflated by ototoxicity. Commonly prescribed pharmacologic agents, including aminoglycoside antibiotics (streptomycin, kanamycin, neomycin, gentamicin, and viomycin), salicylates, diuretics (ethacrynic acid and furosemide), and quinine or chloroquine, are particularly notorious for causing ototoxicity.[6]

Assessing for Hearing Impairment

Simple and accurate methods assess the presence or absence of hearing loss. Some that are commonly used are the whispered voice, a tuning fork, finger rub, a portable audioscope, and the Hearing Handicapped Inventory for the Elderly-Screening (HHIE-S) questionnaire.[7] If the RT suspects that a patient may have significant hearing loss, he or she should inform the nurse and other appropriate members of the patient care team to collectively determine whether further action is appropriate.

Compensating for Hearing Impairment

If a hearing loss is suspected, ask clearly, "Can you hear me?" while facing the patient. If no documented hearing loss exists on the chart, discuss with the nurse the possibility of accumulated earwax or ototoxicity. If the patient has a hearing aid, make sure that it works and that it is in place. If there is no hearing aid, consider using an amplification device if available. Face the patient and speak slowly and clearly, keeping the entire mouth visible. (If you need to wear an isolation mask or have a mustache, the patient may be at a disadvantage.) Lower the pitch of your voice and do not shout.

If you are comfortable with the patient and the situation, you may use your stethoscope as an amplification device by placing the earpieces in the patient's ears and speaking through the bell.

Vision Impairment

Visual impairment is one of the most significant changes associated with aging. Vision is an important part of performing activities of daily living and interaction with society. The patient care team must consider the effect visual impairment has on the geriatric population, including ability to drive a car, read newspapers and books, and identify common objects or people. Given the importance of vision and the impact of vision loss on the patient's well-being, it is important for the clinician to understand the most common causes of vision impairment.

Presbyopia, a normal age-related change in the lens of the eye, usually results in correctable farsightedness. Although presbyopia can occur in adults as early as age 40 years, it is much more common in older adults. More serious disorders of the eye that frequently affect older patients include cataracts, glaucoma, diabetic retinopathy, and macular degeneration. Age is the major risk factor for developing a cataract, an opacity of the lens, that reduces visual acuity. Patients who live to an advanced age are likely to develop cataracts.

Visual impairment has been identified as the second most prevalent disability in adults older than age 65 years.[8] Studies also reveal that sensory impairment diminishes functional status.[4] Thus, RTs need to be aware of assessment techniques and compensatory strategies when caring for patients with vision loss.

Assessing for Vision Impairment

To determine the level of vision loss in older adults, evaluation by an optometrist or ophthalmologist who specializes in low vision is necessary. An evaluation of visual acuity, however, is probably not necessary for providing many forms of respiratory care. Vision impairment generally places the patient at higher risk for falling. As a result, once a clinician suspects that a patient may have a vision problem, especially one that has not previously been detected, appropriate members of the patient care team should be informed, and additional interventions should be considered.

Compensating for Vision Loss or Impairment

Consistency and safety are of primary importance for hospitalized patients with low vision. The old adage "a place for everything and everything in its place" is critical for those with visual impairment.[9] Waste baskets, chairs, and bedside tables that are moved around the room for the convenience of the caregivers may pose a hazard. Knowing on which side the patient is used to getting out of bed will help in properly organizing the hospital room. Paper handkerchiefs, a hairbrush, or a telephone moved from where the patient has placed them will be missed. If the patient wears eyeglasses, make sure they are clean and properly positioned. Older adults with low vision may be able to read words that are enlarged and in bold print. Medicine bottle lids can be marked with a single large letter indicating the name of the medication for when the patient is discharged from the hospital. Words written with puff paint, which is available at craft stores, can help patients distinguish between different metered-dose inhalers (MDIs). Older patients with low vision will require increased illumination. Halogen lighting, if available, provides more illumination than incandescent bulbs. Enhancing contrast also enables elders with low vision to locate and identify objects. The use of coping strategies by older adults with age-related vision loss is associated with better adaptive outcomes.[8]

When patients are blind, verbal communication is extremely important. Speak clearly, and thoroughly explain the procedures you are going to perform until comprehension is evident. If it becomes necessary to move a patient with vision loss, tell him or her what you are going to do, offer an arm as a support and guide, and let the patient initiate the movement.[10]

SIMPLY STATED

Communication barriers that result from sensory deficit may hinder geriatric assessment and compromise patient safety.

Aging of the Organ Systems

The effect of aging on specific organ systems varies widely from one person to another. We spend about one fourth of our lives growing up and another three fourths growing old. Simple observation will attest to the fact that we do not all age at the same rate. Organ systems also age independent of one another. Lifestyle choices and environmental factors influence organ system functioning.[11,12] The combination of these external factors, along with aging and disease processes, alters the body's organ systems in both structure and function.

Age-Related Changes

A brief review of age-related changes in the cardiovascular and pulmonary systems may be helpful before the assessment of an older adult patient. Keep in mind that the following information reflects average changes with age. In older adults, deviation from average is not uncommon. Aging and disease processes also tend to overlap in producing similar signs and symptoms. When evaluating older patients, it is important to understand and recognize the differences.

Cardiovascular System

Diseases of the heart and blood vessels are common in elderly patients. The widespread prevalence of coronary artery disease has presented a challenge for researchers engaged in studying the effect of normal aging on the heart. Evidence regarding aging and human cardiovascular function is generally limited by the need to measure serial cardiac anatomy and physiology noninvasively.[11] Cardiovascular changes have been studied in aging animals; however, translation of animal data to humans cannot be presumed. Many older adults do have some measure of cardiac hypertrophy, but it is generally accepted that in the absence of disease, there is minimal alteration in the size of the heart. As a result of decreased contractile properties in the heart and blood vessels, there is an age-related increase in systolic blood pressure and an elevated left ventricular afterload, which results in left ventricular wall thickening. Arterial walls stiffen with age. Blood vessels lose elastin and smooth muscle fibers and gain collagen and calcium deposits. Left ventricular systolic function remains relatively stable with no significant changes in resting left ventricular ejection fraction, cardiac output, or stroke volume.[11] Left ventricular diastolic function, however, is reduced; this is most likely a result of structural changes in the left ventricular myocardium. The early left ventricular diastolic filling rate progressively slows after the age of 20 years. By the age of 80 years, the filling rate may be reduced by up to 50%.[6]

There is an age-related increase in elastic and collagen tissue in the cardiac conducting system, heart, and arteries, causing the vessels to become more rigid and thick. Researchers have noted a pronounced reduction in the number of pacemaker cells in the sinoatrial (SA) node, estimated by one author to be as high as a 90% decline in SA node cell numbers.[11] The consequence of these age-related losses is an increase in cardiac arrhythmias. Atrial fibrillation is the most common cardiac arrhythmia, occurring in up to 5% of adults older than 80 years of age.[13] Pressure receptor sensitivity declines with age. As a result, older adults have a blunted compensatory response to both hypertensive and hypotensive stimuli.

Calcification of heart valves is more prevalent in elderly people. In elderly patients, the predominant causes of valvular heart disease are degenerative calcification, myxomatous degeneration, papillary muscle dysfunction, and infective endocarditis. One third of patients older than 70 years of age have calcium deposits in the aortic or mitral valves.[6]

Congestive heart failure (CHF) may result from valvular disease, hypertension, cardiomyopathy, or ischemic heart disease. The incidence of CHF doubles for each decade of life between 45 and 75 years.[11] The pressure the ventricles must overcome to pump blood out of the heart can lead to left ventricular failure, right ventricular failure, or biventricular failure. Left- and right-sided failures will both result in reduced cardiac output and an increased heart rate. CHF usually develops gradually and progresses over time. It may not be detected in the early stages, and it has a high morbidity and mortality rate. Some other CHF symptoms are more typically associated with the damaged ventricle, either left or right (Box 13-1).

Box 13-1	Symptoms of Left-Sided Versus Right-Sided Congestive Heart Failure

LEFT-SIDED FAILURE
- Exertional dyspnea, orthopnea
- Possible nocturnal dyspnea
- Cheyne-Stokes breathing
- Pale, cool skin
- Arrhythmias
- Fatigue
- Restlessness, irritability
- Shortened attention span

RIGHT-SIDED FAILURE
- Edema
- Distended neck veins
- Cyanosis
- Dyspnea
- Arrhythmias
- Hepatomegaly
- Occasional ascites

SIMPLY STATED

In persons older than 65 years of age, CHF is the most common medical diagnosis.

Pulmonary System

There are a number of age-related physiologic changes in the pulmonary system. Structurally, the trachea and bronchi become more rigid with age. Smooth muscle fibers in the lungs are progressively replaced with fibrous connective tissue. Alveolar septa gradually deteriorate. Although the number of alveoli does not change, loss of alveolar walls increases the size of the alveoli and reduces surface area for gas exchange. The alveolar-capillary membrane thickens, causing a reduction in diffusion of pulmonary gases. Aging lungs have less elastic recoil. The chest wall becomes stiffer, probably as a result of ossification of the cartilage-rib juncture and progressive dorsal kyphosis. Although loss of elasticity of lung tissue actually increases lung compliance, the rigidity of the thoracic cage reduces compliance enough to result in an overall decrease in lung compliance. The stiffer chest wall and reduction in elastic recoil are factors in an age-related increase in functional residual capacity (FRC) and residual volume (RV).

Physiologically, aging alters both ventilation and gas exchange. Changes in ventilation and gas distribution are primarily related to the altered lung and chest wall compliance. The balance of inward forces (elastic recoil) and outward forces (chest wall and muscles of ventilation) determines lung volumes at rest. At about 55 years of age, respiratory muscle strength begins to weaken.[6] The strength of the diaphragm for a 55-year-old is only about 75% of that for a healthy young adults. The important functional changes that take place with aging of the pulmonary system are reductions in elastic recoil and ventilatory muscle strength. The central control of these activities also changes with increasing years. Cardiac and pulmonary responses to decreased oxygen and elevated carbon dioxide levels diminish with age. Thus, the changes in ventilation and respiration with aging emerge as a complex picture.[14] In the absence of disease, age-related changes in the lungs are inconsequential. However, the combination of age-related and disease-related pulmonary changes puts the patient at risk for increased morbidity and mortality.

Pulmonary Defense Mechanisms

Aging not only alters physiologic functioning of the lung (ventilation and respiration) but also affects the protective function of the lungs. With increasing age, the epithelial cells of the mucous membranes that line the tracheobronchial tree show degenerative changes. The number of cilia is reduced, and ciliary activity slows down. There is a decrease in the phagocytic activity of the macrophages in the mucous membrane. Combined, these changes lead to a reduction in mucociliary clearance. In addition, the loss of an effective cough reflex contributes to the increased susceptibility of older patients to lung infections.

Institutionalized older adults are subject to some conditions that may result in a reduced level of consciousness. Neurologic disorders and pharmacologic agents, such as narcotics or sedatives, can effectively blunt the cough reflex. Aspiration is always a concern. Patients with dysphasia, impaired esophageal motility, or reflux disease are at added risk when the cough mechanism is not working properly.

Immunity

Humoral immunity, which takes place in bodily fluids, is associated with antibody production and B lymphocytes. T cells are primarily related to cell-mediated immunity and constitute about 70% of the lymphoid pool in the blood. Cell-mediated immunity involves a variety of activities designed to restrain or destroy cells that the body recognizes as harmful. With age comes a decrease in cell-mediated immunity. This age-related decline in cellular immunity correlates with an increased frequency of secondary (reactivation) tuberculosis in elderly patients. The acute antibody response to extrinsic antigens, such as pneumococcal and influenza vaccines, is also reduced in old age. Immunizations, although not as effective in older adults, are still strongly recommended.

Research regarding the clinical implications of **immunosenescence**, which is aging of the immune system, is confounded by a number of factors. Within subpopulations of older adults, there is considerable heterogeneity of the immune response. Genetic factors may play a role, as may environmental pollutants, socioeconomic status, and nutrition. Even efforts to increase immune function (nutritional supplements or booster vaccines) may not be equally effective in older adults. Although increased rates of infection and malignancy are associated with the dysregulated immune response common in older adults, these changes have not been causally related to the increased incidence of disease.[15] What does seem reasonable to presume, however, is that the age-related changes in the immune system may impair the older patient's ability to effectively repel bacterial infections and may make them more susceptible to increased morbidity and mortality from pneumonia, sepsis, or other bacterial growths.

Unusual Presentations of Illness

What you see in a 40-year-old patient presenting with an acute condition or exacerbation of a chronic disease may differ from the presenting symptoms of an 80-year-old patient with the same disease. The variations in signs and symptoms can make it difficult to diagnose such common occurrences as pneumonia or a heart attack.

Some older adults will downplay their symptoms, assuming the aches and pains are simply due to old age. However, research indicates that in some cases aging neurons may decrease peripheral sensitivity, causing a reduced sense of pain.[16]

Immune system changes, as previously discussed, put older adults at a higher risk for harboring infectious agents. Changes in the cardiac system may result in blunting of the tachycardiac response to hypoxia or sepsis. Some aging organ systems lose the ability to compensate for injury to other organ systems.

Inflammation is one of the body's first responses to infection or injury. It was once believed that in older adults the diminished febrile response, mild leukocytosis, and weakened local inflammatory response were related to the aging process. New evidence has shown that the same lack of immune response occurs in younger adults with multiple illnesses. Recent data support the theory that it is the accumulation of diseases not the age of the patient that impairs immunity.[6]

Pneumonia

In a patient with pneumonia, typical presentations are cough, fever, and purulent sputum production. These signs can be deceptively subtle in older adults, particularly a lack of an elevated temperature. With a lower base temperature and a reduced ability to mount a febrile response, older adults with pneumonia may be quite ill before the cause is detected. Some older patients with an infection may simply complain of a poor appetite, fatigue, lack of ability to perform daily activities, a generalized weakness, altered mental status, and lethargy. Extrapulmonary symptoms, such as nausea, vomiting, diarrhea, myalgia, and arthralgia, are common. The most sensitive sign of pneumonia in an elderly adult is an increased respiratory rate (>28 breaths/minute).[14]

Chest radiographs may be helpful in diagnosing pneumonia, but this is not the case if the patient is dehydrated. The pneumonic infiltrate may be obscured by pulmonary edema or may not be detectable on the chest film until 24 to 48 hours after the patient has been rehydrated.[17]

Sputum specimens collected for culture and sensitivity are recommended to avoid empirical therapy with a broad-spectrum antibiotic. Unfortunately, obtaining a good sputum specimen from an older debilitated patient is the exception, not the rule. For patients who do not respond to therapy or who relapse after an initial response to therapy, collecting sputum by transtracheal aspiration or a bronchoscopy may be considered. Depending on the pathogenic organism, blood cultures have a diagnostic yield of only about 10% to 20%.[17]

Myocardial Infarction and Congestive Heart Failure

Although the incidence of death from myocardial infarction (MI) has been reduced over the past 30 years, MI remains an important cause of morbidity in the older population. About 50% of patients who die from MI are older than 75 years of age.[18] Unfortunately, the clinical presentation of heart attack may be altered by advanced age. The most common symptom in younger adults is chest pain, but this symptom decreases with age. Also, the pain may be referred or not present at all. Complaints of shoulder, throat, and abdominal pain are common. Some patients may complain of bilateral elbow pain. Other atypical symptoms that can accompany a heart attack are syncope, acute confusion, weakness, fatigue, and restlessness. In the case of silent MI, pain is not a symptom. A prospective study, part of the Bronx Aging Study, showing the magnitude of unrecognized or silent MIs, revealed that the annual incidence of recognized MI was 3.2 per 100 person-years, whereas the incidence of unrecognized MI was 2.4 per 100 person-years.[18] Although atypical presentation may cause diagnostic difficulty, there are many subtle clues that should alert RTs or other members of the patient care team. As a result of the degeneration of the cardiac conduction fibers, if an older patient complains of dizziness, the health care professional should suspect heart problems.

In the United States, heart failure is a major source of chronic disability and the leading indication for hospitalization in adults older than 65 years.[11] In fact, two thirds of patients with CHF are older than 65 years. Cough and wheezing may indicate early left-sided heart failure. Hemoptysis in an older adult may be indicative of heart failure or a pulmonary embolus. Shortness of breath should put the clinician on alert. Dyspnea may be the only complaint from a patient with new-onset CHF.[11]

An awareness of how and why disease can present with unusual symptoms will reduce the chances of missing a diagnosis. Informed clinicians performing good assessments can make a difference in the patient outcome.

Asthma

In older adults, the diagnosis of asthma is not uncommon. It has been estimated that 5% of adults older than 60 years and 7% to 9% of adults older than 70 years have asthma.[19,20] Asthma, unfortunately, is often misdiagnosed or underdiagnosed in the older patient population. Reasons for this are unclear. Perhaps it is because asthma has historically been considered a disease common to children and young adults. Other potential confounding factors may be associated with normal age-related pulmonary changes and a blunted perception of symptoms. It is possible that when asthma and chronic obstructive pulmonary disease (COPD) occur simultaneously, only the COPD is diagnosed. The classic symptoms of asthma—shortness of breath, wheezing, and cough—are also common in diseases such as CHF, emphysema, chronic bronchitis, gastroesophageal reflux, and transbronchial tumors.[20]

Asthma is more common than presumed in older adults, and therapists need to be aware that some presenting symptoms may be atypical. Elderly asthmatic patients are less likely to have a history of allergic disease, less likely to have nocturnal or early morning symptoms, more likely to have a poor immediate response to bronchodilator therapy, and more likely to have a later onset of symptoms. Wheezing, however, remains common. A diagnosis of asthma should be considered in elderly patients with wheezing or dyspnea.

Underdiagnosis of asthma may be more related to the underuse of objective measurement instruments such as spirometers and peak flow meters. Functional ability to do reproducible maneuvers may have been a concern in the past, but according to Enright and associates,[21] about 90% of the elderly participants in the Cardiovascular Health Study Research Group were capable of performing high-quality spirometry tests within 10 minutes. Older adults who experience symptoms and have not been previously assessed for asthma should be considered candidates for pulmonary function screening.

> **SIMPLY STATED**
>
> The diagnosis of asthma should be considered in older adults who are wheezing.

Patient Assessment

Patient assessment represents a skill that is crucial to caring for elderly people. Vital signs, such as temperature, pulse, blood pressure, and respiratory rate, as well as lung sounds and breathing pattern, are noninvasive windows to the health status of the patient. Assessment is truly an art. Given today's climate of managed care, protocols, and clinical practice guidelines, strong assessment skills are vital to good patient care and cost-effective disease management. Patient assessment is the foundation, so the information gathered must be accurate.

One component of assessment that is occasionally overlooked is taking a patient's history. In the case of acute onset dyspnea, a good history and physical examination alone will establish the diagnosis most of the time.[22] Another means of facilitating physical assessment is to try to conceptualize the anatomy. Having a basic knowledge of anatomy and understanding how disease alters both anatomy and physiology are key to accurate assessment.

Vital Signs

Chapter 4 of this text describes techniques involved in obtaining and interpreting vital signs. However, it is important for the RT and other members of the patient care team to keep in mind that age-specific considerations apply when assessing vital signs in elderly patients. The means by which certain vital signs are obtained, normal ranges, and their clinical significance for older adults are often different from other patient populations.

Temperature

As a result of decreased metabolism, the loss of muscle mass, and a reduction in vasoconstriction, older adults have an altered ability to regulate body heat. Older adults usually have lower body temperatures. In patients older than 90 years, body temperatures of 96° and 97° F are not uncommon. Simply taking temperatures in older adults may be a challenge. Oral thermometers are not useful if the elderly patient cannot easily keep his or her mouth closed for 2 or 3 minutes.

The axillary method may not be accurate, particularly in a thin, older adult with a loss of underarm body tissue. Rectal temperatures are accurate but necessitate turning the patient completely to one side, a maneuver that could result in injuring a hip. Tympanic membrane thermometers are generally preferred in older adults and other populations because they are accurate, easy to use, and able to record temperatures within seconds.

Regardless of the method used, it is important to establish a norm for each patient and assess for trends. Once the norm is established, an increase in temperature alerts the health care professional to the possibility of infection. A 95-year-old patient with a temperature of 101° F (whose normal body temperature is 96° F) is in trouble. This patient's temperature is equivalent to 103.6° F in a person whose normal temperature is 98.6° F.

The thermoregulatory mechanism in older adults is blunted, and environmental temperatures may be more influential. During room temperature extremes (hot or cold), monitor the patient's body temperature on a regular basis.

Pulse

The heart rate at rest is regulated by sympathetic and to a greater degree parasympathetic tone. In healthy men, the supine resting heart rate does not change with age. In a sitting position, the heart rate in the same individual will drop slightly from the rate exhibited when supine. In an inactive older adult, the pulse rate may decrease to 50 to 55 beats/minute. In active older adults, although heart rates vary, a normal pulse may range between 60 and 100 beats/minute. Arrhythmias that produce a rapid heart rate are not tolerated well by elderly patients, who may already have a decreased level of daily functioning. If there are any new (not previously noted) irregularities in pulse volume or rhythm, consult a nurse or physician about a follow-up assessment. To most accurately assess pulse in an older patient, use a stethoscope and count beats at the apex.

Blood Pressure

The measurement of blood pressure is essential. Hypertension is an important cardiovascular risk factor in elderly people. Blood pressure and pulse pressure increase progressively with age. In most populations, average diastolic blood pressure increases with age until the sixth decade and then stabilizes, whereas systolic blood pressure continues to rise. As a result, the pulse pressure (the difference between systolic and diastolic pressures) may widen. A normal pulse pressure is anywhere between 50 and 100 mm Hg in older adults. If when documenting blood pressure you note a narrowing of the pulse pressure, it might be wise to monitor the patient. A narrowing pulse pressure can be an early sign of a slow leak tamponade.

Systolic blood pressure rises with aging as a consequence of the loss of elasticity in the peripheral vessels. It is estimated that 60% of older adults have either elevated systolic or diastolic blood pressures or both. Elevation of only the systolic pressure is termed **isolated systolic hypertension (ISH)**. The Systolic Hypertension in the Elderly Program (SHEP) demonstrated that treating ISH in older patients decreased the incidence of stroke.[23] Historically, a sustained systolic pressure of more than 160 mm Hg or a diastolic pressure over 90 mm Hg was thought to constitute hypertension. Additional studies now reveal that the risk for cardiovascular disease rises with increases in both systolic and diastolic blood pressure, approximately doubling for every 20/10 mm Hg incremental increase in blood pressure that occurs within the range of 115/75 to 185/115 mm Hg.[24] Conversely, lowering systolic blood pressure by 10 mm Hg is associated with a reduction in the risk of having a stroke by about 33% regardless of the baseline blood pressure level.[25]

According to a national survey, 70% of Americans with hypertension are aware of their problem. Fifty-nine percent are being treated for the condition, and 34% of those being treated have their blood pressure under control.[26] The current guidelines focus on improving these statistics by recommending interventions and treatments designed to help people regain control of their disease. The recommended treatment guidelines include medication management and lifestyle change.[27]

Blood pressure may be falsely high in older adults because of arterial stiffness. An overestimated blood pressure (**pseudohypertension**) should be suspected in patients with elevated systolic and diastolic pressures but no end-organ damage.

Blood pressure must be measured accurately. Ask the patient to sit quietly for 3 to 5 minutes before taking a measurement, and use a cuff large enough to cover at least one third of the patient's upper arm. Measure pressure in both arms, and note any significant difference. Both supine and standing (or sitting) blood pressures, taken 1 to 3 minutes after the positional change, may reveal the presence of orthostatic hypotension. (Exercise caution, however, when testing volume-depleted patients.) A drop of 20 mm Hg systolic or 10 mm Hg diastolic or an increased heart rate of 20 beats/minute is abnormal. Orthostatic hypotension in older adults is often associated with syncope and falls. Failure to check both supine and standing blood pressure is an oversight in potentially diagnosing an important and often correctable problem. Clearly, obtaining accurate blood pressures is important in the treatment and management of hypertension in elderly people. Remember that emergency department blood pressures are not baseline data. They are measured under less than optimal conditions. Check blood pressure again before acting on a single measurement. Also, document any blood pressure trends. Safe drug therapy may depend on accurate daily blood pressure measurement.

SIMPLY STATED

Emergency department blood pressure measurements are generally not considered reliable baseline data because the setting can cause significant variability.

Respiratory Rate

RV increases almost 50% by the age of 70 years. The total lung capacity remains relatively stable, and the increase in RV comes at the expense of the vital capacity. In older adults, the respiratory rate may increase as a result of a decreased depth of ventilation. Normal respiratory rate in elderly patients ranges from 16 to 25 breaths/minute.

Tachypnea or hyperpnea may be the result of exercise, for example, in a patient who just ambulated in the hallway or returned from therapy. Other factors that could result in an increased rate or depth of breathing are anxiety, fever, pneumonia, hypoxemia, acidemia, or lesions in the pons and medulla. Bradypnea might be secondary to pharmacologic respiratory depressants, or the patient may just be sleeping. When an abnormally slow rate of breathing is noted, other causes could be alkalosis, hypothermia, or hypoglycemia. Older adults are more susceptible to hypothermia. Additionally, older patients with diabetes have a sixfold greater risk for hypothermia, most likely a result of vascular disease that alters the body's thermoregulatory mechanism.[8] In patients being treated with oral antidiabetic agents (sulfonylureas), the incidence of hypoglycemia increases with age or concomitant use of aspirin or sulfonamide antibiotics.[28] Accurate respiratory rates, documented in a timely manner, can assist caregivers in looking for trends and can lead to additional diagnoses. If shallow breathing is noted, respiration may be easier to count by watching the rise and fall of the abdomen instead of the chest. If both the respiratory rate and pulse are elevated (>25 breaths/minute and >100 beats/minute) in an elderly patient for no apparent reason and the patient has other respiratory symptoms, pneumonia should be suspected.[22]

Dyspnea in older adults is abnormal. If a patient with airway disease exhibits significant shortness of breath at rest, the forced expiratory volume in 1 second (FEV_1) is likely less than 50% of predicted.[22] Next to pain, dyspnea is the symptom most feared by patients and clinicians alike. An increased respiratory rate may signal a lower respiratory tract infection, CHF, or another disorder before the appearance of other clinical signs.[6]

Inspection and Palpation

Generally defined as a visual examination of the patient, inspection can be done while taking a patient history, checking vital signs, or auscultating lung sounds. Palpation is the process of using the hands to feel for body movement, lumps, masses, and skin characteristics.

Inspection

Breathing Patterns. Note the pattern of breathing. Is Cheyne-Stokes or periodic breathing perceptible? If so, document the length of the apnea episodes. Older adults with heart disease may demonstrate this pattern of irregular breathing while sleeping. The more common etiologic factors of Cheyne-Stokes breathing include CHF, uremia, decreased blood flow to the respiratory center of the brain, drug-induced respiratory depression, or brain damage. Biot breathing, an irregular breathing pattern, also has characteristic periods of apnea. Again, document the length of apnea episodes in seconds. Biot breathing occurs most often in patients with brain damage and increased intracranial pressure (see Chapter 6).

Cyanosis. Look for cyanosis. If the extremities (i.e., fingers, toes, tip of nose, lips, and earlobes) are bluish in color, the patient has peripheral cyanosis. Peripheral cyanosis is often related to inadequate circulation but may be noted in patients who are cold, are anxious, or have some measure of venous obstruction.

Central cyanosis results from a decreased concentration of oxygen in arterial blood and may be a result of advanced lung disease or CHF.

In older adults, two other manifestations of cyanosis may be noted. Small vessel syndrome can present as local areas of cyanosis or necrosis in a hand or foot that generally has adequate circulation. A number of predisposing conditions, such as disseminated intravascular coagulation

(DIC), essential thrombocytosis, polycythemia, scleroderma, or emboli from arterial aneurysms, can result in small vessel syndrome.[6] Raynaud phenomenon is another syndrome that can present with intermittent cutaneous pallor or cyanosis. It is typically caused by exposure to cold or emotional stimuli and related to peripheral vasospasm. However, older adults may experience the pallor and cyanosis at room temperature.

Skin Turgor. Diminished skin turgor or fullness of the skin is a normal age-related integumentary change. The loss of subcutaneous fat and water, deterioration of elastin, and decreased vascularity can result in wrinkling and loose skin. Pinching the skin to check for tenting used to be a quick check for the presence of dehydration. Now that age-associated structural changes are understood, tenting is no longer used as a valid indicator of dehydration. The condition of the tongue may be a better marker of dehydration rather than the skin.[29] If dehydration in an elderly patient is suspected, appropriate members of the patient care team should be consulted.

SIMPLY STATED

Dehydration should be treated as a potentially life-threatening situation.

Clubbing. The abnormal enlargement of the distal phalanges, most easily noted in the fingers, is not age related. However, the conditions that lead to clubbing are chronic, and older adults have a higher incidence of chronic disease. COPD alone, even in the presence of hypoxemia, does not lead to clubbing. If older adult patients with COPD have clubbing, something other than obstructive lung disease is occurring, such as pulmonary manifestations of connective tissue disease.[14]

Edema. The visible signs of fluid accumulation can signal the presence of a variety of diseases. Check the patient's lower extremities for the presence of edema or swelling. Ask about or check the chart for any recent sudden weight gain. A gain of more than 2 pounds in a day or more than 5 pounds in a week may be fluid retention and could signal CHF.[30] A rapid onset of unilateral leg swelling and dependent edema suggests a diagnosis of deep vein thrombosis.

Unfortunately, because they more commonly exhibit atypical presentations, peripheral edema is not always a reliable indicator of heart failure in elderly people.

Jugular Venous Distention. Peripheral edema may not be a reliable indicator of heart failure, but jugular venous distention (JVD) in older adults is highly suggestive of right heart failure. Chapter 5 contains a detailed description of estimating jugular venous pressure. Hepatojugular reflux, or distention of the jugular vein induced by manual pressure over the liver, is also a reliable indicator of right heart failure in elderly patients.[6] When performing the inspection portion of the physical examination, be sure to make a neck vein assessment.

Palpation

Touching the patient to evaluate for the presence of pathology can assist in the process of assessment. Normally, palpation includes an evaluation for fremitus, including an estimation of thoracic expansion and feeling for crepitus. In older patients, palpation may initially be a scouting maneuver for skin condition, scars, signs of infection, and the presence of bumps or bruises.

When assessing patients whose respiration is being aided with mechanical ventilators, patients who have had thoracic surgery, or patients who have sustained trauma, palpate first for subcutaneous emphysema. Start assessing at the neck and using fingertips, gently "walk" down the sides of the neck from the jaw to the clavicle. **Crepitus** feels like crackling under the skin. Crepitus associated with subcutaneous emphysema is more common in patients who have sustained intrathoracic trauma or barotrauma.

Fremitus consists of palpable vibrations felt on the chest wall when the patient is repeating a sound. The vibrations caused by sound increase over areas of consolidation. Evaluating for fremitus requires a cooperative patient. Likewise, estimating thoracic expansion by palpation requires deep inspiratory and expiratory maneuvers. These maneuvers may be physically difficult for elderly patients to perform. Palpate for chest excursion on a case-by-case basis.

Pulmonary Auscultation

Assessing lung sounds can generate very useful diagnostic information. Abnormal or added lung sounds are referred to as adventitious and can be classified as crackles or wheezes. A few simple questions can be used to classify lung sounds and guide the diagnosis.

QUESTIONS TO ASK

Lung Sounds

When assessing lung sounds, ask yourself the following questions:

- Is the sound continuous or discontinuous?
- Is the sound on one side or both?
- Is the sound on inspiration or expiration?
- Does the sound clear with coughing?

Older adult patients may not always be able to take several consecutive good quality, deep breaths. They may only be able to give you three to four good, deep breaths before they tire. In a quiet environment, with the patient leaning forward, assess posterior lobes first. Position your stethoscope (on skin) midway between the patient's waist and scapula and get four good bilateral breaths. Listen for a full inspiratory-to-expiratory (I/E) cycle. Moving the stethoscope from side to side, compare sounds, and then proceed with anterior and lateral chest assessment. The patient will be taking deeper breaths during the examination, so caution must be exercised to prevent hyperventilation. Ask the patient to report any feelings of dizziness.

Auscultation may reveal diminished breath sounds even in older patients with healthy lungs. An increased anteroposterior (AP) diameter and shallow breathing are common in elderly people and add to the difficulty of hearing normal vesicular breath sounds. However, pathologic conditions still produce characteristic wheezes and crackles. Fine, inspiratory crackles are more likely to represent atelectasis, pulmonary fibrosis, CHF, or an acute inflammatory process in elderly patients.[14] When present, coarse crackles heard on both inspiration and expiration that do not clear with a cough may indicate an upper respiratory infection or severe pulmonary edema. Although very different diseases processes, both CHF and asthma may cause wheezing due to the airway edema that generally accompanies these conditions.

SIMPLY STATED

During auscultation, start on the back and at the lung bases, place the stethoscope on the patient's skin, and listen for a full I/E cycle.

Cardiac Auscultation

The growing population of older patients is presenting a unique challenge for health care providers. Care of adult patients requires at least a working knowledge of cardiac assessment. Cardiac conduction defects, disease, and valvular incompetence can all result in altered heart sounds and murmurs.

Heart Sounds

In about 30% to 40% of elderly patients, you may note an audible splitting of the second heart sound (S_2). Significant splitting of the S_2 that increases with inspiration suggests the presence of right bundle branch block. An S_3 is indicative of ventricular disease in elderly patients and can be auscultated in the same vertical line as S_2, but about 2 inches lower at the fourth intercostal space. It may be one of the earliest markers of CHF. S_4 sounds, when present, can be heard best on the left side, at the fifth intercostal space, midclavicular line. An S_4 is a sign of ventricular disease, as in the patient with CHF or recent MI.

Heart Murmurs

Heart murmurs are a swooshing sound also described as sustained noises (e.g., blowing, harsh, rough, or rumbling sounds). Heart murmurs are most often the result of valvular heart disease and can be caused by stenosis, regurgitation, or valvular incompetence. Murmurs can be further classified as systolic or diastolic. Systolic ejection murmurs, usually in the aortic valve, are detected in about

50% of elderly patients.[12] Some murmurs indicate life-threatening illness. Trauma, infective endocarditis, aortic dissection, papillary muscle, or septal rupture are all acute, severe heart problems and may cause harsh regurgitant murmurs. Urgent attention is indicated.

Infective endocarditis has become more prevalent in older adults despite advances in antibiotic therapy. The increased numbers of older adults accounts for some of the statistical increases. Also factoring into the picture are an increase in the number of older adults with prosthetic valves, a higher prevalence of hospital-acquired bacteremia, and longer survival of persons with a history of rheumatic heart disease. Cardiac murmurs are found in more than 90% of patients with infective endocarditis.[6]

Heart sounds are usually softer in older adults. This may be the result of weakened myocardial function or an increased AP diameter. An increased AP diameter increases the distance between the heart and chest wall and will make detection of the heart sounds more difficult. Take time to listen to heart sounds. The more you listen, the more skilled you will become at distinguishing subtle abnormalities.

SIMPLY STATED

Chest auscultation of an elderly patient can provide a quick and accurate assessment of both the heart and lungs.

Diagnostic Tests

Physiologic and structural changes in the pulmonary system will be manifested as alterations in common diagnostic tests. Arterial blood gases, pulse oximetry, and pulmonary function studies reveal age-associated changes. Age-appropriate norms should be taken into consideration when interpreting diagnostic tests.

Gas Exchange

The effects of pulmonary aging result in a reduced vital capacity and expiratory flow rates as well as reduced partial pressure of arterial oxygenation (Pao_2). To a certain degree, gas exchange is altered even in healthy older adults.

As stated earlier, there is an age-associated loss of alveolar surface area. The alveolar-arterial oxygen partial pressure gradient ($P[A-a]o_2$) is also increased in older adults; this could be a consequence of either intrapulmonary shunting, diffusion limitation of oxygen and carbon dioxide gas exchange, or ventilation-perfusion ($\dot{V}/\dot{Q}$) abnormalities. A study was conducted on normal subjects (lifetime nonsmokers with normal spirometry) aged 18 to 71 years. The age-related increase in $\dot{V}/\dot{Q}$ mismatching was confirmed, but it was not as great as expected. The amount of intrapulmonary shunting was almost negligible (<1% of cardiac output in 90% of cases), and the Pao_2 was reduced but only slightly.[31]

Arterial Blood Gases

Pao_2 (arterial oxygen) declines with age. The linear deterioration of arterial oxygen tension associated with aging is now projected to be about –0.245 mm Hg per year[31] (Table 13-1).

The age-associated decline in Pao_2, although predictable, has been the subject of recent investigation. Some of the traditional arterial oxygenation reference studies did not include adequate samples of subjects older than 60 years, yet these studies were used to extrapolate beyond age 60 years.[32] A newer study conducted in 1995 included a large sample of subjects aged 40 to 90 years. This investigation demonstrated that Pao_2 values clearly declined up to age 75 years and then tended to rise (Fig. 13-2). The mean Pao_2 value for adults older than 75 years was demonstrated to be approximately 83 mm Hg.[33] A more recent study (1999) measured Pao_2 on more than 330 healthy subjects aged 18 to 81 years at two different barometric pressures—sea level and 1400 meters. The decline in Pao_2 in this study (–0.245 mm Hg/year) was consistent with the decline in other studies.[30,34,35]

Arterial oxygenation values are used to determine therapeutic interventions and eligibility for home oxygen therapy; thus, it is important for therapists to understand the effect of body position and gender on Pao_2. A blood gas drawn from an older patient in the supine position on average will produce a Pao_2 about 5 mm Hg less than that produced in the seated position.[30] Interestingly, after age 75 years, Pao_2 also tends to be higher in males than in females.[34]

Even though the Pao_2 is reduced as a result of aging, in the absence of disease, the Pao_2 is adequate to provide for tissue oxygenation. Oxygen consumption declines with age in both males and females as a result of reduced metabolism and the replacement of lean tissue with fat.

Some hypercapnia is occasionally noted in elderly patients, but there does not seem to be a consistent age-related alteration in partial pressure of arterial carbon dioxide ($Paco_2$). Mild hypercapnia in elderly patients could be the result of numerous physiologic changes in the lung seen with age.[34]

Pulse Oximetry

The mild reduction in Pao_2 common to older adults will be consistent with lower oxygen saturation as measured by pulse oximetry (Spo_2), but in a healthy older adult, saturations should be above 93% to 94%. A Pao_2 of 60 mm Hg corresponds to a Spo_2 of about 90%. As long as the patient's Pao_2 values remain on the flat portion of the oxyhemoglobin dissociation curve, the aging process does not significantly decrease the Spo_2.

Some factors that may cause pulse oximeters to inaccurately record Spo_2 are severe or rapid desaturation, hypotension, hypothermia, abnormal hemoglobin, and low perfusion.[35] The presence of a good, measurable pulse is essential to the measurement of Spo_2. Unfortunately, in some older patients with poor perfusion or circulation, obtaining a reading can be a problem.

SIMPLY STATED

Both Pao_2 and Spo_2 decline slightly with age.

Pulmonary Function Studies

After the age of 25 years, pulmonary function in adults starts to decline gradually. The loss of elastic recoil and stiffening of the chest wall shift the balance of lung volumes and capacities. The total lung capacity and tidal volume remain relatively stable throughout the adult life span. The big change is in the RV, which almost doubles with advanced age.

The effect of senescence on pulmonary function measurements has been well documented. When trying to diagnose functional impairment of airflow by

TABLE 13-1	
Estimated Age-Associated Change in Pao_2 by Decade	
Age (yr)	**Estimated Pao_2 (mm Hg)**
10	100
20	97.55
30	95.1
40	92.65
50	90.2
60	87.75
70	85.30
80	82.85
90	80.4
100	77.95

Pao_2, partial pressure of arterial oxygenation.

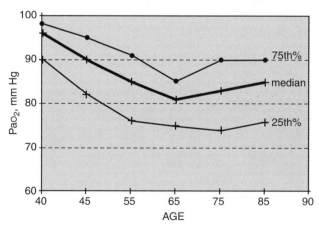

FIGURE 13-2 In healthy people, arterial oxygen (Pao_2) decreases throughout middle age but stabilizes beyond age 65 years. (Redrawn from Hazzard WR, Blass JP, Halter JB, et al, editors: *Principles of geriatric medicine and gerontology*, ed 5, New York, 2003, McGraw-Hill.)

performing pulmonary function studies in older adults, it is important that age-appropriate norms be used as a standard (Box 13-2).

The effect of changes in lung and chest wall mechanics cause forced vital capacity (FVC) and FEV_1 to diminish as early as age 20 years. The mean rate of decline is approximately 30 mL/year for men and 23 mL/year for women.[6]

Diffusing capacity of the lung for carbon monoxide (Dlco) peaks in persons in their early 20s and then gradually decreases. The reduction is estimated to be 2.03 mL/minute per mm Hg per year in men.[6] Women normally have a 10% lower diffusing capacity than men of equal height and weight. As a result of age-related changes in $\dot{V}/\dot{Q}$ and loss of alveolar surface area, the age-related decline in Dlco is not linear. Decremental changes in total pulmonary diffusing capacity become more prominent after 40 years of age.[6]

Standard pulmonary function testing in elderly people requires significant coordination and cooperation on the part of the therapist and patient. Explaining the procedure to the patient may take additional time and require more demonstration. Frequent maneuvers such as repeated breath holding and timed effort-dependent exhalations are required. The extra exertion may be difficult for some patients. After obtaining the best data possible, a consultation with the pulmonologist concerning the patient's level of comprehension and performance may assist in the interpretation of results.

Prediction regression formulas for pulmonary function tests and prediction nomograms for spirometric values are available. The formulas are both age variable and gender specific. The nomograms can accommodate persons aged 20 to 90 years and are also gender specific.

It is important to remember that the predicted values are derived from a statistical analysis of "normal" subjects. These test subjects are classified as normal based on the absence of history or symptoms of lung disease in themselves or their families. Minimal exposure to environmental risk factors (e.g., smoking or pollution) would also be a criterion in selecting these subjects.[36]

Older adults being seen by pulmonary specialists rarely are without a component of lung disease or environmental risk factors. When interpreting pulmonary function studies as part of a geriatric assessment, the age-related deviation from normal must be taken into consideration.

Laboratory Values

Many factors are responsible for the alteration in laboratory values of older adults. Diet, exercise, multisystem disease, and physiologic and structural age-related changes are all variables, which make determination of normal a challenge. The normal value for a laboratory test is its mean value ±2 standard deviations in a population of healthy persons.[6] An abnormal result does not necessarily confirm the presence of disease or disorder. The likelihood of disease is estimated by knowing the test's specificity and sensitivity. Clinicians do not always have precise information on the specificity and sensitivity of tests in elderly patients, and the prevalence of disease often differs in older populations.[6] Chapter 7 outlines clinical laboratory studies, and Box 13-3 shows some laboratory values and the increases and decreases that can result from the aging process.

Box 13-3	Effect of Aging on Laboratory Values

INCREASED VALUES
- Sedimentation rate (mild elevation)
- Glucose
- Cholesterol
- Triglycerides
- Uric acid
- Fibrinogen
- Copper
- Norepinephrine
- Prostate-specific antigen
- Serum potassium (slight increase)

DECREASED VALUES
- Creatinine clearance
- Albumin
- Calcium
- Iron
- Phosphorus
- Zinc
- Vitamins B_6, $B1_2$, and C

UNCHANGED VALUES
- Hemoglobin
- Red blood cell count
- White blood cell count
- Blood urea nitrogen
- Serum creatinine
- Serum electrolytes (sodium, chloride, and bicarbonate)

Data from Abrams WB, Beers MH, Berkow R, editors: *The Merck manual of health and aging*, Whitehouse Station, NJ, 2004, Merck; and Lamy PP: *Prescribing for the elderly*, New York, NY, 1980, PSG.

Box 13-2	Age-Associated Pulmonary Function Test Changes

- Reduced vital capacity, both slow and forced
- Reduced peak expiratory flows
- Reduced inspiratory capacity
- Reduced $FEF_{25-75\%}$
- Reduced FEV_1
- Decreased diffusing capacity
- Increased RV
- Increased FRC

FEF, Forced expiratory flow; FEV_1, forced expiratory volume in 1 second; RV, residual volume; FRC, functional residual capacity.

Hematology

Total hemoglobin in both males and females may remain in the normal range or decrease slightly with age. The decrease is related to the reduced formation and development of blood cells in the bone marrow. In men, reduced hemoglobin may also be a factor of a drop in androgen. Hematocrit may also decrease slightly, which is related to reduced hematopoiesis (see Chapter 7). Aging is not associated with significant changes in the white cell count; however, leukopenia, most frequently neutropenia, occurs in conjunction with a broad spectrum of medical problems. In older adults, leukopenia is likely the result of acquired or secondary disorders, either reactive (e.g., medications, nutritional deficits, infections, or diminished T and B lymphocytes) or malignant.[15]

Blood Chemistry

Age-related albumin reduction is related to a reduced liver size, blood flow, and enzyme production. Low serum albumin can also be a factor of malnutrition. Blood urea nitrogen (BUN) may remain unchanged or may increase when related to compromised renal function. Creatinine (Cr) clearance declines, but serum Cr levels remain stable because elderly persons have less muscle mass. Cr clearance as a measure of kidney function is useful information in prescribing drugs for elderly people. Formulas and nomograms are available for determining age-adjusted normal values for clearance of creatinine. In patients with a reduced Cr clearance, some drugs need to be modified as to dosage to prevent the development of a drug toxicity.

Serum calcium levels will be slightly decreased, whereas potassium will be slightly increased. Fasting glucose increases with age, but values usually remain within the normal range. Glucose tolerance decreases gradually with age. The lack of exercise, obesity, and some medications, however, can exert more influence on glucose tolerance than age alone. When testing for glucose tolerance, there will be a higher peak in 2 hours with a slower decline to base in older adults.[29]

Variability is a hallmark of aging, so it is difficult to extrapolate norms with confidence in elderly people. The establishment of norms for each individual when healthy would be useful to compare with laboratory values when diagnosing a new condition or disease. This, of course, is not feasible with anything except routine tests performed at the time of annual physical examinations. The value of doing an occasional blood screening test in healthy elderly adults is appreciated, however, when facing a challenging disease or diagnosis.

SIMPLY STATED

In older adults, do not assume that variations from the norm are always abnormal or that normal values are always an indicator of health.

Comprehensive Geriatric Assessment

Performing a comprehensive geriatric assessment has become an established component of medical practice, given the growing population of older adults. The needs of many frail elderly patients are too broad to be met by an assessment based only on diagnosis. The symptoms that cause the patient to seek medical attention are not always directly related to the disease, and a more thorough investigation is warranted. For example, a patient may seek help because of an unstable gait and an inability to walk. The underlying diagnosis may be CHF that has produced peripheral edema, causing problems with physical movement before the obvious shortness of breath is noticeable.

Comprehensive geriatric assessment is considered by most geriatricians to be an important and effective form of secondary and tertiary care for elderly patients.[37] Recently, some managed care organizations have realized the potential benefits of preventive intervention. The principal forces driving the managed care of older patients are the U.S. Congress and the Center for Medicare and Medicaid Services (CMS). The Congressional Balanced Budget Act of 1997 mandated that Medicare managed care organizations establish "coordinated care plans, which include health maintenance organizations (HMOs), provider sponsored associations (PSOs), and preferred provider organizations (PPOs), Medicare Medical Savings Account (MSA) plans, private-fee-for-service (PFFS) plans, and Religious Fraternal Benefit (RFB) plans." This was originally known as the Medicare+ Choice program and is currently referred to as Medicare Advantage.[36] Coordinated care planning opens the door to an opportunity to apply principles of geriatric assessment to a large population of older adults.

An improvement in functional ability, rather than a cure, is often the most important goal of geriatric assessment. Geriatric assessment is time consuming. It involves not only physical health but also upper and lower extremity function, nutrition, and mental status. Screening for depression, urinary incontinence, a social support network, the adequacy and safety of the home environment, and functional ability are all components of the comprehensive geriatric assessment (Fig. 13-3).

Functional Ability

Although not usually assessed by RTs, the functional ability of older adults is closely related to a perceived index of health. As a general rule, health in older adults is usually not defined as staying out of the hospital so much as it is retaining the ability to perform daily activities.[38] An often-heard statement from older adults is "I don't feel old as long as I can get around and do things."

Knowing that "health" is so closely correlated with "ability" in older patients, perhaps a brief review of a

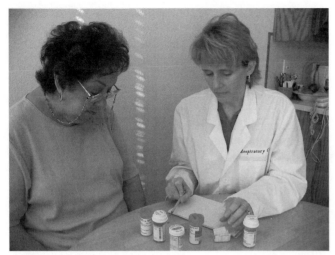

FIGURE 13-3 Ensuring that patients understand their medication regimens is very important.

patient's abilities would be beneficial. How often, as clinicians, do we deal with older patients suffering from hospital psychosis? When patients are out of their familiar environment, away from their usual caregivers, and sick, depression often becomes a problem. Asking simple questions about their abilities may put a more positive focus on what the patients can do versus the temporary losses they are suffering. A positive attitude can have a large impact on a patient's outlook for recovery.

Activities of Daily Living

A number of instruments have been developed for measuring the older adult's ability to complete activities of daily living (ADLs). The basic ADLs usually assessed are mobility and the ability to participate in personal hygiene and grooming, feed oneself, carry out toileting, and dress oneself. To carry out these ADLs, patients must have sufficient range of motion, strength, and endurance.

Instrumental Activities of Daily Living

Some measurement tools, known as instrumental activities of daily living (IADLs), have been designed to evaluate more complex skills. Household management skills, money management, ability to use the telephone, writing skills, and the ability to shop are categorized as IADLs. Only about 5% of adults older than 65 years in the United States are residents of nursing homes, so the hospitalized patient population includes a large percentage of noninstitutionalized older adults with a relatively high degree of functional ability.

Deterioration of functional ability in a previously unimpaired elderly person is an early, subtle sign of illness and is often not accompanied by typical disease signs and symptoms. As soon as functional impairment develops, a thorough clinical evaluation will best serve the patient in maintaining quality of life.

CASE STUDY

A breathing treatment with albuterol has been ordered for an 86-year-old female patient with asthma. She also has macular degeneration, and her vision is very poor. She lives in an assisted living facility and is otherwise fairly functional.

1. What are some of the issues related to medication delivery for this patient that need to be addressed? Will she be able to actuate a metered-dose inhaler (MDI)? Will her inspiratory flow be great enough to use a dry powder inhaler (DPI)? Will she see well enough to manipulate these medication delivery devices? If she is given more than one MDI/DPI, how will she tell them apart? Will a small volume nebulizer (SVN) or handheld nebulizer be the best choice? If an SVN is selected, will she be able to see to dispense the medication into the nebulizer cup?

CASE STUDY—cont'd

2. How common is asthma in older adults? Asthma is a common disease, estimated in the general population to affect 6% to 7% of individuals. Asthma incidence in adults over 70 years old is estimated to be 7% to 9%. Asthma in elderly people has previously been underestimated (often misclassified as COPD). Older adults with asthma also have greater respiratory symptoms and more comorbidities than younger adults (18 to 34 years old).

3. What are some adaptations to the selected medication delivery device that would this patient once she is discharged from the hospital?

   This patient is visually impaired, so careful consideration must be given to what method of aerosol delivery is best. If an MDI or more than one MDI is used, some type of tactile adaptation (e.g., puff paint, 1 dot versus 2 dots on the outside of the inhaler) is needed. Slipping a short length of large-bore flex tubing over the inhaler also gives it a different feel than the smooth inhalers. Therapists can be creative in helping visually impaired patients distinguish among MDIs. If an SVN is ordered, the patient needs to have a supply of unit dose medications and the ability to open the vials and place the medicine in the cup. DPIs might be too much of a challenge for a visually impaired older adult.

CASE STUDY

A 78-year-old retired male executive presents to the clinic with complaints of fatigue and shortness of breath that have worsened over the past weeks to months.

1. What are some possible diagnoses based only on this information?

   Fatigue and dyspnea are abnormal in older adults and should be investigated. Many times, older adults falsely presume that these are just normal old-age symptoms and tend to ignore them. Presenting symptoms of dyspnea and fatigue may be cardiac related (e.g., CHF) or pulmonary related (e.g., pneumonia, fungal disease, or pulmonary hypertension). Depression should also be ruled out because that may also manifest as dyspnea and fatigue.

   Physical examination reveals the following: temperature, 98.4° F; blood pressure, 200/110 mm Hg; pulse, 100 beats/minute; respiratory rate, 28 breaths/minute; height, 6 feet, 1 inch; weight, 66 kg. The patient is alert and in no obvious distress, but on further questioning, he admits to having a lot of heartburn, the inability to walk as far as he used to, and sleeping at night with two or three pillows or in his recliner.

2. Based on this information, what abnormalities are noted, and what diagnosis should be considered?

   The elevated blood pressure, increased respiratory rate, and orthopnea suggest CHF. Although the patient has a seemingly normal body temperature, understanding that body temperatures are lower in older adults should lead to a consideration that 98.4° F may be an elevated temperature in this patient. A chest radiograph to rule out pneumonia might be a good idea. "Heartburn" may be

masking pathology and needs to be investigated. Clinicians should also recognize that this patient's calculated ideal body weight is about 84 kg, whereas his real weight is 66 kg. Malnourishment adds another complicating factor when considering a diagnosis.

ASSESSMENT QUESTIONS

See Appendix for answers.

1. Which of the following is true about communicating with older adult patients?
   a. It is waste of time if they cannot respond
   b. It is unnecessary; just check their ID band
   c. It is a time-consuming task if done appropriately
   d. It is impossible when they cannot see or hear well

2. Which of the following statements reflect an ageist attitude?
   a. Many older adults have poor vision.
   b. Most older adults are sick and frail.
   c. Many older adults have some measure of hearing loss.
   d. Most older adults have some degree of cardiac hypertrophy.

3. Which of the following medications may cause ototoxicity?
   a. Theophylline
   b. Atropine sulfate
   c. Antihistamines
   d. Aspirin

4. The major risk factor associated with development of cataract is?
   a. Age
   b. Smoking
   c. Alcohol consumption
   d. Overexposure to bright light

5. Normal age-related restructuring of the heart results in an enlargement of what structure?
   a. Left ventricular
   b. Right ventricular
   c. Left atrial
   d. Right atrial

6. Typical symptoms of right-sided heart failure include all of the following except which one?
   a. Jugular venous distention
   b. Cheyne-Stokes breathing
   c. Cyanosis
   d. Hepatomegaly

7. Which of the following is not an age-related pulmonary change?
   a. Loss of elastic recoil
   b. Increase in FRC
   c. Increase in total lung compliance
   d. Decrease in vital capacity

8. Blunted cell-mediated immunity in older adults is one factor in the increased incidence of:
   a. Pneumonia
   b. Leukemia
   c. Emphysema
   d. Tuberculosis

9. A 90-year-old patient is admitted to the hospital with a diagnosis of pneumonia. Based on your knowledge of pneumonia in older adults, the clinical presentation would most likely include:
   a. An increased respiratory rate
   b. A productive cough
   c. An elevated body temperature
   d. Radiating chest pain

10. Which of the following is the definition of pulse pressure?
    a. A palpable apical pulse
    b. A pulse felt over the point of maximal impulse
    c. The sum of systolic and diastolic pressures
    d. The difference between systolic and diastolic pressures

11. Syncope associated with standing up quickly may be the result of which of the following?
    a. Hyperthermia
    b. Orthostatic hypertension
    c. Orthostatic hypotension
    d. Pulmonary hypertension

12. Which of the following is an abnormal heart sound in older adults that may be an early sign of CHF?
    a. S_1
    b. S_2
    c. S_3
    d. S_4

13. Which serum value may decrease as a result of the normal aging process?
    a. Glucose
    b. Calcium
    c. Creatinine
    d. Cholesterol

14. Which of the following activities is classified as an IADL?
    a. Combing one's own hair
    b. Walking from the bedroom to the kitchen
    c. Calling the neighbor on the telephone
    d. Getting dressed by oneself

15. Based on current data, which of the following is the projected Pao_2 of a healthy 74-year-old person?
    a. 74.4 mm Hg
    b. 80.8 mm Hg
    c. 84.2 mm Hg
    d. 87.2 mm Hg

16. Approximately what percentage of adults older than 65 years of age in the United States live in a nursing home?
    a. 5%
    b. 10%
    c. 15%
    d. 20%

17. A normal Spo_2 percent for a healthy active older adult should be no lower than which of the following?
    a. 98
    b. 96
    c. 94
    d. 92

18. Lower systolic blood pressure in an adult will cause which of the following?
    a. Increased risk for stroke
    b. Decreased risk for stroke
    c. Orthostatic hypotension
    d. Syncope

19. Ageism is defined as which of the following?
    a. A study of the effects of aging on older adults
    b. Sociologic consequences of aging and how they affect individuals
    c. A discriminatory attitude against older adults
    d. The realization that all older adults are sick and frail

References

1. *National Association for Area Agencies on Aging Policy Priorities.* Washington, DC: The Association; 2011.
2. United States Census. *Statistical Abstract of the United States.* www.census.gov:2012 Accessed March 21.
3. Siedman MD, Ahmad N, Bai U, et al. Molecular mechanisms of age-related hearing loss. *Ageing Res Rev* 2002;**1**:331.
4. Keller BK, Morton JL, Thomas VS, et al. The effect of visual and hearing impairment on functional status. *J Am Geriatr Soc* 1999;**47**:1319.
5. Noell CA, Meyerhoff WL. Tinnitus: diagnosis and treatment of this elusive symptom. *Geriatrics* 2003;**58**:28.
6. Beers MH. *The Merck manual of health and aging.* Whitehouse Station, NJ: Merck; 2004.
7. Mulrow CD, Lichtenstein MJ. Screening for hearing impairment in the elderly: rationale and strategy. *J Gen Intern Med* 1991;**6**:249.
8. Brennan M, Cardinali G. The use of preexisting and novel coping strategies in adapting to age-related vision loss. *Gerontologist* 2000;**40**:327.
9. Stevenson MR, Hart PM, Montgomery AM, et al. Reduced vision in older adults with age-related macular degeneration interferes with ability to care for self and impairs role as carer. *Br J Ophthalmol* 2004;**88**:1125.
10. Warnecke P. A caregiver's eye on elders with low vision. *CARING Magazine* 2003;**11**:25.
11. Oxenham H, Sharpe N. Cardiovascular aging and heart failure. *Eur J Heart Failure* 2003;**5**:427.
12. Kaloustian K. Effects of exercise on the cardiovascular system, Presented at the Association for Gerontology in Higher Education Annual Meeting. *San Jose, CA* February 2001;**9**:22.
13. Waktare JEP. Atrial fibrillation. *Circulation* 2002;**106**:14.
14. Connolly MJ. *Respiratory disease in the elderly.* London: Chapman & Hall; 2007.
15. Halter J. *Hazzard's principles of geriatric medicine and gerontology.* 6th ed. New York, NY: McGraw-Hill; 2009.
16. Emmett KR. Nonspecific and atypical presentation of disease in the older patient. *Geriatrics* 1998;**53**:50.
17. Feldman C. Pneumonia in the elderly. *Clin Chest Med* 1999;**20**:563.

18. Ham RJ, Sloane PD, Warshaw GA. *Primary care geriatrics.* 4th ed. Saint Louis: Mosby; 2002.

19. Huss K, Travis P. Prevalence, severity of asthma continues to rise in the elderly. *Acad News Am Acad Allerg Asthma Immunol* February/March 1997.

20. Braman SS. Asthma in the elderly. *Clin Geriatr Med* 2003;**19**:57.

21. Enright PL, McClelland RL, Newman AB, et al. Underdiagnosis and undertreatment of asthma in the elderly. Cardiovascular Health Study Research Group. *Chest* 1999;**116**:603.

22. Petty TL, Seebass JS. *Pulmonary disorders of the elderly: diagnosis, prevention and treatment.* Philadelphia: American College of Chest Physicians; 2007.

23. Perry Jr HM, Davis BR, Price TR, et al. Effect of treating isolated systolic hypertension on the risk of developing various types and subtypes of stroke: the Systolic Hypertension in the Elderly Program (SHEP). *JAMA* 2000;**284**:465–71.

24. Lewington S, Clarke R, Qizilbash N, et al. Age-specific relevance of usual blood pressure to vascular mortality: a meta-analysis of individual data for one million adults in 61 prospective studies. *Lancet* 2002;**360**:1903.

25. Goldstein LB, Hankey GJ. Advances in primary stroke prevention. *Stroke* 2006;**37**:317.

26. Griffth RW. High blood pressure: new guidelines are out!. *Health and Age* 2003:June 5.

27. Chobanian AV, Bakris GL, Black HR, et al. The Seventh Report of the Joint National Committee on Prevention, Detection, Evaluation, and Treatment of High Blood Pressure: the JNC 7 report. *JAMA* 2003;**289**:2560.

28. Skidmore-Roth L. *Nurses drug reference.* Saint Louis: Mosby-Elsevier; 2011.

29. Emlet CA, Crabtree JL, Condon V, et al. *In home assessment of older adults: an interdisciplinary approach.* Gaithersburg, Md: Aspen Publishers; 1996.

30. Hardie JA, Morkve O, Ellingsen I. Effect of body position on arterial oxygen tensions in the elderly. *Respiration* 2002;**69**:123.

31. Cardús J, Burgos F, Diaz O, et al. Increase in pulmonary ventilation-perfusion inequality with age in healthy subjects. *Am J Respir Crit Care Med* 1997;**156**:648.

32. Cerveri I, Zoia MC, Fanfulla F, et al. Reference values of arterial oxygen tension in the middle-aged and elderly individuals. *Am J Respir Crit Care Med* 1995;**152**:934.

33. Crapo RO, Jensen RL, Hegewald M, et al. Arterial blood gas reference values for sea level and an altitude of 1,400 meters. *Am J Respir Crit Care Med* 1999;**160**:1525.

34. Hardie JA, Vollmer WM, Buist S, et al. Reference values for arterial gases in the elderly. *Chest 125* 2004:2053.

35. Jensen LA, Onyskiw JE, Prasad NG, et al. Meta-analysis of arterial oxygen saturation monitoring by pulse oximetry in adults. *Heart Lung* 1998;**27**:387.

36. Thorson JA. *Aging in a changing society.* Belmont, CA: Wadsworth; 1995.

37. Bickeley L, Szilagyi P. *Bates' guide to physical examination and history taking.* Philadelphia: Lippincott Williams &Wilkins; 2009.

38. Saxon SV, Etten MJ, Perkins EA. *Physical change and aging.* New York, NY: Springer; 2010.

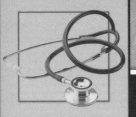

Chapter 14

Respiratory Monitoring in Critical Care

DAVID L. VINES*

CHAPTER OUTLINE

Ventilatory Assessment
  Lung Volumes and Flows
  Airway Pressures
  Integrating Pressure, Flow, and Volume
  Fractional Gas Concentrations
Evaluation of Oxygenation
  Evaluation of Oxygen Transport
  Monitoring the Adequacy of Arterial
    Oxygenation
**Monitoring Tissue Oxygen Delivery
  and Utilization**
  Oxygen Delivery and Availability
  Oxygen Consumption

Mixed Venous Oxygen Tension
Mixed Venous Oxygen Saturation
Arterial-to-Mixed Venous Oxygen Content
  Difference
Oxygen Extraction Ratio
Blood Lactate
Regional Tissue Oxygenation (Near Infrared
  Spectroscopy)

LEARNING OBJECTIVES

After reading this chapter, you will be able to:
1. Identify the methods, normal values, and significance of measuring the following lung volumes in the intensive care unit:
   a. Tidal volume
   b. Rapid-shallow breathing index
   c. Vital capacity
   d. Functional residual capacity
2. Identify the methods, normal values, and significance of measuring the following airway pressures or related indices in the intensive care unit:
   a. Peak pressure
   b. Plateau pressure
   c. Compliance
   d. Airway resistance
   e. Mean airway pressure
   f. Maximum inspiratory pressure
3. List the definition, methods of detection, and methods of minimizing auto-PEEP.
4. Describe the value of monitoring pressure, volume and flow waveforms, and pressure-volume curves in mechanically ventilated patients.
5. Describe the methods and significance of measuring the fraction of inspired oxygen and exhaled carbon dioxide in the intensive care unit.
6. List the components of oxygen transport and their significance.
7. List the components involved in the clinical evaluation of oxygenation and their significance.
8. Explain how the following parameters can be used to evaluate tissue oxygen delivery and utilization:
   a. Oxygen delivery and availability
   b. Oxygen consumption
   c. Mixed venous oxygen tension

*Michael H. Terry and Tom Malinowski contributed some of the content for this chapter as contributors of a prior edition of this text.

LEARNING OBJECTIVES—cont'd

    d. Venous saturation
    e. Arterial-to-mixed venous oxygen content difference
    f. Oxygen extraction ratio
    g. Blood lactate
    h. Regional tissue oxygenation
  9. Describe the value and limitations of pulse oximetry in monitoring oxygenation and oxygen delivery.
10. Identify the techniques for monitoring tissue oxygenation and utilization.

KEY TERMS

airway resistance	dynamic hyperinflation	oxygen consumption
alveolar dead space	end-tidal P_{CO_2}	oxygen content
anatomic dead space	Fick principle	oxygen delivery (D_{O_2})
arterial-to-alveolar tension ratio	functional residual capacity (FRC)	oxygen extraction ratio ($C(a - \bar{v})_{O_2}/C_{aO_2}$)
arterial-to-mixed venous oxygen content difference ($C(a - \bar{v})_{O_2}$)	iatrogenic	oxygen transport
	intrapulmonary shunt ($\dot{Q}_s/\dot{Q}_t$)	oxyhemoglobin dissociation curve
auto–positive end-expiratory pressure (auto-PEEP)	lower inflection point	peak inspiratory pressure (PIP)
	maximum inspiratory pressure ($P_I max$)	
barotrauma	mean airway pressure ($P_{\overline{aw}}$)	physiologic dead space
capnography	mixed venous oxygen saturation ($S\bar{v}_{O_2}$)	plateau pressure
capnometry		pressure-volume loop
carbon dioxide production	mixed venous oxygen tension ($P\bar{v}_{O_2}$)	rapid-shallow breathing index (RSBI)
compliance	monitoring	static compliance
dead space–to–tidal volume ratio (V_D/V_T)	near infrared spectroscopy (NIRS)	upper inflection point
dynamic compliance		volutrauma

Monitoring has been defined as "repeated or continuous observations or measurements of the patient, his or her physiologic function, and the function of life support equipment, for the purpose of guiding management decisions, including when to make therapeutic interventions, and assessment of those interventions."[1]

Respiratory monitoring refers to the process of continuously evaluating the cardiopulmonary status of patients for the purpose of improving clinical outcomes. The goals of monitoring include alerting clinicians to changes in the patient's condition and improving our understanding of pathophysiology, diagnosis, and cost-effective clinical management. These goals are accomplished through the use of physical examination, monitoring equipment, measurements, calculations, and alarms.

The goals of this chapter are to introduce the most common forms of respiratory monitoring in the intensive care unit (ICU), describe the information they provide, and discuss their application. Some of the information that normally would be included under respiratory monitoring, such as physical assessment, blood gas interpretation, and hemodynamic monitoring, is reviewed in other chapters of this book.

Ventilatory Assessment

Arterial pressure of carbon dioxide (Pa_{CO_2}) is traditionally thought of as the standard for assessing ventilation (see Chapter 8). However, changes in the patient's metabolism, lung mechanics, ventilatory efficiency, and equipment function will occur before changes are seen in the blood gases. It is therefore important to monitor the ventilatory parameters in addition to the blood gases. Table 14-1 provides a list of frequently used ventilatory parameters and their commonly cited reference ranges and critical values, with the critical value representing the threshold for *insufficiency*. In general, the respiratory therapist (RT) should not judge a patient's status based on a single critical value, but instead should assess these parameters in combination with each other.

The ventilatory measurements that can be monitored at the bedside in the ICU routinely include the following:
- Lung volumes and flows
- Airway pressures
- Fractional gas concentrations

Lung Volumes and Flows

Ventilation is the process of moving gases between the atmosphere and the lung. These gases occupy spaces

TABLE 14-1

Common Parameters Used for Ventilatory Assessment

Parameter	Common Reference Range	Critical Value
Tidal volume (V_T)	5-8 mL/kg PBW	<4-5 mL/kg or <300 mL
Frequency (fb)	12-20 breaths/min	>30-35 breaths/min
Rapid shallow breathing index (RSBI)		>105 without PS or CPAP
Dead space–to–tidal volume ratio (V_D/V_T)	0.25-0.40	>0.60
Minute volume ($\dot{V}_E$)	5 to 6 L/min	>10 L/min
Vital capacity (VC)	65 to 75 mL/kg	<10-15 mL/kg
Maximum inspiratory pressure ($P_I$max)	−80 to −100 cm H_2O	0 to −20 cm H_2O

CPAP, continuous positive airway pressure; PBW, predicted body weight; PS, pressure control.

commonly called *lung volumes*. Although lung volumes have been described and their measurement discussed in Chapter 9, their importance to the critical care clinician is emphasized here.

Why Monitor Lung Volumes?

The reasons that lung volumes are important to the clinician are as follows:
- They affect gas exchange in the lung.
- They reflect changes in the patient's clinical status (improvement or deterioration).
- They indicate response to therapy.
- They signal problems with the patient-ventilator interface (i.e., circuitry or ventilator settings).
- They help ascertain the patient's ability to breath spontaneously or be weaned from mechanical ventilation.

Who Should Be Monitored for Lung Volumes?

Following is a list of the most common circumstances in which patients will benefit from the monitoring of lung volumes:
- Intubated patients
  - Patients being considered for mechanical ventilation
  - Patients receiving and being weaned from mechanical ventilation
  - Patients with an abnormal breathing pattern
- Nonintubated patients
  - Preoperative evaluation (especially upper abdominal and thoracic surgery)
  - Adult patients with respiratory rates greater than 30 breaths/minute
  - Patients with neuromuscular disease
  - Patients with central nervous system (CNS) depression
  - Patients with deteriorating blood gases
  - Patients receiving noninvasive positive-pressure ventilation

What Do We Measure?

Tidal volume (V_T) is defined as the volume of air inspired or passively exhaled in a normal respiratory cycle. V_T for a healthy person varies with each breath but usually ranges between 5 to 8 mL/kg of predicted body weight.[2]

V_T has two components: alveolar volume (V_A), or the portion of V_T that effectively exchanges with alveolar-capillary blood, and dead space volume (V_D), or the portion of V_T that does not exchange with capillary blood. The common reference range cited for V_D is 25% to 40% of the V_T. The conductive airways and alveolar units that are ventilated but not perfused create the true or **physiologic dead space**. If the dead space exceeds 60% of the V_T, the patient may need ventilator support to help with the associated increase in the work of breathing.[2]

In healthy, spontaneously breathing people, the V_T occasionally increases to three or four times normal levels. These larger tidal breaths are known as *sighs* and normally occur about 6 to 10 times each hour. In acutely ill patients, there is often a loss of the sigh, and the size of the patient's V_T tends to diminish.[3] A V_T less than 5 mL/kg may indicate the onset of a respiratory problem.[2] Impending respiratory failure causes V_T to become more irregular.[4] If shallow breathing without occasional sighing is maintained for prolonged periods, atelectasis and pneumonia may result, especially in patients breathing high oxygen concentrations or having compromised mucociliary clearance.

SIMPLY STATED

Rapid and shallow breathing in a critically ill patient at rest may indicate impending respiratory failure.

Conditions that may cause the V_T to be reduced include pneumonia, atelectasis, chest or abdominal surgery, chest trauma, acute exacerbation of chronic obstructive pulmonary disease (COPD), congestive heart failure (CHF), pulmonary edema, acute restrictive diseases such as acute respiratory distress syndrome (ARDS), neuromuscular diseases, and CNS depression (especially of the respiratory centers). Larger than normal V_T may be seen with metabolic acidosis, sepsis, or severe neurologic injury.

Critically ill patients without an artificial airway may not tolerate the measurement of V_T. To accurately measure V_T, a facemask or mouthpiece is required. Patients often change their breathing patterns when a mask or mouthpiece is applied, which alters their V_T.

Patients receiving continuous mechanical ventilation (CMV) are routinely ventilated with V_T of 8 to 10 mL/kg, approximately two times the normal spontaneous V_T. When normal spontaneous V_T is used during CMV without positive end-expiratory pressure (PEEP), there is a reduction in **functional residual capacity (FRC)**, an increase in intrapulmonary shunt, and a fall in partial pressure of arterial oxygen (Pa_{O_2}). These potentially harmful conditions can be reversed in part or totally by increasing the V_T or by applying PEEP.[5]

The use of higher V_T ventilation can cause complications, particularly in patients with severe respiratory failure.[6-9] Evidence exists that lung injury may occur with a high V_T that increases alveolar pressures (plateau pressure) beyond 30 cm H_2O.[6,9] The use of high-V_T ventilation may predispose patients to **volutrauma**, a lung injury that occurs from overdistention of the terminal respiratory units. Volutrauma often develops in nondependent lung regions and is a main reason why lung damage persists after recovery from severe protracted ARDS.[10] To avoid this lung injury, patients at risk for developing ARDS should be ventilated with mechanical V_T of 6 mL/kg or less at a higher frequency (breaths per minute) to maintain an acceptable acid-base balance (pH > 7.30).[9] Unfortunately, patients receiving low V_T (4 mL/kg) who have a strong respiratory drive may experience breath "stacking."[11] The stacking results from a patient trying to inhale a V_T greater than set, decreasing their airway pressure and triggering an additional breath on top of the previous V_T.

When using a smaller V_T, the application of PEEP maintains FRC and prevents the fall in Pa_{O_2}. Although no single approach to setting PEEP has been adopted, a recent review recommends setting the PEEP level to that resulting in the best compliance and lowest driving pressure.[6]

Monitoring V_T during mechanical ventilation of a critical ill patient is crucial. Discrepancies between set and measured V_T are often seen in these patients. Most of the time, the differences are not clinically significant, and the clinician can make small adjustments in the V_T settings to meet the patient's delivered V_T needs. The differences are often caused by the compressible volume of the ventilator circuit or environmental factors at the different locations of the inspiratory and expiratory flow sensors (i.e., heated, humidified gases or differing flow profiles). Compressible volume is an important consideration in neonatal and pediatric patients and in patients with higher peak airway pressures and lower V_T. Most of today's ventilators will correct for volume loss to the ventilator circuit and humidifier if circuit compliance correction is selected and performed before the ventilator and circuitry are connected to the patient. Other sources that may cause a difference between set and measured V_T include leaks in the ventilator circuit, a leaky endotracheal (ET) tube cuff, and bronchopleural fistula.

A low measured V_T also can be caused by severe air trapping or **dynamic hyperinflation**, which is a problem seen with severe airway obstruction. If not enough time is allowed for exhalation before the next breath is initiated by the ventilator, the subsequent V_T will stack on top of the previous breath. This problem creates higher peak airway pressure, and pressure injury to the lung or **barotrauma** may result. Increasing expiratory time, administering bronchodilators, or decreasing the V_T may help resolve the problem. Expiratory time is increased by reducing ventilator rate (if inspiratory time remains constant), increasing inspiratory flow rate, or decreasing inspiratory time.

If the circuit compliance feature is not used, then corrected tidal volume will need to be calculated. The corrected or delivered V_T is determined by calculating the compressible volume of the ventilator circuit and subtracting it from the exhaled V_T. To calculate the compressible volume of the ventilator circuit, the clinician needs to know the compliance of the ventilator circuit being used. If the circuit's compliance is unknown, then it can be determined by increasing the high pressure limit to 120 cm H_2O, setting PEEP to 0 cm H_2O, and setting a V_T of 100 mL. Then divide the 100 mL by the resulting peak inspiratory pressure to obtain circuit compliance. The compliance of the adult ventilator circuit varies with the structure and diameter of the tubing but is generally 1 to 3 mL/cm H_2O. If the patient is being ventilated with high airway pressures, a significant portion of the V_T is lost to tubing expansion, and erroneous respiratory system compliance measurements would be computed if this loss were not considered.

$$Corr\ V_T = (V_T - [(PIP - EEP) \times CF])$$

where

Corr V_T = corrected or delivered tidal volume

V_T = exhaled tidal volume

PIP = peak inspiratory pressure

EEP = total-end expiratory pressure (defined later)

CF = circuit compliance factor (mL/cm H_2O)

Where V_T is monitored often plays an important role in data interpretation. Proximal volume monitoring eliminates the loss of compressible volume to the circuit and may reflect a more accurately delivered V_T than does expiratory limb monitoring. This is particularly true during conditions of low V_T, low lung compliance, and high **airway resistance** (R_{aw}). Proximal monitoring is not without drawbacks. Proximal sensing makes the measuring device more susceptible to condensate and secretions, potentially reducing reliability and accuracy. It also may increase circuit resistance and dead space, increasing the patient's imposed work of breathing.

Air trapping and dynamic hyperinflation often occur in mechanically ventilated patients with severe airway obstruction. One technique that can measure the degree of dynamic hyperinflation is to measure the volume of gas exhaled during an expiratory hold on a ventilator. This maneuver measures the additional trapped gas above the patient's normal FRC. Ventilatory adjustments that reduce minute ventilation ($\dot{V}_E$), V_T, and lengthen expiratory time should reduce the degree of air trapping.

SIMPLY STATED

V_T for mechanically ventilated patients should be adjusted for clinical conditions. Some patients, including those at risk for air trapping and dynamic hyperinflation or ARDS, should be ventilated with a lower V_T of 6 mL/kg and adjusted down to 4 mL/kg to keep plateau pressure less than 30 cm H_2O or eliminate dynamic hyperinflation.

Box 14-1	Criteria Indicating Failure of a Spontaneous Breathing Trial (SBT)

- Twenty percent increase or decrease in blood pressure or heart rate
- Oxygen saturation via pulse oximetry (SpO_2) ≤ 85%-90%
- Respiratory rate greater than 35 breaths/minute
- Change in patient's mental status, accessory muscle use, or the onset of diaphoresis

Patients receiving synchronous intermittent mandatory ventilation (SIMV) are allowed to breathe spontaneously through the ventilator circuit between mechanical breaths. As a result, their spontaneous V_T may differ in size from the mechanical V_T being delivered by the ventilator. It is important for the clinician to distinguish between spontaneous and mechanical V_T during weaning so that a true assessment of the patient's ventilatory status can be made.

When a patient is ready to be weaned from mechanical ventilation, a spontaneous breathing trial (SBT) should be attempted. The patient should be monitored for gas exchange, respiratory distress, and hemodynamic stability during this trial. Box 14-1 outlines the criteria used to define SBT failure.[12] V_T also may decrease if the patient fatigues during the SBT, as indicated by breath volumes below 300 mL or less than 4 mL/kg.[12] Usually more than one of these signs is present when a patient fails an SBT.

The **rapid-shallow breathing index (RSBI)** incorporates this spontaneous breathing rate change and measures the ratio of respiratory frequency (fb) to V_T.

$$RSBI = f\,(breaths/min)/V_T\,(L)$$

RSBI values greater than 105 have been reported to be strong prognostic indicators of weaning failure.[13] More predictive than a single measurement is the progressive change in RSBI. Patients who demonstrate a significant increase in their RSBI on ventilator removal are very likely to fail weaning.[14,15] Serial measurements of the RSBI during a period of spontaneous breathing may more accurately predict the ability to be successfully weaned from mechanical ventilator support.[15] However, early measures of RSBI during a spontaneous breathing trial appear to be of little value in predicting weaning outcomes in COPD patients.[16]

$\dot{V}_E$ is the product of V_T and respiratory rate or frequency and represents the total volume of gas inspired or exhaled by the patient in 1 minute. The average $\dot{V}_E$ for a normal healthy adult is 5 to 6 L/minute.[2] As with V_T, approximately 25% to 40% of $\dot{V}_E$ is dead space ventilation. $\dot{V}_E$ is often increased in the early stages of respiratory failure; it is not until later stages of failure that $\dot{V}_E$ begins to fall.

$Paco_2$ is considered an indicator of the adequacy of ventilation. The relationship of $\dot{V}_E$ to $Paco_2$ indicates the efficiency of ventilation. A $\dot{V}_E$ of 6 L/minute is usually associated with a $Paco_2$ of approximately 40 mm Hg in a

healthy person with a normal metabolic rate. If a higher than normal $\dot{V}_E$ occurs with a normal $Paco_2$ in a patient with a normal metabolic rate, there must be an increase in dead space ventilation. This is usually associated with hypovolemia, pulmonary embolism, or obstructive disease.

An increase in carbon dioxide production caused by an increased metabolism (as occurs with trauma or fever) or high carbohydrate loading accompanying parenteral feedings may result in an increased in $\dot{V}_E$ with a normal $Paco_2$ (see Chapter 18). The elevated production of CO_2 requires an increase in ventilation to maintain the $Paco_2$ in normal range. Patients with varying metabolic rates should be ventilated with modes that allow them to set their own frequency of breathing and thereby vary $\dot{V}_E$ as needed to maintain a normal $Paco_2$.

A resting spontaneous $\dot{V}_E$ of 10 L/minute or less during an SBT is often considered an acceptable weaning criterion. $\dot{V}_E$ may fluctuate widely both during traditional T-piece weaning and during low-rate SIMV. Many therapeutic activities also can alter $\dot{V}_E$. A good example is the postoperative administration of opiates to control pain. Opiates like morphine can blunt the respiratory drive sufficiently to cause a sudden onset of hypoventilation.

For these reasons, $\dot{V}_E$ should be monitored frequently before and during weaning. A sudden rise or drop in $\dot{V}_E$ should be investigated because both may signal ventilatory failure. If a $\dot{V}_E$ greater than 10 L/minute is needed for a mechanically ventilated patient to maintain a normal $Paco_2$, weaning is not likely to be successful. The elevated $\dot{V}_E$ indicates that the patient's respiratory muscles will probably fatigue when the mechanical ventilation is discontinued. Compared with the RSBI, however, a patient's spontaneous $\dot{V}_E$ is a much less reliable predictor of weaning success.[12,13]

Vital capacity (VC) is the maximum volume of gas that can be expired from the lungs following a maximal inspiration. The typical reference range for healthy subjects is 65 to 75 mL/kg of predicted body weight.[2] The VC maneuver depends on the patient's effort and position; the largest values usually are recorded with the patient in the upright position.

The VC is an excellent measurement of ventilatory reserve in the cooperative patient. It reflects the respiratory muscle strength and volume capacity of the lung while the patient is performing a maximal inspiratory and expiratory maneuver. These are of paramount importance in maintaining an adequate cough to clear secretions and in guaranteeing periodic inflation of alveoli that may be prone to collapse.

As described in Chapter 9, VC can be measured as either a forced maneuver (FVC) or a slow maneuver (SVC). The SVC maneuver may be much easier for the patient to perform, especially if the patient is lethargic, medicated, or experiencing pain or has obstructive airway disease.

The accuracy and repeatability of the values depend on the patient's effort and the coaching skills of the therapist. It is important that the patient understand how to perform the maneuver correctly. A tight seal around the mouthpiece or mask is crucial. The patient may perform better if able to observe the tracing generated by the effort or to receive some similar visual feedback.

During preoperative evaluation of a patient's lung function, an $FEV_1\%$ (ratio of FEV in 1 second to the FVC) less than 50% of normal or an FVC of less than 20 mL/kg indicates that the patient may be at high risk for developing pulmonary complications in the postoperative period. Factors that influence the degree of decrease in VC during the postoperative period and the incidence of postoperative pulmonary complications include the surgical site, smoking history, age, nutritional status, obesity, pain, type of anesthesia, and type of narcotics used for pain control.

Although many factors can contribute to a reduction in VC postoperatively, one of the most important is the incision site. Thoracic and abdominal surgeries produce a significant fall in VC postoperatively, and this reduction may persist for a week or more.[17,18] Operative procedures below the umbilicus are associated with fewer pulmonary complications.

A VC of 10 to 15 mL/kg is usually needed for effective deep breathing and coughing. Values below this range are usually associated with impending respiratory failure.[2] Values greater than 15 mL/kg usually indicate adequate ventilatory reserve and the possibility of discontinuing CMV and extubation.

VC also is measured to follow the responsiveness of the patient to various respiratory therapies such as incentive spirometry or intermittent positive-pressure breathing (IPPB). A common goal of both these maneuvers is to promote lung expansion.

SIMPLY STATED

Serial, not individual, measurements of weaning indices (RSBI, VC, and V_T) are most likely to predict success or failure.

FRC is the volume of gas remaining in the lungs at the end of a normal passive exhalation. It is rarely measured in the ICU. The FRC is continuously in contact with pulmonary capillary blood and undergoing gas exchange. It is composed of a combination of residual volume (RV) and expiratory reserve volume (ERV). Normally, FRC is about 40 mL/kg of predicted body weight, or about 35% to 40% of total lung capacity (TLC). FRC can vary from breath to breath by as much as 300 mL in healthy people.[19] Changes in body position affect FRC, with the greatest values being recorded in the upright position.[20] These changes in FRC between 30-degree Fowler and supine positions may not occur in overweight or obese patients.[21] When alveolar volume falls, as with atelectasis, FRC is reduced, and there are regional changes in alveolar pressure-volume curves. Initially, as FRC decreases, dependent alveoli collapse and

require higher distending pressures to inflate. Because the apical alveoli remain at least partially open, they are more compliant and require less pressure to inflate. Subsequently, during mechanical ventilation, the inspired volumes are preferentially distributed to the apices. This distribution of inspired volumes to nondependent, poorly perfused alveoli contributes to the abnormal gas exchange seen in patients with decreased FRC. Dependent atelectatic alveoli open throughout inspiration as alveolar pressure increases and collapse during expiration. Experimental evidence now demonstrates that repeated collapse and reinflation of alveoli leads to alveolar damage, capillary rupture, and considerable lung injury. The application of PEEP prevents alveolar collapse and may reduce the extent of acute lung injury.[22-24] Therapeutic modalities, such as PEEP or continuous positive airway pressure (CPAP), increase FRC. This is the primary benefit to patients with atelectasis and refractory hypoxemia.

Airway Pressures

It is important to monitor airway pressures for the following reasons:

- To help determine the need for mechanical ventilation and the patient's readiness for weaning
- To help determine the site and thereby the cause of impedance to mechanical ventilation
- To evaluate elastic recoil and compliance of the intact thorax
- To help estimate the amount of positive airway pressure being transmitted to the heart and major vessels
- To help assess the patient's respiratory muscle strength

Airway pressures should be measured as closely as possible to the ET tube. This prevents resistance caused by the ventilator circuit from influencing the peak pressure measurement. On certain occasions, as when using high-frequency ventilation or tracheal gas insufflation (TGI), the pressure should be measured at the distal tip of the ET tube.

Peak Pressure

Peak inspiratory pressure (PIP) is the maximum pressure attained during the inspiratory phase of mechanical ventilation (Fig. 14-1). It reflects the amount of force needed to overcome opposition to airflow into the lungs. Causes of this opposition to flow include resistance generated by the ventilator circuit, the artificial airway (ET tube), and the patient's airways and elastic recoil of the thoracic cage and the lungs. Sudden increases in PIP or peak airway pressure should alert the clinician to the possible presence of a patient-ventilator interface problem. Potential causes of an increase in peak pressure are listed in Box 14-2.

An increase in PIP while the plateau pressure (explained later) remains unchanged suggests an increase in Raw. Common causes include bronchospasm, airway secretions, and mucous plugging. As a result of the relationship between PIP and R_{aw}, monitoring the PIP provides

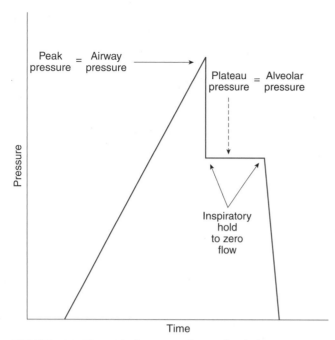

FIGURE 14-1 Theoretical pressure-time scalar during constant flow volume control ventilation. The *solid-lined arrow* indicates peak airway pressure; the *dotted-lined arrow* indicates theoretical alveolar pressure. The difference between the dotted and solid line is the resistive component of the ventilator circuit, endotracheal tube, and airways. Notice that alveolar pressure equates to airway pressure only during the static, no-flow period.

valuable information about the bronchodilator-induced changes in lung function of the mechanically ventilated patient.[25,26] It is important to note that whenever changes in the PIP are used for evaluating Raw, no changes in the inspiratory flow, flow pattern, or V_T should be made.

High PIP may cause barotrauma.[23,27] However, evidence suggests that high peak alveolar pressures from overdistention lead to alveolar rupture, or volutrauma.[23,28] Conditions that raise the PIP may not affect alveolar pressure because of increased inspiratory resistance during mechanical ventilation. Static pressure (plateau pressure) more accurately reflects alveolar pressure than does peak pressure and should be used as the primary indicator of the risk for alveolar rupture.[28]

Plateau Pressure

To determine the cause of an elevated peak pressure, it is beneficial to separate the resistance component from the elastic recoil of the combined lung and chest wall. This can be accomplished by measuring the **plateau pressure**. The plateau pressure (also referred to as *static pressure*) is the pressure required to maintain a delivered V_T in a patient's lungs during a period of no gas flow (see Fig. 14-1). Plateau pressure is measured by occluding an exhalation valve immediately after the set V_T has been delivered and holding the exhalation valve closed until a plateau pressure is observed. In patients with airway obstruction, achievement of a stable plateau pressure may take several seconds. Any

Box 14-2	Potential Causes of Increased Peak Pressure

RESISTANCE FACTORS

PATIENT AIRWAYS
- Bronchospasm
- Peribronchiolar edema
- Retained secretions
- Airway obstruction caused by foreign body

ARTIFICIAL AIRWAY
- Internal diameter of tube too small
- Kinking of endotracheal tube
- Mucous plugging
- Cuff herniation
- Tube impinging on tracheal wall

VENTILATOR CIRCUIT
- Water in tubing
- Kinking of circuit tubing
- High inspiratory flow rates (mechanical)

ELASTIC RECOIL

THORACIC CAGE
- Chest wall deformity
- Obesity
- Abdominal distention, compression, or herniation
- Diaphragmatic and intercostal muscle dyscoordination
- Active expiration, restlessness, pain
- Patient placement in lateral or prone position
- Chest wraps or casts

LUNG INVOLVEMENT
- Acute respiratory failure
- Pneumonia
- Acute respiratory distress syndrome
- Atelectasis
- Pneumothorax
- Fibrosis

patient effort to inhale or exhale during the inspiratory hold can invalidate the measurement (Fig. 14-2).

During the period of no gas flow, the Raw component of ventilation is eliminated, leaving the elastic recoil component as the force required to maintain inflation. If the volume maintained inside the lungs during this plateau period is known, the effective static or respiratory system compliance can be determined.

Mean Airway Pressure

Mean airway pressure ($P_{\overline{aw}}$) is the average pressure recorded during the positive-pressure and spontaneous phases of a respiratory cycle. $P_{\overline{aw}}$ is calculated to determine the average airway pressure being applied to the lungs. Ventilator measurements affecting $P_{\overline{aw}}$ include CPAP and PEEP levels, inspiratory time (flow rate and flow patterns), peak pressure, and rate. A simple method of estimating $P_{\overline{aw}}$ is as follows:[29]

$$P_{\overline{aw}} = [1/2(\text{PIP} - \text{PEEP}) \times (\text{inspiratory time/total cycle time})] + \text{PEEP}$$

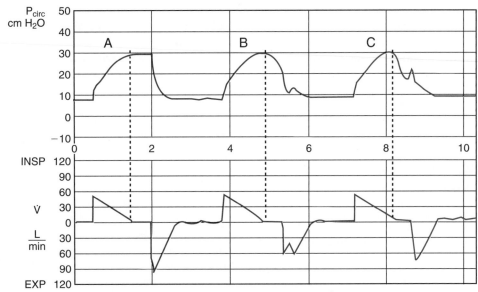

FIGURE 14-2 Plateau pressure measurement during decelerating flow volume control ventilation. The *dashed lines* indicate the point at which the inspiratory hold begins. **A,** Notice that the pressure-time waveform flattens and then squares as expiration begins, providing an accurate measure of plateau pressure. **B** and **C,** The pressure-time waveform dips, indicating patient effort during the inspiratory hold. Breathing efforts during the hold will cause inaccurate plateau pressure measurements. These inaccuracies are more common when low tidal volume strategies are used.

Increases in $P_{\overline{aw}}$ are usually associated with an improvement in Pa_{O_2} but can cause barotrauma and a reduction in cardiac output. When examining the aforementioned formula, it is easier to understand the greater impact that increasing PEEP and CPAP levels have on $P_{\overline{aw}}$ and thus oxygenation compared with increases in inspiratory time or inspiratory-to-expiratory (I/E) ratio. $P_{\overline{aw}}$ is often considered to be equivalent to mean alveolar pressure, but these values are not always equal. Discrepancies between the two values may be caused by imbalances in inspiratory and expiratory resistance, variable flow resistance, leakage of gas volume, and measurement error.[30] Currently, no studies have shown a correlation between specific levels of $P_{\overline{aw}}$ and barotrauma in the adult population, but caution should be used when applying greater than 20 cm H_2O.[31] Clinicians may need to adjust $P_{\overline{aw}}$ levels when switching from one ventilator modality to another. This is particularly important when switching to high-frequency oscillatory (HFO) ventilation. Typically, we use a $P_{\overline{aw}}$ 3 to 5 cm H_2O higher when switching to HFO.

Maximum Inspiratory Pressure

Maximum inspiratory pressure ($P_I$max), sometimes called the *negative inspiratory force (NIF)*, is the maximum inspiratory pressure the patient's ventilatory pump is capable of generating against a closed airway. The following factors influence the patient's ability to produce a normal $P_I$max:

- Respiratory muscle strength
- Patient effort

- Ventilatory drive
- Lung volume
- Phrenic nerve function
- Nutritional status
- Oxygenation status
- Acid-base status

Because $P_I$max is intended to be a measure of respiratory muscle strength, these variables must be considered when interpreting $P_I$max.

$P_I$max can be measured even if an artificial airway is not in place by using a mask or mouthpiece and an external pressure manometer. The alert patient should be asked to exhale to a volume between FRC and RV because this will improve the mechanical advantage of the inspiratory muscles. At the end of exhalation, the airway is occluded while the patient makes a maximal inspiratory effort.

Marini[32] has reported a standardized approach to measuring $P_I$max in uncooperative critically ill patients. The patient is prepared for the maneuver by careful explanation of the procedure, proper positioning, and thorough suctioning with hyperoxygenation. Next, a one-way valve is placed in the expiratory path of a rigid T tube to allow exhalation but not inhalation. This technique reduces lung volume to a level between FRC and RV. $P_I$max is usually generated within 20 seconds of occlusion. Careful explanation of the procedure is important because occlusion of the airway can be frightening.

A normal individual can generate a $P_I$max between −80 and −100 cm H_2O.[2] Values more negative than −30 cm H_2O have been used to predict successful weaning; however, there is limited agreement on this criterion.[12] Although $P_I$max is useful in measuring the patient's respiratory muscle strength, it provides little information about muscle endurance. Most importantly, $P_I$max should never be used as the sole respiratory factor for predicting a patient's ability to wean. In combination with increasing respiratory rate and decreasing V_T, however, a low $P_I$max (0 to −20 cm H_2O) may indicate impending respiratory failure.[2]

> ### SIMPLY STATED
>
> Mechanical ventilation is usually indicated in patients with neuromuscular disease (Guillain-Barré syndrome or myasthenia gravis) when serial measurements of VC decrease to less than 10 mL/kg or less than 1 L, and the $P_I$max/NIF has dropped into the threshold range of 0 to −20 cm H_2O.

Auto–Positive End-Expiratory Pressure

If mechanically ventilated patients do not complete exhalation before inspiration begins, they will develop **auto–positive end-expiratory pressure (auto-PEEP)**. This can result from airways obstruction that increases during exhalation and causes insufficient time for exhalation. Therefore, exhalation of each successive V_T is incomplete, and a positive alveolar pressure occurs. The rise in alveolar pressure results in a PEEP-like effect, hence the term *auto-PEEP*. Auto-PEEP is not detected by the ventilator pressure indicator unless the expiratory valve is occluded at the end of expiration. When the flow is stopped at end-exhalation, pressure equilibrates throughout the closed system and registers on the pressure indicator.

Auto-PEEP is defined as the difference between the total PEEP (obtained by expiratory hold maneuver) and the ventilator's set PEEP value.[33] All patients receiving mechanical ventilation should be assessed for the presence of auto-PEEP. It can be detected through observation, palpation, and auscultation of the patient's chest during exhalation to determine whether flow ends before the onset of the next inhalation. More accurately, the flow-time waveform can be examined to determine whether expiratory flow returns to baseline before the subsequent inhalation.

If auto-PEEP is detected, measurement of total PEEP should be attempted. It is not always possible to make accurate measurements of total PEEP because the patient must not inhale or exhale during the expiratory hold maneuver and the circuit cannot have any leaks. Many modern ventilators incorporate the ability to impose an expiratory pause that allows the measurement of total PEEP.

When auto-PEEP is caused by dynamic airway compression, the patient may be unable to trigger ventilator breaths despite spontaneous efforts. Forceful inspiratory efforts or the inability to trigger the ventilator will be seen. Increasing PEEP to slightly below the level of the measured total PEEP will reduce the inspiratory efforts needed to trigger the breaths. PIP will increase if the set PEEP level exceeds the resulting auto-PEEP. If this occurs, the set PEEP level should be decreased until PIP returns to its previous value.[34]

Auto-PEEP varies with the time allowed for exhalation, the elastic recoil of the lung, and the resistance to flow of the airways, ET tube, and expiratory limb (exhalation valve) of the ventilator circuit. Bronchodilator therapy, decreased inspiratory time, and a reduction in the mandatory breath rate have been shown to reduce the amount of auto-PEEP. The most effective method to reduce auto-PEEP during conventional ventilation is through the reduction of $\dot{V}_E$. Strategies that alter V_T, ventilator rate, or inspiratory time without reducing $\dot{V}_E$ do little to reduce auto-PEEP.

Compliance

Compliance is defined as volume change per unit of pressure change, or the amount of lung volume achieved per unit of pressure. Two forms of compliance are commonly reported: effective dynamic compliance and static compliance. **Dynamic compliance** represents the total impedance to gas flow into the lungs, and it is determined by dividing delivered or corrected V_T by the peak airway pressure minus the positive end-expiratory pressure (PEEP):

$$\text{Dynamic compliance} = \text{Corr } V_T / \text{PIP} - \text{PEEP}$$

where Corr V_T = corrected or delivered tidal volume.

Dynamic compliance incorporates both the flow-resistive characteristics of the airways and ventilator circuit and the elastic components of the lung and chest wall. Dynamic compliance curves are seen most commonly on ventilator graphic screens through the pressure-volume loops.

Static compliance, also called *respiratory system compliance*, is the lung volume change per unit of pressure during a period of no gas flow. Static compliance is reflection of the combination of chest wall and lung compliance. It is calculated clinically by dividing delivered V_T by the plateau pressure minus PEEP:

$$\text{Static compliance} = \text{Corr } V_T / P_{plateau} - \text{PEEP}$$

where Corr V_T = corrected or delivered tidal volume and $P_{plateau}$ = plateau pressure.

In practice, static calculations should be based on at least three breaths. It is important to use the corrected or delivered V_T (discussed earlier) to more accurately reflect the compliance of the lung-thorax unit.

Effective static compliance measurements can be useful in monitoring patients receiving mechanical ventilation. Lung diseases such as pulmonary edema, pneumothorax, pneumonia, and ARDS increase lung recoil and the observed static pressure. As a result, the static compliance is reduced in these situations.

The textbook normal values for static compliance of 100 mL/cm H_2O are rarely seen in mechanically ventilated patients because even patients with normal lungs usually develop a decrease in lung volume and compliance after receiving positive-pressure ventilation for a few hours. Thus, normal static compliance values in patients receiving mechanical ventilation range from 40 to 80 mL/cm H_2O. Patients with static compliance values less than 20 to 25 mL/cm H_2O may be hard to remove from ventilatory support[13,35] and difficult to withdraw from PEEP.

Airway Resistance

Airway resistance (Raw) is the opposition to airflow by the inelastic forces of the lung. True Raw is not measured routinely in the ICU. A reliable estimate of the flow-restrictive components of Raw can be made by subtracting the static or plateau pressure from the PIP and dividing by flow in liters per second:

$$Raw = PIP(cm\ H_2O) - P_{plateau}(cm\ H_2O)/Flow\ (L/sec)$$

The typical reference range cited for Raw is 1 to 3 cm H_2O/L/sec. Raw can be elevated by numerous factors (discussed earlier). Increased Raw can cause problems not only during positive-pressure breathing but also during spontaneous breathing. A small-diameter ET tube will significantly increase the work of breathing for a spontaneously breathing patient. High flow rates from a continuous-flow SIMV system or high base flow through a demand valve system can increase expiratory work by forcing the patient to exhale the delivered V_T against the expiratory valve and the high continuous flow through the patient's circuit.

Integrating Pressure, Flow, and Volume
Evaluating the Patient-Ventilator Interface

The RT is often called on to evaluate the integration of the ventilator to the patient. Most often this consists of a sequential evaluation starting with the patient (use of accessory muscles, color, diaphoresis, heart rate, and respiratory rate) and airway (type, size, integrity, and stability), progressing down both limbs of the ventilator circuit (leaks, temperature, and condensate), and terminating with the ventilator settings and patient-monitoring panel. The RT also can observe the synchrony of the patient's breathing pattern and respiratory effort. This approach is beneficial at the beginning of the shift, after any ventilator-related event, and before and after adjustment of ventilator settings. The RT should then focus on the patient, ventilator settings, measured parameters, and when available, ventilator graphics.

Monitoring Pressure, Flow, and Volume in the Intensive Care Unit

Most ventilators manufactured today are equipped with a graphic display screen. This screen allows clinicians to review large amounts of patient ventilation data. Three of the most important parameters to follow are the pressure, flow, and volume tracings. The data can be displayed as a single parameter in a continuous tracing over time, called a *scalar*, or in combination with other parameters, called a *loop*. The individual parameters may be indexed to each other in a **pressure-volume loop** or a *flow-volume loop*. The integration of these three parameters provides a wealth of information important for proper ventilator management.

Pressure-Time Waveforms. The continuous display of the airway pressure waveform provides the opportunity to visually evaluate the following (Fig. 14-3):

- Airway pressure levels
- Characteristics of the airway pressure curve during all breath cycles
- Mode of ventilation
- Estimated respiratory work
- Adequacy of inspiratory flow pattern and peak flow
- Inspiratory resistive load (peak-plateau pressures)
- Gross estimates of patient inspiratory effort
- Estimations of the level of synchrony between the patient and ventilator

The pressure display on a ventilator graphic screen traces the rise and fall in airway pressure as measured within the ventilator circuit or at the airway opening. The clinician must remember that this tracing is a reflection of airway circuit pressure, ET tube resistance, airway resistance, and lung and chest wall compliance. If the ET tube is small or airway resistance is high, the tracings will not reflect alveolar pressures (intrapulmonary). In fact, only during a period of zero airflow (inspiratory or expiratory hold) does the ventilator airway pressure waveform reflect the actual intrapulmonary pressure (see Fig. 14-1).

The airway pressure waveform is helpful in setting rise time during pressure-limited modes. In adjusting rise time, the RT is setting how fast the airway pressure rises to the set pressure limit. If airway pressure rises too rapidly, then overshoot of the airway pressure curve may occur. This overshoot appears as a dog ear on the left side of the pressure-time curve (Fig. 14-4). This problem is corrected by decreasing the rise time until this left-sided dog ear disappears. If airway pressure rises too slowly, then the patient will feel air hungry, and patient comfort and synchrony will be compromised. This situation may increase the patient's work of breathing. The clinician should avoid a rise time that results in overshoot or increases work of breathing.[36] If possible, communicating with the patient to determine whether the breath feels comfortable can help the RT achieve the optimal setting.

Airway pressure tracings also are beneficial in adjusting the percentage of peak flow that cycles a pressure-supported breath (PS cycle %) into expiration. The lower this percentage is set, the greater the exhaled V_T delivered for a given pressure-support level. This increase in volume results from an increase in inspiratory time due to the lower PS cycle %. Patients with high Raw typically need a higher PS cycle % setting in order to prevent active muscle effort to force expiration. If this occurs, the RT will likely see the

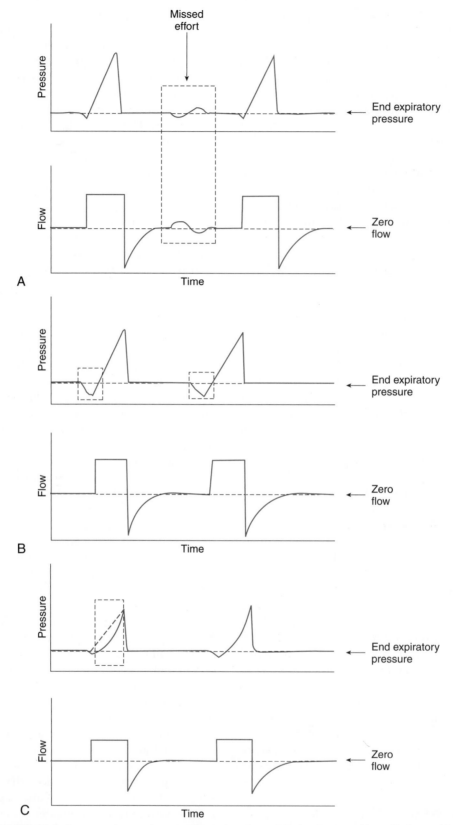

FIGURE 14-3 Pressure-time scalars. **A**, The patient is receiving assist/control ventilation, and the ventilator fails to sense the patient's inspiratory effort on the second attempt-missed effort. The trigger method and sensitivity should be adjusted to avoid missed efforts. **B**, Delayed onset of flow resulting from lack of sensitivity results in excessive trigger work. **C**, Scooping of the inspiratory pressure curve from inadequate flow relative to the patient's inspiratory flow demand. The *dotted line* represents the expected path of rise in inspiratory pressure.

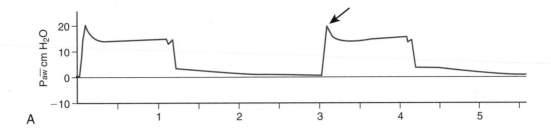

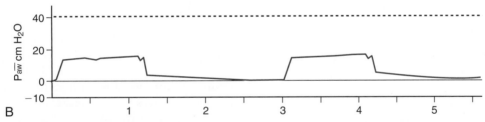

FIGURE 14-4 Pressure-time curves can be used to set rise time during pressure-support and pressure-control ventilation. **A**, The rise time is too fast and results in pressure overshoot that appears as a left dog ear on the curve (*arrow*). **B**, The rise time is set more appropriately, and the overshoot is no longer occurring.

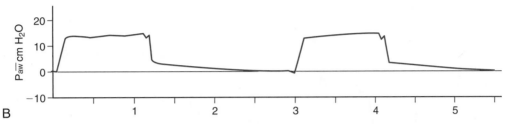

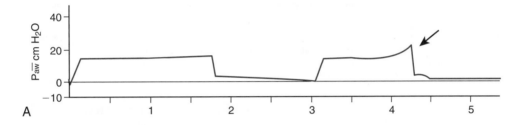

FIGURE 14-5 In this patient with an obstructive disease process, the pressure-time curves can be used to set the percentage of peak flow that cycles a pressure support breath (PS cycle %). **A**, The patient is exhaling against the pressure support breath to cycle it into expiration. This expiratory effort by the patient creates the dog ear on the right side of the pressure-time curve (*arrow*). **B**, The inspiration has been shortened by increasing the PS cycle %, and the patient is more synchronous.

abdominal muscles contract to push against the delivered pressure support and force the breath into exhalation. On the pressure-time waveform, this extra expiratory effort will appear as a dog ear on the *right side* of the pressure-time curve (Fig. 14-5). If these conditions are occurring, then the RT should increase the PS cycle % setting until the right-sided dog ear disappears or the patient is no longer using accessory muscles to force exhalation. If a targeted V_T is desired during pressure-support ventilation, an increase in pressure-support level may be required after this setting is increased.

During pressure-limited modes that are time cycled, such as pressure control (PC) and pressure-regulated volume control (PRVC), pressure-time waveforms are useful in determining if inspiratory time is too long. Prolonged inspiratory time can result in the patient breathing against or fighting the sustained inspiratory pressure (Fig. 14-6). Reducing the inspiratory time until the patient no longer opposes the sustained pressure should improve patient-ventilator synchrony. If shortening of inspiratory time causes inspiratory flow to no longer reach zero, then delivered V_T may be reduced (discussed later).

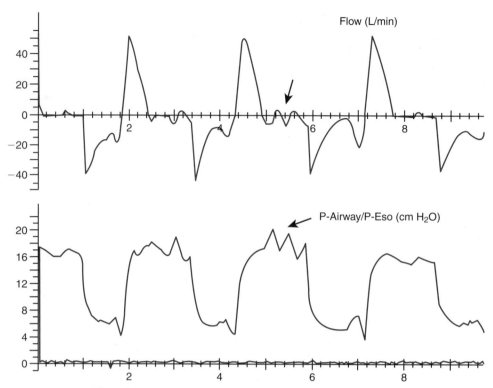

FIGURE 14-6 In these flow-time and pressure-time waveforms, the patient is breathing against or fighting (*arrows*) the sustained inspiratory pressure during pressure-control ventilation. To correct this problem, the inspiratory time should be shortened.

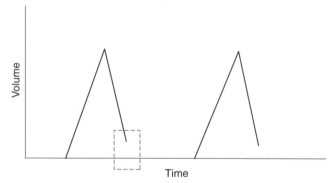

FIGURE 14-7 Volume-time scalar. The inspiratory volume is greater than the expiratory volume because of a leak in the patient-ventilator system, possibly from a bronchopleural fistula, endotracheal tube leak, or ventilator circuit leak.

Volume-Time Waveforms. The volume-time waveform is most often used to compare the inspiratory and expiratory delivered volumes. This can be particularly useful in checking for leaks within the ventilator circuit system or in determining the amount of leak around the ET tube or through a chest tube (Fig. 14-7).

Flow-Time Waveforms

The flow-time waveform allows the clinician to evaluate the following:
- Both inspiratory and expiratory flow rates
- Characteristics of the flow profile during all breath cycles

- Presence of air trapping (i.e., auto-PEEP)
- Estimations of inspiratory effort
- Estimations of the level of synchrony between the patient and ventilator

The inspiratory flow profile provides information about how the ventilator breath is entering the patient. This profile is influenced by the flow pattern selected, mode of ventilation being used, and level of patient effort. During pressure-limited ventilation, the resistive and elastic forces of the chest also affect this profile, but the flow pattern usually assumes a decelerating appearance as set pressure equilibrates with alveolar pressure. The inspiratory flow rate and pattern should match the patient's efforts and breathing demands, demonstrating patient-ventilator synchrony. During volume ventilation, the set inspiratory flow and pattern chosen should create a smooth, consistent rise in airway pressure. If the set flow rate is too slow, the pressure-time waveform will show a dip or become concave (see Fig. 14-3C). Excessive flow rate creates a sharp, sudden rise in airway pressure. Some patients, particularly those with significant dyspnea, may require a higher inspiratory flow rate. Flow rate and flow profiles are particularly important to monitor during volume-limited modes of ventilation because the RT sets the pattern and determines a finite flow rate. The RT should evaluate the inspiratory flow profile periodically and make necessary adjustments when using volume-limited modes of ventilation.

SIMPLY STATED

Scooping of the pressure-time waveform and a figure-of-eight pattern of the pressure-volume loop during volume-controlled ventilation indicate the need for higher peak inspiratory flows.

During pressure-limited ventilation, such as pressure support (PS), PC, PRVC, and volume support (VS), the inspiratory flow rate is determined by the resistive and elastic forces of the lungs and patient inspiratory effort. This flow pattern shows a rapid rise to a maximum flow rate, followed by a gradual tapering to a point of flow termination. This pattern is usually well matched to any changes in patient effort and allows the patient to determine the flow rate of the inspiratory phase of the breath. Adjusting rise time setting (previously discussed) also affects the peak flow rate and flow pattern created during pressure-limited ventilation.

During pressure-control ventilation, flow-time waveforms can be used to estimate inspiratory time needed for the set inspiratory pressure to equilibrate in the lung. When the inspiratory flow profile decreases to zero before expiration begins, the inspiratory pressure equilibrates throughout the lung, and maximum delivery V_T for set pressure will have been achieved. Using an inspiratory time that does not allow inspiratory flow to reach zero will result in a lowered delivered V_T (Fig. 14-8). If inspiratory flow is reaching baseline, further increases in inspiratory time will only result in a pause or inspiratory hold that increases $P_{\overline{aw}}$. Unless the ventilator has an active exhalation valve that allows spontaneous breathing during the inspiratory phase, prolonged inspiratory time can result in severe patient dyssynchrony with the ventilator (see Fig. 14-6).

The expiratory flow profile displays how gas is leaving the lung and indicates the level of expiratory resistance and the expiratory time required to return to zero flow. The expiratory flow profile is used routinely to determine the presence of air trapping. When air trapping or auto-PEEP occurs, flow continues throughout expiration, and the onset of inspiration occurs before exhalation is complete (Fig. 14-9). However, a quantitative calculation of auto-PEEP cannot be made from an examination of the expiratory flow profile unless accompanied by a pressure-time tracing with an expiratory hold to zero flow.

SIMPLY STATED

If the expiratory flow of a flow-time waveform does not return to zero before inspiration begins, air trapping and auto-PEEP are occurring.

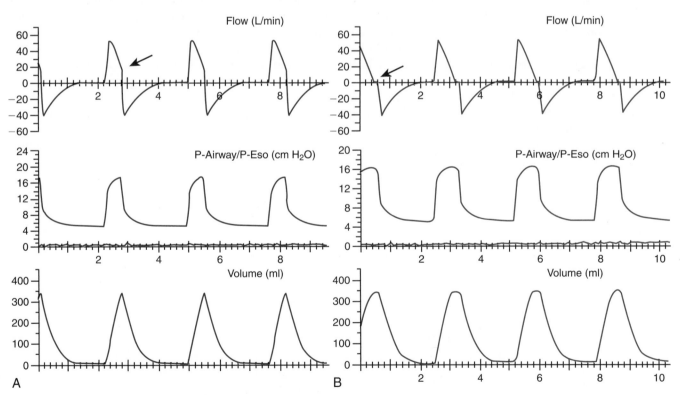

FIGURE 14-8 During pressure control ventilation, the flow-time waveform can be used to set inspiratory time. **A,** Inspiratory time is not long enough for inspiratory flow to reach zero (see *arrow*), which indicates that the set inspiratory pressure has not equilibrated in the lung. **B,** Inspiratory time has been increased, and inspiratory flow has reached zero (see *arrow*), which indicates that the set inspiratory pressure has equilibrated in the lung. In this pediatric patient, the increase in inspiratory time has resulted in a slightly larger tidal volume caused by the equilibration of set and alveolar pressures.

Pressure/Volume Curves. The integration of pressure and volume data produces a useful tool: the pressure-volume loop. Pressure is most often displayed on the X-axis and volume on the Y-axis. The angle of the inspiratory and expiratory curves is known as the *slope* of the tracings. At normal inspiratory flows, the pressure-volume curve is a display of the dynamic compliance. It reflects both the resistive and elastic components of the circuit-patient interface. A typical tracing during constant inspiratory flow reveals a slightly concave inspiratory tracing, with the expiratory curve being slightly convex. The flatter the slope of the tracing, the less compliant the system. Lower compliance tracings are most often seen with restrictive conditions such as ARDS and lung consolidation (Fig. 14-10). The wider the curve or the greater the difference between its inspiratory and expiratory limbs, the greater the airway resistance (Fig. 14-11). However, proper interpretation of pressure-volume loop width must take into account the ventilator flow pattern. For example, as depicted in Figure 14-12, a decelerating inspiratory flow pattern typically causes the inspiratory limb of the loop to bulge downward due to the higher initial flow.

The pressure-volume loop also can be helpful in setting inspiratory flow during volume-limited ventilation. The inspiratory limb should be slightly curved outward, as mentioned earlier. The tracings should move in a counterclockwise fashion. If the patient's effort exceeds the set inspiratory flow rate, then the width of the curve will narrow and in some cases create a figure-of-eight appearance (Fig. 14-13). In such cases, the inspiratory flow should be increased until the curve resumes its normal shape. When using low V_T strategies to prevent lung injury in patients with an increased drive to breathe, the pressure-volume curve can be inverted and move in the clockwise instead of counterclockwise motion. If this happens, the patient's work of breathing would be significantly elevated. An increase in both V_T and flow may be needed to correct this problem.

Remember that plateau pressure should remain below 28 to 30 cm H_2O in patients with acute lung injury or ARDS.

Titrating PEEP and Tidal Volume with the Pressure-Volume Curve. Some investigators have advocated using a static pressure-volume curve to titrate PEEP and V_T. It is not routinely used in the ICU, mainly because it is time consuming and cumbersome, but it can be valuable for some patients, particularly those with acute lung injury. This technique, which incorporates a supersyringe filled with 100% oxygen and a pressure manometer, requires the sequential delivery of specific volumes to the airway. The volumes are delivered to the lung and held for a few seconds to allow equilibration and a static condition to occur. Sometimes the lung is inflated to a maximal level and then emptied in the same stepwise fashion. The corresponding pressures and volumes are recorded and plotted to form a curve. The initial points of the curve are fairly flat, indicating increasing pressure with minimal alveolar recruitment. As one moves up the curve, the compliance points change their slope. This is seen as a greater change in lung volume per unit of pressure. The point on the curve at which a significant upslope first occurs is known as the **lower inflection point**. This point's corresponding pressure plus 2 cm H_2O is considered to be the minimum PEEP that should be applied to the lung. As the remainder of the volume is delivered into the lungs, the corresponding line increases at the same slope unless compliance changes. Eventually, the slope flattens again, indicating that more pressure is being required to deliver the given volume. This upper flattening characteristic identifies the **upper inflection point** and is referred to as *beaking*. Its presence in an apneic mechanically ventilated patient indicates a significant decrease in compliance caused by overdistention of the lung. The static pressure-volume curve can be used to adjust the minimum PEEP required to recruit and maintain open alveoli

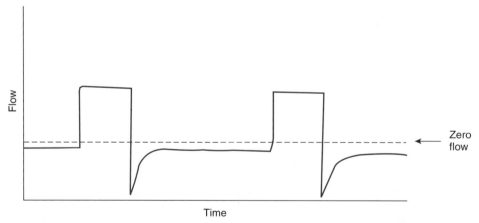

FIGURE 14-9 Flow-time scalar. The expiratory flow fails to return to baseline before the onset of the next inhalation. This demonstrates the presence of air trapping and auto-PEEP. The shape of the expiratory tracing demonstrates a prolonged expiratory time with low expiratory flow consistent with significant expiratory resistance in either the patient or the ventilator circuit.

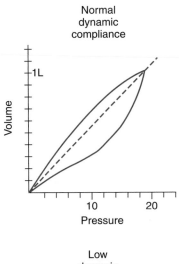

Normal dynamic compliance

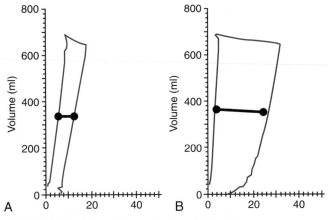

FIGURE 14-11 The difference in the width of the pressure-volume loop between **A** and **B** is due to airway resistance.

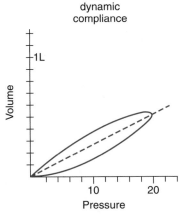

Low dynamic compliance

Constant flow

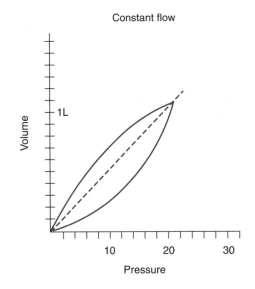

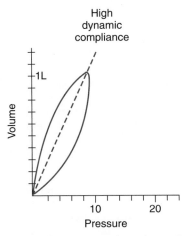

High dynamic compliance

FIGURE 14-10 Dynamic pressure-volume loops. The slope of the curve represents the dynamic compliance of the system (*dashed lines*).

(lower inflection point)[23,24] and to determine the maximal pressure level to limit the possibility of overdistention (upper inflection point) (Fig. 14-14).

The dynamic pressure-volume curves commonly displayed on ventilators in the ICU are different from the static curves just described. Because the pressure-volume points are being taken while the ventilator is delivering the

Nonconstant flow

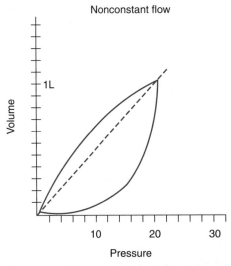

FIGURE 14-12 Dynamic pressure-volume loops. Nonconstant flow (decelerating ramp) changes the appearance of the pressure-volume loop. The decelerating inspiratory flow seen with pressure-limited ventilation will cause the inspiratory curve to bulge downward.

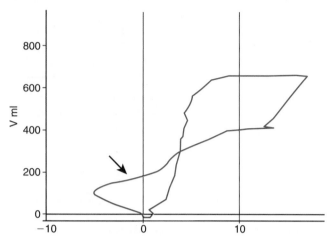

FIGURE 14-13 Pressure-volume loop indicating inadequate flow during volume control ventilation. The inward curve of the inspiratory limb of the loop, and especially a figure-of-eight appearance, indicate that the patient's inspiratory flow is exceeding the set flow rate.

breath, the ventilator tracings are incorporating the resistive and elastic characteristics of the ventilator circuit and the lungs. Consequently, the lower inflection point is typically higher than the minimal level of PEEP.

Quasi-static pressure-volume curves using specific settings have been advocated as a simple and reliable technique to determine the lower and upper inflection points.[37] Inflation of the lungs is accomplished with a constant, low flow (<10 L/minute) from FRC through the set V_T range. The pressure-volume curve for this inflation is frozen on the screen for assessment. Patients must be sedated and paralyzed in order to obtain accurate lower and upper inflection points. It is thought that maintaining breath delivery above the lower infection point and below the upper inflection point protects the lungs against ventilator-associated lung injury.[23,24] Some ventilator manufacturers have incorporated this as an executable maneuver in their software.

SIMPLY STATED

Graphic displays of ventilator pressure, volume, and flow waveforms are invaluable in the titration of ventilator settings and the assessment of patient-ventilator synchrony.

Fractional Gas Concentrations

The ability to monitor inspired oxygen concentrations is crucial for many respiratory procedures. Monitoring of exhaled gas concentrations also can be useful in patient management. These measurements can provide information about changes in gas exchange, tissue perfusion, ventilation-perfusion ($\dot{V}/\dot{Q}$) relationships, metabolic rate, and equipment function. This section discusses oxygen concentration and carbon dioxide analysis and their use in the ICU.

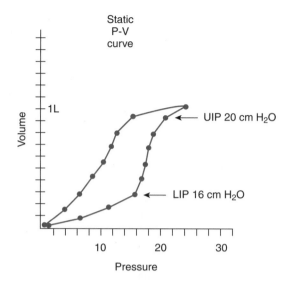

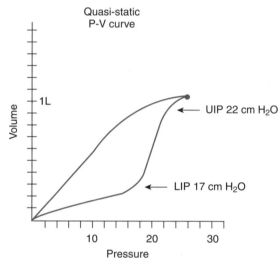

FIGURE 14-14 Static and quasi-static pressure loops. The static pressure-volume loop is constructed by serial injection of aliquots of volume with a pause to zero flow and recording the resultant pressure. The volume and pressure data points are plotted through both inhalation and exhalation. The lower and upper inflection points (LIP, UIP) can often be determined by this method. It can be difficult to accomplish in the unstable, critically ill patient. The quasi-static method uses a constant, low flow (<10 L/min) inhalation with continuous recording of the volume and pressure data points. Although there is a small error related to the pressure being recorded during flow, the error is fairly constant, and the inflection points can be approximated with this method. For both methods, the patient must remain completely passive, and attention to detail is critical in obtaining reliable results.

Fraction of Inspired Oxygen Concentration

Measurement of the fraction of inspired oxygen (F_IO_2) is essential to the modern ICU. Various oxygen delivery devices require at least intermittent analysis of F_IO_2 to ensure that the appropriate oxygen concentration is being delivered and to interpret blood gases. If the F_IO_2 is inappropriately low, hypoxia may result; an inappropriate elevation of F_IO_2

may lead to oxygen toxicity. Moreover, accurate measurement of both the inspired and expired O_2 concentration is required to conduct metabolic evaluations.[38]

Exhaled Carbon Dioxide

Carbon dioxide is one of the by-products of tissue metabolism, and its elimination is a prime function of ventilation. Monitoring of exhaled carbon dioxide with either **capnometry** (simple measurement) or **capnography** (graphing the measurement against time) can detect changes in the following:

- Metabolic rate as a result of cardiac output and body temperature changes, shivering, seizures, trauma, and high carbohydrate infusion
- Ventilator function such as a patient disconnection or apnea
- Efficiency of ventilation (by looking at the increase and decrease in dead space)
- Transport of carbon dioxide as a result of changes in perfusion

Exhaled CO_2 analysis may be done on a breath-by-breath basis or by sampling mean concentration. The most common systems in current use employ infrared analysis (absorption of a specific wavelength of infrared radiation). Sampling can be done either by aspiration through a sample line or by placement of the sensor between the ventilator circuit wye and ET tube. Typically expired CO_2 is plotted against time. However, CO_2 levels also can be plotted against volume by incorporating a flow transducer. The latter technique allows the clinician to estimate dead space.

A single breath capnograph tracing for CO_2 concentration against volume is illustrated in Figure 14-15. The tracing has three phases. Phase I contains no CO_2 and represents gas coming exclusively from dead space. Phase II shows a rapid increase in CO_2 concentration because alveolar gas begins mixing with the remaining dead space gas. In phase III, the CO_2 concentration begins to plateau with gas now coming mainly from the ventilated alveolar region.

The peak CO_2 concentration in phase III normally occurs at end-exhalation and is referred to as the **end-tidal P_{CO_2}** (P_{ETCO_2}). The commonly cited reference range for P_{ETCO_2} in normal subjects is 30 to 43 mm Hg, or about 2 to 5 mm Hg less than the P_{aCO_2}. In individuals with healthy lungs, therefore, the difference between the arterial and end-tidal P_{CO_2} (the arterial-P_{ETCO_2} gradient) ranges between 2 and 5 mm Hg, the P_{ETCO_2} provides a good estimate of P_{aCO_2}.

However, CO_2 elimination depends on many factors, including cardiac output, regional $\dot{V}/\dot{Q}$ ratios and the emptying times of different areas of the lung. These factors commonly are seen among critically ill patients (e.g., mechanical ventilation, pulmonary disease, poor perfusion) and typically have the effect of altering $\dot{V}/\dot{Q}$ relationships and increasing the arterial-P_{ETCO_2} gradient.[39,40] For this reason, among critically ill patients, the P_{ETCO_2} should never be used as a substitute for direct measurement of the P_{aCO_2}.[40]

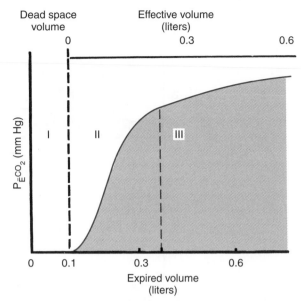

FIGURE 14-15 Single-breath tracing for exhaled carbon dioxide.

Even among the critically ill, capnometry and capnography can be used to assess both equipment function and effectiveness of therapy. Current guidelines recommend that some form of P_{ETCO_2} measurement be used to confirm proper placement of both ET tubes and supraglottic airway devices such as the laryngeal mask airways.[40] In terms of detecting equipment malfunction, Figure 14-16 depicts several good examples of abnormal capnography waveforms indicating specific equipment-related problems. Last, capnography is now considered a standard of care during cardiopulmonary resuscitation, both to confirm proper airway placement and to assess circulatory function.[41] Specifically, during cardiopulmonary resuscitation, P_{ETCO_2} levels below 10 mm Hg indicate poor circulation and the need to improve the quality of compressions.[40] Moreover, an abrupt and sustained increase in P_{ETCO_2} is a good indicator of return of spontaneous circulation (ROSC).[41]

SIMPLY STATED

During cardiopulmonary resuscitation, capnography should be used both to confirm proper airway placement and assess circulatory function.

Carbon dioxide production ($\dot{V}_{CO_2}$) is the carbon dioxide produced and excreted over 1 minute. The $\dot{V}_{CO_2}$ values provide information about changes in metabolic rate and transport of carbon dioxide. The formula for calculating $\dot{V}_{CO_2}$ is as follows:

$$\dot{V}_{CO_2} = F_{\bar{E}CO_2} \times \dot{V}_E$$

where $F_{\bar{E}CO_2}$ = mean fraction of expired carbon dioxide and $\dot{V}_E$ = minute volume exhaled at standard temperature and pressure dry (STPD).

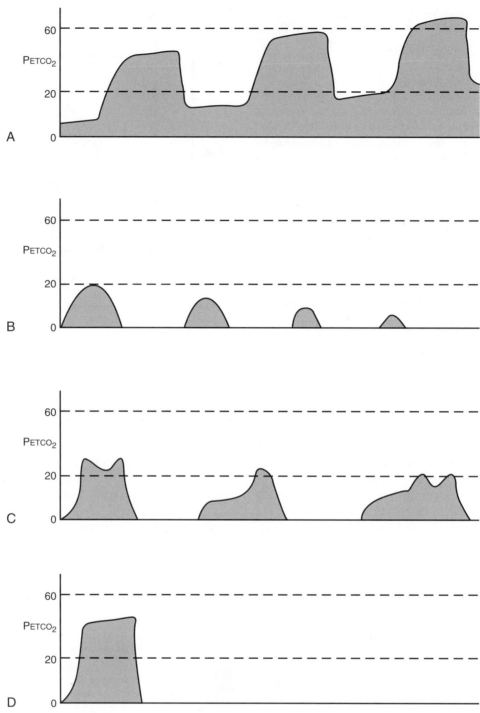

FIGURE 14-16 Examples of abnormal capnograms. **A,** Progressive rebreathing causing a rise in baseline P_{ETCO_2}. **B,** Placement of endotracheal (ET) tube in esophagus, causing a drop in P_{ETCO_2} to 0. **C,** Leak in sample line or around ET tube cuff, resulting in low and variable P_{ETCO_2} levels. **D,** Ventilator disconnect, causing an abrupt drop in P_{ETCO_2} to 0.

The formula assumes that there is no carbon dioxide in inspired air. $\dot{V}_{CO_2}$ is often increased in fever (10% increase per 1° C body temperature increase), trauma, peritonitis (25% to 50% increase), head trauma, rewarming after hypothermia, and high carbohydrate loading with total parenteral nutrition. A rapid decrease in $\dot{V}_{CO_2}$ or carbon dioxide elimination accompanies a low cardiac output and a fall

in tissue perfusion, decreased right ventricular output, decreased venous return, or pulmonary embolism.

Dead Space/Tidal Volume Ratio. V_D is the inspired volume that does not come in contact with pulmonary capillary blood. The **dead space–to–tidal volume ratio** (V_D/V_T) expresses the relationship between V_D and total V_T, or the portion of the V_T that is "wasted." V_D has two components: **anatomic dead space** and alveolar dead space. Anatomic dead space is made up of the conducting airways and is normally about 1 mL/kg of predicted body weight. **Alveolar dead space** is classically defined as alveoli that are ventilated but not perfused. The combination of anatomic and alveolar dead space is called physiologic dead space. V_D/V_T is traditionally calculated by the Enghoff modification of the Bohr equation, as follows:

$$V_D/V_T = Pa_{CO_2} - P_{\bar{E}CO_2}/Pa_{CO_2}$$

where Pa_{CO_2} = arterial P_{CO_2} and $P_{\bar{E}CO_2}$ = P_{CO_2} of mixed exhaled gas.

The patient is stabilized for 20 minutes, and arterial blood and exhaled gases are sampled simultaneously. $P_{\bar{E}CO_2}$ should be provided by a capnometer as one of its measures, or the exhaled gases may be collected in a Douglas bag. Factors that may contaminate or dilute the $P_{\bar{E}CO_2}$, such as compressible gas volume from the patient ventilator circuit or gases from a continuous flow SIMV system, should be eliminated by double exhalation valves.[42,43]

The common normal reference range for V_D/V_T in healthy subjects is 25% to 40% and is position dependent. Patients receiving positive-pressure ventilation usually have a higher V_D/V_T while they are upright or in the lateral position than when they are in the supine position.[44] During anesthesia, V_D/V_T is usually increased because of an overall reduction in lung volume. In patients receiving mechanical ventilation, higher inspiratory flow rates or small VT's usually is associated with an increase in V_D/V_T.[45] Variations in the inspiratory waveforms, tapered wave, sine waves, and end-inspiratory pause maneuvers may decrease V_D/V_T.[46] Changes in the pulmonary perfusion caused by emboli, hypoperfusion, and precapillary constriction may result in an increased V_D/V_T.

Evaluation of Oxygenation

Inappropriate oxygenation is a common occurrence in critically ill patients. The recognition and correction of this problem are crucial to the patient's well-being. Respiratory care maneuvers, pharmacologic and fluid therapy, and diagnostic procedures often affect tissue oxygenation. The bedside clinician must be able to monitor and determine the effect of these activities.

This section describes the concepts and techniques used in the assessment of oxygenation. It includes the components of oxygen transport and the measurements used to monitor oxygenation. This section also discusses the indices of pulmonary gas exchange and indicators of systemic and regional tissue oxygenation.

The potential causes of hypoxemia and hypoxia are diverse. Hypoxic episodes can be **iatrogenic** (complication due to a procedure) in origin, as with suctioning or equipment failure. Progressive disease or a new problem

can make oxygenation more difficult. Therefore, the bedside clinician must be able to identify the causes of these problems, select the appropriate therapy or therapies, and monitor the outcome. Causes of impaired oxygenation in critically ill patients are listed in Box 14-3. Haldane, the physiologist, said it best almost a century ago: "Anoxia not only stops the machine but wrecks the machinery."[47]

Evaluation of Oxygen Transport

Oxygen transport is the essential mechanism by which oxygen is carried from the lungs to the capillary bed. Equally important is how oxygen is used by the tissues, a process known as **oxygen consumption or utilization**. The majority of cellular oxygen is used for the production of adenosine triphosphate (ATP). Recent evidence shows that other activities, such as cell wall stabilization and chemical synthesis, are extremely oxygen dependent and sensitive to minor fluctuations in oxygen tension. Box 14-4 lists some of the crucial factors that determine **oxygen delivery (D_{O_2})** and oxygen utilization.

Oxygen Reserves

In the critically ill patient, an increase in oxygen consumption or decrease in D_{O_2} to the tissues must be compensated for by an increase in one or more of the reserve systems:

- Cardiac output and distribution
- Pa_{O_2} and oxygen saturation (Sa_{O_2}) values
- Functional hemoglobin levels

Patients with two compromised reserve systems are at high risk for inadequate D_{O_2} and subsequent tissue hypoxia. Critically ill patients often have compromised reserve systems. Low cardiac output (shock), blood flow maldistribution, anemia, and ventilatory failure do not allow adequate compensation to occur. As the abnormal situation persists, it becomes more difficult to correct. The longer oxygenation is compromised, the more profoundly the "machinery" is damaged.

Oxygen content is defined as the total amount of oxygen carried in the blood as described in Chapter 8 and is calculated by summing its component parts:

$$O_2 \text{ content} = O_2 \text{ chemically bound to Hb} \\ + O_2 \text{ dissolved in plasma}$$

$$O_2 \text{ content} = (Hb \text{ content} \times 1.34 \times \% \ HbO_2) \\ + (Pa_{O_2} \times 0.003)$$

Under normal conditions, Hb is responsible for carrying 99% or more of the O_2 in the blood, with the remainder (<1%) dissolved in plasma, and is measured as the Pa_{O_2}. Pa_{O_2} is important because it reflects the degree of saturation of Hb and the driving pressure of oxygen between systemic capillary blood and the tissues.

Traditional respiratory care has focused on the physiologic mechanisms causing inadequate oxygenation of the

Box 14-3	Causes of Impaired Oxygenation in Critically Ill Patients

EQUIPMENT-RELATED PROBLEMS, LOW- OR HIGH-FLOW OXYGEN DELIVERY DEVICES
- Loose tubing connection, cannula
- Loose humidifier, nipple connector
- Inadequate flow to meet patient peak inspiratory flow, air entrainment
- Blender malfunction

VENTILATOR-RELATED PROBLEMS
- Endotracheal: tracheostomy tube malfunctions
- Ventilator and circuit malfunctions
- Improper settings, modes of ventilation

PROGRESSION OF UNDERLYING DISEASE PROCESS
- Acute respiratory distress syndrome
- Cardiogenic pulmonary edema
- Pneumonia
- Airway obstruction, asthma, chronic obstructive pulmonary disease

ONSET OF A NEW CLINICAL PROBLEM
- Pneumothoraces: simple, tension, loculated
- Lobar atelectasis
- Gastric aspiration
- Artificial airway problems: stenosis, fistula, malacia
- Nosocomial pneumonia
- Fluid overload
- Microatelectasis
- Bronchospasm
- Retained secretions
- Shock
- Sepsis
- Additional organ failure

INTERVENTIONS AND PROCEDURES
- Endotracheal tube suctioning
- Position changes
- Chest physiotherapy
- Bronchoscopy
- Thoracentesis
- Peritoneal dialysis
- Hemodialysis
- Transport
- Diagnostic procedures
- Line or tube placement

MEDICATIONS
- Bronchodilators
- Vasodilators
- Inotropic agents

MISCELLANEOUS
- Leukocytopenia
- Intralipids

Data from Glauser FL, Polatty RC, Sessler CN: Worsening oxygenation in the mechanically ventilated patient. *Am Rev Respir Dis* 138:458-465, 1988.

Box 14-4	Factors that Determine Oxygen Delivery and Utilization

OXYGEN TRANSPORT
Oxygen content of the blood
Cardiac output
Distribution of cardiac output
Oxyhemoglobin dissociation curve

OXYGEN UTILIZATION
Metabolic rate (disease, trauma, sepsis, nutrition)
Cell integrity (organ injury, sepsis)
Oxygen availability
Level of cellular toxins, by-products (organ injury, sepsis)

pulmonary capillary blood (hypoxemia). Causes of hypoxemia include the following:
- $\dot{V}/\dot{Q}$ mismatch (most common cause)
- Diffusion block (rare cause)
- Hypoventilation
- Shunt (extreme $\dot{V}/\dot{Q}$ mismatch)

Details on the differential assessment of these causes of hypoxemia are provided in Chapter 8.

SIMPLY STATED

Oxygen transport depends primarily on the following three components:
   Cardiac output and distribution
   Pa_{O_2} and Sa_{O_2} values
   Sufficient levels of functional hemoglobin
   A compromise in any of the three parameters must be compensated for by the other components. Patients with two compromised components are at high risk for inadequate D_{O_2} and subsequent tissue hypoxia.

Cardiac Output

The techniques used to assess cardiac output are described in Chapter 16. D_{O_2} is extremely dependent on cardiac output and systemic distribution of blood flow. The major determinant of cardiac output is metabolic activity, whereas peripheral distribution of blood flow depends on regional oxygen consumption, temperature, humoral agents, and other factors. Cardiac output is not sensitive to moderate changes in oxygen tension (P_{O_2}) and usually does not increase until the Pa_{O_2} drops below 50 mm Hg.[48] In the patient with shock, blood flow is redirected away from the low-oxygen-consuming regions of the body, such as the skin, to the vital organs, such as the heart and brain, in response to an increase in sympathetic tone.

Oxyhemoglobin Dissociation Curve

Another factor influencing D_{O_2} is the **oxyhemoglobin dissociation curve**. This curve graphically depicts the relationship between Pa_{O_2} and Hb saturation. The clinical significance of the curve is that large changes in Pa_{O_2} may have little effect on the oxygen content or Hb saturation of arterial blood on the upper, flat portion of the curve (Pa_{O_2} > 70 mm Hg), but dramatic changes occur in oxygen content or Hb saturation on the steep portion of the curve (Pa_{O_2} < 70 mm Hg). At P_{O_2} below 70 mm Hg, large volumes of oxygen can be unloaded at the cellular level with relatively small changes in Pa_{O_2}.

O_2 loading and unloading also are affected by the position of the curve. The position of the curve is measured by the P_{50}, which equals the P_{O_2} at which Hb is 50% saturated with O_2. A normal P_{50} is approximately 27 mm Hg. A shift of the curve to the left decreases the P_{50}, whereas a shift to the right increases the P_{50}. Shifts of the curve to the left cause O_2 to bind more tightly to Hb, which can impair unloading at the tissues. A left shift can be caused by massive transfusion of stored blood, rapid correction of acidosis that has been present for hours or days, or severe hyperventilation resulting in respiratory alkalosis. Other less commonly seen causes of a left-shifted curve are hypothermia and hypophosphatemia. Conversely, shifts of the curve to the right decrease Hb affinity for O_2 and improve its delivery to the tissues.[49] Acidosis, hypercapnia, and fever all shift the curve to the right.

The normal compensatory mechanism for a left-shifted curve is an increase in the cardiac output. Patients with compromised reserve systems who are not capable of increasing cardiac output or who cannot tolerate a further reduction in tissue oxygenation are at great risk for hypoxia if they have a significantly left-shifted curve.

To show how efficient the position of the curve is in improving D_{O_2}, consider the following theoretical clinical situation. A patient with a normal fixed oxygen consumption of 250 mL/minute, a cardiac output of 5.4 L/minute, a mixed venous oxygen tension ($P\overline{v}_{O_2}$) of 36 mm Hg, and a P_{50} of 27 mm Hg develops a clinical condition in which the curve shifts to the left and reduces the P_{50} to 20 mm Hg. This patient would need to increase cardiac output by 50% to deliver the equivalent volume of O_2 to the tissues. However, if P_{50} were increased from 27 mm Hg to 30 mm Hg, the patient would require 20% less cardiac output.[50] If such a patient had heart damage and was unable to increase cardiac output, the significant shift to the left of curve could be very serious.

Monitoring the Adequacy of Arterial Oxygenation
Partial Pressure of Arterial Oxygen

Pa_{O_2} is used universally in the ICU as a measure of pulmonary gas exchange, but it is not specific or sensitive enough to be used exclusively in the estimation of oxygen transport. Practitioners must keep this in mind when treating the critically ill patient who is hemodynamically unstable.

Pa_{O_2} is an excellent value to follow to identify which therapies are effective to manage a pulmonary gas exchange problem (e.g., asthma) that is not associated with other complications. However, it should not be relied on in assessing systemic oxygen transport for the following reasons. First, it is a gas tension and does not directly reflect delivered oxygen. Second, Pa_{O_2} reflects partial pressure available at the systemic bed, not what is used. Third, factors that may improve oxygen transport by improving cardiac output may cause Pa_{O_2} to fall because of an increase in intrapulmonary shunt.[51,52] It is not uncommon for multiple deficiencies to exist that adversely affect the oxygen transport system but are not directly related to pulmonary gas exchange.

Under most clinical conditions, Pa_{O_2} should be kept within a range of 60 to 80 mm Hg. This usually ensures an arterial saturation of at least 90%. Pa_{O_2} values greater than 80 mm Hg are usually unnecessary except in situations such as carbon monoxide poisoning and during periods of severe anemia or cardiogenic shock. A higher than normal Pa_{O_2} does not necessarily improve oxygen transport. A Pa_{O_2} greater than 125 mm Hg has been shown to cause a reduction of blood flow to both the kidneys and the brain, probably as a result of vasoconstriction.[49]

Alveolar-to-Arterial Oxygen Tension Difference

The alveolar-to-arterial oxygen tension difference [$P(A-a)_{O_2}$] has commonly been used as an indication of gas exchange efficiency. Its major limitation is that it changes with alterations in $F_{I_{O_2}}$.[53] See Chapter 8 for guidance on interpreting the $P(A-a)_{O_2}$.

Ratio of Pa_{O_2} to $P_{A_{O_2}}$ (a/A Ratio)

The **arterial-to-alveolar tension ratio** ($Pa_{O_2}/P_{A_{O_2}}$, or a/A ratio) is a more useful index of pulmonary gas exchange than the $P(A-a)_{O_2}$ because it remains relatively stable with changes in $F_{I_{O_2}}$.[54] The a/A ratio is most stable when $F_{I_{O_2}}$ is greater than 0.30 and Pa_{O_2} is less than 100 mm Hg.

An example computation is as follows. Given a Pa_{O_2} of 50 mm Hg and a Pa_{CO_2} of 40 mm Hg while breathing an $F_{I_{O_2}}$ of 0.6, you would first compute the $P_{A_{O_2}}$:

$$P_{A_{O_2}} = [0.6 \times (760 - 47)] - (1.25 \times 40) = 378 \text{ mm Hg}$$

Then divide the $P_{A_{O_2}}$ into the Pa_{O_2}:

$$Pa_{O_2}/P_{A_{O_2}} = 50/378 = 0.13$$

The lower limit of normal of the a/A ratio is 0.77 to 0.82, with values below 0.20 to 0.25 (as above) indicating the presence of significant intrapulmonary shunting and acute lung injury.

The a/A ratio also can be used to predict the $F_{I_{O_2}}$ required for a desired Pa_{O_2}.[55] In the above example, were we to increase the $F_{I_{O_2}}$ to 0.7, we could estimate the new Pa_{O_2} as follows:

$$\text{New } P_{A_{O_2}}(70\% \ O_2) = [0.7 \times (760 - 47)] - (1.25 \times 40)$$
$$= 449 \text{ mm Hg}$$

$$\text{a/A ratio} = 0.13 \text{ (given)}$$

$$\text{a/A ratio} \times \text{new } P_{AO_2} = \text{estimated new } Pa_{O_2}$$
$$0.13 \times 449 = 58 \text{ mm Hg}$$

Because the a/A ratio requires calculation of the alveolar P_{O_2}, many clinicians prefer one of two other simpler measures of oxygenation, the P/F ratio or the oxygenation index (OI).

Ratio of Pao₂ to F₁O₂ (P/F Ratio)

The $Pa_{O_2}/F_{I_{O_2}}$ or P/F ratio is computed simply by dividing the arterial P_{O_2} by the decimal value of the $F_{I_{O_2}}$. Using the same patient example above, the P/F ratio would be calculated as:

$$Pa_{O_2}/F_{I_{O_2}} = 50/0.6 = 83$$

A "normal" P/F ratio breathing room air would be 95/0.21 or about 450. The 1994 American-European Consensus Conference on ARDS used the P/F ratio as one of the criteria to define and distinguish between acute lung injury (ALI) and ARDS. A P/F ratio between 200 and 300 mm Hg is associated with ALI, whereas a P/F ratio of less than 200 is associated with ARDS. The other criteria required by both were acute onset, bilateral infiltrates, and a pulmonary artery wedge pressure of 18 mm Hg or less.[56]

Note that although simpler to compute, the P/F ratio does not take into account changes in Pa_{CO_2}. Moreover, unlike the a/A ratio, it cannot be used to predict the Pa_{O_2} resulting from changes in $F_{I_{O_2}}$.

Oxygenation Index

The OI was initially developed as an index of ventilatory oxygenation support for a neonatal surfactant trial[57] and then adapted as a prognostic index for morbidity and mortality for infants requiring extracorporeal membrane oxygenation (ECMO).[58] The OI is defined as the reciprocal of P/F ratio multiplied by the mean airway pressure ($P_{\overline{aw}}$) times 100:

$$OI = F_{I_{O_2}}/Pa_{O_2} \times P_{\overline{aw}} \times 100$$

Again using our prior patient as an example (Pa_{O_2} of 50 mm Hg with $F_{I_{O_2}} = 0.6$) and assuming $P_{\overline{aw}} = 15$ cm H_2O, the patient's OI would be computed as follows:

$$OI = F_{I_{O_2}}/Pa_{O_2} \times P_{\overline{aw}} \times 100$$
$$OI = 0.60 / 50 \times 15 \times 100$$
$$OI = 18$$

In general, OI values less than 5 are considered acceptable. Values in the 10 to 20 range indicate impaired oxygenation, with an OI above 25 associated with a severe oxygenation disturbance and poor clinical outcomes.[58]

SIMPLY STATED

Parameters that incorporate ventilator settings (oxygenation index) are helpful in determining severity of illness and can guide the initiation of other forms of care (i.e., if OI ≥ 25 for 4 hours, consider lung-protective ventilation strategies).

Intrapulmonary Shunt

Intrapulmonary shunting ($\dot{Q}_s/\dot{Q}_t$) is a major contributor to hypoxemia in critically ill patients. An intrapulmonary shunt occurs when there is perfusion to alveolar regions that lack ventilation. Clinical states that increase $\dot{Q}_s/\dot{Q}_t$ include atelectasis, pneumonia, ARDS, pulmonary edema, and, rarely, congenital heart anomalies or arteriovenous anastomosis. The $\dot{Q}_s/\dot{Q}_t$ and $\dot{V}/\dot{Q}$ relation may be measured by tracer gas techniques[59] or radioactive gas and microsphere techniques,[20] but the calculation most often used in the ICU is the following classic shunt equation:

$$\dot{Q}_s\dot{Q}_t = \frac{Cc'_{O_2} - Ca_{O_2}}{Cc'_{O_2} - C\overline{v}_{O_2}}$$

where Cc'_{O_2} = end-capillary oxygen content (an idealized value computed using the $P_{A_{O_2}}$), Ca_{O_2} = arterial oxygen content, and $C\overline{v}_{O_2}$ = mixed venous oxygen content.

Note that this measurement requires simultaneous collection of both arterial and mixed venous blood samples and thus necessitates having a pulmonary artery catheter in place (see Chapter 15).

$\dot{Q}_s/\dot{Q}_t$ is often measured while the patient is breathing 100% oxygen. However, breathing 100% oxygen for 30 minutes can lead to nitrogen washout and collapse of low $\dot{V}/\dot{Q}$ units.[60-62] This phenomenon of alveolar collapse appears to be caused by poor ventilation of low $\dot{V}/\dot{Q}$ units so that oxygen uptake by the blood exceeds oxygen delivered to the alveoli by means of ventilation. The resulting microatelectasis increases the shunt fraction. Regional blood flow is usually reduced to areas of the lung with low $\dot{V}/\dot{Q}$ as a protective mechanism.[61] Breathing 100% oxygen alters this natural autoregulation,[63] causing increased shunt.

Pulmonary vasodilation[63] and inotropic agents (e.g., dopamine) increase cardiac output but also can increase $\dot{Q}_s/\dot{Q}_t$.[51,52] If oxygen transport is improved with this pharmacologic support, its use may be indicated regardless of the increased shunt.

In patients without pulmonary artery catheters, an estimation of $\dot{Q}_s/\dot{Q}_t$ can be made by substituting the value of 3.5 mL/dL for the actual measured arteriovenous difference in the denominator (a typical value in a critically ill patients). Compared with the other previously described oxygenation indices, this method for estimating the shunt fraction correlates best with the actual measured $\dot{Q}_s/\dot{Q}_t$.[64] This is because all the other oxygenation indices fail to account for the mixed venous O_2 content and, except for the a/A ratio, ignore the effects of alveolar ventilation.[65]

Pulse Oximetry

The principles of measurement, clinical use, interpretation, and limitations of HbO_2 saturation measured by pulse oximetry are detailed in Chapter 8. Because pulse oximetry is quick and noninvasive and can be used for continuous monitoring, it has become a standard of care in critical care units, in operating and emergency rooms, and during transport and special procedures such as bronchoscopy, computed tomography (CT), sleep studies, exercise testing, and weaning from supplemental oxygen and mechanical ventilation. Oximetry also can be helpful in the ambulatory care settings to support pulmonary rehabilitation and justify and monitor home oxygen therapy.

Many studies have been performed to compare the accuracy and responsiveness of pulse oximeters to direct measures of HbO_2 saturation.[66-69] Studies of healthy and critically ill patients with adequate cardiac output generally show a high degree of accuracy and correlation compared with direct arterial saturation, as long as saturation exceeds 65%. However, as described in Chapter 8, numerous factors can cause erroneous SpO_2 readings and must be taken into account when interpreting this measurement.

Selecting the monitoring site can be crucial to obtaining accurate measurement of SpO_2. Pulse oximetry sensors are primarily applied to the thumb or a finger of the hand if available. Unfortunately, use of the digits increases the likelihood of motion artifact that can interfere with good signal acquisition. Secondarily, the great toe of the foot, an earlobe, or the forehead can be used with the appropriate equipment. Earlobe and forehead sensors are specifically designed for those sites and less prone to motion artifact. Forehead and ear sensors also may be less affected than the extremities by poor perfusion. Fortunately, ongoing improvements in pulse oximetry technology have resulted in better artifact filtration and pulse signal recognition. These changes enable pulse oximeters to more accurately provide SpO_2 readings during periods of movement and during low perfusion states.[70,71]

Pulse oximetry can be a useful tool in the ICU, but also is prone to overuse and misinterpretation. Normal pulse oximetry values do not guarantee adequate DO_2 to the tissues. The anemic patient may be adequately saturated, but hypoxia may be present because of the low arterial oxygen concentration (CaO_2). In addition, the pulse oximeter does not measure PCO_2 or acid-base status. Abnormalities in these variables can be just as life threatening as hypoxia yet may go undetected when the SpO_2 reads normal.

Monitoring Tissue Oxygen Delivery and Utilization

Oxygen Delivery and Availability

Oxygen deliver (DO_2) is calculated as follows:

$$DO_2 (mL/min) = CO\ (L/min) \times CaO_2 (mL/dL) \times 10$$

The delivered oxygen value reflects the total amount of oxygen carried in the blood per unit of time. Adjusted for body surface area, the reference range for DO_2 for normal subjects is 550 to 650 mL/m^2 per minute. The delivered oxygen often is elevated with hyperdynamic states such as septic shock. Reduced values indicate low cardiac output, or decreased CaO_2. Measuring DO_2 is one way to see whether the overall effect of a specific therapy is positive

or negative. For example, increasing the PEEP level of a patient with acute lung injury may well increase the PaO_2, SaO_2, and CaO_2, but this improvement may be offset by a fall in cardiac output due to higher $P_{\overline{aw}}$ and resulting impaired venous return.

Oxygen Consumption

Oxygen consumption ($\dot{V}O_2$) is defined as the oxygen consumed by the entire body in milliliters per minute. The reference range is 2.86 to 4.29 mL/kg per minute at STPD or 100 to 140 mL/m^2 per minute of body surface area. If one thinks of DO_2 as the supply, then the $\dot{V}O_2$ is the utilization. Adequate supply does not always ensure proper utilization.

Many factors determine tissue $\dot{V}O_2$. $\dot{V}O_2$ can be limited by decreased oxygen availability because of a decrease in regional perfusion or a decrease in oxygen content.[72-74] Demand may exceed supply, as in a hypermetabolic state, or cellular metabolism may be impaired, as in cyanide poisoning.

$\dot{V}O_2$ can be measured directly, through the analysis of inspired and exhaled gas volumes and concentrations, or indirectly, by multiplying the cardiac output by the arteriovenous oxygen content difference (Fick calculation). The formula for calculating $\dot{V}O_2$ using the direct method is as follows:

$$\dot{V}O_2 = ([\ (1 - F_{\overline{E}}O_2/1 - F_IO_2) \times F_IO_2] - F_{\overline{E}}O_2) \times \dot{V}_E$$

All volumes are converted to STPD conditions. Fraction of exhaled gas that is oxygen (F_EO_2) is measured directly. The formula assumes that nitrogen is an inert (nonreactive) gas and that no other gases are present. The presence of nitrous oxide (a gas used in surgery by anesthesiologists) may introduce a considerable error if the patient's $\dot{V}O_2$ is measured immediately after anesthesia.

Another direct technique requires that the patient breathe a specific concentration of gas through a closed-circuit system that incorporates a carbon dioxide absorber. $\dot{V}O_2$ can be measured by the following formula:

$$\dot{V}O_2 = \text{Change in volume at STPD} \times F_IO_2$$

Direct $\dot{V}O_2$ measurement techniques are extremely demanding. The circuit must be completely free of leaks. Gas volumes and concentrations must be accurately collected and measured. The F_IO_2 must remain stable with minimal fluctuation. Technologic advances allow $\dot{V}O_2$ to be monitored continuously in critically ill patients during continuous mechanical ventilation.[75]

The indirect calculation of $\dot{V}O_2$ is based on the **Fick principle**:

$$\dot{V}O_2 (mL/min) = CO(L/min) \times C(a - \overline{v})O_2 (mL/dL) \times 10$$

The Fick principle is used often in the ICU because of its convenience more than its accuracy. Variations between Fick calculations and direct measurement of $\dot{V}O_2$ may be clinically significant, primarily because of errors in venous gas sampling and cardiac output analysis.[76,77] This error is greatest in patients with high cardiac output.

When Do_2 is adequate, $\dot{V}o_2$ is determined by the metabolic demands of the patient. $\dot{V}o_2$ will stay constant as long as the delivered oxygen is greater than a critical threshold of approximately 8 to 10 mL/kg per minute in anesthetized humans.[78] This critical threshold is significantly elevated in ARDS and sepsis[79] (Fig. 14-17). In patients with ARDS, $\dot{V}o_2$ is linearly related to Do_2 up to 21 mL/kg per minute.[80] ICU patients often exhibit alterations in $\dot{V}o_2$ caused by trauma, sepsis, shock, changes in body temperature, anesthesia, therapeutic modalities such as chest physiotherapy, and ventilator settings. $\dot{V}o_2$ has been shown to be an excellent predictor of survival in patients with trauma and shock and is helpful in determining the adequacy of resuscitation.[73,79] It also has been advocated as an index of the cost of breathing in terms of oxygen use and therefore is useful in predicting the patient's ability to be weaned from mechanical ventilation.[75,81]

$\dot{V}o_2$ values of 100% to 150% of normal after trauma or shock are associated with a better prognosis and have been identified as appropriate therapeutic goals for the high-risk surgical patient.[82] Values less than 100% may be the result of decreased oxygen availability, as with low cardiac output or oxygen content, or with decreased use, as in hypothermia. In patients with severe injury, values greater than 150% may indicate a poor prognosis. If Do_2 is increased for any reason, increased availability may lead to increased consumption. This phenomenon has been observed in patients with ARDS, cardiogenic pulmonary edema, COPD, and pneumonia.[72,83,84]

SIMPLY STATED

Oxygen consumption is partially influenced by oxygen availability. In many critically ill patients, as Do_2 goes, so goes oxygen consumption.

Mixed Venous Oxygen Tension

Mixed venous oxygen tension ($P\bar{v}o_2$) is a measure of the partial pressure of oxygen in mixed venous blood and is an indication of oxygen use by the entire body. Factors that influence oxygen transport and consumption invariably affect $P\bar{v}o_2$. The normal reference range is 38 to 42 mm Hg. Low $P\bar{v}o_2$ may result from the following:

- Inadequate cardiac output
- Anemia
- Significant hypoxia
- "Affinity" hypoxia (low $P\bar{v}o_2$ with increased $S\bar{v}o_2$)

A $P\bar{v}o_2$ of less than 27 mm Hg is usually associated with lactic acidosis. Increased $P\bar{v}o_2$ (>45 mm Hg) may result from the following:

- Poor sampling technique (pulmonary artery catheter in wedge position)
- Left-to-right shunt

- Septic shock
- Increased cardiac output
- Cyanide poisoning

Because $P\bar{v}o_2$ reflects the components of the supply-demand balance in perfused tissues, it is possible to have normal values of $P\bar{v}o_2$ and still have inadequate Do_2 to certain organs (e.g., kidneys). Organs with poor perfusion make a minimal contribution to venous return; therefore, $P\bar{v}o_2$ may remain in the normal range even though an oxygen deficit exists, as in the vasodilated, septic patient with normal cardiac output.

$P\bar{v}o_2$ may not reflect changes in Do_2 and cardiac output. Because variations in $\dot{V}o_2$ also affect the balance between supply and demand, elevated $P\bar{v}o_2$ may indicate inadequate tissue oxygen utilization and marked maldistribution in systemic blood flow. This is common in septic shock. A low $P\bar{v}o_2$ is expected when the tissues are using the available oxygen effectively but the supply is insufficient.

$\dot{V}o_2$ is particularly high for the heart and the brain, so the $P\bar{v}o_2$ of these organs is extremely critical. A fall in perfusion would require a compensatory mechanism to maintain blood flow and oxygen to these organs.

The mixed venous sample is obtained by slowly aspirating, over about 1 minute, 3 to 5 mL of blood from the distal port of a pulmonary artery catheter. Central venous blood samples may trend well if the catheter is properly positioned, but generally there is a difference of 2 to 3 mm Hg between the Po_2 of central venous and pulmonary artery samples. The technique used for mixed venous gas analysis is important because errors in sampling may result in erroneous readings. The pressure waveform should be inspected before the sample is aspirated to ensure that the catheter is not wedged. Wedging may result in aspirating postcapillary blood and thus produce an erroneously high

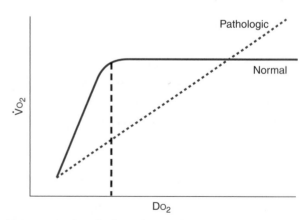

FIGURE 14-17 Supply dependence of oxygen consumption ($\dot{V}o_2$). Under normal conditions (*solid line*), $\dot{V}o_2$ will increase until a critical threshold (*dashed line*) of delivered oxygen (Do_2) is reached. Beyond this critical threshold, $\dot{V}o_2$ remains stable, despite the increase in Do_2. In pathologic conditions (*dotted line*), such as acute respiratory distress syndrome (ARDS), $\dot{V}o_2$ may not plateau but will continue to rise, as Do_2 increases, until well past the normal critical threshold.

measurement of $P\bar{v}o_2$. Air bubbles in the sample are also a possible cause of falsely elevated values.

Mixed Venous Oxygen Saturation

Mixed venous oxygen saturation ($S\bar{v}o_2$) is measured from a mixed venous blood sample. Small changes in $P\bar{v}o_2$ lead to large changes in $S\bar{v}o_2$ and therefore large changes in mixed venous oxygen content ($C\bar{v}o_2$). As a result, the

measurement is a sensitive index of cardiac output and tissue perfusion if $\dot{V}o_2$ is stable (Table 14-2). Like $P\bar{v}o_2$, $S\bar{v}o_2$ is a means of monitoring the general supply-and-demand differences in Do_2, not the use of oxygen at a specific site.

$S\bar{v}o_2$ can be monitored continuously through a fiberoptic system incorporated in a five-lumen pulmonary artery catheter. The system incorporates the principle of *reflection spectrophotometry* (traditional oximetry uses transmission spectrophotometry). An optical module transmits light through the blood by means of a fiberoptic monofilament. Reflected light is transmitted by a separate monofilament to a photodetector in the module. Because reduced Hb and oxygenated Hb absorb different wavelengths of light, a microprocessor can quantify the reflected wavelengths and calculate $S\bar{v}o_2$ (Fig. 14-18). When the catheter is properly positioned and calibrated, values correlate well with benchmark saturation measurements.[85] Continuous monitoring has the advantage of providing immediate feedback for purposes of evaluating therapy. The continuous measurement of central venous oxygen saturation ($Scvo_2$) has been shown to be comparable to $S\bar{v}o_2$ monitoring,[86] although others question its reliability.[87]

TABLE 14-2	
Interpretation of Venous Oxygen Saturation ($S\bar{v}o_2$)	
$S\bar{v}o_2$	**Interpretation**
68% to 77%	Normal
>77%	Sepsis, left-to-right shunt, excessive cardiac output, hypothermia, cell poisoning, wedged catheter
<60%	Cardiac decompensation
<50%	Lactic acidosis
<30%	Unconsciousness
<20%	Permanent damage

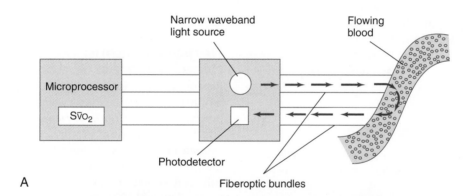

A

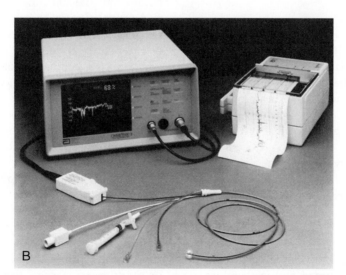

B

FIGURE 14-18 A, Principles of reflection spectrophotometry. **B**, Fiberoptic catheter system used for continuous monitoring of venous oxygen saturation ($S\bar{v}o_2$). (**A**, From Ruppel GL: *Manual of pulmonary function testing*, ed 9, St Louis, 2009, Mosby. **B**, Courtesy Hospira, Inc., Lake Forest, IL.)

Various factors, such as suctioning, shivering, pharmacologic intervention, extubation, weaning, and positive-pressure therapy, can decrease the $S\bar{v}_{O_2}$ measurement, signifying a deterioration in pulmonary gas exchange, an increase in $\dot{V}_{O_2}$, or a reduction in cardiac output.

Arterial-to-Mixed Venous Oxygen Content Difference

The **arterial-to-mixed venous oxygen content difference $[C(a - \bar{v})o_2]$** reflects the difference in oxygen content between arterial and venous blood. It is derived after simultaneous arterial and mixed venous blood gases are drawn. The normal reference range is 4 to 6 vol%.

Values greater than 6 vol% may be the result of the following:

- Low cardiac output
- Increasing $\dot{V}_{O_2}$

Values less than 4 vol% may be the result of the following:

- Septic shock
- Increased cardiac output
- Anemia
- Increased oxygen affinity caused by a left-shifted oxyhemoglobin dissociation curve

The $C(a - \bar{v})o_2$ is useful in determining the effects of mechanical ventilation and PEEP on cardiac output[88] and evaluating the need for additional circulatory support. It has a slight advantage over the $P\bar{v}_{O_2}$ measurement in that it reflects content differences instead of partial pressure.

> **SIMPLY STATED**
>
> Traditional parameters, such as pulse oximetry and Pa_{O_2}, reflect the adequacy of pulmonary oxygenation, not tissue oxygenation.

Oxygen Extraction Ratio

The **oxygen extraction ratio $[C(a - \bar{v})o_2/Ca_{O_2}]$** expresses the relationship between available oxygen (Ca_{O_2}) and oxygen extracted $[C(a - \bar{v})o_2]$. The normal reference range is 25% to 30%. Values greater than 30% indicate one of the following:

- Increased extraction caused by low cardiac output
- Increased $\dot{V}_{O_2}$
- Decreased oxygen availability caused by decreased Ca_{O_2}

Values less than 25% indicate that supply is out of proportion to demand, which may be a result of the following:

- High cardiac output
- Sepsis with systemic shunts

The $C(a - \bar{v})o_2/Ca_{O_2}$ ratio identifies the portion of the delivered oxygen actually consumed and is therefore an index of the efficiency of circulation.

Blood Lactate

If oxygen transport or its use by the tissues is insufficient for metabolic demands, anaerobic metabolism occurs and lactic acid is produced. Clinically this is seen as a metabolic acidosis with an elevation in blood lactate concentrations. The degree of lactic acidosis corresponds to the severity of oxygen deficit and is therefore a good indicator of prognostic outcome in patients with shock and multisystem organ dysfunction syndrome.[89,90] The reference range for normal blood lactate is less than 1.7 to 2.0 mM/L. In patients with shock, lactate levels greater than 3.83 mM/L are associated with 67% mortality, and values greater than 8 mM/L are associated with greater than 90% mortality.[89,91] β-Adrenergic stimulator drugs increase lactate levels because of glycolysis, and β-blockers decrease blood lactate levels.[92] Patients with lactic acidosis are often treated with alkaline solutions such as sodium bicarbonate. This alkalinization may increase blood lactate levels because of a redistribution of extracellular and intracellular lactate, but does not indicate a worsening metabolic acidosis.[93]

Patients with cirrhosis have a reduced ability to clear peak lactate concentrations after periods of increased production. As a result, lactate is useful in confirming the presence of tissue hypoxia in these patients, but it is not a useful prognostic index.[94]

Regional Tissue Oxygenation (Near Infrared Spectroscopy)

Recent advances in technology now provide the means to monitor regional tissue oxygenation noninvasively. The principle is basically the same as that used for estimating arterial O_2 saturation by pulse oximetry (see Chapter 8).[95] Instead of using visible light however, tissue oxygenation monitors use near infrared light, a technique called **near infrared spectroscopy (NIRS)**. Light in the NIR spectrum (700 to 1100 nm) can penetrate tissues and bone to a depth of several centimeters. As with pulse oximetry, using different wavelengths of light allows quantification of the relative differences in the amount of oxygenated and deoxygenated hemoglobin present and thus provides a measure of HbO_2 saturation in the tissues. This measure is commonly abbreviated as either St_{O_2} or Sr_{O_2} (regional O_2 saturation). In addition to St_{O_2}, some tissue oxygenation monitors also can provide an estimate of the Hb concentration that correlates well with *in vitro* blood Hb measurement.

The most common application of NIRS has been to assess cerebral oxygenation during surgery. NIRS monitors and sensors designed to assess peripheral tissue oxygenation are now being used in critical care. Sampling sites include the thenar eminence (group of muscles on the palm of the hand at the base of the thumb) or the inner surface of the forearm (Fig. 14-19).[95] As a measure of regional oxygenation, the St_{O_2} reflects not

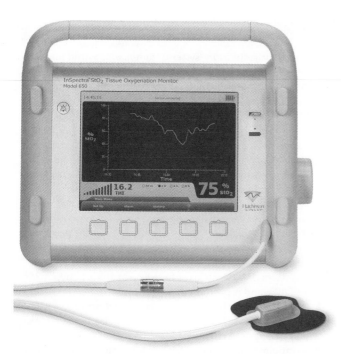

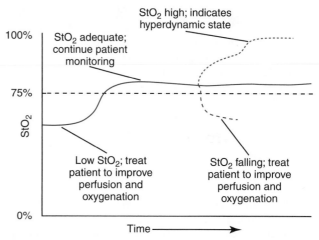

FIGURE 14-20 Example of trend monitoring of Sto₂. Goal-directed therapy (e.g., fluid resuscitation, pharmacologic therapy) aims to maintain the Sto₂ at or above the threshold value of 75%. Note that higher than normal Sto₂ values can occur in hyperdynamic states such as septic shock.

FIGURE 14-19 Tissue oxygenation monitor (InSpectra Sto₂ Monitor) used to measure regional HbO₂ saturation, in this case using a probe placed over the thenar eminence. (Photograph courtesy of Hutchison Technology, Inc., BioMeasurement Division, Hutchison, MN.)

only the HbO₂ saturation but also the matching of O₂ delivery to O₂ utilization of the underlying tissues, including the extent of peripheral vasoconstriction and regional ischemia that occurs in shock-like states. Often not detectable using central venous blood measures, regional ischemia is associated with poor outcomes among critically ill patients. Because Sto₂ levels fall well before standard markers of tissue hypoxia such as blood lactate, tissue oxygenation monitors can provide an early warning of potential perfusion deficits. In addition to providing early detection of regional ischemia or hypoxia, tissue oxygenation monitors can help guide therapy to treat it.

Among patients suffering from trauma or sepsis, keeping Sto₂ levels above 75% decreases the likelihood of organ dysfunction.[96] Indeed, mortality has been shown to increase as much as two- to three-fold when the Sto₂ remains significantly below this level and cannot be restored.[95-97] For this reason, an Sto₂ of 75% has been recommended as the threshold for intervention (Fig. 14-20).[96] The addition of a vascular occlusion test (VOT) improves the ability of Sto₂ to identify tissue hypoperfusion.[98,99] To perform a VOT, blood flow to the arm is rapidly stopped by inflating a sphygmomanometer cuff to 30 mm Hg above systolic pressure either for 3 minutes or until the forearm or thenar Sto₂ drops to a defined minimal value (usually 40%), followed by rapid release

of the cuff and restoration of perfusion. The slope of the fall in Sto₂ with arterial occlusion is termed the *deoxygenation rate* (Deo₂), which reflects the metabolic rate of the underlying tissues. The slope of the rise in Sto₂ with restoration of blood is termed the *reoxygenation rate* (Reo₂), which is a measure of local cardiovascular reserve and microcirculatory flow.

Because maintenance of adequate tissue oxygenation is a primary goal of respiratory care, RTs must become more involve in both the collection and interpretation of relevant data like that now being provided through noninvasive monitoring of this critical parameter. In addition, because various respiratory care interventions can affect both systemic and local perfusion, RTs should incorporate the information provided by this new technology into their clinical decision making.

KEY POINTS

▶ The ventilatory measurements that can be monitored at the bedside in the ICU routinely include lung volumes and flows, airway pressures, and fractional gas concentrations

▶ V_T for a healthy person varies with each breath but typically ranges from 5 to 8 mL/kg of predicted body weight.

▶ If shallow breathing without occasional sighing is maintained for prolonged periods, atelectasis and pneumonia may result, especially in patients breathing high oxygen concentrations or having compromised mucociliary clearance.

▶ Conditions that may cause the V_T to be reduced include pneumonia, atelectasis, the postoperative period after chest and abdominal surgeries, chest trauma, acute exacerbation of COPD, CHF, acute restrictive diseases such

KEY POINTS—cont'd

as ARDS, neuromuscular diseases, and CNS depression (especially of the respiratory centers).

▶ The use of high V_T ventilation may predispose patients to volutrauma, a lung injury that occurs from overdistention of the terminal respiratory units.

▶ A low measured V_T also can be caused by "stacking" or dynamic hyperinflation, a problem seen with severe airway obstruction. If not enough time is allowed for exhalation before the next breath is initiated by the ventilator, the subsequent V_T will "stack" on top of the previous breath.

▶ When a patient is ready to be weaned from mechanical ventilation, a spontaneous breathing trial (SBT) should be attempted. The patient should be monitored for gas exchange, respiratory distress, and hemodynamic stability during this trial.

▶ If a higher than normal $\dot{V}_E$ is associated with a normal Pa_{CO_2} in a patient with a normal metabolic rate, there must be an increase in wasted or dead space ventilation.

▶ If a spontaneous $\dot{V}_E$ greater than 10 L/minute is needed for a mechanically ventilated patient to maintain a normal Pa_{CO_2}, weaning is not likely to be successful.

▶ VC is the maximal volume of gas that can be expired from the lungs following a maximal inspiration. The normal reference range for healthy persons is 65 to 75 mL/kg of predicted body weight.

▶ A VC of 10 to 15 mL/kg is usually needed for effective deep breathing and coughing.

▶ PIP is the maximal pressure attained during the inspiratory phase of mechanical ventilation. It reflects the amount of force needed to overcome opposition to airflow into the lungs.

▶ If the PIP increases while the plateau pressure is unchanged, an increase in Raw is probably occurring. Common causes include bronchospasm, airway secretions, and mucous plugging.

▶ The plateau pressure (also referred to as static pressure) is the pressure required to maintain a delivered V_T in a patient's lungs during a period of no gas flow.

▶ P_Imax, sometimes called the NIF, is the maximal inspiratory pressure the patient's ventilatory pump is capable of generating against a closed airway.

▶ A normal P_Imax or NIF is approximately −80 to −100 cm H_2O. A P_Imax of −30 cm H_2O may be useful when used in conjunction with other parameters in predicting successful weaning.

▶ If mechanically ventilated patients do not complete exhalation before inspiration begins, they will develop auto-PEEP. This can result from airway obstruction that increases during exhalation and causes insufficient time for exhalation.

▶ Auto-PEEP varies with the time allowed for exhalation, the elastic recoil of the lung, and the resistance to flow of the airways, ET tube, and expiratory limb (exhalation valve) of the ventilator circuit. Bronchodilator therapy, decreased inspiratory time, and a reduction in the mechanical frequency have been shown to reduce the amount of auto-PEEP.

KEY POINTS—cont'd

▶ Static (or respiratory system) compliance is the lung volume change per unit of pressure during a period of no gas flow. Static compliance reflects a combination of chest wall and lung compliance.

▶ Most ventilators manufactured today are equipped with a graphic display screen. Three of the most important parameters to follow are the pressure, flow, and volume tracings of mechanically ventilated patients. The individual parameters may be indexed to each other, as in a pressure-volume loop or a flow-volume loop.

▶ V_D is the inspired volume that does not come in contact with pulmonary capillary blood. The V_D/V_T ratio expresses the relationship between V_D and total V_T, or the portion of the V_T that is "wasted." V_D has two components: anatomic dead space and alveolar dead space.

▶ The normal V_D/V_T ratio for healthy persons is between 25% and 40% and is position dependent.

▶ Oxygen delivery to the tissues is a function of Ca_{O_2} and cardiac output. If either component fails, tissue hypoxia may occur.

▶ Intrapulmonary shunt ($\dot{Q}_s/\dot{Q}_t$) is a major contributor to hypoxemia in most critically ill patients and represents the proportion of blood flow perfusing the lungs that does not pass by ventilated alveoli.

▶ Pulse oximetry is a noninvasive technique for measuring HbO_2 saturation in the arterial blood.

▶ $\dot{V}_{O_2}$ is defined as the oxygen consumed by the entire body in milliliters per minute. The normal reference range is 2.86 to 4.29 mL/min/kg at STPD or 100 to 140 mL/min/m² of body surface area.

▶ $P\bar{v}_{O_2}$ is a measure of the O_2 partial pressure in mixed venous blood and is an indication of oxygen use by the entire body; the normal reference range of $P\bar{v}_{O_2}$ is 38 to 42 mm Hg, with low values associated with low cardiac output or reduced Ca_{O_2} in a patient with limited cardiac reserve.

▶ Keeping noninvasively monitored tissue O_2 saturation (Sto_2) levels above 75% decreases the likelihood of organ dysfunction and mortality among shock and trauma patients.

CASE STUDY

Lucy is a 30-year-old woman with asthma who presented to the emergency room with shortness of breath, respiratory distress, and wheezing. She has been given steroids and bronchodilators for the past 3 hours. The following data were recently collected: arterial blood gas (ABG) values (pH, 7.36; Pa_{CO_2}, 44 mm Hg; Pa_{O_2}, 65 mm Hg; Sa_{O_2}, 91%; $F_{I}O_2$, 0.40); respiratory rate, 30; and V_T, 220 mL. Lucy is using abdominal muscles to force exhalations and is wheezing and appears severely dyspneic. She was unable to perform bedside spirometry and weighs 60 kg.

CASE STUDY—cont'd

Interpretation

Even though the pH and $Paco_2$ are normal, we would expect this patient with an asthma exacerbation and mild hypoxemia to be hyperventilating (see Chapter 8). The fact that this patient's $Paco_2$ is 44 mm Hg is a sign of fatigue and impending respiratory failure. The high respiratory rate and V_T of less than 4 mL/kg are also signs of fatigue and impending respiratory failure. When these factors are combined with the patient's severe respiratory distress, the need for mechanical ventilation and admission to the ICU is apparent.

CASE STUDY

When assessing a patient with COPD who requires mechanical ventilation, the RT notices that the patient is using his abdominal muscles when exhaling and that he appears to be in some respiratory distress. When assessing the ventilator, she found the following parameters and graphics: PS, 15 cm H_2O; PEEP, 0 cm H_2O; F_IO_2, 0.40; PS cycle %, 10%; flow trigger, 2 L/min; PIP, 18 cm H_2O; spontaneous respiratory rate, 20; and spontaneous V_T, 420 mL. The pressure-time waveform is as follows:

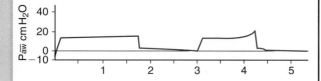

Interpretation

When assessing this pressure-time waveform, the inspiratory time during PS is too long on the first breath, and the second breath ends earlier because of the patient exhaling against the set PS level. The RT's observation of the patient confirms that the patient has some expiratory dyssynchrony and the patient's work of breathing is elevated.

This type of dyssynchrony is most likely to occur in patients with obstructive lung disease with high PS levels and low set PS cycle %. To correct this patient's dyssynchrony, the PS cycle % of 10% would need to be increased until the dog ear on the right side of the pressure-time waveform disappears. A PS cycle % of 30% to 40% will usually correct the problem.

ASSESSMENT QUESTIONS

See Appendix for answers.

1. Which of the following patients is *least* likely to benefit from having their lung volumes monitored?
   a. A patient receiving mechanical ventilation through an ET tube
   b. A patient with neuromuscular disease
   c. A patient with mild to moderate hypoxemia
   d. A patient with CNS depression

2. Which of the following is true regarding the measurement of V_T as a means of ventilatory assessment in intensive care?
   a. It is normally 3 to 4 mL/kg of predicted body weight
   b. It should be at least 450 mL before weaning from mechanical ventilation
   c. It may decrease after abdominal or thoracic surgery
   d. It should be increased to keep plateau pressures above 30 cm H_2O

3. Which of the following conditions is most likely to cause an increase in a patient's V_T?
   a. Metabolic acidosis
   b. Pneumonia
   c. Atelectasis
   d. CHF

4. What is the primary concern with ventilating patients using larger V_T?
   a. Heart failure
   b. Volutrauma
   c. Atelectasis
   d. Aortic rupture

5. What diagnosis is most likely to lead to dynamic hyperinflation during mechanical ventilation?
   a. ARDS
   b. CHF
   c. COPD
   d. Pneumonia

6. What would be the corrected or delivered V_T using the following data: set V_T, 600 mL; exhaled V_T, 590 mL; frequency, 10 breaths/min; PIP, 25 cm H_2O; plateau, 20 cm H_2O, PEEP, 5 cm H_2O; spontaneous V_T, 400 mL; spontaneous frequency, 6 breaths/min; and circuit compliance, 2 mL/cm H_2O.
   a. 550 mL
   b. 560 mL
   c. 570 mL
   d. 590 mL

7. You are attending to a 45-year-old man weighing 80 kg who has been mechanically ventilated for 3 days as a result of bilateral pneumonia. The physician asks you to check his spontaneous breathing parameters, and you find the spontaneous V_T to be 250 mL with a respiratory rate of 30 breaths/minute. What is your advice about proceeding with weaning?
   a. The patient is ready
   b. The patient is not ready
   c. The patient needs a higher F_IO_2
   d. The patient needs a PEEP level

8. Which of the following would reduce air trapping or auto-PEEP during mechanical ventilation?
   a. Increasing the inspiratory flow
   b. Increasing the machine rate
   c. Increasing the set V_T
   d. Increasing the I/E ratio

9. An increased $\dot{V}_E$ with a normal Pa_{CO_2} indicates which of the following?
   a. Shunt
   b. Decreased metabolic rate
   c. Increased dead space
   d. Atelectasis

10. Which of the following is true regarding the measurement of vital capacity in the ICU?
    1. The measured value depends on patient position and effort
    2. It reflects the ventilatory reserve of the patient
    3. A value less than 10-15 mL/kg suggests respiratory failure
    a. 1 and 2
    b. 2 and 3
    c. 3 only
    d. 1, 2, and 3

11. Which of the following increases FRC?
    a. Long expiratory times
    b. High tidal volumes
    c. Air trapping and auto-PEEP
    d. High inspiratory flows

12. Which of the following would cause peak airway pressures to decrease on a mechanical ventilator?
    a. Partial airway obstruction
    b. Tension pneumothorax
    c. High inspiratory flow setting
    d. Leak in the ventilator circuit

13. Given a peak pressure of 50 cm H_2O, a static pressure of 35 cm H_2O, a PEEP of 5 cm H_2O, and a delivered V_T of 850 mL, what is the effective static compliance?
    a. 2 mL/cm H_2O
    b. 18 mL/cm H_2O
    c. 24 mL/cm H_2O
    d. 28 mL/cm H_2O

14. Which of the following is true regarding auto-PEEP?
    a. It normally is not detected by airway pressure monitoring
    b. It can be reduced by decreasing the inspiratory flow
    c. Administration of bronchodilators worsens the condition
    d. It decreases the patient's work of breathing

15. Given a peak airway pressure of 40 cm H_2O, a static pressure of 32 cm H_2O, a PEEP of 7 cm H_2O, a V_T of 675 mL, and an inspiratory flow of 60 L/minute, what is the Raw?
    a. 2 cm H_2O/L/sec
    b. 5 cm H_2O/L/sec
    c. 8 cm H_2O/L/sec
    d. 12 cm H_2O/L/sec

16. Which of the following ventilator graphic displays would be most useful in adjusting the level of PEEP applied to a patient with acute lung injury?
    a. Flow-pressure loop
    b. Volume-time scalar
    c. Pressure-volume loop
    d. Pressure-time scalar

17. The pressure-time ventilator graphic display can be used to assess all of the following, *except:*
    a. Mode of ventilation
    b. Estimate of patient effort
    c. Adequacy of inspiratory flow
    d. Presence of circuit leaks

18. Which of the following is true regarding the measurement of V_D/V_T in the ICU?
    a. It is calculated using the Pa_{O_2} and Pa_{CO_2}
    b. It is often increased during mechanical ventilation
    c. It is normally ranges between 50% and 60%
    d. It requires that the patient be fully preoxygenated

19. What is the normal range for V_D/V_T?
    a. 10% to 25%
    b. 15% to 30%
    c. 25% to 40%
    d. 30% to 60%

20. Which of the following would most likely result in a significant decrease in oxygen transport to the tissues?
    a. Cardiac output of 6 L/min
    b. Arterial saturation of 75%
    c. Hb level of 15 g/dL
    d. Arterial Po_2 of 60 mm Hg

21. Which of the following clinical indices denotes poor oxygenation?
    a. Pa_{O_2} of 80 mm Hg
    b. $Pa_{O_2}/F_{I_{O_2}}$ ratio of 400
    c. $P(A-a)o_2$ of 55 mm Hg on room air
    d. Oxygen index of 10

22. Which of the following would cause a low $P\bar{v}_{O_2}$?
    a. Left-to-right shunt
    b. Increased cardiac output
    c. Septic shock
    d. Hypoxia

23. Which of the following is true regarding the measurement of blood lactate?
    1. It corresponds to the level of oxygen deficit
    2. It is usually a result of anaerobic metabolism
    3. It can be increased by the administration of β-adrenergic drugs
    a. 2 only
    b. 1 and 2
    c. 2 and 3
    d. 1, 2, and 3.

24. Which of the following oxygen delivery values falls within the normal reference range?
    a. 200 mL/min/m^2
    b. 300 mL/min/m^2
    c. 500 mL/min/m^2
    d. 600 mL/min/m^2

25. What is the effect of cyanide poisoning on the body?
    a. Reduced oxygen consumption
    b. Reduced oxygen content
    c. Increased oxygen delivery
    d. Decreased $P\bar{v}_{O_2}$

26. What is the normal reference range for $P\bar{v}o_2$?
    a. 26-30 mm Hg
    b. 38-42 mm Hg
    c. 44-58 mm Hg
    d. 56-60 mm Hg

27. Your patient has a $P\bar{v}o_2$ of 55 mm Hg. Which of the following may explain the finding?
    a. Low cardiac output
    b. Septic shock
    c. Lung disease
    d. Renal failure

28. At what level of regional tissue HbO_2 saturation (Sto_2) should intervention to improve O_2 delivery be recommended?
    a. <95%
    b. <85%
    c. <75%
    d. <65%

References

1. Hudson LD. Monitoring of critically ill patients: conference summary. *Respir Care*. 1985;**30**:628.

2. Aboussouan LS. Respiratory failure and the need for ventilatory support. In: Kacmarek RM, Stoller JK, Heuer AL, editors. *Egan's fundamentals of respiratory care*. 10th ed. St Louis: Mosby; 2013.

3. Askanazi J, Silverberg PA, Hyman AI, et al. Patterns of ventilation in postoperative and acutely ill patients. *Crit Care Med*. 1979;**7**:41–6.

4. Wysocki M, Cracco C, Teixeira A, et al. Approximate entropy of respiratory rate and tidal volume during weaning from mechanical ventilation. *Crit Care Med*. 2006;**34**(8):2076–83.

5. Visick WD, Fairley HB, Hickey RF, et al. The effects of tidal volume and end-expiratory pressures on pulmonary gas exchange during anesthesia. *Anesthesiology*. 1973;**19**:285–90.

6. Hess DR. Approaches to conventional mechanical ventilation of the patient with acute respiratory distress syndrome. *Respir Care*. 2011;**56**(10):1555–72.

7. Peck MD, Koppelman T. Low-tidal-volume ventilation as a strategy to reduce ventilator-associated injury in ALI and ARDS. *J Burn Care Res*. 2009;**30**:172–83.

8. Dreyfuss D, Soler P, Basset G, Saumon G. High inflation pressure pulmonary edema: respective effects of high airway pressure, high tidal volume, and positive end-expiratory pressure. *Am Rev Respir Dis*. 1988;**137**:1159–64.

9. ARDS Network. Ventilation with lower tidal volumes as compared with traditional tidal volumes for acute lung injury and the acute respiratory distress syndrome. *N Engl J Med*. 2000;**342**(18):1301–8.

10. Finfer S, Rocker G. Alveolar overdistention is an important mechanism of persistent lung damage following severe protracted ARDS. *Anaesth Int Care*. 1996;**24**(5):569.

11. Pohlman MC, McCallister KE, Schweickert WD, et al. Excessive tidal volume from breath stacking during lung-protective ventilation for acute lung injury. *Crit Care Med*. 2008;**36**(11):3019–29.

12. MacIntyre NR, Cook DJ, Ely EW, et al. Evidence-based guidelines for weaning and discontinuing ventilatory support: a collective task force facilitated by the American College of Chest Physicians; the American Association for Respiratory Care; and the American College of Critical Care Medicine. *Chest*. 2001;**120**(6):375S–95S.

13. Yang KL, Tobin MJ. A prospective study of indexes predicting the outcome of trials of weaning from mechanical ventilation. *N Engl J Med*. 1991;**324**:1445.

14. Vassilakopoulos T, Zakynthinos S, Roussos C. The tension-time index and the frequency/tidal volume ratio are the major pathophysiologic determinants of weaning failure and success. *Am J Respir Crit Care Med*. 1998;**158**(2):378.

15. Segal LN, Oei E, Oppenheimer BW, et al. Evolution of pattern of breathing during a spontaneous breathing trial predicts successful extubation. *Intensive Care Med*. 2010;**36**:487–95.

16. Bouton AK, Abatzidou F, Tryfon S, et al. Diagnostic accuracy of the rapid shallow breathing index to predict a successful spontaneous breathing trial outcome in mechanically ventilated patients with chronic obstructive pulmonary disease. *Heart Lung*. 2011;**40**(2):105–10.

17. Craig DG. Postoperative recovery of pulmonary function, anaesthesia and analgesia. *Anaesthesia*. 1981;**60**:46.

18. Ragnarsdottir M, Kristjánsdóttir Á, Ingvarsdóttir I, et al. Short-term changes in pulmonary function and respiratory movements after cardiac surgery via median sternotomy. *Scand Cardiovasc J*. 2004;**38**:46.

19. Wessell HU, Stout RL, Abstainer CK, et al. Breath-by-breath variation of FRC: effect on Vo_2 and Vco_2 measured at the mouth. *J Appl Physiol*. 1979;**46**:1122–6.

20. West JB. Regional differences in the lung. *Chest*. 1978;**74**:426.

21. Benedik PS, Baun MM, Keus L, et al. Effects of body position on resting lung volume in overweight and mildly to moderately obese subjects. *Respir Care*. 2009;**54**(3):334–9.

22. Dreyfuss D, Saumon G. Role of tidal volume, FRC, and end-inspiratory volume in the development of pulmonary edema following mechanical ventilation. *Am Rev Respir Dis*. 1993;**148**(5):1194.

23. Verbrugge SJC, Lachmann B, Kesecioglu J. Lung protective ventilatory strategies in acute lung injury and acute respiratory distress syndrome: from experiment findings to clinical application. *Clin Physiol Funct Imaging*. 2007;**27**:67–90.

24. Amato MB, Barbas CS, Medeiros DM, et al. Effect of a protective-ventilation strategy on mortality in the acute respiratory distress syndrome. *N Engl J Med*. 1998;**338**:347–54.

25. Gay PC, Rodarte JR, Tayyab M, et al. Evaluation of bronchodilator responsiveness in mechanically ventilated patients. *Am Rev Respir Dis*. 1987;**138**:880–5.

26. Duarte AG. Inhaled bronchodilator administration during mechanical ventilation. *Respir Care*. 2004;**49**(6):623–34.

27. Haake R, Schlichtig R, Ulstad DR, et al. Barotrauma: pathophysiology, risk factors, and prevention. *Chest*. 1987;**91**:608–13.

28. Pierson DJ. Alveolar rupture during mechanical ventilation: role of PEEP, peak airway pressure, and distending volume. *Respir Care*. 1988;**33**:472.

29. Pilbeam SP, Cairo JM. Improving oxygenation and management of ARDS. In: Cairo JM, editor. *Pilbeam's mechanical ventilation: physiological and clinical applications*. 5th ed. St Louis: Mosby; 2012.

30. Marini JJ, Ravenscraft SA. Mean airway pressure: physiologic determinants and clinical importance. Part 2: clinical implications. *Crit Care Med*. 1992;**20**:1604.

31. Broccard AF, Hotchkiss JR, Suzuki S, et al. Effects of mean airway pressure and tidal excursion on lung injury induced by mechanical ventilation in an isolated perfused rabbit lung model. *Crit Care Med*. 1999;**27**(8):1533–41.

32. Marini JJ. Estimation of inspiratory muscle strength in mechanically ventilated patients: the measurement of maximal inspiratory pressure. *Crit Care Med*. 1986;**1**:32.

33. Brochard L. Intrinsic (or auto-) PEEP during controlled mechanical ventilation. *Intensive Care Med*. 2002;**28**:1376.

34. Blanch L, Bernabé F, Lucangelo U, et al. Measurement of air trapping, intrinsic positive end-expiratory pressure, and dynamic hyperinflation in mechanically ventilated patients. *Respir Care.* 2005;**50**(1):110–23.

35. Aboussouan LS, Lattin CD, Anne VV, et al. Determinants of time-to-weaning in a specialized respiratory care unit. *Chest.* 2005;**128**(5):3117–26.

36. Hess DR. Ventilator waveforms and the physiology of pressure support ventilation. *Respir Care.* 2005;**50**(2):166.

37. Lu Q, Rouby JJ. Measurement of pressure-volume curves in patients on mechanical ventilation: methods and significance. *Crit Care.* 2000;**4**:91–100.

38. Browning JA, Linberg SE, Turney SZ, et al. Effect of a fluctuating FIO_2 on metabolic measurement in mechanically ventilated patients. *Crit Care Med.* 1982;**10**:82–5.

39. McSwain SD, Hamel DS, Smith PB, et al. End-tidal and arterial carbon dioxide measurements across all levels of physiologic dead space. *Respir Care.* 2010;**55**(3):288–93.

40. AARC Clinical Practice Guideline. Capnography/capnometry during mechanical ventilation, 2011 revision and update. *Respir Care.* 2011;**56**(4):503–9.

41. Neumar RW, Otto CW, Link MS, et al. Part 8: adult advanced cardiovascular life support: 2010 American Heart Association guidelines for cardiopulmonary resuscitation and emergency cardiovascular care. *Circulation.* 2010;**122**(18 Suppl 3):S729–67.

42. Sinha P, Flower O, Soni N. Deadspace ventilation: a waste of breath! *Intensive Care Med.* 2011;**37**:735–46.

43. Craig K, Pierson DJ. Expired gas collections for deadspace calculations: a comparison of two methods. *Respir Care.* 1979;**24**:435.

44. Rehder K, Knopp TJ, Sessler AD, et al. Regional intrapulmonary gas distribution in awake and anaesthetized-paralyzed prone man. *J Appl Physiol.* 1977;**45**:528–35.

45. Fairley HB, Blenkarm GD. Effect on pulmonary gas exchange of variations in inspiratory flow rate during IPPV. *Br J Anaesth.* 1966;**38**:320.

46. Dammann JF, McAslan TC, Maffeo CJ, et al. Optimal flow pattern for mechanical ventilation of the lungs. *Crit Care Med.* 1978;**6**:293–310.

47. Haldane JS. Symptoms, causes, and prevention of anoxemia. *Br Med J.* 1919:65–72.

48. Finch CA, Lenfant C. Oxygen transport in man. *N Engl J Med.* 1972;**286**:407–15.

49. Bryant-Brown CW. Blood flow to the organs: parameters for function and survival in critical illness. *Crit Care Med.* 1988;**16**:170.

50. Scadding JG, Cumming G. *Scientific foundations of respiratory medicine.* Philadelphia: Saunders; 1981.

51. Berk JL, Hagen JF, Tong RK, et al. The use of dopamine to correct the reduced cardiac output resulting from positive end expiratory pressure. *Crit Care Med.* 1977;**5**:269.

52. Russell WJ, James MF. The effects on arterial haemoglobin oxygen saturation and on shunt of increasing cardiac output with dopamine and dobutamine during one-lung ventilation. *Anaesth Intensive Care.* 2004;**32**(5):644–8.

53. Kanber GJ, King FW, Eshchar YR, et al. The alveolar-arterial oxygen gradient in young and elderly men during air and oxygen breathing. *Am Rev Respir Dis.* 1968;**97**:376–81.

54. Gilbert R, Keighley JF. The arterial-alveolar oxygen tension ratio: an index of gas exchange applicable to varying inspired oxygen concentrations. *Am Rev Respir Dis.* 1974;**109**(1):142–5.

55. Maxwell C, Hess D, Shefet D, et al. Use of the arterial/alveolar oxygen tension ratio to predict the inspired oxygen concentration needed for a desired arterial oxygen tension. *Respir Care.* 1984;**29**:1135–9.

56. Villar J. What is the acute respiratory distress syndrome? *Respir Care.* 2011;**56**(10):1539–45.

57. Hallman M, Merritt TA, Jarvenpaa AL, et al. Exogenous human surfactant for treatment of severe respiratory distress syndrome: a randomized prospective clinical trial. *J Pediatr.* 1985;**106**:963–9.

58. Bartlett H. Extracorporeal membrane oxygenation (ECMO) in neonatal respiratory failure. *Ann Surg.* 1986;**204**:236.

59. Dantzker DR. Ventilation-perfusion distributions in the adult respiratory distress syndrome. *Am Rev Respir Dis.* 1979;**120**:1039.

60. West JB. Pulmonary gas exchange in the critically ill patient. *Crit Care Med.* 1974;**2**:171.

61. Suter PM, Fairley HB, Schlobohm RM, et al. Shunt, lung volume and perfusion during short periods of ventilation with oxygen. *Anesthesiology.* 1975;**43**:617–27.

62. Edmark L, Auner U, Enlund M, et al. Oxygen concentration and characteristics of progressive atelectasis formation during anaesthesia. *Acta Anaesthesiol Scand.* 2010;**55**:75–81.

63. Domino KB, Wetstein L, Glasser SA, et al. Influence of mixed venous oxygen tension on blood flow to atelectatic lung. *Anesthesiology.* 1983;**59**:428–34.

64. Cane RD, Shapiro BA, Templin R, et al. Unreliability of oxygen tension-based indices in reflecting intrapulmonary shunting in critically ill patients. *Crit Care Med.* 1988;**16**:1243–5.

65. Coetzee A, Swanevelder J, van der Spuy G, Jansen J. Gas exchange indices: how valid are they? *S Afr Med J.* 1995;**85**(11 Suppl):1227–32.

66. Milner QJW, Mathews GR. An assessment of the accuracy of pulse oximeters. *Anesthesia.* 2012;**67**:396–401.

67. Feiner JR, Severinghaus JW, Bickler PE. Dark skin decreases the accuracy of pulse oximeters at low oxygen saturation: the effects of oximeter probe type and gender. *Anesth Analg.* 2007;**105**:S18–23.

68. Falconer RJ, Robinson BJ. Comparison of pulse oximeters: accuracy at low arterial pressure in volunteers. *Br J Anaesth.* 1990;**65**(4):552.

69. Yamaya Y, Bogaard HJ, Wagner PD, et al. Validity of pulse oximetry during maximal exercise in normoxia, hypoxia, and hyperoxia. *J Appl Physiol.* 2002;**92**:162–8.

70. Petterson MT, Begnoche VL, Graybeal JM. The effect of motion on pulse oximetry and its clinical significance. *Anesth Analg.* 2007;**105**(6 Suppl):S78–84.

71. Graybeal JM, Petterson MT. Adaptive filtering and alternative calculations revolutionizes pulse oximetry sensitivity and specificity during motion and low perfusion. *Conf Proc IEEE Eng Med Biol Soc.* 2004:75363–7536.

72. Mohsenifar Z, Amin D, Jasper AC, et al. Dependence of oxygen consumption on oxygen delivery in patients with chronic congestive heart failure. *Chest.* 1987;**92**(3):447–50.

73. Shoemaker WC, Appel PL, Kram HB, et al. Tissue oxygen debt as a determinant of lethal and nonlethal postoperative organ failure. *Crit Care Med.* 1988;**16**:1117–20.

74. Caille V, Squara P. Oxygen uptake-to-delivery relationship: a way to assess adequate flow. *Crit Care.* 2006;**10**(3):S4.

75. Miwa K, Mitsuoka M, Takamori S, et al. Continuous monitoring of oxygen consumption in patients undergoing weaning from mechanical ventilation. *Respiration.* 2003;**70**(6):623–30.

76. Nelson LD, Houtchens BA, Westenskow DR, et al. VO_2 and PEEP in acute respiratory failure. *Crit Care Med.* 1982;**10**:857–62.

77. Bizouarn P, Blanloeil Y, Pinaud M, et al. Comparison between oxygen consumption calculated by Fick's principle using a continuous thermodilution technique and measure by indirect calorimetry. *Br J Anaesth.* 1995;**75**:719–23.

78. Cain SM. Peripheral oxygen uptake and delivery in health and disease. *Clin Chest Med.* 1983;**4**:139.

79. Astiz ME, Rackow EC, Kaufman B, et al. Relationship of oxygen delivery and mixed venous oxygenation to lactic acidosis in patients with sepsis and acute myocardial infarction. *Crit Care Med.* 1988;**16**:655-8.

80. Mohsenifar Z. Relationship between O_2 delivery and O_2 consumption in ARDS. *Chest.* 1983;**84**:267.

81. Harpin RP, Baker JP, Downer JP, et al. Correlation of the oxygen cost of breathing and length of weaning from mechanical ventilation. *Crit Care Med.* 1987;**15**:807-12.

82. Shoemaker WC, Appel PL, Kram HB, et al. Prospective trial of supranormal values of survivors as therapeutic goals in high-risk surgical patients. *Chest.* 1988;**94**:1176-86.

83. Danek SJ, Lynch JP, Weg JG, et al. The dependence of oxygen uptake on oxygen delivery in ARDS. *Am Rev Respir Dis.* 1980;**122**:387-95.

84. Yu M, Burchell S, Takiguchi SA, et al. The relationship of oxygen consumption measured by indirect calorimetry to oxygen delivery in critically ill patients. *J Trauma.* 1996;**41**(1):41-8.

85. Baele PL, McMichan JC, Marsh HM, et al. Continuous monitoring of mixed venous oxygen saturation in critically ill patients. *Anesth Analg.* 1982;**61**:513-28.

86. Molnar Z, Umgelter A, Toth I, et al. Continuous monitoring of ScvO2 by a new fibre-optic technology compared with blood gas oximetry in critically ill patients: a multicentre study. *Intensive Care Med.* 2007;**33**:1767-70.

87. Baulig W, Dullenkopf A, Hasenclever P, et al. In vitro evaluation of the CeVOX continuous central venous oxygenation monitoring system. *Anaesthesia.* 2008;**63**:412-7.

88. Downs JB, Klein EF, Modell JH, et al. The effect of incremental PEEP on Pao2 in patients with respiratory failure. *Anesth Analg.* 1973;**52**:210-5.

89. Rashkin MC, Bosken C, Baughman RP, et al. Oxygen delivery in critically ill patients: relationship to blood lactate and survival. *Chest.* 1985;**87**:580-4.

90. Jansen TC, Bommel JV, Bakker J. Blood lactate monitoring in critically ill patients: a systemic health technology assessment. *Crit Care Med.* 2009;**37**:2827-39.

91. Cady LD Jr, Weil MH, Afifi AA, et al. Quantitation of severity of critical illness with special reference to blood lactate. *Crit Care Med.* 1973;**1**:75.

92. Berk J, Sampliner JE. *Handbook of critical care medicine.* 2nd ed. Boston: Little, Brown; 1982.

93. Sabatini S, Kurtzman NA. Bicarbonate therapy in severe metabolic acidosis. *J Am Soc Nephrol.* 2009;**20**(4):692-5.

94. Clemmesen JO, Høy CE, Kondrup J, et al. Splanchnic metabolism of fuel substrates in acute liver failure. *J Hepatol.* 2000;**33**(6):941-8.

95. Scheeren TW, Schober P, Schwarte LA. Monitoring tissue oxygenation by near infrared spectroscopy (NIRS): background and current applications. *J Clin Monit Comput.* 2012;**26**(4):279-87.

96. Mesquida J, Masip J, Gili G, et al. Thenar oxygen saturation measured by near infrared spectroscopy as a noninvasive predictor of low central venous oxygen saturation in septic patients. *Intensive Care Med.* 2009;**35**(6):1106-9.

97. Vorwerk C, Coats TJ. The prognostic value of tissue oxygen saturation in emergency department patients with severe sepsis or septic shock. *Emerg Med J.* 2012;**29**(9):699-703.

98. Lipcsey M, Woinarski NC, Bellomo R. Near infrared spectroscopy (NIRS) of the thenar eminence in anesthesia and intensive care. *Ann Intensive Care.* 2012;**2**(1):11.

99. Pinsky MR, Payen D. Probing the limits of regional tissue oxygenation measures. *Crit Care.* 2009;**13**(Suppl 5):S1.

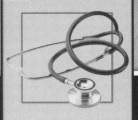

Chapter **15**

Vascular Pressure Monitoring

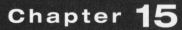

KENNETH MILLER AND CRAIG L. SCANLAN*

CHAPTER OUTLINE

Arterial Pressure Monitoring
    Indications for Arterial Pressure Monitoring
    Arterial Catheter Insertion Sites
    Equipment Set-Up
    Procedure for Inserting an Arterial Line
    Arterial Pressure Waveforms
    Interpretation of Arterial Pressure
      Measurements
    Complications Associated with Arterial Lines
Central Venous Pressure Monitoring
    Indications for CVP Monitoring
    CVP Catheters and Insertion Sites

    Procedure for Inserting a CVP Catheter
    Central Venous and Atrial Pressure Waveforms
    Interpretation of CVP Measurements
    Complications of CVP Monitoring
Pulmonary Artery Pressure Monitoring
    Indications for Pulmonary Artery Pressure
      Monitoring
    Pulmonary Artery Catheters and Insertion Sites
    Placement of the Pulmonary Artery Catheter
    Interpretation of Pulmonary Artery Pressures
    Complications of Pulmonary Artery Catheters
Central Line Bundle

LEARNING OBJECTIVES

After reading this chapter, you will be able to:
  1. Describe the following regarding arterial cannulation:
    a. Indications for placing an A line
    b. Common insertion sites
    c. Monitoring equipment set-up
    d. Procedure for placement of the catheter
    e. Interpretation of arterial pressure waveforms
    f. Pressures measured and their interpretation
    g. Potential complications
  2. Describe the following regarding central venous pressure (CVP) monitoring:
    a. Indications for placing a CVP catheter
    b. Catheter description and insertion sites
    c. Procedure for placement of the catheter
    d. Interpretation of the CVP waveform
    e. Interpretation of pressures measured
    f. Relationship of CVP to left and right ventricular function
    g. Potential complications
  3. Describe the following regarding pulmonary artery pressure monitoring:
    a. Indications for placing a pulmonary artery catheter
    b. Catheter description and insertion sites
    c. Procedure for placement of the catheter
    d. Interpretation of pulmonary artery waveforms
    e. Interpretation of pressures measured
    f. Relationship between pulmonary artery diastolic pressure and pulmonary artery wedge pressure (PAWP)
    g. Techniques for obtaining an accurate PAWP reading

---

*Dr. Robert Wilkins and Dr. James Dexter contributed some of the content for this chapter as coeditors of the prior edition of this text.

LEARNING OBJECTIVES—cont'd

    h. Relationship between transmural pressure and PAWP

    i. Effect of positive end-expiratory pressure on PAWP measurements

    j. Potential complications of using the pulmonary artery catheter

  4. Outline the key interventions recommended to minimize central line–associated bloodstream infections (the central line bundle)

KEY TERMS

central venous pressure (CVP)

dicrotic notch

inotropic agent

mean arterial pressure (MAP)

phlebostatic axis

pulmonary artery occlusion pressure (PAOP)

pulmonary artery wedge pressure (PAWP)

pulmonary capillary wedge pressure (PCWP)

pulse pressure

transmural pressure

Hemodynamic monitoring often plays an important role in the assessment and treatment of critically ill patients. It is performed to evaluate intravascular fluid volume by measuring central venous pressure (CVP); cardiac function by measuring arterial blood pressure, pulmonary artery wedge pressure (PAWP), and cardiac output (CO); and vascular function by measuring systemic and pulmonary vascular resistance. Ideally, the information will be easily obtained, continuously available, and reliable, and the process of obtaining the information will not harm the patient.

Invasive hemodynamic monitoring is needed because basic clinical assessments such as evaluating jugular venous distention or heart sounds alone may not accurately reflect patients' hemodynamic status. Before a catheter is placed in a patient, however, clinicians must consider the risk-to-benefit ratio of invasive monitoring. The risk for invasive hemodynamic monitoring is minimized when properly trained clinicians insert and maintain the system. The complications associated with placing a catheter in a major blood vessel are detailed throughout this chapter.

Bedside monitors acquire and calculate physiologic data in real time and often transfer the data automatically to computers for trend analysis. However, monitors may not always provide accurate information. Therefore, optimal invasive monitoring requires not only knowledge of the procedural complications and use of the information but also understanding and control of the factors affecting the validity of the data. Therapeutic decision making based on the numbers alone is never adequate and can be dangerous.

This chapter provides an introduction to the hemodynamic pressures most often monitored invasively in critically ill patients: arterial pressure, CVP, and pulmonary artery pressures (Box 15-1). Indications and complications of invasive monitoring, normal and abnormal pressure waveforms, and clinical applications are discussed.

Table 15-1 summarizes the common reference ranges and the abbreviations for the pressures discussed in this chapter. Although intracardiac pressures are essentially the same in adults and children, heart rate and blood pressure vary significantly by age. Table 15-2 lists the common reference ranges for heart rate and blood pressure for children from infancy through 16 years of age. Remember that reference ranges are obtained from studies on healthy people and may be neither normal nor desirable for a specific patient. Nevertheless, knowledge of these reference ranges is essential in the interpretation and application of hemodynamic data.

Arterial Pressure Monitoring

Indications for Arterial Pressure Monitoring

The attending physician may place or order placement of an arterial catheter into a patient with significant hemodynamic instability or a patient who will require frequent arterial blood sampling. Patients with severe hypotension (shock), severe hypertension, or unstable respiratory failure (acute respiratory distress syndrome [ARDS]) are likely candidates to have continuous arterial pressure monitoring. Patients in need of medications that affect blood pressure (e.g., vasodilators or **inotropic agents**) may benefit from arterial pressure monitoring.

Arterial Catheter Insertion Sites

Arterial catheters may be placed in the radial, ulnar, brachial, axillary, or femoral arteries. The radial site is preferred because it is readily accessible and usually has adequate collateral circulation through the ulnar artery. The radial site is easy to monitor and provides a stable location for blood sampling. The femoral artery provides pressure measurements that are less affected by peripheral vasoconstriction, but significant leakage of blood into the surrounding tissue can occur without detection. The femoral site also is more prone to contamination than the other locations.

| Box 15-1 | The Heart as Two Pumps: An Overview of Hemodynamic Pressure Relationships |

When discussing hemodynamic parameters, it is necessary to think of the heart as two separate pumps. The right heart receives blood from the venous system (venous return) and pumps blood to the pulmonary system. The left heart receives blood from the pulmonary system and pumps blood to the systemic circulation. In normal states, both hearts pump at the same time and move the same amount of blood.

Both atria are filling chambers for the ventricles. Their pressures are about equal, and they have the same waveform. When the atrioventricular valves open (tricuspid and mitral), the pressures in the atrium and ventricle are equal; therefore, atrial pressure usually reflects the ventricle's filling pressure (end-diastolic pressure).

Both ventricles pump blood into arterial systems and create two waveforms: ventricular and arterial. Their waveforms have the same shape characteristics, but their pressures are significantly different. The right heart pumps to a low-resistance circuit, the lungs, and thus produces a lower pressure. The left heart pumps to a high-pressure circuit, the body, so it has to produce a high pressure.

Alterations in blood flow and resistance to flow are reflected backward through the cardiopulmonary circuit as pressure changes. Pulmonary hypertension causes pressure to increase in the right heart and eventually the venous system.

$$\uparrow \text{Lung pressure} \rightarrow \uparrow \text{PAP} \rightarrow \uparrow \text{CVP} \rightarrow \uparrow \text{Venous congestion}$$

A failing left ventricle will cause blood to "dam up" in the left heart, then the lungs, and eventually alters the entire circuit.

$$\rightarrow \uparrow \text{LAP} \rightarrow \uparrow \text{PAWP} \rightarrow \uparrow \text{PAP} \rightarrow \uparrow \text{CVP} \rightarrow \uparrow \text{Venous congestion}$$

The following simple diagram illustrates the dynamic relationship between the two hearts and shows where pressures are measured. Marking a patient's pressure changes helps clarify where there is and is not a problem (e.g., increased PAWP with normal PAP and CVP indicates a left heart problem that has not altered the lungs or right heart).

Pressures:	CVP			PAP	PAWP	LAP				Arterial BP	
Venous system		RA	RV		Lungs	LA		LV		Aorta	Arterial circulation
Blood flow →						← Alterations in resistance and flow are reflected backward					

AV, arteriovenous; BP, blood pressure; CVP, central venous pressure; LA, left atrium; LAP, left atrial pressure; LV, left ventricle; PAP, pulmonary artery pressure; PAWP, pulmonary artery wedge pressure; RA, right atrium; RV, right ventricle; vertical bars indicate heart valves.

TABLE 15-1		
Reference Ranges for Hemodynamic Pressures		
Pressure	**Abbreviation**	**Normal Value (mm Hg)**
Arterial pressure	BP	Systolic 100-140 Diastolic 60-90 120/80 (90/60 in teenage girls)
Mean arterial pressure	MAP	70-105
Central venous pressure	CVP	2-6 (mean)
Right atrial pressure	RAP	2-6 (mean)
Right ventricular pressure	RVP	Systolic 15-30 Diastolic 2-8
Right ventricular end-diastolic pressure	RVEDP	2-6
Pulmonary artery pressure	PAP	Systolic 15-30 Diastolic 8-15
Mean pulmonary artery pressure	MPAP or PAP	9-18
Pulmonary artery wedge pressure	PAWP, PCWP, PAOP	6-12
Left atrial pressure	LAP	4-12
Left ventricular pressure	LVP	Systolic 100-140 Diastolic 0-5
Left ventricular end-diastolic pressure	LVEDP	5-12

TABLE 15-2			
Reference Ranges for Heart Rate and Blood Pressure in Children			
	Blood Pressure Average for Males (Females 5% Lower)	**Heart Rate***	
Age		**Average**	**Range**
Neonate	75/50	140	100-190
1-6 mo	80/50	145	110-190
6-12 mo	90/65	140	110-180
1-2 yr	95/65	125	100-160
2-6 yr	100/60	100	65-130
6-12 yr	110/60	80	55-110
12-16 yr	110/65	75	55-100
	Range: ±20%		

*Heart rates rounded to nearest 5.
Data from Rubenstein JS, Hageman JR: Monitoring of critically ill infants and children. *Crit Care Clin* 4:621, 1988.

Equipment Set-Up

Figure 15-1 shows the basic equipment used for an indwelling vascular line, in this case a brachial artery catheter. Once inserted, the catheter connects to a disposable continuous flush device by low-compliance tubing. The flush device keeps the line open by providing a continuous

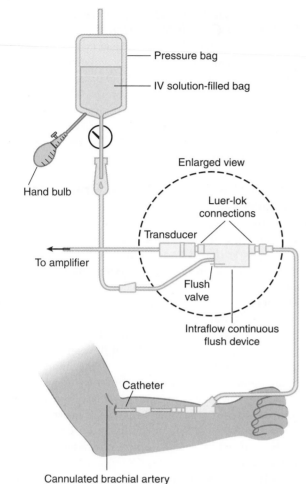

FIGURE 15-1 An indwelling vascular line system (brachial artery catheter) used to monitor blood pressures and obtain blood samples. See text for description. (From Kacmarek R, Stoller J, Heuer A: *Egan's fundamentals of respiratory care*, ed 10, St. Louis, 2013, Mosby-Elsevier.)

Box 15-2	Key Elements in Arterial Line Insertion Procedure

- Ensure that a "time out" is performed before the procedure.
- Obtain patient written consent if required (some institutions).
- Ensure that monitoring system is set up and calibrated, with lines properly flushed.
- Restrain arm with the wrist dorsiflexed using an armboard or towel.
- Assess adequacy of ulnar collateral blood flow by Allen test.
- Decontaminate hands and don personal protection equipment (use sterile gloves).
- Scrub the insertion area using chlorhexidine (30 seconds) and allow to dry.
- Drape the area per proper aseptic technique.
- Apply local anesthetic agent (as needed).
- Locate pulsating artery by palpation.
- Puncture skin at 30-degree angle, with needle bevel and hub arrow up.
- Advance catheter into position (direct cannulation or Seldinger technique).
- Connect catheter system to transducer tubing and flush.
- Confirm proper arterial waveform on monitor (neither overdampened or underdampened).
- Reposition catheter if waveform is inadequate or dampened.
- Cleanse area, apply benzoin, and let dry.
- Secure line to prevent traction on catheter.
- Cover line insertion point with clear sterile dressing.
- Dispose of infectious waste and sharps and decontaminates hands.
- Recheck for adequacy of distal blood flow and patient comfort.
- Instruct patient on line use and safety considerations.
- Record pertinent data in chart and departmental records.

---

low flow of fluid (2 to 4 mL/hour) through the system. To maintain continuous flow, the intravenous bag supplying these systems must be pressurized, usually by a hand bulb pump. A pressure transducer, connected to the flush device, provides an electrical signal to an amplifier or monitor, which displays the corresponding pressure waveform. A sampling port (not shown) typically is included to allow blood withdrawal. CVP and pulmonary artery monitoring systems use the same basic set-up.

Procedure for Inserting an Arterial Line

Box 15-2 outlines the key procedural steps for inserting a radial artery line. Note that if the Allen test for collateral circulation is negative, the opposite wrist should be assessed. If collateral circulation cannot be confirmed on either side, the brachial site typically is used.

There are two common arterial line insertion methods: direct cannulation and the guidewire (Seldinger) technique. The direct cannulation method uses a puncture needle sheathed with the catheter. Using this approach, once a flash of blood is observed in the needle hub, the catheter sheath is advanced over the needle into the artery, and the needle is then removed.

With the Seldinger technique, a needle is used to penetrate the artery, with a soft-tipped guidewire then threaded through the needle into the vessel. Next, the needle is removed, leaving the guidewire in place. Finally, the indwelling catheter is advanced over the guidewire into position, and the guidewire is removed.

Arterial Pressure Waveforms

An arterial pressure waveform should have a clear upstroke on the left, with a **dicrotic notch** representing aortic valve closure on the downstroke to the right (Fig. 15-2). If the dicrotic notch is not visible, the pressure tracing is dampened and probably inaccurate, and the measured pressures likely lower than the patient's actual values. The dicrotic notch disappears in some patients when the systolic pressure drops below 50 or 60 mm Hg.

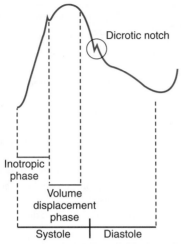

FIGURE 15-2 Arterial pressure waveform. Increase of circulating catecholamines can cause the inotropic phase to become steeper and form a point that may be higher than in the volume displacement phase. The *circle* marks the dicrotic notch that results from closure of the aortic valve. If the dicrotic notch cannot be visualized and the patient's systolic pressure is greater than 50 mm Hg, the measuring system likely is dampened.

Arterial pressure waves take on many different configurations (Fig. 15-3). The left side of the pressure wave may become straight and even pointed on the top when there is an increase in circulating catecholamines that increase cardiac contractility (a positive inotropic response). A tall, narrow pressure wave is also seen in patients with a stiff aorta due to arteriosclerotic vascular disease. In these patients, the diastolic pressure may also fall, producing an exaggerated tall and narrow complex. Increases in heart rate and vascular resistance increase diastolic pressure. On the other hand, vasodilation decreases vascular resistance and can cause a fall in diastolic pressures. Because approximately 70% of coronary artery perfusion occurs during diastole, coronary artery perfusion may be compromised if the diastolic pressure falls below 50 mm Hg.

Respiratory Variations

Respiratory variations in the arterial pressure waveform normally go unnoticed because arterial pressures are substantially higher than intrathoracic pressure changes during breathing. Also, the monitor scale usually is set to a pressure range of 0 to 300 mm Hg, making changes of 10 mm Hg barely visible. When respiratory variations in the arterial pressure waveform are seen, the possibility of cardiac tamponade or other causes of paradoxical pulse must be considered (see Chapter 4). Increases in arterial pressure during inspiration (reverse pulsus paradoxus) are seen after heart surgery and in patients with left ventricular failure who are mechanically ventilated with techniques that produce high mean airway pressures, such as positive end-expiratory pressure (PEEP). Dysrhythmias and *pulsus alternans* also cause variations in the height and shapes of the arterial pressure waveform.

Use of Arterial Pressure Waveform to Estimate Cardiac Output

Recently, monitors have been developed that use sophisticated software algorithms to calculate and display continuous beat-to-beat stroke volume and CO based on the shape and area of the arterial pressure waveform. This method is called arterial pulse contour (APC) analysis and is among the most commonly used minimally invasive methods to measure CO in critically ill patients. Chapter 16 provides details on the use of these systems.

Interpretation of Arterial Pressure Measurements

Normal arterial pressure in the adult is approximately 120/80 mm Hg and increases gradually with age. Systolic pressures greater than 140 and diastolic pressures greater than 90 are considered hypertensive (see Chapter 4 for the current classification of hypertension). A pressure below 90/60 mm Hg in adults is termed *hypotension*.

Although arterial pressure is one of the most frequently monitored vital signs, it reflects only the general circulatory status. Pressure is the product of flow and resistance. Because neurovascular compensatory mechanisms can maintain blood pressure by vasoconstriction while flow is decreasing, low blood pressure is a late sign of hypovolemia or impaired cardiac function. Earlier evidence of decreased blood volume or CO includes cold, clammy extremities caused by catecholamine-mediated peripheral vasoconstriction.

Arterial pressure decreases in the following circumstances:
- With hypovolemia from fluid or blood loss (most commonly, bleeding)
- During cardiac failure and shock (most commonly, heart attack)
- With vasodilation (most commonly, sepsis or anesthetic agents)

Diastolic pressure must be watched carefully during the administration of vasodilators such as sodium nitroprusside, which may reduce diastolic pressure more rapidly than systolic or mean pressure. Diastolic pressure less than 50 mm Hg and mean pressure less than 60 mm Hg in an adult may result in compromised coronary perfusion.

Arterial pressure increases with the following:
- Improvement in circulatory volume and function
- Sympathetic stimulation (e.g., fear or medications)
- Vasoconstriction
- Administration of vasopressors

Administration of inotropic agents may or may not increase blood pressure. If a positive inotropic drug stimulates the heart under conditions of inadequate myocardial oxygenation or hypovolemia, the pressure may fall. Additionally, if the inotropic agent also causes vasodilation, the pressure may stay the same or fall as the medication is increased. In addition to systolic and diastolic blood pressure, arterial pressure monitoring allows assessment of pulse and mean arterial pressure.

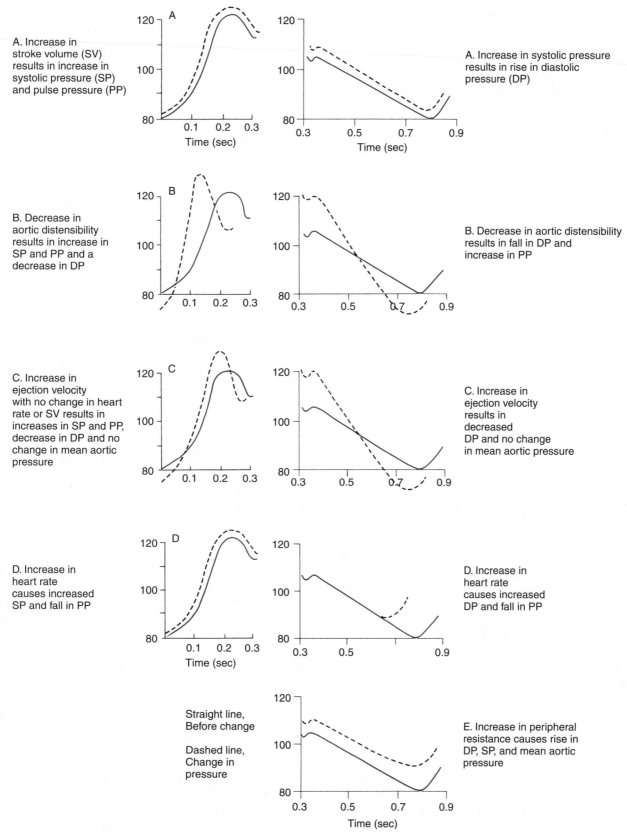

A. Increase in stroke volume (SV) results in increase in systolic pressure (SP) and pulse pressure (PP)

A. Increase in systolic pressure results in rise in diastolic pressure (DP)

B. Decrease in aortic distensibility results in increase in SP and PP and a decrease in DP

B. Decrease in aortic distensibility results in fall in DP and increase in PP

C. Increase in ejection velocity with no change in heart rate or SV results in increases in SP and PP, decrease in DP and no change in mean aortic pressure

C. Increase in ejection velocity results in decreased DP and no change in mean aortic pressure

D. Increase in heart rate causes increased SP and fall in PP

D. Increase in heart rate causes increased DP and fall in PP

Straight line, Before change

Dashed line, Change in pressure

E. Increase in peripheral resistance causes rise in DP, SP, and mean aortic pressure

FIGURE 15-3 Determinants of aortic pressures. Diagrams indicate general tendencies when other factors are held constant. (Modified from Smith JJ, Kampine JP: *Circulatory physiology: the essentials,* Baltimore, 1980, Williams & Wilkins.)

The **pulse pressure** is the difference between the systolic and diastolic pressure. Normal pulse pressure is 30 to 40 mm Hg and is a reflection of left ventricular stroke volume (SV) and arterial system compliance. A decreasing pulse pressure is a sign of low SV. An increasing SV in a patient receiving fluid therapy is consistent with improved preload.

> **SIMPLY STATED**
>
> A pulse pressure lower than 30 mm Hg indicates low left ventricular SV. If the pulse pressure increases with fluid therapy, the patient was probably hypovolemic.

Mean arterial pressure (MAP) is an average of pressures in the systemic circulation and thus the pressure best associated with the adequacy of tissue perfusion. The normal reference range for MAP is 70 to 105 mm Hg. MAP is not an arithmetic average of systolic and diastolic pressures because the cardiac cycle spends about twice as long in diastole as in systole when the heart rate is normal. Most monitors compute MAP and display it digitally. MAP can be estimated mathematically by either of the following formulas:

$$MAP = 1/3 \text{ Pulse pressure} + \text{Diastolic pressure}$$

or

$$MAP = \frac{\text{Systolic pressure} + (\text{diastolic pressure} \times 2)}{3}$$

Circulation to the vital organs (i.e., kidneys, coronary arteries, and brain) may be compromised when MAP falls below 60 mm Hg. In such cases, the patient may need fluid therapy or medications to increase left ventricular contractility (inotropics) or to increase vascular resistance. Elevated MAP is associated with increased risk for stroke and heart failure. Pharmacologic treatment of elevated MAP may include vasodilators or negative inotropic agents. MAP is used in calculating derived hemodynamic variables such as systemic vascular resistance, left ventricular stroke work, and cardiac work (see Chapter 16).

Complications Associated with Arterial Lines
Ischemia
Ischemia resulting from embolism, thrombus, or arterial spasm is the major complication of direct arterial monitoring. It is evidenced by pallor distal to the insertion site and usually is accompanied by pain and paresthesia (numbness and tingling). Ischemia can proceed to tissue necrosis if the catheter is not repositioned or removed. Thrombosis is prevented by irrigation with diluted heparinized solution. Bolus irrigation is done in very small amounts because flushing the line can result in retrograde flow and cerebral embolization.

Hemorrhage
Hemorrhage is possible if the line becomes disconnected or a stopcock is left open; therefore, the tubing should be kept on top of the bed sheets, where it can be observed. Blood flow through an 18-gauge catheter is sufficient to allow a 500-mL blood loss per minute, and exsanguination can occur. Bleeding and hematoma at the insertion site can also occur, especially if the catheter was placed through a needle. Sites should be assessed regularly while the catheter is in place and after its removal.

Infection
As with all invasive lines, the presence of an arterial catheter increases the risk for infection. The incidence of infection increases over time and is directly related to the care of the lines and transducers; frequency of dressing, tubing, and solution change; to-and-fro motion of the catheter; and altered host defenses. Fever in any patient with invasive lines must trigger questions about the necessity of the lines and their role as a cause of the infection process. More detail on preventing catheter-associated infections is provided later in this chapter.

> **SIMPLY STATED**
>
> All invasive hemodynamic monitoring lines are a potential source of infection, bleeding, hematoma, embolus, thrombus, and impaired circulation. Fever in any patient with invasive lines must trigger questions about the necessity of the lines and their role in an infectious process.

Central Venous Pressure Monitoring

Central venous pressure (CVP) is the pressure of the blood in the right atrium or vena cava, where the blood is returned to the heart from the venous system. Because the tricuspid valve is opened between the right atrium and ventricle during diastole (ventricular filling), CVP also represents the end-diastolic pressure in the right ventricle (RVEDP) and reflects right ventricular preload (filling volume). To obtain a CVP measurement, a venous catheter is placed in a major vein (see the later section on insertion).

Indications for CVP Monitoring
CVP monitoring is indicated to assess the circulating blood volume (adequacy of cardiac filling), adequacy of venous return, or right ventricular function. Patients who have had major surgery or blood loss caused by trauma and those suspected of severe dehydration may benefit from placement of a CVP catheter to guide fluid replacement therapy. Patients with either cardiogenic or noncardiogenic pulmonary edema also need CVP monitoring to guide fluid therapy. In addition, CVP measurements are useful in evaluating patients suspected of having right ventricular damage due to myocardial infarction. Once the catheter is in place, the line can be used for rapid infusion of fluids or medications and to obtain blood samples for measurement of routine laboratory studies (e.g., complete blood counts and electrolytes).

CVP Catheters and Insertion Sites

The most common central venous catheters are 7-French, triple-lumen catheters with one distal port and two ports 3 to 4 cm from the distal end of the catheter (Fig. 15-4). The multiple-lumen catheter allows infusion of blood and various medications and solutions through different ports and permits aspiration of blood samples or injections for CO measurements without interrupting the infusion of medication. Catheters with walls that are impregnated with antibiotics are less commonly associated with infection than standard catheters.

Common sites for introduction of central venous catheters include the subclavian and internal jugular veins (Fig. 15-5). An advantage of the subclavian vein approach is that it results in a much more stable catheter after placement. Disadvantages of the subclavian vein approach are that it is technically more difficult because the vein is harder to find and the catheter guidewire does not follow the subclavian vein as easily as it turns to form the superior vena cava. The subclavian vein is close to the subclavian artery, which is easily punctured, and the mediastinum can hold a fair amount of blood without external evidence of blood loss. The pleural surface is not far below the vein, so pneumothorax is a potential complication of the procedure.

The internal jugular vein approach is easier because there is nearly a straight shot for the guidewire to reach the superior vena cava and less risk for pneumothorax, and hematomas are easier to see and control. Disadvantages of the internal jugular vein approach are that the catheter is much less stable after placement and is subject to kinking, breakage, and accidental removal.

A chest radiograph should be performed after central venous line insertion to ensure proper placement and to rule out pneumothorax.

Procedure for Inserting a CVP Catheter

Central venous line kits commonly include a needle for venous penetration, a stiff plastic dilator, and a guidewire coiled in a plastic sheath with a "J" tip to prevent venous wall penetration. The J tip is held straight by a small separate sheath to accommodate entry into the hub of the insertion needle.

The technique is nearly identical for subclavian and internal jugular line insertions. Normally, the head of the patient's bed is lowered, which increases venous pressure and causes the vein to swell, making it easier to penetrate and thread the guidewire. This also decreases the risk for inadvertent air embolism. The subclavian vein is entered from an insertion site at the edge of the distal third of the clavicle. The internal jugular vein can be entered from the head of the clavicle or a site behind the brachial artery.

The catheter lumens are flushed with heparinized saline, and the cap is removed from the lumen with the distal port. The guidewire is inserted and threaded, and the needle

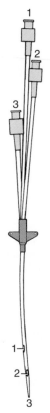

FIGURE 15-4 Triple-lumen central venous pressure catheter designed for placement through the internal or external jugular vein. The tip ends in the right atrium. The catheter does not have a balloon; air is never injected into ports.

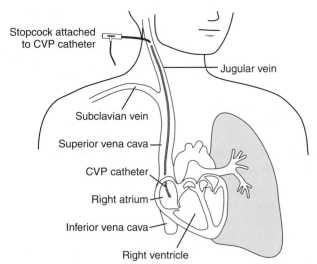

FIGURE 15-5 Central venous pressure (CVP) catheter inserted through the jugular vein with the tip positioned in the right atrium.

withdrawn. A dilator is inserted over the guidewire and removed, and the distal port of the CVP catheter is threaded onto the guidewire. It is advanced to a depth that should leave the tip in the superior vena cava. The guidewire is then removed, the hub replaced, the port flushed with heparinized saline, and the catheter secured in position. A chest

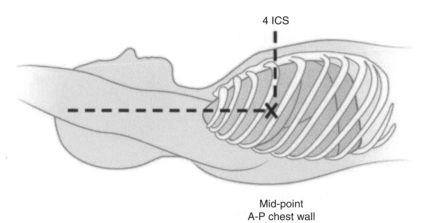

4 ICS

Mid-point
A-P chest wall

FIGURE 15-6 The phlebostatic axis at the intersection of the fourth intercostal space (ICS) and midaxillary line corresponds with the location of the right atrium. Central venous pressure and pulmonary artery transducers need to be level with this point. AP, anteroposterior. (From Sole ML, Klein D, Moseley M: *Introduction to critical care nursing*, ed 5, St. Louis, 2008, Saunders-Elsevier.)

radiograph typically is taken after insertion to verify the tip of the catheter is in the superior vena cava just above the right atrium.

Once inserted and secured, the CVP catheter is attached to a flushed and calibrated monitoring system like that used for pressure measurement through an arterial line (see Fig. 15-1). However, because central venous pressures typically are much lower than arterial pressures, two key differences in the procedure are required. First, the monitor scale for CVP measurement should be set to the low range, typically 0 to 30 mm Hg. Second, to assure accuracy in measurement and interpretation, the pressure transducer must be placed level with the patient's right atrium, identified externally at the **phlebostatic axis.** As indicated in Figure 15-6, the phlebostatic axis is located at the intersection of the fourth intercostal space and midaxillary line. Positioning of the transducer below the phlebostatic axis will result in erroneously high CVP readings, whereas positioning the transducer above this level will cause the reading to be lower than the patient's actual value.

Central Venous and Atrial Pressure Waveforms

The CVP waveform reflects pressure changes in the right atrium and normally consists of three waves for each cardiac cycle: a, c, and v (Fig. 15-7).

The a wave results from atrial contraction and occurs during ventricular diastole. When there is no atrial contraction (atrial fibrillation), there is no a wave. Conversely, when the atrium contracts against a closed valve, as occurs during atrioventricular (AV) dissociation or with some junctional or ventricular pacemaker rhythms, large a waves called *cannon waves* occur. The downslope of the a wave (X descent) results from the decrease in atrial pressure as the blood moves into the ventricle and ends with the closure of the tricuspid valve (tricuspid on right, mitral on left).

The c wave occurs at the completion of AV valve closure. It represents the movement or bulging of the AV valve back toward the atrium during ventricular contraction.

The v wave results from atrial filling while the AV valve is closed during ventricular systole. The downslope of the v wave (Y descent) occurs when the tricuspid and mitral valves open and the ventricle begins to fill with blood. When an AV valve does not close all the way (incompetent or leaky valve), some of the blood is ejected backward into the atrium during systole (tricuspid regurgitation), creating exaggerated v waves and an elevated CVP measurement.

Respiratory Variations

Respiratory-induced pressure changes are normal on CVP waveforms. In fact, the absence of respiratory oscillations on a CVP tracing indicates a measurement error that requires troubleshooting. The most likely cause of absent respiratory oscillations is a kink or air in the tubing, a stopcock turned in the wrong direction, or a small clot or kink in the catheter. Rarely, when a hypovolemic patient is breathing spontaneously at small tidal volumes, respiratory oscillations may not be apparent and the typical a, c, and v wave pattern may not be seen. If the patient is asked to take a deep breath, the waveform should fall below baseline as intrathoracic pressure falls with inspiration. The catheter and tubing should still be checked carefully for air and other causes of dampened pressure traces.

Because the CVP decreases with spontaneous inspiration and increases with delivery of positive pressure breaths, accurate determination of this parameter can be problematic. For spontaneously breathing patients who are awake and cooperative, having them briefly suspend their breathing for a few cardiac cycles can yield an accurate CVP measurement. For patients receiving positive-pressure ventilation, it is best to view a simultaneous tracing of CVP with the airway pressure and record the CVP value that most closely corresponds to the average end-expiratory

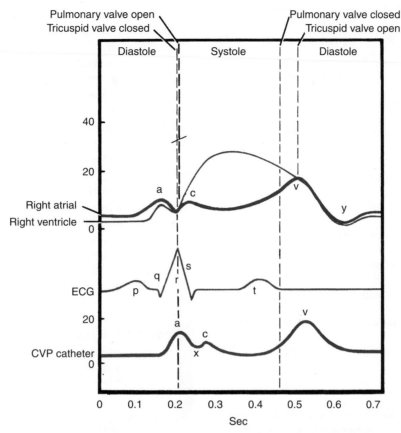

FIGURE 15-7 Central venous pressure (CVP) and right atrial pressure traces with a, c, and v waves shown in relation to the electrocardiogram (ECG) and ventricular pressure waves. When traces are recorded from long catheters, especially pulmonary artery catheters, there is usually a time delay in visualizing the pressure waveform so that the a wave coincides with the QRS complex rather than preceding it slightly, as occurs with the right atrial pressure trace. a, atrial contraction; b, closure of the AV valve; v, ventricular contraction.

pressure over several respiratory cycles. Most protocols recommend against removing patients from the ventilator to measure the CVP, especially if PEEP is in use.

Interpretation of CVP Measurements

CVP is regulated by a balance between the volume of blood being returned to the heart (venous return) and the ability of the right heart to pump this blood out into the pulmonary circulation. In general, any peripheral factor that decreases the amount of blood returning to the heart decreases CVP, and any factor that increases venous return increases CVP. When the pumping capacity of the right heart is increased, more blood is moved out of the right ventricle, and CVP decreases. Conversely, any impairment to the pumping ability of the right heart tends to increase CVP. Box 15-3 summarizes the common causes of increased and decreased CVP.

In patients with poor perfusion and a low CVP, a fluid challenge may be given to determine whether the cause is hypovolemia. A fluid challenge involves the rapid administration of 200 to 500 mL of intravenous fluid over a short time period, such as 10 minutes. If the CVP does not change after a fluid challenge, this indicates that the poor perfusion is due to hypovolemia, with the administration of additional fluid warranted. However, if the CVP increases by 2 mm Hg or more during the challenge, hypovolemia is unlikely, and additional fluid should be administered with caution. It is important to note that with more and better ways to monitor cardiac function, the CVP fluid challenge has fallen out of favor. Real-time measures of stroke volume and CO in response to a fluid challenge are now considered the best predictor of hemodynamic response to changes in circulating blood volume. Details on these methods are provided in Chapter 16.

Note also that a normal CVP does not necessarily indicate normal circulating volume or cardiac function. For example, if a patient is hypovolemic but has pulmonary hypertension with decreased right ventricular function, the balance of these opposing factors may result in a normal CVP. This is most commonly seen in patients with

Box 15-3	Causes of Changes in Central Venous Pressure

INCREASED PRESSURE

- Volume overload or fluids being given more rapidly than the heart can tolerate
- Increased intrathoracic pressure (CVP increases with positive-pressure breath or tension pneumothorax)
- Compression around the heart: constrictive pericarditis or cardiac tamponade
- Pulmonary hypertension (primary or secondary)
- Right ventricular failure (e.g., myocardial infarction or cardiomyopathy)
- Left heart failure severe enough to cause right heart failure
- Pulmonary valvular stenosis
- Tricuspid valvular stenosis or regurgitation
- Pulmonary embolism
- Increased large vessel tone throughout the body, resulting in venoconstriction
- Arteriolar vasodilation that increases the blood supply to the venous system
- Infusion of solution into the CVP line (especially by infusion pumps)
- Placement of the transducer below the patient's right atrium and phlebostatic axis

DECREASED PRESSURE

- Vasodilation (drugs hyperpyrexia, sepsis)
- Inadequate circulating blood volume (hypovolemia) caused by dehydration, blood loss, gastrointestinal loss, wound drainage, perspiration, urine output (diuresis), insensible losses (high temperature, low humidity), and losses to the interstitial space (edema, third spacing)
- Spontaneous inspiration
- Placement of the transducer above the patient's right atrium and phlebostatic axis
- Air bubbles or leaks in the pressure line

cor pulmonale who become dehydrated and hypovolemic. In such cases, correcting the hypovolemia will cause an abnormal elevation in the CVP.

> **SIMPLY STATED**
>
> CVP rises as the efficiency of the right heart to move blood through the lungs decreases. When the CVP is elevated and accurately measured while pulmonary artery pressures are normal or low, the cause of the problem resides in the right heart (e.g., right ventricular infarction or tricuspid stenosis and regurgitation). If both CVP and pulmonary artery pressures are elevated while the left-sided filling pressures are normal, the problem probably resides in the lung.

CVP as a Reflection of Left Ventricular Function

Can CVP be used to estimate left ventricular filling pressures and performance? Yes, it can, under some circumstances. In patients with an ejection fraction greater than

0.50 (50% of the left ventricular end-diastolic volume (LVEDV) and no cardiopulmonary disease, excellent correlation has been found between central venous, left atrial, and pulmonary artery wedge pressures.

CVP is an acceptable option for management of intraoperative fluid levels, postoperative fluid levels, or volume replacement in young patients with no history of heart disease or hypertension. However, in patients with valvular heart disease or coronary artery disease and in critically ill patients, CVP may not correlate well with left heart filling pressures.

In a patient with pulmonary disease, the left heart pressures remain normal or may even be decreased, whereas the pulmonary artery pressure and therefore right heart pressures are significantly elevated. Therefore, a patient with pulmonary hypertension may benefit from monitoring of both the left and right heart pressures.

> **SIMPLY STATED**
>
> Patients with pulmonary hypertension have increased pulmonary vascular pressures and CVP resulting from the pulmonary disease process; therefore, CVP is not a good reflection of volume status. It is necessary to look more directly at left heart filling pressure to determine whether the patient's volume status is adequate.

Complications of CVP Monitoring

Complications of using a CVP catheter can occur during placement or during its use over time. Placement of the catheter can cause problems such as bleeding or pneumothorax. Bleeding is often minimal because of the low pressures characterizing the venous system. Bleeding is more likely if the patient is taking heparin or has low platelet counts. Bleeding also can be severe if the subclavian artery is accidentally penetrated. Pneumothorax is uncommon but can occur if the catheter punctures the pleural lining. The most common complication associated with use of the catheter over time is infection (see Central Line Bundle section presented later in chapter). A less common complication is development of thrombus around the catheter. Accidental opening of the central venous line stopcock could allow air to enter the vein and result in an air embolus.

Pulmonary Artery Pressure Monitoring

The development of the pulmonary artery catheter (PAC) by Drs. Swan and Ganz in the late 1960s began a new era in assessment of left ventricular function and hemodynamic performance. Placement of a flow-directed PAC into the patient's pulmonary artery allows assessment of the filling pressures of the left side of the heart. Before the PAC was developed, measurement of left-sided filling pressures required cardiac catheterization, with bedside care estimates based on the CVP measurement. However, as previously mentioned, many critically ill patients have factors present that make CVP a poor estimate of left heart filling pressures. Thus, the PAC provides better assessment of left-sided heart function. In addition, a PAC provides the means to assess CO and tissue oxygenation.

These values allow assessment of the following (Box 15-4):
- Left ventricular preload through measurement of the **pulmonary artery wedge pressure (PAWP)**
- Cardiac output and its related computations (stroke volume and cardiac index)
- Pulmonary vascular resistance (PVR) through measurement of pulmonary artery pressure, wedge pressure, and CO
- Mixed venous O_2 content (reflecting tissue oxygenation) and the AV oxygen content difference
- Proportion of left-to-right shunted pulmonary blood flow
- Patient's response to therapy with vasoactive agents, fluid, and positive-pressure ventilation

Indications for Pulmonary Artery Pressure Monitoring

Insertion of the PAC represents increased risk compared with the CVP catheter. The additional risk is present because the catheter must pass through the right side of the heart and into the pulmonary artery. The procedure may cause dysrhythmias or other serious complications (see later discussion). As a result, the PAC must be inserted only in those patients in whom the anticipated benefit outweighs the potential risks. Unfortunately, there is no specific diagnosis or group of patients in which PAC placement is an absolute indication. Rather, the decision to place a PAC is individualized on a case-by-case basis. Common factors to consider include the following:
- Experience of the attending physician
- Availability of proper equipment and personnel to insert and maintain the catheter
- Diagnosis of the patient
- Cardiac history of the patient
- Pulmonary history of the patient

The common situations in which PAC monitoring is considered include the following:
- Diagnosis and treatment of patients with severe cardiogenic pulmonary edema, especially if the patient has unstable angina, has ventricular pathology, or does not respond to initial therapy
- Diagnosis and treatment of patients with severe ARDS who are hemodynamically unstable
- Monitoring of patients who have had major thoracic surgery (e.g., coronary bypass surgery) with a recent history of myocardial infarction or poor ventricular function
- Diagnosis and treatment of patients in cardiogenic or septic shock

---

Box 15-4	Interpreting Pulmonary Artery Pressure

Pulmonary artery pressure is the product of the volume ejected by the right ventricle and resistance of flow through the pulmonary vasculature.

Pulmonary artery pressure measures right heart function and reflects the following:
- Preload and end-diastolic filling pressure
- Ability of the right heart to move blood through the lungs and left heart

Pulmonary artery pressure can reflect left heart filling pressure in young patients with no hypertension, cardiac disease, or pulmonary disease.

Pulmonary artery pressure increases with the following:
- Increased venous return (volume)
- Increased intrathoracic pressure
- Increased PVR

Pulmonary artery pressure decreases with the following:
- Decreased venous return (volume)
- Decreased intrathoracic pressure
- Decreased PVR

Normal pulmonary artery pressure is as follows:
- Systolic: 15 to 30 mm Hg
- Diastolic: 8 to 15 mm Hg*
- Mean: 9 to 18 mm Hg

If pressure is abnormally low or falling, think of the following:
- Inadequate volume, volume loss
- Vasodilation (could be fever or medications)
- Plumbing or measurement problem

If pressure is abnormally high or climbing, think of the following:
- Increased PVR
- Constriction, obstruction, compression of pulmonary vasculature (e.g., ↑ intrathoracic pressure, pulmonary hypertension, or cardiac tamponade)
- Backpressure from high left heart pressures
- Volume overload
- Technical problem or not reading at end-expiration

Pulmonary diastolic pressure can be used instead of wedge pressure if the diastolic is higher than the wedge and if none of the following is present:
- Tachyarrhythmia
- Vasoconstriction, increased pulmonary resistance
- Pulmonary emboli
- Fluctuating PVR

---

*Normal pulmonary artery diastolic pressure is 2 mm Hg higher than wedge pressure.

PVR, pulmonary vascular resistance.

SIMPLY STATED

A PAC should be inserted only in a patient in whom the anticipated benefits clearly outweigh the potential risks. Diagnosis alone is usually not sufficient to support its use.

Pulmonary Artery Catheters and Insertion Sites

PACs, also called *Swan-Ganz catheters*, are made of radiopaque polyvinylchloride, with the adult version being about 110 cm long (marked in 10-cm increments) and tipped with a small inflatable balloon. The balloon is used both to float the catheter into position and to obtain wedge pressure measurements. A 5-French catheter typically is used with children up to 20 kg, with 7- and 8-French versions selected respectively for large children/small adults and average-sized adults.

Typically, the catheter has at least three lumens connecting to three external ports: a proximal CVP/atrial lumen, a distal pulmonary artery lumen, and a balloon lumen

(Fig. 15-8). Other connectors may include those for a CO computer, atrial and ventricular pacemakers, and a mixed venous O_2 sensor (not shown).

The proximal lumen ends approximately 30 cm back from the tip of the catheter and normally rests in the right atrium when the catheter is properly placed. The proximal port is used for aspirating blood samples, measuring CVP, injecting drugs, and injecting the thermal bolus used for thermodilution CO measurements (see Chapter 16). Some catheters have two lumens ending in the right atrium: one for routine infusion of drugs or continuous pressure monitoring, the other for infusion of thermodilution materials and other periodic injections.

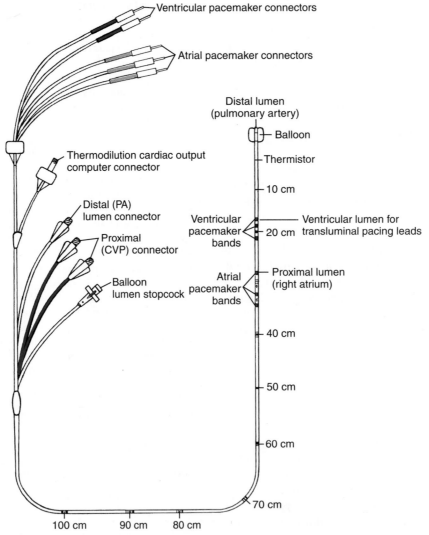

FIGURE 15-8 Idealized pulmonary artery (PA) catheter showing many of the features available; no catheters have all the features shown. Distal lumen opens into the PA. Fiberoptic filaments used for $S\bar{v}O_2$ monitoring (see Fig. 14-18) and the balloon are also located at the tip. The thermistor bead is located 1.5 inches from the tip and is connected by a wire through the catheter to the connector for the thermodilution cardiac output computer. The proximal lumen located 30 cm back from the tip opens into the right atrium. Catheters are available for ventricular, atrial, or atrioventricular sequential pacing using either pacemaker bands positioned on the catheter or pacing leads, which are passed through the lumen. Ventricular bands or lumens are located 20 cm from the tip; atrial, 30 cm from the tip. CVP, central venous pressure.

The distal lumen terminates at the tip of the catheter and is used for measuring pulmonary artery pressures, aspirating mixed venous blood samples, and injecting medications.

The balloon lumen exits inside of the balloon just behind the tip of the catheter. This lumen is used only to inflate/deflate the balloon. Most balloons hold approximately 1.5 mL of air when fully inflated. To help the catheter float through the right side of the heart and into the pulmonary artery, the balloon is fully inflated during insertion. Once the catheter is properly positioned, the balloon is deflated and maintained in that state except when obtaining wedge pressure measurements.

PACs used for thermodilution CO measurement have a thermistor bead located approximately 4 cm from the tip of the catheter. The thermistor senses temperature changes in the blood and is used for obtaining body core temperature as well as CO measurements.

PACs are available with bands for atrial, ventricular, or AV sequential cardiac pacing. The pacemaker bands must stay in contact with the wall of the atrium or ventricle to work effectively. Another type of pulmonary artery pacing catheter has a ventricular lumen 20 cm back from the tip in addition to the proximal (atrial) lumen. Specially designed pacing leads can be passed through the lumen and positioned more securely against the wall of the chamber. The pacer leads are then connected directly to the pacemaker. If cardiac pacing is not required, the lumen can be used for infusions and blood sampling.

The insertion sites for the PAC are the same as those for the CVP catheter, with the subclavian route being the most common site used in the intensive care unit (ICU).

Placement of the Pulmonary Artery Catheter

The PAC can be positioned using fluoroscopy but is more often floated into place using pressure waveforms to indicate the catheter's position. The distal lumen of the catheter is connected to the same basic transducer-monitoring system depicted in Figure 15-1. Before insertion, both the proximal and distal lumens are flushed with sterile saline to make sure they are free of air bubbles, and then the catheter is placed through an introducer. The clinician placing the catheter usually inflates the balloon on the tip of the catheter when it reaches the superior vena cava or the right atrium. The clinician observes the pressure waves transmitted through the distal lumen as displayed on the bedside monitor. As the catheter passes through the various anatomic structures (e.g., right atrium, right ventricle, and pulmonary artery), distinct waveforms are observed (Fig. 15-9). Based on these waveforms, the clinician placing the catheter can know when the tip passes into the pulmonary artery and is near the wedge position. The wedge position is reached when the balloon arrives at an artery that is too small to allow further advancement of the catheter. The waveforms generated by the catheter as it is inserted are briefly discussed in the next sections according to anatomic site.

Right Atrium

When the tip of the catheter reaches the superior vena cava, a typical CVP waveform appears on the monitor, with its characteristic a, c, and v waves (see Fig. 15-9). The balloon is fully inflated while the catheter is still in the superior

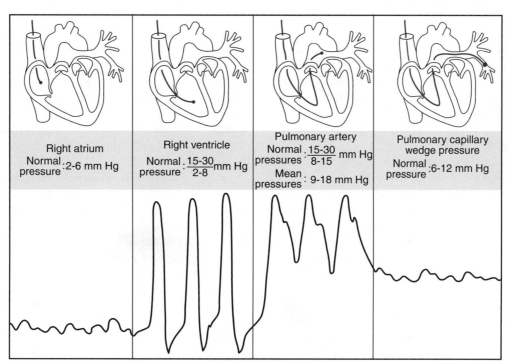

FIGURE 15-9 Schematic of waveforms and normal pressures visualized as the pulmonary artery catheter is floated into position.

vena cava or atrium. This encourages the catheter to follow the blood flow into the right ventricle and then into the pulmonary artery.

Right Ventricle

When the catheter passes through the tricuspid valve into the right ventricle, a rapid increase in the height of the pressure waveform occurs (see Fig. 15-9). This almost always provides a landmark in catheter insertion. Exceptions are patients with severe tricuspid regurgitation that produces marked pressure waves in the superior vena cava, or patients with right ventricular failure causing markedly decreased contractility. The right ventricular waveform is easily distinguished from the pulmonary artery waveform because the waveform downstroke drops straight down to near zero as the ventricle relaxes during diastole. As soon as the ventricle relaxes, the tricuspid valve opens and blood begins to flow into the ventricle, causing the pressure wave to increase gradually. End-diastolic pressure occurs just before the upstroke created by ventricular contraction (see Fig. 15-9).

The catheter is supposed to float easily from the right ventricle into the pulmonary artery; however, achieving proper catheter placement can take from minutes to more than an hour. Difficult insertions are caused by a large, dysfunctional right ventricle, tricuspid regurgitation, and pulmonary hypertension with pulmonary valve incompetence. Placement is often most difficult in patients who would most benefit from its use. Under these circumstances, it is often necessary to position the catheter visually using fluoroscopy.

In most adults, insertion of the catheter through the subclavian or jugular vein to the 50-cm marker is sufficient to reach the pulmonary artery. If the insertion depth exceeds 50 cm and no pulmonary artery waveform is observed, it is generally assumed that the catheter is curling in the atrium or ventricle or is going down the inferior vena cava. In these cases, the clinician deflates the balloon and withdraws the catheter until the tip is in the atrium. The balloon is then reinflated and the catheter repositioned.

Pulmonary Artery

Entry into the pulmonary artery is recognized by a change in the diastolic portion of the waveform (see Fig. 15-9). The pulmonary artery maintains pressure throughout the cardiac cycle so that the baseline pressure usually increases to 8 to 15 mm Hg over right ventricular diastolic pressures. The pulmonary artery waveform is a miniature of the peripheral arterial waveform, with a dicrotic notch and a gradual diastolic runoff that does not drop to zero.

Wedge Position

When the catheter wedges in a smaller branch of the pulmonary artery, the forward flow of the pulmonary arterial blood is occluded. With pulsatile arterial blood flow stopped, the tip of the catheter "reflects" the backpressure from the pulmonary venous system and left atrium, and the

waveform takes on the appearance of an atrial/CVP pressure waveform with its typical a, c, and v waves (Fig. 15-10). The pulmonary artery waveform should return when the balloon is deflated. Adjustments in catheter placement are often needed to keep the catheter tip in position to easily wedge but to avoid a permanently wedged position. Care should be taken to inflate the balloon only enough to provide a wedge reading because overdistention of the pulmonary artery could cause rupture of the artery, which could be fatal.

Interpretation of Pulmonary Artery Pressures

As seen in the previous discussion, the PAC provides numerous measurements, including pulmonary artery systolic and diastolic pressures and the wedge pressure. Interpretation of each is discussed in the following sections.

Pulmonary Artery Systolic Pressure

Pulmonary artery systolic pressure is the highest pressure created when the right ventricle ejects blood through the pulmonary valve and into the lungs. Like systemic arterial pressure, pulmonary artery pressure is a product of the volume of blood ejected by the ventricle and the resistance of the pulmonary circulation. Normal pulmonary artery systolic pressure is 15 to 30 mm Hg.

Pulmonary artery pressures decrease when the volume of blood ejected by the right ventricle decreases or when the pulmonary vasculature relaxes or dilates (decreased PVR).

Pulmonary artery pressures increase when pulmonary blood flow increases or when PVR increases. The right ventricle pumps increased amounts of blood into the lungs with volume overload or when it receives excess blood from left-to-right intracardiac shunts (e.g., atrial or ventricular septal defects or patent ductus arteriosus).

Resistance to pulmonary flow (increased PVR) can be caused by constriction, obstruction, or compression of the pulmonary vasculature or by backpressure from the left heart. Examples of conditions that can cause increased PVR include the following:
- Pulmonary emboli
- Acute or chronic lung disease that causes pulmonary vasoconstriction in response to hypoxia
- Cardiac tamponade or increased intrathoracic pressure compressing the vasculature and impeding forward flow
- Left heart failure and mitral valve regurgitation causing backpressure from the left heart into the lungs

Pulmonary arterial pressures average about 25/12 mm Hg, with a mean pressure of about 16 mm Hg. However, with pulmonary disease, it is not uncommon for the systolic pressure to exceed 45 mm Hg and the mean pulmonary pressure to exceed 35 mm Hg. Advanced pulmonary hypertension can result in pressures approaching systemic artery pressures. Such severe pulmonary hypertension can impair right ventricular function, which in turn decreases

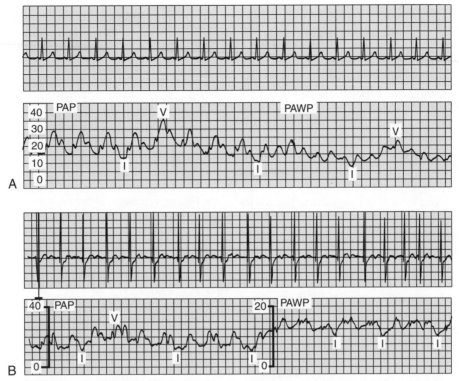

FIGURE 15-10 Pulmonary artery pressure (PAP) trace converting to wedge pressure. **A**, Patient is on intermittent mandatory ventilation of 12 and positive end-expiratory pressure (PEEP) of 5 cm H_2O. Note respiratory swing in pressure wave. Heart rate: 98/min, normal sinus rhythm; PAP, 27/15 mm Hg; wedge pressure (PAWP), 13 mm Hg. **B**, Note difference in appearance of waveforms in patient with atrial fibrillation. Heart rate: 87 to 102/min; PAP: 23/14 mm Hg; PAWP: 13 mm Hg. I, spontaneous inspiration; V, intermittent ventilator breath.

right ventricular output. With less blood moving forward, left ventricular preload is decreased, and subsequently left ventricular SV and systemic oxygen transport may also decrease.

Pulmonary Artery Diastolic Pressure

Pulmonary artery diastolic pressure (PADP) normally ranges between 8 and 15 mm Hg and under normal conditions reflects pulmonary venous, left atrial, and left ventricular end-diastolic pressure (the mitral valve is open during diastole). Additionally, pulmonary capillary resistance and impedance to flow normally are minimal. Therefore, in the absence of severe pulmonary vascular changes, marked tachycardia, pulmonary embolism, and mitral valve stenosis or regurgitation, PADP can be used to monitor left ventricular filling pressure. Unfortunately, such ideal conditions are uncommon in the ICU, and PADP is often unreliable as a measure of left ventricular filling pressure.

Normally, PADP is approximately 2 mm Hg higher than wedge pressure, but elevated PVR increases the gradient. In fact, a PADP-PAWP gradient that is greater than 5 mm Hg is characteristic of ARDS, sepsis, excessive PEEP, or other conditions that increase PVR. In contrast, pulmonary hypertension caused by left ventricular failure is characterized by a normal PADP-PAWP gradient (<5 mm Hg). With heart rates greater than 120/minute, the time for diastolic

runoff is shortened, and diastolic pressure and the gradient increase.

> **SIMPLY STATED**
>
> Pulmonary artery diastolic pressure may reflect filling pressures of the left ventricle if the mitral valve of the patient is normal and the PVR is normal. In most ICU patients, however, these conditions are not present.

Wedge Pressure

Normal PAWP is 6 to 12 mm Hg. Wedge pressure is lower than mean pulmonary artery pressure and is usually about 2 mm Hg lower than PADP. These normal pressure relationships are easier to remember by keeping in mind that blood flows from higher pressure to lower pressure. Wedge pressure is also called **pulmonary capillary wedge pressure (PCWP)** or **pulmonary artery occlusion pressure (PAOP)**.

The PAWP reading is used to monitor left ventricular filling during diastole. Under normal conditions (e.g., healthy heart) the filling pressure correlates well with the volume of blood filling the ventricle (preload). However, when the heart is damaged, healthy myocardium often is replaced with scar tissue, resulting in the ventricles becoming stiffer than normal. When the ventricle is stiff or noncompliant, the same filling volume results in a higher filling pressure.

As a result, the PAWP reading must be interpreted in light of the patient's medical history.

Optimal PAWP values for any one patient depend on the condition of the left ventricle. In the normal heart, an optimal SV is obtained with a PAWP of 10 to 12 mm Hg. In the patient with left ventricular hypertrophy, a PAWP of 18 mm Hg or higher may be needed to optimize SV. Thus, optimal PAWP varies from patient to patient and is identified by construction of left ventricular function curves for each patient. The function curves are created by measuring the SV at various PAWP readings. This allows determination of the pressure readings that result in the best CO. PAWP readings above or below this range cause the SV to decrease.

PAWP increases for a variety of reasons. Left ventricular failure is a common cause. The lack of forward flow out of the left ventricle causes the left ventricle to dilate and blood to back up into the pulmonary circulation, resulting in an elevated PAWP. In some cases, the PAWP is markedly elevated, indicating overstretching of the left ventricle. This overstretching of the left ventricle causes the SV to decrease and adds to the problem. In these cases, diuretics usually are needed, along with other therapy to reduce the PAWP and optimize left ventricular function. PAWP also increases with mitral valve regurgitation and when the pulmonary venous circulation is obstructed with a tumor. In these cases, the elevated PAWP tends to overestimate the filling volume of the left ventricle. Additional physiologic conditions and technical problems in which the wedge pressure tends to overestimate left ventricular filling volume are outlined in Box 15-5.

The most common cause for a reduction in PAWP is hypovolemia. This is common after major surgery or trauma in which blood loss is significant. Severe dehydration can also lead to a reduction in PAWP.

SIMPLY STATED

The most common cause of an elevated PAWP is left ventricular failure.

Obtaining an Accurate Wedge Pressure. The accuracy of the wedge pressure reading is related to numerous factors, including technical issues and position of the catheter within the chest. Table 15-3 summarizes the criteria used to ensure that the pressure measured is really wedge pressure.

The technical aspects of setting up a pressure monitoring system include calibrating the monitor and transducer, positioning the transducer and patient, verifying and maximizing frequency response and dampening characteristics, and recording the pressures at end-expiration. Attention to proper management of the technical steps is vital to obtaining accurate pulmonary artery and wedge pressure measurements.

Box 15-5	**Conditions in which PAWP Overestimates Left Ventricular Filling Volume**

PHYSIOLOGIC CONDITIONS
- Pulmonary venous obstruction and compression (e.g., lung or mediastinal tumors, left atrial myxoma)
- Mitral valve stenosis or occlusion
- Mitral valve insufficiency: large v waves
- Decreased left ventricular compliance
- Inotropic drugs, hypertension
- Acute cardiac dilation
- Myocardial ischemia, hypertrophy, injury, infarction, infiltrate
- Pericardial disease or tamponade
- Increased intrathoracic pressure
- High mean airway pressures (e.g., PEEP >10 cm H_2O or APRV)

TECHNICAL PROBLEMS
- Overinflation of balloon
- Incomplete wedging
- Catheter fling
- Underdampened trace
- Occluded catheter tip (e.g., clot, vessel wall, embolism)
- Transducer below left atrial level and phlebostatic axis
- Reading not made at end-expiration
- Tubing or patient movement
- Cough or Valsalva maneuver during measurement

APRV, airway pressure release ventilation; PEEP, positive end-expiratory pressure.

Another key point related to obtaining an accurate PAWP reading is the position of the catheter tip in relation to the heart. For wedge pressure to reflect pulmonary venous and therefore left atrial pressure, blood flow must be uninterrupted between the catheter tip and the left heart. This condition exists only in what is termed zone III, an area of the lung where both pulmonary arterial and venous pressures exceed alveolar pressure.

As depicted in Figure 15-11, zone I theoretically has no blood flow because alveolar pressure exceeds both pulmonary venous and pulmonary artery (PAP) pressures. In zone II, alveolar pressure exceeds venous pressure but is less than PAP. Because breathing (inspiration and expiration) and pulmonary artery pressure (systolic and diastolic) are phasic, flow is intermittent. Thus, a catheter located in zone II measures pulmonary arterial pressure with the balloon deflated but reflects alveolar pressure when it is wedged.

The lung zones are not anatomically fixed but rather are functional, gravity-dependent areas that are altered by position, blood flow, blood pressure, and ventilatory status (mean airway pressure, air trapping). Zone II conditions dominate in supine patients. However, because the catheters are flow directed, they tend to advance to areas of continuous blood flow. Nevertheless, the location of the catheter tip at or below the left atrium should be verified by a lateral chest film.

TABLE 15-3

Criteria for Wedge Pressure that Represents Left Heart Filling Pressure

Criteria	Characteristics
Distinct and valid pulmonary artery pressure trace before inflation	Frequency response not overdampened or underdampened
	Transducer calibrated at left atrial level (phlebostatic axis)
	Patient supine, head of bed ≤45 degrees
Catheter tip in zone III	At or below left atrial level with lateral radiograph
PADP > PAWP	If PADP < PAWP, consider non-zone III, tachycardia >120/min, and increased PVR
Distinct PAWP trace immediately on wedge	Clearly visible a and c waves
	Elevated v waves suggest mitral regurgitation; may also be seen with MI and mitral stenosis
Free flow with catheter wedged	No overinflation (climbing wave)
	Easy withdrawal of blood
	Nondampened tracing
Change in PAWP <½ change in airway pressure	Applies to both increase and decrease of PEEP or CPAP
Aspiration of "arterialized" blood from distal port while catheter is wedged	$P_wO_2 - Pa_{O_2} \geq 19$ mm Hg
	$Pa_{CO_2} - P_wCO_2 \geq 11$ mm Hg
	$pH_w - pH_a \geq 0.08$
Pressure reading using the a wave at end-expiration	Obtain from paper recording to ensure accuracy
	If monitor has algorithm to find end-expiration and if digital and paper recording agree:
	• Use systolic pressure for spontaneous breathing
	• Use diastolic pressure for positive-pressure breathing

CPAP, continuous positive airway pressure; MI, myocardial infarction; Pa_{CO_2}, arterial carbon dioxide tension; PADP, pulmonary artery diastolic pressure; Pa_{O_2}, arterial oxygen tension; PAWP, pulmonary artery wedge pressure; PEEP, positive end-expiratory pressure; pH_a, arterial pH; pH_w, wedge pH; P_wCO_2, wedge pressure, carbon dioxide; P_wO_2, wedge pressure, oxygen.

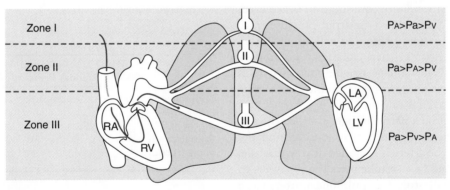

FIGURE 15-11 Pulmonary artery catheter wedged in zone III, where both pulmonary arterial pressures are greater than alveolar pressure, resulting in uninterrupted blood flow to the left heart and a wedge pressure that reflects pulmonary venous and left heart pressures. Relationship of pressures is shown at the right. See text for explanation of West zones I, II, and III. LA, left atrium; LV, left ventricle; PA, alveolar pressure; Pa, pulmonary arterial pressure; Pv, pulmonary venous pressure; RA, right atrium; RV, right ventricle.

To measure left heart pressure accurately, the catheter tip must be in zone III. When intravascular volume decreases (diuresis, hypovolemia, hemorrhage) or alveolar pressure increases (PEEP), zone III areas can convert to zone I or II. Catheters located at or below the left atrium are less likely to be affected by these changes. The following observations indicate inappropriate catheter positioning in zones I or II:
• PADP < PAWP
• Smooth trace: no a or v waves

• With changes in PEEP:
  • PAWP increase >50% of PEEP increase
  • PAWP decrease >50% of PEEP reduction
• With catheter wedged:
  • Inability to withdraw blood
  • Mixed venous blood rather than "arterialized" blood
  • Catheter tip above left atrial level on lateral chest film

Alterations in ventilatory patterns cause fluctuations in intrapleural pressure. End-expiration minimizes the influence of the pressure swings for both spontaneous and mechanical ventilation, provided the patient is not exhaling against positive pressure. Ideally, the pressure will be recorded from a calibrated paper trace that also records the ventilatory pattern so that the end-expiratory pressures are clearly identified over several respiratory cycles.

Wedging the Balloon. Ideally, the catheter ends up in a portion of the pulmonary artery that is at or below the left atrial level, where a wedge trace with very clear a and v waves is obtained. Locating the catheter tip in a slightly larger segment of the artery reduces the risk associated with catheter migration and decreases the likelihood of overinflation and eccentric balloon inflation. Subsequently, the balloon should be inflated with the minimum amount of air needed to obtain a clear wedge reading. Placing too much air in the balloon (hyperinflation) results in a pressure waveform without clearly distinguishable a and v waves that gradually climbs upward across the screen. Rarely, hyperinflation may produce a waveform that gradually declines, without clearly distinguishable a and v waves.

The wedge position is verified first by visualizing the waveform. Before balloon inflation, there should be a clear pulmonary artery trace with systolic, dicrotic notch, and diastolic segments. The balloon is then inflated, but only long enough to obtain a good wedge trace. Normally, 5 to 20 seconds are required for equilibration of the left heart and pulmonary pressures. Once equilibration is achieved, the waveform should convert to an atrial pressure trace resembling a CVP pressure pattern. On balloon deflation, the waveform should convert back to a crisp pulmonary artery pattern. To avoid damage to the balloon (which would require catheter reinsertion), it should deflate passively rather than by aspiration.

It is possible to obtain a partial wedge, in which the systolic pressure is high enough to push blood around the inflated balloon but the artery is occluded during diastole. The trace is recognized by a systolic wave that converts to a wedge trace during diastole: half pulmonary artery trace and half wedge trace. This waveform produces a pressure that is higher than true wedge pressure.

Wedge pressure readings normally are about 2 mm Hg lower than pulmonary diastolic pressure readings because blood flows from high pressure to low pressure. If the wedge pressure were higher, blood would be flowing backward. In fact, that does occur with mitral valve regurgitation, in which the valve does not close completely during systole and blood is ejected backward into the left atrium. On a wedge tracing, this problem is evident as giant v waves, which are more than 10 mm Hg higher than the a waves. In these cases, recording the waveform on paper and using the a wave (atrial systole) at end-expiration result in a more consistent and accurate reflection of LVEDV.

Relationship Between Transmural Pressure and Wedge Pressure. **Transmural pressure** is the net distending pressure within the ventricle. It provides a true estimation of LVEDV filling because the effect of pressure around the heart is considered. Transmural pressure cannot be measured directly but is calculated by subtracting the pressure around the heart from the measured filling pressure in the heart.

Wedge pressure is used to estimate left ventricular filling pressure inside the heart. Intrapleural or esophageal pressure is used to approximate the pressure pushing on the heart from the outside.

During spontaneous breathing, intrapleural pressure is nearly zero at end-expiration. Therefore, as shown in the example that follows, end-diastolic pressure and transmural pressure are approximately equal, and wedge pressure is a good estimator of left ventricular filling pressure in the patient during normal spontaneous breathing. However, positive-pressure ventilation, labored respiratory effort, coughing, and the Valsalva maneuver cause large swings in intrapleural pressure. These pressure fluctuations can cause wedge pressure to overestimate or underestimate left ventricular filling pressure. The following example shows how a PAWP of 12 mm Hg can occur with very different transmural pressures. Remember that left ventricular filling pressure (PAWP) minus pressure around the heart (pleural pressure) equals pressure distending the left ventricle (transmural pressure).

	PAWP	(minus)	Pleural Pressure	(equals)	Transmural Pressure
Spontaneous breathing	12	–	0	=	12 mm Hg
20 cm PEEP	12	–	10	=	2 mm Hg
Partial airway obstruction	12	–	−10	=	22 mm Hg

The relationship between wedge and transmural pressures must be kept in mind in interpreting the numbers. The example "20 cm PEEP" shows how transmission of positive pleural pressure can cause the wedge pressure reading on the monitor or on paper to appear normal (12 mm Hg) while, in fact, the patient is really hypovolemic, with a transmural pressure of 2 mm Hg. The example "partial airway obstruction" shows how filling pressure can appear to be normal (12 mm Hg) when the true filling pressure would be high (22 mm Hg).

Clinically, PEEP levels less than 10 cm H_2O have a limited effect on intrapleural pressure. However, when PEEP exceeds 15 cm H_2O, the effect of PEEP on transmural pressure is uncertain and is altered by lung compliance and changing venous return. As lung compliance decreases, the lung gets stiffer, and a smaller amount of the positive pressure is passed to the pleural space. This has led to the practice of estimating the effect of PEEP on wedge pressure by converting PEEP to millimeters of mercury (1.36 cm H_2O = 1 mm Hg) and subtracting part of PEEP from wedge pressure as follows:

- Compliant lungs: subtract one half of PEEP from PAWP
- Noncompliant lungs: subtract one fourth of PEEP from PAWP

The effects of PEEP on transmural pressure also can be assessed by measuring pleural pressure. In practice, esophageal pressure is measured with a fluid-filled tube while the patient is in the lateral decubitus position. The esophageal pressure, which is essentially the same as pleural pressure, is then subtracted from the wedge pressure.

Removing the patient from PEEP while the wedge pressures are obtained has been suggested. However, this maneuver alters the pressure gradient for venous return to the thorax and may result in sudden "autotransfusion." In addition, sudden removal of PEEP has been reported to cause deterioration in gas exchange that is not readily corrected. In patients with left ventricular dysfunction, removal from mechanical ventilation with PEEP may be associated with increased pulmonary artery pressure, hypoxemia, and deterioration in cardiac function. For these reasons, removal of patients from mechanical ventilation with PEEP to obtain pressure readings is not recommended.

Complications of Pulmonary Artery Catheters

PAC has been associated with multiple complications. During cannulation of a central vein, it is possible for pneumothorax, hydrothorax, hemothorax, air embolism, and damage to the vein, nearby arteries, or nerves to occur. Movement of the catheter inside the heart can trigger bundle branch block and supraventricular or ventricular dysrhythmia. Hypoxemia, acidosis, hypokalemia, hypocalcemia, and hypomagnesemia increase the likelihood of a dysrhythmia. In addition, perforation of the heart or pulmonary artery is possible.

The PAC, like all other invasive lines, is a source of embolus, thrombus, bleeding, hematoma, site infection, and sepsis. The constant movement of the catheter with heartbeat, breathing, and patient movement can result in catheter migration. It should be remembered that a balloon left inflated or a catheter that migrates into wedge position acts like a pulmonary embolus.

Pulmonary infarction and even pulmonary artery rupture can result from overfilling the balloon while obtaining a wedge pressure, as well as from catheter migration.

Pulmonary infarction should be suspected and assessed whenever a patient with a PAC coughs up blood-tinged sputum. An overfilled balloon can rupture, causing possible fragment or air embolism.

Catheter movement and catheter removal can trigger dysrhythmia, as well as looping of the catheter in the ventricle, with possible knotting and valve damage. Lidocaine and emergency resuscitation equipment should be immediately available at both insertion and removal. Blood gases and serum electrolytes should be optimized to decrease the risk for dysrhythmia. Catheter resistance during removal is not normal and is an indication for obtaining a chest radiograph to assess the cause.

Central Line Bundle

As discussed throughout this chapter, a common complication associated with all intravascular lines is infection. Indeed, it is estimated that each year more than 80,000 catheter-related bloodstream infections occur in the nation's ICUs, with as many as 28,000 deaths associated with this serious complication of medical management. In addition to mortality, catheter-related bloodstream infections increase morbidity, length of stay, and hospital costs.

Reducing the incidence of these infections requires a multidisciplinary approach among all those caring for patients with intravascular lines. Because respiratory therapists (RTs) are part of the multidisciplinary critical care team, they must be active contributors to this effort.

As with ventilator-associated pneumonia, a "bundle" of evidence-based interventions for patients with intravascular catheters has been established that, when implemented together, can reduce the incidence of catheter-related infections. Although the bundle focuses on central lines (i.e., those with the tip terminating in a great vessel), it applies equally to arterial line insertion and maintenance. The five key components in a bundle include the following:

1. Hand hygiene
2. Maximal barrier precautions
3. Chlorhexidine skin antisepsis
4. Optimal catheter site selection
5. Daily review of line status

Box 15-6 outlines the specific actions involved in applying each of the bundle's components. Given their active participation in the use of intravascular lines among the critically ill patients they care for, RTs must assume major responsibility for implementing and assuring application of these important infection-control strategies.

| Box 15-6 | Central Line Bundle |

HAND HYGIENE

Hand hygiene involves washing hands or using an alcohol-based waterless hand cleaner.

- When caring for central lines, appropriate times for hand hygiene include:
  - Before and after palpating catheter insertion sites
  - Before and after inserting, replacing, accessing, repairing, or dressing an intravascular catheter
- When hands are obviously soiled or if contamination is suspected:
  - Before and after invasive procedures
  - Between patients
  - Before donning and after removing gloves
  - After using the bathroom

MAXIMAL BARRIER PRECAUTIONS

- Strict compliance with hand hygiene (above)
- Wear a cap, mask, sterile gown, and sterile gloves; consider protective eyewear for arterial line insertion
- Cover the insertion area with a sterile fenestrated drape
- Use a sterile sleeve to protect pulmonary artery catheters during insertion
- Wear either clean or sterile gloves when changing the dressing on intravascular catheters
- Use either sterile gauze or sterile, transparent, semipermeable dressing to cover the catheter site
- Replace catheter site dressing if the dressing becomes damp, loosened, or visibly soiled
- Avoid using topical antibiotic ointment or creams on insertion sites (can promote fungal infections)
- Replace gauze dressings every 2 days and transparent dressings at least every 7 days
- Scrub access port and diaphragm with antiseptic (e.g., chlorhexidine, povidone iodine, 70% alcohol) and access only with sterile devices

CHLORHEXIDINE SKIN ANTISEPSIS

The technique, for most kits, is as follows:

- Prepare skin with antiseptic-detergent chlorhexidine 2% in 70% isopropyl alcohol
- Pinch wings on the chlorhexidine applicator to break open the ampule (when ampule is included)
- Hold the applicator down to allow the solution to saturate the pad
- Press sponge against skin, using a back-and-forth friction scrub for at least 30 seconds
- Let solution dry completely before puncturing the site (about 2 minutes)
- If chlorhexidine is contraindicated, use tincture of iodine, an iodophor, or 70% alcohol

  Note: Palpation of the insertion site should not be performed after antiseptic application.

OPTIMAL CATHETER SITE SELECTION

- Whenever possible, avoid the femoral site in adults
- For central venous pressure and pulmonary artery catheters, prioritize the subclavian site over the jugular
- Avoid brachial site for arterial lines in children

DAILY REVIEW OF CENTRAL LINE STATUS

- Remove the arterial catheter as soon as it is no longer needed
- Evaluate the catheter insertion site daily by palpation and inspection
- Monitor the catheter sites visually when changing the dressing
- If the patient has local tenderness or other signs of infection, remove dressing and visually inspect the site
- Do not routinely replace catheters to prevent catheter-related infections; replace only when there is a specific indication
- Encourage patients to report any changes in their catheter site or any new discomfort to their provider
- Replace tubing assembly, continuous flow device, and transducers every 96 hours

KEY POINTS

- Patients with severe hypotension (shock), severe hypertension, or unstable respiratory failure are likely candidates for continuous arterial pressure monitoring.
- An arterial waveform should have a clear upstroke on the left, with a dicrotic notch representing aortic valve closure on the downstroke to the right.
- Normal arterial pressure in the adult is approximately 120/80 mm Hg and increases gradually with age. Systolic pressures greater than 140 mm Hg and diastolic pressures greater than 90 mm Hg are considered hypertensive. A pressure below 90/60 mm Hg in adults is known as hypotension.
- Arterial pressure decreases with hypovolemia from fluid or blood loss (most commonly, bleeding), during cardiac failure and shock (most commonly, heart attack), and with vasodilation (most commonly, sepsis).
- Normal MAP is considered to be 70 to 105 mm Hg.
- Ischemia resulting from embolism, thrombus, or arterial spasm is the major complication of direct arterial monitoring.

KEY POINTS—cont'd

- As with all invasive lines, the presence of an arterial catheter increases the risk for infection.
- CVP is the pressure of the blood in the right atrium or vena cava, in which the blood is returned to the heart from the venous system.
- CVP monitoring is indicated to assess the circulating blood volume (adequacy of cardiac filling) or the degree of venous return or to evaluate right ventricular function.
- Patients who have had major surgery or blood loss caused by trauma and those suspected of severe dehydration may benefit from placement of a CVP catheter to guide fluid replacement therapy.
- CVP is regulated by a balance between the ability of the heart to pump blood out of the right atrium and ventricle and the amount of blood being returned to the heart by the venous system (venous return).
- Elevations of CVP occur under the following conditions:
  - Volume overload or fluids being given more rapidly than the heart can tolerate

· CVP catheter
· PAC

KEY POINTS—cont'd

- ▶ Increased intrathoracic pressure (CVP increases with positive-pressure breath or tension pneumothorax)
- ▶ Compression around the heart: constrictive pericarditis or cardiac tamponade
- ▶ Pulmonary hypertension (primary or secondary)
- ▶ Right ventricular failure (e.g., myocardial infarction or cardiomyopathy)
- ▶ Left heart failure severe enough to cause right heart failure
- ▶ Pulmonary valvular stenosis
- ▶ Tricuspid valvular stenosis or regurgitation
- ▶ Pulmonary embolism
- ▶ Causes of decreased CVP include vasodilation and inadequate circulating blood volume (hypovolemia).
- ▶ Complications of using a CVP catheter can occur during placement or during its use over time. Placement of the catheter can cause problems such as bleeding or pneumothorax. Infection is the most common side effect over time.
- ▶ Insertion of the PAC represents increased risk compared with the CVP catheter. The additional risk is present because of the need for the catheter to pass through the right side of the heart and into the pulmonary artery.
- ▶ The PAC may be helpful in monitoring selected patients with cardiogenic or septic shock and ARDS.
- ▶ Normal PAWP is 6 to 12 mm Hg.
- ▶ The lack of forward flow out of the left ventricle causes the left ventricle to dilate and blood to back up into the pulmonary circulation, resulting in an elevated PAWP.
- ▶ The most common cause of a decreased PAWP is hypovolemia.
- ▶ Pulmonary artery catheterization has been associated with multiple complications. During cannulation of a central vein, it is possible for pneumothorax, hydrothorax, hemothorax, air embolism, and damage to the vein, nearby arteries, or nerves to occur.
- ▶ To help catheter-related bloodstream infections, RTs must work together with the critical care team to implement the components of the central line bundle, including hand hygiene, barrier precautions, chlorhexidine skin antisepsis, optimal catheter site selection, and daily review of line status.

CASE STUDY

A 32-year-old man is brought to the emergency department (ED) after a motor vehicle accident in which he suffered a broken femur, multiple lacerations, and a possible ruptured spleen. The paramedics state that the patient lost several units of blood at the scene, but the bleeding was stopped before he was transported to the ED. On entering the ED, he is semiconscious and has the following vital signs: pulse, weak and 122/min; respirations, 34/min; blood pressure, 80/60 mm Hg; body temperature, normal. A CVP catheter is placed, and the initial reading is 0 mm Hg.

CASE STUDY—cont'd

1. What is your assessment of the patient at this point?

The CVP reading of 0 mm Hg and the blood pressure of 80/60 mm Hg indicate significant hypovolemia. The narrow pulse pressure is consistent with a low stroke volume, probably the result of poor preload of the heart. The patient is suffering from hypovolemic shock.

2. Should a PAC be placed?

A PAC is not needed at this time. The patient can be managed with volume replacement using the CVP readings before taking him to the operating room to repair the ruptured spleen.

CASE STUDY

A 55-year-old woman was admitted to the cardiac unit for chest pain and dyspnea. Her hospital stay has been complicated by severe pulmonary edema and a poor response to initial therapy with inotropic agent. The attending physician decided to place a PAC to assist with treatment. Initial findings after placement of the PAC are as follows:

Pulse: 98/min
Respirations: 28/min
Blood pressure: 90/60 mm Hg
SpO_2: 92% on F_IO_2 of 0.40
CO: 2.3 L/min
CI: 1.5 L/min/m$_2$
PVR: 310 dynes/sec/cm^5
SVR: 1700 dynes/sec/cm^5
PAWP: 22 mm Hg
CVP: 8 mm Hg
PAP: 38/28 mm Hg

1. What is your interpretation of the PVR and the SVR? What could cause these findings?

The PVR and SVR are both elevated. The increase in PVR is probably related to the pulmonary edema and hypoxemia. The increase in SVR is caused by the peripheral vasoconstriction in response to a reduced CO.

2. What is the patient's SV? How do you interpret it?

The SV is determined by dividing the CO by the heart rate. In this case, it is 23.5 mL, which is markedly reduced.

3. What is your interpretation of the PAWP and CO? What is probably causing the overall hemodynamic picture?

The PAWP is increased, and the CO is reduced; these indicate that the left ventricle is not pumping blood forward effectively, causing a backup of blood into the pulmonary circulation and increasing the hydrostatic pressure in the pulmonary capillaries. The high hydrostatic pressure in the pulmonary capillaries is the cause of her pulmonary edema. The overall clinical picture is one of cardiogenic shock.

ASSESSMENT QUESTIONS

See Appendix for answers.

1. What is the preferred site for insertion of an arterial catheter for continuous pressure monitoring?
   a. Femoral artery
   b. Brachial artery
   c. Radial artery
   d. Ulnar artery

2. A patient with which of the following conditions is least likely to need placement of an indwelling arterial catheter?
   a. Septic shock
   b. Cardiogenic shock
   c. ARDS
   d. Pneumonia

3. Just after insertion of a radial arterial catheter, you note that the pressure waveform appears dampened. All connecting tubing is secure and free of air. Which of the following actions is appropriate at this time?
   a. Remove the catheter and cannulate the other wrist
   b. Increase the sensitivity setting on the monitor
   c. Withdraw and then reinject 5 mL of blood
   d. Reposition the catheter while observing the waveform

4. The dicrotic notch on the arterial pressure waveform represents closure of which of the following heart valves?
   a. Pulmonic
   b. Aortic
   c. Tricuspid
   d. Mitral

5. Which of the following will cause a tall, narrow arterial pressure waveform?
   a. A stiff aorta
   b. Vasodilation
   c. Mitral valve stenosis
   d. Ventricular hypertrophy

6. What change in the arterial pressure waveform is normally seen with respiration?
   a. A large decrease with inspiration
   b. A large increase with inspiration
   c. A large increase with expiration
   d. Minimal changes with inspiration and expiration

7. Which of the following will cause the arterial pressure to decrease?
   1. Vasodilators
   2. Cardiac failure
   3. Hypovolemia
      a. 1 and 2
      b. 2 and 3
      c. 2 only
      d. 1, 2, and 3

8. Which of the following is true about MAP?
   1. It normally ranges between 70 and 105 mm Hg.
   2. It is the arithmetic average of the systolic and diastolic pressures.

3. Organ perfusion is reduced if MAP is less than 60 mm Hg.
   a. 1 and 3
   b. 2 and 3
   c. 1 only
   d. 1, 2, and 3

9. Which of the following are possible complications of arterial cannulation?
   1. Infection
   2. Arterial spasm
   3. Thromboembolism
      a. 1 and 2
      b. 2 and 3
      c. 1 only
      d. 1, 2, and 3

10. CVP is a reflection of which of the following?
    a. Right ventricular filling volume
    b. Left ventricular filling volume
    c. Left atrial pressure
    d. Pulmonary artery diastolic pressure

11. A patient with which of the following conditions is least likely to need placement of a CVP catheter?
    a. Cardiogenic pulmonary edema
    b. Noncardiogenic pulmonary edema
    c. Large pleural effusion
    d. Major trauma

12. Which of the following is true about the CVP catheter?
    1. It is commonly inserted by way of the subclavian vein.
    2. The catheter can have multiple lumens.
    3. A balloon is located on the distal end.
       a. 1 and 2
       b. 2 and 3
       c. 1 only
       d. 1, 2, and 3

13. The c wave of a CVP waveform represents which of the following?
    a. Atrial contraction
    b. Ventricular contraction
    c. Atrial filling
    d. Ventricular filling

14. In which of the following conditions would an elevated CVP be expected?
    a. Pneumonia
    b. Hypovolemia
    c. Cor pulmonale
    d. Pleural effusion

15. Which of the following is the correct method of measuring CVP in a patient receiving mechanical ventilation with PEEP?
    a. At end-inspiration on the ventilator
    b. At end-inspiration off the ventilator
    c. At end-expiration on the ventilator
    d. At end-expiration off the ventilator

16. What is the normal value for CVP?
    a. 2 to 6 mm Hg
    b. 6 to 8 mm Hg
    c. 8 to 12 mm Hg
    d. 12 to 18 mm Hg
17. Which of the following causes the CVP to increase?
    a. Vasodilator therapy
    b. Spontaneous inspiration
    c. Fluid overload
    d. Air in the pressure-sensing line
18. What size catheter typically is used for adults to monitor pulmonary artery pressures?
    a. 2 French
    b. 4 French
    c. 6 French
    d. 8 French
19. The proximal port of a pulmonary artery catheter can be used for all of the following *except:*
    a. Measuring the CVP
    b. Withdrawing blood samples
    c. Injecting medications
    d. Measuring stroke volume
20. What is the approximate amount of air required to fill the balloon on a pulmonary artery catheter?
    a. 0.5 mL
    b. 1.5 mL
    c. 2.5 mL
    d. 3.5 mL
21. During insertion of a pulmonary artery catheter, when is the balloon inflated?
    a. Immediately after inserted into the venous site
    b. When the catheter enters the superior vena cava and right atrium
    c. When the catheter passes through the tricuspid valve and enters the right ventricle
    d. When the catheter passes through the pulmonic valve and enters the pulmonary artery
22. What would be considered a normal value for pulmonary artery pressure?
    a. 15/4 mm Hg
    b. 18/10 mm Hg
    c. 25/12 mm Hg
    d. 36/22 mm Hg
23. Which of the following would increase pulmonary artery pressure?
    1. Severe hypoxemia
    2. Thromboembolism
    3. Acidosis
       a. 1 and 2
       b. 2 and 3
       c. 1 and 3
       d. 1, 2, and 3
24. Which of the following statements is true about pulmonary artery wedge pressure?
    1. It is normally 6 to 12 mm Hg.
    2. It is normally higher than PADP.

3. It reflects left ventricular preload.
    a. 1 only
    b. 1 and 3
    c. 2 and 3
    d. 1, 2, and 3
25. What clinical condition is most likely to cause the PAWP to be elevated?
    a. ARDS
    b. Left heart failure
    c. Cor pulmonale
    d. Pneumonia
26. Which of the following could cause PAWP to be overestimated?
    1. PEEP or CPAP greater than 10 cm H_2O
    2. Mitral valve stenosis
    3. Reduced left ventricular compliance
       a. 1 only
       b. 2 only
       c. 1 and 3
       d. 1, 2, and 3
27. Your patient has a pulmonary artery catheter in place and suddenly starts coughing up bloody sputum. What is the most likely cause of this?
    a. Pneumothorax
    b. Pulmonary infarction
    c. Mitral valve stenosis
    d. Myocardial infarction
28. What complication is most likely to occur during removal of a pulmonary artery catheter?
    a. Pneumothorax
    b. Pulmonary infarction
    c. Pulmonary embolism
    d. Dysrhythmias
29. Which of the following personal protective equipment should be worn when inserting an arterial line?
    1. Cap
    2. Mask
    3. Sterile gown
    4. Sterile gloves
       a. 2 and 4
       b. 1, 2, and 3
       c. 3 and 4
       d. 1, 2, 3, and 4
30. When obtaining an arterial blood sample from an arterial line, you note that the patient complains of significant tenderness at the insertion site. You should recommend which of the following to the patient's nurse?
    a. Removal of the dressing and inspection of the site
    b. Immediate removal of the catheter
    c. Replacement of the catheter with a new one
    d. Application of an antibiotic cream to the insertion site

Bibliography

Augusto JF, Teboul JL, Radermacher P, et al. Interpretation of blood pressure signal: physiological bases, clinical relevance, and objectives during shock states. *Intensive Care Med.* 2011;**37**(3):411–9.

Bridges EJ. Arterial pressure-based stroke volume and functional hemodynamic monitoring. *J Cardiovasc Nurs.* 2008;**23**(2):105–12.

Bridges EJ. Pulmonary artery pressure monitoring: when, how, and what else to use. *AACN Adv Crit Care.* 2006;**17**(3):286–303.

Burchell PL, Powers KA. Focus on central venous pressure monitoring in an acute care setting. *Nursing.* 2011;**41**(12):38–43.

Cole E. Measuring central venous pressure. *Nursing Standard.* 2007;**22**(7):40–2.

Frazier SK, Skinner GJ. Pulmonary artery catheters: state of the controversy. *J Cardiovasc Nurs.* 2008;**23**(2):113–21.

Healthcare Infection Control Practices Advisory Committee. *Guidelines for the prevention of intravascular catheter-related infections, 2011.* Atlanta, GA: Centers for Disease Control and Prevention; 2011.

Hofer CK, Cecconi M, Marx G, et al. Minimally invasive haemodynamic monitoring. *Eur J Anaesthesiol.* 2009;**26**(12):996–1002.

Husain S, Pamboukian SV, Tallaj JA, et al. Invasive monitoring in patients with heart failure. *Curr Cardiol Rep.* 2009;**11**(3):159–66.

Institute for Healthcare Improvement. *How-to guide: prevent central line-associated bloodstream infections.* Cambridge, MA: Institute for Healthcare Improvement; 2012.

Marik PE. Techniques for assessment of intravascular volume in critically ill patients. *J Intensive Care Med.* 2009;**24**(5):329–37.

Marik PE, Baram M. Noninvasive hemodynamic monitoring in the intensive care unit. *Crit Care Clin.* 2007;**23**(3):383–400.

Marik PE, Baram M, Vahid B. Does central venous pressure predict fluid responsiveness? A systematic review of the literature and the tale of seven mares. *Chest.* 2008;**134**(1):172–8.

Montenij LJ, de Waal EE, Buhre WF. Arterial waveform analysis in anesthesia and critical care. *Curr Opin Anaesthesiol.* 2011;**24**(6):651–6.

Polanco PM, Pinsky MR. Practical issues of hemodynamic monitoring at the bedside. *Surg Clin North Am.* 2006;**86**(6):1431–56.

Richard C, Monnet X, Teboul JL. Pulmonary artery catheter monitoring in 2011. *Curr Opin Crit Care.* 2011;**17**(3):296–302.

Wiener B, Chacko S, Cron SG, et al. Guideline development and education to insure accurate and consistent pulmonary artery wedge pressure measurement by nurses in intensive care units. *Dimens Crit Care Nurs.* 2007;**26**(6):263–8.

Wong FW. Where is end expiration? Measuring PAWP when the patient is on pressure support ventilation. *Dynamics.* 2010;**21**(1):11–6.

Chapter 16

Cardiac Output Measurement

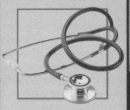

RUBEN D. RESTREPO

CHAPTER OUTLINE

Cardiac Output
Venous Return
Measures of Cardiac Output and Pump Function
  Cardiac Index
  Cardiac Work
  Ventricular Stroke Work
  Ventricular Volume
  Ejection Fraction

Determinants of Pump Function
  Heart Rate
  Preload
  Afterload
  Contractility
Methods of Measuring Cardiac Output
  Invasive Methods
  Noninvasive Methods

LEARNING OBJECTIVES

After reading this chapter, you will be able to:
1. Define cardiac output, cardiac index, stroke volume, and venous return.
2. Describe the method of calculation, common reference range, and effect of sympathetic nervous stimulation on cardiac output.
3. Describe the effects of metabolism and reduced oxygen availability on the regulation of blood flow through organs.
4. Explain the effect of blood loss (hypovolemia) on circulatory function.
5. Describe the effect of mechanical ventilation on cardiac output and blood flow.
6. Explain the significance of the following indicators of cardiac output:
    a. Cardiac index
    b. Ejection fraction
    c. Stroke volume
    d. End-diastolic volume
    e. Cardiac work
    f. Ventricular stroke work
7. List the most important factors that regulate cardiac preload, afterload, and cardiac contractility.
8. Calculate systemic and pulmonary vascular resistance
9. Describe the technique for obtaining cardiac output through the following invasive methods:
    a. Fick
    b. Thermodilution (pulmonary artery and transpulmonary)
    c. Pulse contour analysis
    d. Doppler ultrasound
10. Describe the noninvasive methods for evaluating cardiac performance:
    a. Transthoracic electrical bioimpedance
    b. Echocardiography
    c. Radionuclide cardiac imaging
    d. Partial carbon dioxide rebreathing

KEY TERMS

afterload	cardiac work index	end-diastolic pressure
cardiac index	central venous pressure	end-diastolic volume
cardiac output	contractility	negative inotropic effect
cardiac work	ejection fraction	positive inotropic effect

KEY TERMS—cont'd

preload	pulse pressure	venous return
pulmonary capillary wedge pressure	rate-pressure product	ventricular compliance
	stroke volume	ventricular function curves
pulmonary vascular resistance	systemic vascular resistance	ventricular stroke work

Cardiac output monitoring provides essential information regarding the adequacy of perfusion and helps guide the management of patients at increased risk for developing cardiac complications. Adequacy of perfusion is the most important factor in the assessment of the cardiovascular system's ability to meet the body's metabolic demands. Early detection of key circulatory function derangements allows the clinician to begin proactive therapeutic interventions. This is important because most patients do not succumb to their disease but to vital organ failure.

The aim of this chapter is to describe the physiologic principles used to measure cardiac output and the most common techniques used to assess it. Chapter 15 describes the specific vascular pressure parameters used in the intensive care unit (ICU) to monitor patients with circulatory issues.

Cardiac Output

The amount of blood pumped out of the left ventricle in a minute is known as **cardiac output** (CO). It is the product of heart rate (HR) and **stroke volume** (SV), which is the volume of blood ejected by the ventricle by a single heartbeat (Box 16-1). Normal SV for adults is 60 to 130 mL/beat and is roughly equal for both the left and right ventricles. The average CO for men and women of all ages is approximately 5 L/minute at rest (reference range is 4 to 8 L/minute); however, the normal CO for an individual varies with age, sex (10% higher in men), body size, blood viscosity (hematocrit), and the tissue demand for oxygen.[1]

The normal heart is capable of pumping approximately 10 to 13 L/minute and twice that amount when stimulated by the sympathetic nervous system. A well-trained athlete's

---

Box 16-1	Cardiac Output: An Overview

CARDIAC OUTPUT (CO)
Amount of blood pumped by the heart per minute:
   CO = HR × SV
Varies with age, gender, body size, blood viscosity, and tissue demand for oxygen
Adult reference range for cardiac output: 4-8 L/min

CARDIAC INDEX (CI)
Ratio of cardiac output to body surface area (m²): CO/BSA
Reference range for cardiac index: 2.5-4.0 L/min/m²

STROKE VOLUME (SV)
Volume of blood ejected with each beat, determined by the following:
   Preload: stretch on ventricle at filling before contraction volume, venous return, compliance
   Afterload: resistance to ventricular emptying, vasoconstriction versus vasodilation, blood viscosity, ventricular wall tension, negative intrathoracic pressure
   Contractility: strength of ventricular contraction sympathetic stimulation, inotropes, depressants, coronary flow, heart muscle damage

FRANK-STARLING MECHANISM (VENTRICULAR FUNCTION CURVE)
Defines a characteristic relationship between:
   Volume filling the ventricle (end-diastolic volume/preload) and volume ejected per contraction (ventricular stroke volume): ↑ filling volume → ↑ muscle stretch → ↑ energy → ↑ output
   If the ventricle becomes too large, overdistention: → ↓ SV

VENTRICULAR FILLING VOLUME AND FILLING PRESSURE ARE CLOSELY RELATED
Filling pressure is used to evaluate ventricular filling volume.
Atrial pressures approximate ventricular end-diastolic pressure.
   Right atrial pressure (RAP or CVP) for right heart filling
   Left atrial pressure (LAP) for left heart filling
Pulmonary artery wedge pressure (PAWP), also known as **pulmonary capillary wedge pressure** (PCWP), approximates LAP and left heart filling pressure in most patients (see Chapter 15). For consistency throughout the chapter, the acronym PAWP is used.

CARDIAC OUTPUT CAN BE USED TO DETERMINE VASCULAR RESISTANCE
Resistance = pressure/flow
↑ Vascular resistance → ↑ heart work
↓ Vascular resistance (vasodilation) → ↓ heart work
Right heart: Pulmonary vascular resistance (PVR)
Left heart: Systemic vascular resistance (SVR)
   Ventricular filling pressure, volume, vascular resistance, and blood pressure can be manipulated by fluids and drugs to optimize CO and perfusion of oxygen and nutrients to the tissues.

CVP, central venous pressure; HR, heart rate.

heart enlarges sometimes as much as 50% and is capable of pumping up to 35 L/minute.[1] Under normal conditions, the heart plays a passive role in CO and pumps whatever amount of blood is returned to it. When the diseased or damaged heart can no longer pump the amount of blood returned to it, it is said to be failing.

Venous Return

The volume of blood returning to the right atrium is known as the **venous return**. The resting blood flow through an organ is determined by the metabolic needs of the organ. As the organ's demand for oxygen increases, perfusion to the organ increases. The muscles, liver, and kidneys receive the greatest amount of blood flow in the resting state because of their high metabolic needs. When the metabolic activity of the tissues increases (as during exercise) or when the availability of oxygen to the tissues decreases (as occurs at high altitudes or with carbon monoxide or cyanide poisoning), vasodilation allows more blood to flow to the tissues.

The concentration of oxygen, carbon dioxide (CO_2), hydrogen ions, electrolytes, and other humoral substances regulate capillary blood flow. The presence of low oxygen concentration and increased levels of hydrogen ions and CO_2 at the tissue level causes vasodilation and increases blood flow to the affected area.

In addition to providing tissue regulatory control of CO, the venous system acts as a reservoir of blood. Normally about two thirds of the total blood volume resides in the venous system. When blood volume to vital organs decreases, the veins and the spleen constrict and redistribute volume to maintain venous return and cardiac pressures. In fact, 20% to 25% of the total blood volume can be lost without altering circulatory function and pressures.[2] In cases of severely reduced CO such as heart failure, the central nervous system (CNS) elicits a sympathetic stimulation that increases vasoconstriction. As the heart fails, this compensatory mechanism reduces blood flow to the liver, kidneys, and other body areas to maintain perfusion to the most vital organs (heart and brain).

SIMPLY STATED

- The adequacy of perfusion is the most important factor in the assessment of the cardiovascular system's ability to meet the body's metabolic demands.
- Blood flow to tissues can be inadequate when blood pressure is too low, but a normal blood pressure does not always indicate optimal blood flow to the tissues.
- The venous system serves as a reservoir for the entire circulatory system and through vasoconstriction can compensate for loss of up to one fourth of the total blood volume.

Measures of Cardiac Output and Pump Function

Cardiac Index

Because CO, like most other hemodynamic measurements, varies with body size, **cardiac index** (CI) is often used to describe flow output. CI is obtained by dividing CO by body surface area (BSA) and is reported as liters per minute per square meter (L/minute/m²). BSA is calculated using the patient's weight and height and the DuBois nomogram (Fig. 16-1). The advantage of using an index is that values are standardized and comparisons can be made among patients of different heights and weights.

A commonly cited resting CI reference range for patients of all ages is 2.5 to 4.0 L/minute/m², with the average for

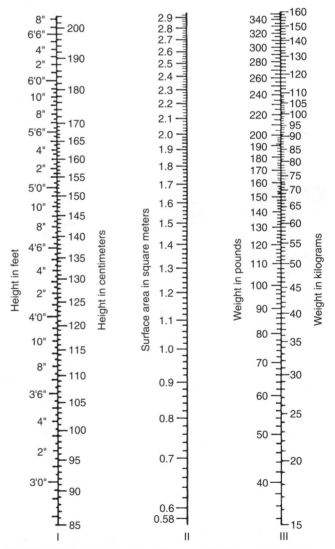

FIGURE 16-1 DuBois body surface area (BSA) nomogram. BSA is found by locating the patient's height on scale I and weight on scale III and placing a straight edge between the two points. The line intersects scale II at the patient's BSA. (From DuBois EF: *Basal metabolism in health and disease*, Philadelphia, 1936, Lea & Febiger.)

adults being about 3.0 L/minute/m² (Table 16-1). The CI is highest at 10 years of age and decreases with age to approximately 2.4 L/minute/m² at age 80 years.[2]

Cardiac Work

Cardiac work is a measure of the energy the heart uses to eject blood against the aortic or pulmonary pressures (resistance). It increases as the end-diastolic ventricular size increases and correlates well with the oxygen requirements of the heart. Although the left and right ventricles eject the same volume of blood, the left ventricle must eject against the mean aortic pressure (MAP), which is about six times greater than the mean pulmonary artery pressure (MPAP). Therefore, the work performed by the left ventricle is much greater than that performed by the right ventricle. This is evident in comparing the **cardiac work index** for each ventricle (LCWI and RCWI). This index measures the work per minute per square meter for each ventricle and is calculated using the following formulas:

$$LCWI = CI \times MAP \times 0.0136 = 3.4 - 4.2 \text{ kg/min/m}^2$$
$$RCWI = CI \times MPAP \times 0.0136 = 0.4 - 0.66 \text{ kg/min/m}^2$$

where 0.0136 is a conversion factor for changing pressure to work.

Ventricular Stroke Work

Ventricular stroke work is a measure of myocardial work per contraction. It is the product of the stroke volume index (SVI) times the pressure across the vascular bed. Normal left ventricular stroke work index (LVSWI) and right ventricular stroke work index (RVSWI) values are as follows:

$$LVSWI = SVI \times MAP \times 0.0136 = 50\text{-}60 \text{ g/min/m}^2/\text{beat}$$
$$RVSWI = SVI \times MPAP \times 0.0136 = 7.9\text{-}9.7 \text{ g/min/m}^2/\text{beat}$$

Ventricular Volume

End-diastolic ventricular size can be assessed by the **end-diastolic volume** (EDV), defined as the amount of blood in the ventricle at the end of filling (diastole). The most common indirect method of measuring the end-diastolic ventricular size is the measurement of the **end-diastolic pressure** (EDP). Further discussion of the EDV and EDP relationship is found in the Ventricular Function Curves section.

Ejection Fraction

Ejection fraction (EF) represents the percentage of the EDV that is ejected with each beat. EF is either measured directly or calculated from the following formula:

$$EF = SV/EDV$$

TABLE 16-1

Hemodynamic Variables, Example Reference Ranges, and Formulas[3,4]

Variable	Example Reference Range*	Formula
Cardiac output (CO)	4-8 L/min	CO = direct measurement
Cardiac index (CI)	2.5-4.0 L/min/m²	CI = CO/BSA
Stroke volume (SV)	60-130 mL/beat	SV = CO/HR or EDV – ESV
Stroke volume index (SVI)	30-50 mL/m²	SVI = CI/HR or SV/BSA
Ejection fraction (EF)	65%-75%	EF = SV/EDV or direct measurement
End-diastolic volume (EDV)	120-180 mL/beat	EDV = direct measurement
End-systolic volume (ESV)	50-60 mL	ESV = direct measurement
Rate-pressure product (RPP)	<12,000 mm Hg	RPP = systolic BP × HR
Coronary perfusion pressure (CPP)	60-80 mm Hg	CPP = diastolic BP – PAWP
Left cardiac work index (LCWI)	3.4-4.2 kg/min/m²	LCWI = CI × MAP × 0.0136†
Right cardiac work index (RCWI)	0.4-0.66 kg/min/m²	RCWI = CI × MPAP × 0.0136†
Left ventricular stroke work index (LVSWI)	50-60 g/min/m²/beat	LVSWI = SI × MAP × 0.0136†
Right ventricular stroke work index (RVSWI)	7.9-9.7 g/min/ m²/beat	RVSWI = SI × MPAP × 0.0136‡
Pulmonary vascular resistance (PVR)	<2 units	PVR = (MPAP – PAWP)/CO
	110-250 dynes-sec/cm⁵	PVR = (MPAP – PAWP)/CO × 80§
Pulmonary vascular resistance index (PVRI)	225-315 dynes-sec/cm⁵/m²	PVRI = (MPAP – PAWP)/CI × 80§
Systemic vascular resistance (SVR)	15-20 units	SVR = (MAP – CVP)/CO × 80
	900-1400 dynes-sec/cm⁵	
Systemic vascular resistance index (SVRI)	1970-2400 dynes-sec/cm⁵/m²	SVRI = (MAP – CVP)/CI × 80§

*Commonly cited references ranges for adults. Sources vary somewhat in the ranges reported.
†Conversion factor to convert L/mm Hg to kg/min/m²; 0.0144 is used by some sources.[4]
‡Conversion factor to convert mL/mm Hg to g/min/m²; 0.144 is used by some sources.[4] An alternative version of the formula includes subtraction of the filling pressures: LVSWI = SV × (MAP – PAWP) × 0.0136; RVSWI = SV × (MPAP – CVP) × 0.0136.[2,3]
§Conversion factors of 79.92 and 79.96 may also be used.[3,4]
BP, blood pressure; BSA, body surface area; CVP, central venous pressure (mm Hg); HR, heart rate; MAP, mean arterial pressure (mm Hg); MPAP, mean pulmonary artery pressure (mm Hg); PAWP, pulmonary artery occlusion pressure (mm Hg).

Normal EF is 65% to 70%. The EF declines as cardiac function deteriorates. When the EF falls to the 30% range, a patient's exercise tolerance is severely limited because of the heart's inability to maintain an adequate CO.

Determinants of Pump Function

The performance ability of the heart (CO) is determined by both HR and SV. SV is determined by three factors: preload, afterload, and contractility (Fig. 16-2).

Heart Rate

HR normally does not play a large role in control of CO in the adult except when it is outside the normal range or when a dysrhythmia is present.

Bradycardia is an HR less than 60 beats/minute in an adult; however, low HR does not drop CO if the heart can compensate with increased SV. A well-trained athlete may have a resting pulse rate below 50 beats/minute but still maintain normal blood pressure. However, if a patient has a damaged heart that cannot alter SV to compensate for bradycardia, CO will fall.

Tachycardia (adult HR >100 beats/minute) is the body's way of maintaining CO when compensatory mechanisms to increase SV are inadequate. In the resting patient, CO may begin to decline at rates of 120 to 130 beats/minute. Because diastole is shortened by increased rates, the time for ventricular filling is decreased. In addition, maintaining the higher rate requires an increased oxygen consumption that the patient with coronary artery disease may not be able to provide. In subjects with a healthy heart who undergo exercise and sympathoadrenal stimulation, the CO does not decline until the HR reaches about 180

beats/minute. Premature heartbeats (premature ventricular contractions and premature atrial contractions) also alter the time for ventricular filling and may decrease CO.

Preload

Preload is the stretch on the ventricular muscle fibers before contraction. Preload is created by the EDV. In 1914, Starling found that up to a critical limit, the force of a muscle contraction was directly related to the initial length of the muscle before contraction. His theory is known as *Starling's law of the heart.* Simply stated, the greater the stretch on the resting ventricle, the greater the strength of contraction within physiologic limits. When the physiologic limits are exceeded, greater stretching of the muscles does not result in an increased force of contraction.

Ventricular Function Curves

Figure 16-3 shows **ventricular function curves** (often called *Starling curves*) for the right and left ventricles. The horizontal

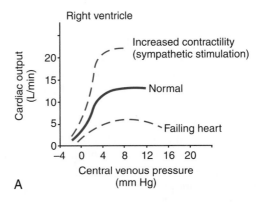

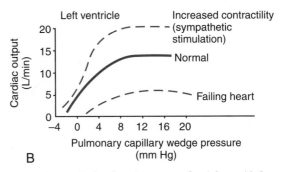

FIGURE 16-3 Ventricular function curves for right and left ventricles. Note that filling pressures are used to represent end-diastolic volume. **A,** Ventricular function curves for the right ventricle. Upstroke of curve shows rapid change in cardiac output for small change in end-diastolic volume initially, but the curve then plateaus, with little change in output for large changes in right atrial pressure. *Dashed curves* show change in output for given pressure occurring with altered contractility from sympathetic stimulation (as occurs with exercise or fear) and heart failure. **B,** Ventricular function curves for left ventricle. End-diastolic volume can be used for plotting horizontal axis. Cardiac index, stroke volume, or left ventricular stroke work index can be graphed on the vertical axis rather than cardiac output. Output begins to decline after pulmonary capillary wedge pressure reaches 20 mm Hg unless ventricular compliance is abnormal.

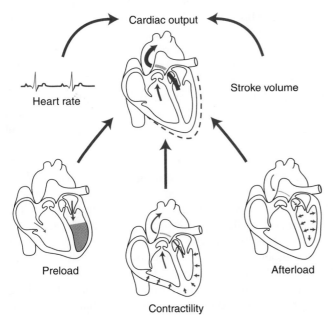

FIGURE 16-2 Cardiac output is determined by stroke volume and heart rate. Stroke volume is determined by preload, afterload, and contractility.

axis represents the volume (preload), and the vertical axis is a measure of the heart's output: CO, CI, SV, stroke index, or ventricular SWI. Increasing the volume increases output. However, when the pump becomes overstretched, it can no longer eject all of its blood efficiently and CO begins to fall.

Continuously measured EDV is the ideal but time-consuming way to assess preload. Most critical care units only measure ventricular volumes on a periodic basis using echocardiography or radionuclide imaging. Therefore, atrial pressures, which can be measured continuously, are used to reflect EDV. During diastole, the atrioventricular valves (tricuspid and mitral) are open. If there is no narrowing or dysfunction of the valves, the pressures in the atrium and ventricle should be the same at end-diastole. The filling pressure for the right heart is right atrial pressure, commonly measured as the **central venous pressure** (CVP). The filling pressure for the left heart is left atrial pressure, commonly measured as pulmonary artery wedge pressure (PAWP). How these pressures are measured is discussed in Chapter 15. Because a nonlinear relationship exists between the EDV and EDP, filling pressure does not always reflect ventricular volume in the critically ill patient when ventricular compliance is altered. An example in which EDP does not accurately reflect EDV is in patients with increased ventricle chamber stiffness (e.g., myocardial infarction). In these cases, EDP may remain constant as EDV decreases.

Ventricular Compliance

It is important to understand that pressure is the result of the volume, space, and compliance of the chamber the volume is entering. Forcing 100 mL of water into a small, rigid chamber takes more pressure than filling a compliant balloon with 100 mL of water. Figure 16-4 shows how ventricular pressure is affected by changes in volume and **ventricular compliance** (distensibility). When compliance is reduced, a much higher pressure is generated for a given volume. Pressure also increases more rapidly as the ventricle fills; thus, the ends of the curves rise more abruptly as the ventricle becomes full and tension is developed in the ventricular walls.

Factors that decrease ventricular compliance and therefore cause the pressure to increase out of proportion to the volume include the following:
- Myocardial ischemia and infarction
- Hemorrhagic and septic shock
- Pericardial effusions
- Right ventricular dilation and overload (causing the septum to shift to the left and impinge on the left ventricle)
- Positive end-expiratory pressure (PEEP) or continuous positive airway pressure (CPAP)
- Inotropic drugs (increase the strength of myocardial contraction)

Factors that increase ventricular compliance include the following:
- Relief of ischemia
- Vasodilator drugs (nitroprusside or nitroglycerin)
- Cardiomyopathies

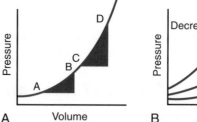
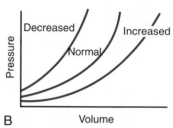

FIGURE 16-4 Compliance can be altered along a single pressure-volume relationship or by a change in the rate of increase in diastolic pressure. **A,** Small rise in pressure (point A to point B) for given change in end-diastolic volume is in contrast to large increase in pressure seen from point C to point D with the same (or smaller) change in end-diastolic volume. Therefore, the ventricle described by A to B is more compliant than the ventricle described by C to D. **B,** Ventricular compliance curves. Not only may compliance fall along the ascending curve, but disease and drugs may also effect a change in the compliance curve up and to the left (reduced compliance) or down and to the right (increased compliance). (From Sibbald WJ, Driedger AA: Right and left ventricular preload and diastolic ventricular compliance: implications for therapy in critically ill patients. In Shoemaker WC, Thompson WL, editors: *Critical care: state of the art, vol 3,* Fullerton, CA, 1982, Society for Critical Care Medicine.)

Factors that Affect Venous Return, Preload, and Cardiac Output

The three main factors affecting the amount of blood returned to the heart are the following:
1. Changes in circulating blood volume
2. Changes in the distribution of the blood volume
3. Atrial contraction

Circulating Blood Volume. Circulating blood volume is obviously altered by bleeding but is also decreased by loss of other body fluids. Excessive urine output (as occurs with diuretics), wound drainage, diarrhea, perspiration, and gastric secretions can result in a large decrease in blood volume (hypovolemia). Fluid can also shift into the interstitial space. Sepsis, burns, and shock may result in tremendous amounts of fluid being moved into this so-called "third space." On the other hand, fluids ingested or given intravenously increase the circulating blood volume. Administration of colloids (large-molecular-weight solutions) pulls water from the interstitial space to "dilute out" the large molecules, resulting in an increase in blood volume. Use of continuous bland aerosols or even heated humidification to overcome a patient's humidity deficit can also cause a net fluid gain, especially in small children.

Distribution of the Blood Volume. Distribution of the blood volume is altered not only by third spacing but also by changes in body position, venous tone, intrathoracic pressure, and, rarely, obstruction of the large veins returning to the heart. As the body changes position, blood tends to move to dependent areas. Standing decreases venous return; conversely, raising the legs of a patient who is lying down increases venous return.

Venous tone also alters the distribution of blood in the body. Venous tone may increase (vasoconstriction) as a compensatory mechanism and shift more blood to the vital organs (heart, lungs, and brain). Vasodilation therapy relaxes vascular tone and may decrease venous return.

Raised intrathoracic pressure decreases venous return. Tension pneumothorax, the Valsalva maneuver, breath holding in children, prolonged bouts of coughing, and positive-pressure ventilation increase intrathoracic pressure and thereby decrease venous return.

Atrial Contraction. Atrial contraction contributes approximately 30% of the subsequent SV and total CO by loading the ventricle at the end of diastole. When a patient develops atrial fibrillation, atrioventricular dissociation, or third-degree heart block or is being paced by a ventricular pacemaker, this so-called "atrial kick" is lost and CO may fall.

Clinical Applications of Ventricular Function Curves

Preload is the major determinant of contractility, but ideal filling pressures vary greatly with cardiac compliance and the patient's condition. Ventricular function curves may be constructed to find a patient's ideal filling pressure at a given time and provide information about ventricular compliance. Most commonly, they are used when large amounts of fluid are administered; however, they may also be used to monitor CO response to changes in filling pressure resulting from volume unloading (diuresis) and administration of intravenous cardiopulmonary drugs such as inotropes and vasodilators.

To construct a ventricular function curve, CI, CO, SV, or another measure of heart output is plotted on the vertical axis. Filling pressure (usually pulmonary artery diastolic or PAWP) is plotted on the horizontal axis. A baseline CO measurement is obtained, and the point corresponding to the CO reading and simultaneous pressure reading is plotted (Fig. 16-5A). A fluid challenge is administered, and another set of output and pressure measurements is obtained. Pressure is again plotted against output. As the plotting continues, a Starling (or ventricular function) curve is created. When satisfactory CO is achieved or when CO begins to decline as the filling pressure increases, the fluid challenge is stopped. The pressure that corresponds to the highest CO reading obtained is used to indicate optimal preload. Volume can then be administered as needed to maintain this optimal pressure. It is important to remember that the venous system will begin to "relax" and expand as the volume status is corrected, so it is necessary to follow the patient carefully and reassess the need for additional volume.

Effects of Mechanical Ventilation on Preload and Venous Return

Normal Spontaneous Breathing. During normal spontaneous inspiration, contraction of the diaphragm and enlargement of the thoracic cage reduce the intrapleural pressure to approximately −6 cm H_2O. The drop in intrapleural pressure increases the negative gradient between the intrathoracic and extrathoracic vessels. This higher gradient favors the movement of blood into the chest and heart, thus increasing venous return. Because the negative inspiratory pressure is also transferred to the heart, more blood is pulled in the right atrium, which augments preload.

During spontaneous expiration, the reverse occurs. Recoil of the thoracic cage causes the intrathoracic pressure to rise, augmenting CO and creating the slight rise in arterial blood pressure that is normally seen with expiration. Thus, spontaneous inspiration functions as a circulatory assist pump for the heart. During labored breathing, as often seen in the patient having a severe asthma attack, these pressure swings are exaggerated and may result in a *paradoxical pulse*, which is a drop in blood pressure of more than 10 mm Hg during inspiration.

Increased Intrapleural Pressure. Increased intrapleural pressure, as occurs during the Valsalva maneuver, decreases venous returns and thereby may decrease CO. Increased intrapleural pressure also occurs with loss of spontaneous breathing, disruption of the chest wall, collection of fluid or air in the pleural space, or positive-pressure ventilation.

Positive-Pressure Ventilation and Compliance. The effect of positive-pressure ventilation on venous return depends on how much of the airway pressure is transferred to the pleural space. When lung and thorax compliances are equal, only about half of the change in airway pressure is transmitted to the pleural space. If the lung compliance decreases, as occurs with certain types of respiratory failure, less positive pressure is transmitted to the pleural space; thus, these patients can tolerate positive-pressure ventilation better and may experience little effect on cardiovascular function.

When chest wall compliance decreases, as commonly seen with abdominal distention or after thoracic or abdominal surgery, more airway pressure is transmitted to the pleural space. If chest wall compliance is decreased while lung compliance is increased (e.g., chronic obstructive pulmonary disease), even more of the elevated airway pressure is transmitted to the pleural space. These patients are more likely to develop problems of both decreased venous return and increased pulmonary vascular resistance during positive-pressure ventilation, with the potential result being a reduction in CO.

PEEP and CPAP. Positive expiratory pressures, including auto-PEEP (intrinsic PEEP), exaggerate the inspiratory effects of positive-pressure ventilation and maintain increased intrapleural pressure throughout expiration, thus having an even greater potential for decreasing venous return. It has been shown that venous return is affected most by continuous mechanical ventilation (CMV) with PEEP. However, if intravascular volume is maintained or increased to offset the ventilator-induced reduction in venous return, CO may not be affected when positive airway pressure is used. The effect of mechanical ventilation on vascular pressure measurements is discussed in Chapter 15.

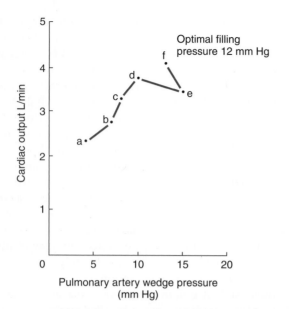

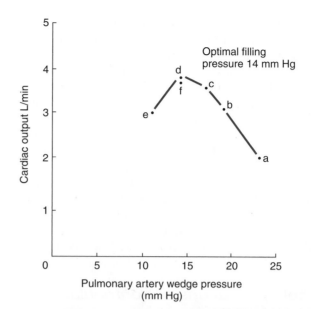

#	PAWP (mm Hg)	CO (L/min)	IV Fluid Challenge in response to hemodynamics
a	4	2.4	200 ml × 10 min
b	7	2.8	200 ml × 10 min
c	8	3.3	200 ml × 10 min
d	10	3.8	200 ml × 10 min
e	16	3.5	stop challenge, monitor
f	12	4.1	monitor

A

#	PAWP (mm Hg)	CO (L/min)	Rx or Fluid Challenge in response to hemodynamics
a	23	2.2	furosemide 40 mg IV
b	19	3.3	furosemide 40 mg IV
c	17	3.8	monitor
d	14	3.9	monitor
e	11	3.0	100 ml × 10 min
f	14	3.9	monitor

B

FIGURE 16-5 Ventricular function curves constructed to determine optimal filling pressure using pulmonary artery wedge pressure (PAWP, mm Hg) as the filling pressure measurement and cardiac output (CO, L/min) as the heart output measurement. **A,** Fluid challenge curve for a patient with low output (CO 2.4 L/min) and low filling pressure (PAWP 4 mm Hg) treated with four intravenous (IV) fluid challenges. Administrations of the first three fluid challenges (a-c) were followed by increases in filling pressure and output (↑ PAWP to 8, ↑ CO to 3.3). After the fourth challenge (d), filling pressure continued to increase, but output began to fall (e) (↑ PAWP to 16, ↓ CO to 3.5), suggesting volume overload. The fluid challenge was stopped. Subsequent measurements confirmed that output increased as the filling pressure dropped back toward normal (f) (↓ PAWP to 12, ↑ CO to 4.1). An optimal filling pressure near 12 mm Hg using PAWP was suggested. B, Diuresis curve for a heart failure patient with low cardiac output (2.2 L/min) and high filling pressure (PAWP 23 mm Hg) treated with two doses of IV furosemide. Diuresis after the first dose of furosemide decreased the filling pressure with a corresponding improvement in heart output (b) (↓ PAWP to 19, ↑ CO to 3.3). A second dose of furosemide was given to further unload the ventricle and improve pulmonary congestion. Filling pressure decreased toward the normal range and output improved (c-d) (↓ PAWP to 14, ↑ CO to 3.9). However, continuing diuresis caused the filling pressure and the output to drop (e) (↓ PAWP to 11, ↓ CO to 3.0). A fluid challenge was given to increase filling pressure and output improved (f) (↑ PAWP to 14, ↑ CO to 3.9). An optimal filling pressure near 14 mm Hg using PAWP was suggested.

SIMPLY STATED

Because the heart is inside the chest, it is subject to the pressure changes occurring in the chest:
- Positive pressures around the heart push on the heart, making it harder for blood to enter the heart (decrease venous return) but easier for blood to be ejected.
- Negative pressures around the heart pull blood toward the heart (increase venous return and preload) but make it more difficult for blood to leave the heart.

Afterload

Afterload, the resistance or sum of the external factors that oppose ventricular ejection, has the following two components:
1. Ventricular wall stress
2. Peripheral vascular resistance

Ventricular Wall Stress

Ventricular wall stress is directly related to the tension on the wall of the ventricle (ventricular pressure × radius) and inversely related to the wall thickness. Cardiac factors that decrease ventricular emptying include the following:

- Ventricular overdistention
- Abnormally high intraventricular pressure
- Thinning of the ventricular wall
- Negative intrathoracic pressure

Increased Afterload. When the ventricle is distended from too much volume and pressure, tension in the muscle increases, and more oxygen and energy are required for contraction. Thus, afterload increases. Similarly, as intrathoracic pressure becomes more negative, the vacuum-like effect favors the opening and filling of the ventricle but increases resistance to ventricular emptying.

Decreased Afterload. Positive intrathoracic pressure favors compression of the ventricle, decreases the pressure gradient across the ventricular wall, and decreases resistance to ventricular emptying but opposes right ventricular filling. Positive-pressure ventilation with PEEP may compress the heart during inspiration, reducing diastolic filling but at the same time enhancing systolic emptying. This combination may be beneficial for many patients in congestive heart failure.

Peripheral Resistance

The peripheral component of afterload is determined by the following:

- Elasticity (compliance) of the vessels
- Size (radius) of the vessels
- Viscosity of the blood
- Driving pressure (changes in pressure from one end of the vessel to the other)

Increased Vascular Resistance. The radius of the vessels is the greatest determinant of peripheral resistance to blood flow. In the presence of vasoconstriction, the heart must exert more energy to eject the blood. As afterload increases, the myocardial oxygen demands on the heart also increase. When the heart is receiving an inadequate supply of oxygen (as occurs with coronary artery disease), it is not able to produce the amount of energy needed to eject efficiently against the afterload, and failure worsens. A downward cycle of cardiac failure ensues if afterload is not decreased; inadequate CO causes vasoconstriction, which causes increased work for the heart, resulting in less CO and more vasoconstriction, and so on. The cycle is broken by maximizing cardiac oxygenation and performance and decreasing the afterload, either by vasodilator therapy or with a cardiac assist device such as an intra-aortic balloon pump.

Afterload also increases as the viscosity of the blood increases. This is an important consideration in some patients with chronic pulmonary disease because the concentration of red blood cells often rises above normal in order to increase their oxygen-carrying capacity (see Chapter 7). When hematocrit levels exceed 60%, CO often decreases. Conversely, one of the causes of high CO (hyperdynamic state) is anemia (low hematocrit).

Blood flow is also dependent on a pressure gradient. When the backpressure in the venous system increases, as occurs when the right heart is not able to pump blood efficiently, the pressure gradient across the capillary beds decreases. Blood flow from the arteries through the capillaries to the venous system slows. This damming effect causes the afterload to increase, which can lead to left heart failure.

Decreased Vascular Resistance. It is important to remember that although vasodilator therapy decreases afterload and therefore decreases the energy demands on the heart, it also increases the size of the "vascular container." If the container is made larger but the volume in the container stays the same, the amount of blood returning to the heart (venous return) decreases, and preload decreases. Conversely, when the volume in the ventricle is more than the ventricle can pump effectively, decreasing the preload can unload the ventricle and improve CO. However, if the venous return decreases too much, the stretch on the ventricle (preload) will be inadequate, and CO will fall. In addition, if vasodilation causes the arterial diastolic pressure to fall below 50 mm Hg or MAP to fall below 60 mm Hg, perfusion to the coronary arteries may decrease, and CO will be compromised even further.

Calculating Systemic and Pulmonary Vascular Resistance

Calculated values for **systemic vascular resistance** (SVR) and **pulmonary vascular resistance** (PVR) are helpful in evaluating the vascular component of afterload for each of the ventricles. The values typically are reported as absolute resistance units (dynes-sec/cm^5), or divided by CI and reported as an index.

Elevated SVR is associated with clinical conditions that cause vasoconstriction, such as cold, inadequate perfusion, hypertension, or administration of vasopressors such as norepinephrine (Levophed), methoxamine (Vasoxyl), or epinephrine (Adrenalin). Warming a hypothermic patient to normal temperature or administering vasodilators such as nitroprusside decreases SVR.

PVR is increased by conditions that decrease blood flow through the pulmonary artery, such as constriction, obstruction (e.g., emboli), or compression of the pulmonary vasculature. In addition, hypoxemia, acidosis, and release of histamine from an allergic response also cause vasoconstriction of the pulmonary vasculature and thus increase in PVR. Over time, increased PVR causes changes in the pulmonary vasculature, resulting in pulmonary hypertension and eventually right heart failure or cor pulmonale (Table 16-2).

SIMPLY STATED

CO may decrease by one third before a significant drop in arterial blood pressure occurs. Because systemic arterial pressure is the product of SVR and CO, reflex vasoconstriction may increase SVR and maintain a normal or increased blood pressure despite the decreasing CO. However, once compensatory vasoconstriction is maximized, the patient may suddenly "crash" because this mechanism may no longer be able to maintain an adequate blood pressure.

TABLE 16-2

Causes of Pulmonary Hypertension and Cor Pulmonale[5]

Mechanisms	Related Disorders
Loss of pulmonary vasculature and tissue (blockage, compression, destruction)	Primary pulmonary hypertension, multiple pulmonary emboli, pulmonary thrombosis Malignant metastasis, collagen vascular diseases Inflammatory and fibrotic disease of the lung (diffuse interstitial pneumonia, sarcoidosis, pneumonoconiosis)
Pulmonary vasoconstriction resulting from hypoxemia and/or acidosis	COPD (emphysema, bronchitis, asthma) Neuromuscular disorders (e.g., myasthenia gravis, Guillain-Barré syndrome, poliomyelitis) Extreme obesity (pickwickian syndrome) Thoracic spine and chest wall deformities
Increased pulmonary venous pressure	Mitral valve stenosis, left atrial embolus or tumor, rheumatic heart disease Idiopathic veno-occlusive disease
Increased pulmonary blood flow	Ventricular septal defect, patent ductus arteriosus
Increased blood viscosity	Polycythemia

COPD, chronic obstructive pulmonary disease. (Modified from Margulies DM, Thaler MS: The physician's book of lists, New York, 1983, Churchill Livingstone)

Contractility

The third primary factor determining CO is **contractility**, which is a measure of myocardial contraction strength. The strength of a cardiac contraction is modified by the following two major influences:

1. Change in the initial muscle length caused by stretch of the cardiac muscle (preload)
2. Change in contractility or inotropic state of the heart at any given amount of muscle stretch

For all practical purposes, contractility represents the force generated when myocardial muscle fibers shorten during systole, independent of preload or afterload. In Figure 16-3, an increase in contractility is shown to be associated with an increase in CO, despite no change in the preload. Conversely, heart failure is usually accompanied by decreased contractility with a downward shift of the ventricular function curve and a lowering of CO for a given preload.

Factors Related to Contractility

Myocardial contractility is affected by the following factors:

- Sympathetic nerve stimulation
- Inotropic drugs
- Physiologic depressants
- Damage to the heart
- Coronary blood flow

Sympathetic Nerve Stimulation. Sympathetic nerve stimulation with release of norepinephrine and other circulating catecholamines increases the strength and the rate of cardiac contraction (the "fight-or-flight response"). Conversely, inhibiting the sympathetic nervous system with a drug or by total spinal anesthesia depresses contractility. Parasympathetic stimulation (vagal stimulation) also decreases contractility.

Inotropic Drugs. Inotropic drugs are medications that affect the force or energy of muscular contraction. A drug with a **positive inotropic effect** increases the strength of contraction of the myocardial fibers, most often by increasing intracellular calcium levels. These drugs also increase myocardial oxygen consumption because cells are pushed beyond their metabolic rate to increase the force of contraction. Positive inotropic drugs include calcium, digitalis, epinephrine, norepinephrine, dopamine, dobutamine, amrinone, isoproterenol, and caffeine. If a positive inotropic drug is used to strengthen the heart when there is inadequate preload, myocardial oxygen supply and demand can become increasingly mismatched and even result in myocardial infarction. Therefore, it is necessary to maximize preload before "driving" the heart with these drugs.

Drugs with a **negative inotropic effect** decrease the strength of contraction but may also decrease the myocardial oxygen demand. Negative inotropic drugs include β-blockers, barbiturates, and many antidysrhythmic agents such as procainamide and quinidine. In a patient with angina resulting from myocardial ischemia, negative inotropic agents, such as β-blockers, may be used to enhance the relationship of myocardial oxygen supply to demand.

Physiologic Depressants. Physiologic depressants of cardiac contractility include hypoxia, hypercapnia, and acidosis. Decreased extravascular calcium and elevated potassium and sodium levels can severely depress myocardial contractility. An excess of calcium ions has the opposite effect, causing the heart to go into spastic contraction. Low potassium and sodium levels are associated with conduction disturbances and dysrhythmia associated with decreased cardiac performance.

Damage to the Heart. Damage to the myocardium, valves, or conduction system reduces the pumping ability of the heart. Loss of ventricular tissue results in decreased contractility because of the reduced effectiveness of muscle contraction, as in cardiomyopathy, myocardial ischemia, and myocarditis. The muscle in the area of a myocardial infarction typically loses contractile ability or, over time, may even balloon out and develop into a ventricular aneurysm.

Chronic increase in myocardial work will result in enlargement of the chambers and hypertrophy of the muscle.

Coronary Blood Flow. The flow of blood through the myocardium is influenced by myocardial oxygen demand. When myocardial oxygen demand increases, coronary blood flow increases. This autoregulation of coronary blood occurs within a MAP range of 60 to 180 mm Hg. Coronary blood flow continues throughout the cardiac cycle but is depressed during systole and increased during diastole. When MAP or diastolic pressure falls, coronary artery perfusion may be compromised, resulting in decreased myocardial oxygen delivery and a subsequent fall in contractility.

Normal coronary perfusion pressure (CPP) is 60 to 80 mm Hg and is calculated as follows:

$$CPP = \text{Diastolic arterial blood pressure} - PAWP$$

SIMPLY STATED

Decreased contractility generally is caused by loss of contractile muscle mass resulting from injury, disease, dysrhythmias, drugs, or poor perfusion. Increased contractility can be caused by sympathetic nerve stimulation or inotropic drugs.

Variables Used to Assess Contractility

Unfortunately, it is not possible to directly conclude that the cause of low CO is decreased contractility. In addition, there is no definitive hemodynamic measure of contractility.

SV is a good indicator of ventricular performance and is directly related to the degree of myocardial fiber shortening and circumferential ventricular size. Other variables used to describe ventricular performance and pumping efficiency include EF, cardiac work, stroke work, and their indices, which were described earlier in this chapter. These calculations are used to describe the work the heart can do and thereby indicate its contractile ability.

Rate-pressure product is a simplified approach to evaluating cardiac work. It is obtained by multiplying the easily measured variables of HR and systolic blood pressure, based on the well-established fact that increases in HR and blood pressure result in increases in myocardial oxygen demand. Values greater than 12,000 are thought to indicate increased myocardial work and increased oxygen demand.

Echocardiography and radionuclide cardiac imaging can provide visual assessment of ventricular volumes and function. Transthoracic electrical bioimpedance, a noninvasive method of measuring cardiac performance variables, also can be used to assess the ventricular contractile state. These three methods for assessing contractility are discussed later in this chapter.

SIMPLY STATED

CO is determined by a complex set of interrelated physiologic variables, including the volume of blood in the heart (preload), the downstream resistance to ejecting blood from the heart (afterload), the contractility and compliance of the heart muscle, and the metabolic requirements of the body. A single measurement of CO represents the interaction of all the variables. CO reflects not only heart function but also the response of the circulatory system to acute and chronic disease and the effect of therapeutic interventions (Table 16-3).

Methods of Measuring Cardiac Output

Accurate clinical assessment of the circulatory status is particularly desirable in critically ill patients in the ICU and in patients undergoing cardiac, thoracic, or vascular interventions. Invasive techniques are still considered the gold standard for measuring CO. However, greater emphasis now is being placed on minimally invasive and noninvasive techniques.[6] The ideal CO monitoring techniques should be accurate, reproducible or precise, fast responding, noninvasive, operator independent, easy to use, continuous, cost-effective, cheap, and safe. None of the methods currently used meet all these criteria.[7]

SIMPLY STATED

The ideal characteristics for CO monitoring techniques are accuracy, reproducibility or precision, fast response time, operator independence, ease of use, continuous use, noninvasive access, cost-effectiveness, and safety.

Invasive Methods
Fick Cardiac Output

The Fick method of CO measurement is based on a method described by Adolph Fick in 1870. This principle indicates that the CO of the heart can be calculated if the oxygen uptake ($\dot{V}O_2$) is measured and the amount of oxygen in each volume of arterial blood (CaO_2) and mixed venous blood ($C\bar{v}O_2$) is known. Thus, the CO can be calculated as follows:

$$CO \ (mL/min) = \frac{\text{Whole body } O_2 \text{ consumption (mL/min)}}{\text{Arterial} - \text{mixed } O_2 \text{ content difference (mL/dL)} \times 10}$$

Or, symbolically:

$$CO \ (L/min) = \frac{\dot{V}O_2}{C(a - \bar{v})O_2 \times 10}$$

Using a normal or expected value of oxygen consumption and measuring the arteriovenous oxygen difference,

TABLE 16-3

Conditions Associated with Alteration in Hemodynamic Measurements Used to Evaluate Low Cardiac Output

Normal Hemodynamics	Altered Hemodynamics	Conditions	Corrective Therapy
Preload			
Right heart CVP and RAP = 2-6 mm Hg or 4-12 cm H_2O Left heart LAP, PAWP, PADP 8-15 mm Hg EDV = 120-180 mL/beat	Low pressure or EDV ↓ CVP, ↓ PAWP, and ↓ urine output ↓ PAWP	1. Inadequate vascular volume 2. ↓ SVR (vasodilation) from drugs, spinal anesthetic, fever, sepsis 3. SVR may ↑ (vasoconstriction) to maintain MAP and CO if significant hypovolemia has developed	1. Volume expansion: intravenous solutions, blood, albumin 2. Stop vasodilators; volume expansion, vasoconstriction 3. Volume expansion; if SVR does not ↓, vasodilation and additional volume may be needed
Urine output 30 mL/hr	High pressure or EDV poor pump/too much volume		
	1. ↑ CVP or PAWP	1. a. Cardiac failure b. Cardiac tamponade	1. a. Inotropic drugs, diuretics b. Volume expansion and isoproterenol until correction of tamponade
	2. ↓ CVP and ↑ PAWP	2. Left heart failure, intraoperative myocardial infarction, left heart valve malfunction	2. Inotropic drugs, vasodilate to ↓ SVR, surgical correction
	3. ↑ CVP and ↓ PAWP	3. a. Right heart failure/valve malfunction b. Chronic pulmonary disease c. Pulmonary embolism	3. a. Inotropic drugs, surgical correction b. ↓ PVR, watch for hypovolemia with low PAWP c. Heparin, inotropic drugs, vasopressors, surgical correction
Afterload			
SVR = <20 units or 900-1400 dyne-sec/cm^5	1. ↑ SVR, ↓ CVP and PAWP	1. Vasoconstriction: body's natural response to maintain perfusion to vital organs when BP drops; ↓ temperature	1. Volume expansion; warm to normal temperature, watch for hypovolemia with vasodilation from warming
Urine output Adult = 30 mL/hr Pediatric = ≥1 mL/kg/hr	2. ↑ SVR and ↑ PAWP	2. ↑ SVR is compensation for failing pump; if uncorrected, will proceed to downward cycle of cardiac failure to cardiogenic shock	2. Vasodilators, diuretics, inotropic drugs
Extremities warm Capillary refill = <3 sec	3. ↓ SVR	3. Vasodilation: spinal anesthetic, ↑ temperature, vasovagal response, sepsis	3. Stop vasodilators/diuretics; consider volume expansion; inotropic drugs, possible vasoconstrictors
Contractility			
CI = 2.5-4.0 L/min/m^2	Causes of decreased contractility:		
SV = 60-130 mL SVI = 30-50 mL/m^2 RVSWI = 7.9-9.7 g/min/m^2 LVSWI = 50-60 g/min/m^2	1. ↓ Volume	1. Dehydration	1. Volume expansion; in some failing hearts, PAWP must be kept at 15 mm Hg or higher to maintain contractility
MAP = 70-105 mm Hg (see Table 16-2 for formulas)	2. Inadequate coronary perfusion/ heart muscle	2. Inadequate diastolic pressure; coronary stenosis, occlusion; myocardial ischemia, infarction; ventricular aneurysm, congenital defects, surgery	2. Maintain MAP >60 mm Hg, diastolic pressure >50 mm Hg (watch for drop in diastolic pressure with vasodilators) Angioplasty, surgery Inotropic drugs when volume is adequate (driving heart when volume is low could lead to myocardial infarction). Low-dose inotropic support may be used continuously for 24-48 hr after surgery to support a weak myocardium

TABLE 16-3

Conditions Associated with Alteration in Hemodynamic Measurements Used to Evaluate Low Cardiac Output—cont'd

Normal Hemodynamics	Altered Hemodynamics	Conditions	Corrective Therapy
	3. HR >100 beats/min HR <60 beats/min		3. ↓ HR: ensure adequate volume; β-blockers, calcium antagonists ↑ HR: atropine; rarely, isoproterenol Pacemaker (CO may ↓ if loss of atrial kick)
	4. Dysrhythmia	4. ↓ K$^+$, Ca^2, O$_2$ Drug-induced Other	4. Replace K$^+$, Ca^2, maintain adequate Pa$_{O_2}$ Withdraw/change medication Treat with antidysrhythmics, cardioversion, pacemaker
	5. Hypotension	5. Negative inotropic drugs β-Blockers (propranolol), antiarrhythmics, barbiturates	5. Decrease or discontinue medication; inotropic drugs as needed
	6. ↑ SVR (heart must work harder to pump against vasoconstriction)		6. Vasodilators with volume expansion if necessary; inotropic drugs
	7. ↓ PO$_2$, pH, K$^+$, Na$^+$, Ca^2; ↑ PCO$_2$, K$^+$, Na$^+$	7. ARDS, pulmonary edema	7. Correct oxygenation electrolytes, acid-base balance

BP, blood pressure; CPP, cerebral perfusion pressure; CVP, central venous pressure; LAP, left atrial pressure; PADP, pulmonary artery diastolic pressure; PAWP, pulmonary artery wedge pressure; RAP, right atrial pressure; SVR, systemic vascular resistance. For other abbreviations, see text.

an estimated Fick CO reading can be obtained in the ICU setting. The following three steps are required:

1. Calculate the expected oxygen consumption ($\dot{V}O_2$). The normal range of $\dot{V}O_2$ is 120 to 160 mL/minute/m^2, with an average of 125 mL/minute/m^2. $\dot{V}O_2$ for a patient with a body surface area of 2 m^2 would be calculated as follows:

$$\dot{V}O_2 = 125 \text{mL/min/m}^2 \times 2\text{m}^2 = 250 \text{ mL/min}$$

2. Calculate the arterial and mixed venous oxygen contents and arteriovenous oxygen difference. For example, given a hemoglobin of 14 g/dL, an arterial oxygen saturation (Sa$_{O_2}$) of 90%, and a mixed venous oxygen saturation (S$\bar{v}_{O_2}$) of 60%, the C(a − $\bar{v}$)$_{O_2}$ is computed as:

Arterial O$_2$content = 14g/dL × 1.34mL/g × 0.90 = 16.9 mL/dL
Venous O$_2$content = 14g/dL × 1.34mL/g × 0.60 = 11.3 mL/dL
C(a − $\bar{v}$)$_{O_2}$ = 5.6 mL/dL

The normal range for the C(a − $\bar{v}$)$_{O_2}$ is 3.0 to 5.5 mL/dL. The lower the C(a − $\bar{v}$)$_{O_2}$, the smaller the amount of oxygen removed per 100 mL of blood passing through the capillaries. Low values are seen when the following occurs:

- Well-oxygenated blood moves rapidly through the capillaries (high CO)
- Cells extract less oxygen (septic shock)
- Oxygen is not released from hemoglobin (left-sided shift in the oxyhemoglobin dissociation curve)

Higher values indicate more oxygen was removed, as when the following occurs:

- Blood flow is slow (low CO), *or*
- Tissue extraction of oxygen is high (increased oxygen consumption)

3. Calculate the CO

$$CO\ (L/min) = \frac{\dot{V}O_2}{C(a - \bar{v})O_2 \times 10}$$
CO (L/min) = 250 mL/min/5.6 mL/dL × 10
CO (L/min) = 250 mL/min/56 mL/L
CO (L/min) = 4.46 L/min

If carefully performed, the Fick method is accurate; however, it is not practical in the routine clinical setting. To derive actual O$_2$ consumption, the expired gas volume over a known time and the difference in O$_2$ concentrations between this expired gas and inspired gas must be measured. Accurate collection of the gas is difficult unless the patient is intubated. Analysis of the gas is straightforward if the inspired gas is air, but if it is oxygen-enriched air, there are two problems: (1) potential fluctuations in the inspired O$_2$ concentration (F$_I$O$_2$), and (2) difficulty in measuring small changes in O$_2$ concentrations at high F$_I$O$_2$. Moreover, measurement of mixed venous blood O$_2$ contents is required, which can only be obtained from the distal port of a pulmonary artery catheter. Indeed, if pulmonary artery catheter placement is needed, other simpler methods to compute CO are available and used.

Pulmonary Artery Thermodilution Cardiac Output

The pulmonary artery (PA) catheter thermodilution method is considered the most accurate and reproducible method for CO determination and the one to which all other methods are compared.[8,9] However, thermodilution CO measurement (TDCO) requires placement of a PA catheter and thus carries with it all the potential complications of central venous access. For this reason, PA catheter use has decreased substantially during the past two decades,[10] mostly owing to the lack of evidence demonstrating improved patient outcomes.[11]

The indicator measured for TDCO is change in blood temperature. Sterile dextrose in water or normal saline solution at least 2° C colder than blood temperature is injected into the proximal port (right atrium) of the PA catheter. The resultant cooling is detected by a thermistor bead located just behind the balloon of the catheter, which is positioned in the pulmonary artery (Fig. 16-6). A temperature-time curve is recorded by the computer, with the CO inversely proportional to the area under the curve (Steward-Hamilton equation). As with all indicator-dilution methods, TDCO measurement makes three major assumptions: (1) complete mixing of blood and indicator, (2) no loss of indicator between place of injection and place of detection, and (3) constant blood flow. Errors in measurement are primarily related to the violation of these conditions.

Acceptable Variations in Thermodilution Injection Technique. Accurate TDCO results can be achieved using iced, refrigerated, or room-temperature injectant in most patients.[9,12] Injection can be through the proximal injectant port, proximal infusion port, right atrial port, venous infusion port, or side port of the introducer catheter. Because SV can vary significantly with intrapleural pressures, an average of multiple determinations with injections equally spaced throughout the respiratory cycle has been shown to provide the best estimate of mean CO. Manual injection at end-exhalation may not accurately reflect the average CO, especially in mechanically ventilated patients. Use of an injection gun and a connecting system that measures the injectant temperature as it enters the catheter produces more consistent TDCO readings.

Accuracy and reproducibility of results depend on extremely careful attention to detail and technique.[13]

Indicators must be measured precisely and injected as a bolus in less than 3 seconds. Computers must be calibrated, carefully maintained by biomedical engineers, and balanced before each measurement. Catheters must be properly located and patent, and tips must be away from the wall of the vessel. The cardiac monitor should be watched during CO measurements because dysrhythmias may alter the CO. When a significant dysrhythmia does occur, the CO should be recorded separately (not averaged into the set) and noted to occur with the identified dysrhythmia. Then, another output measurement is obtained, averaged into the set, and recorded as CO without the presence of dysrhythmia.

> ### SIMPLY STATED
>
> Despite the introduction of various less-invasive concepts of CO measurement, pulmonary arterial thermodilution is still considered the gold standard technique of measuring CO.

Transpulmonary Indicator Dilution Cardiac Output

As a result of the numerous complications associated with the placement and presence of a PA catheter, alternative less-invasive ways to measure CO have been developed. One approach is to use the same indicator-dilution method as with a PA catheter, but instead inject the indicator into a central vein and measure the change through an arterial line placed in a large artery. This technique is referred to as the *transpulmonary indicator-dilution CO method*. CO determination by this method is reliable and agrees well with the results from pulmonary artery thermodilution. Because most critically ill patients already have CVP and arterial lines in place, this method is not only less risky than PA thermodilution but also more practical. As with PA thermodilution, repeated measurements are possible. Moreover, transpulmonary indicator dilution methods are less influenced by respiratory variations than CO measured by PA thermodilution.

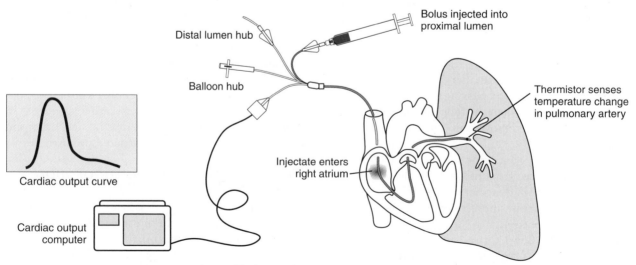

FIGURE 16-6 Thermodilution cardiac output measurement. See text for details.

Two methods are in current use: (1) transpulmonary thermodilution (PiCCO, Pulsion Medical Systems) and (2) transpulmonary lithium dilution (LiDCO, LiDCO Group). Both methods also are used to calibrate CO measurement through arterial pulse contour analysis, discussed subsequently.

PiCCO. The PiCCO system is based on the injection of a cold fluid bolus into a central vein. A thermistor located in the tip of a catheter inserted into a large artery (usually femoral) is used to measure blood temperature changes. A thermodilution curve is created, and CO is computed using the same basic Steward-Hamilton equation as applied with pulmonary artery thermodilution.[14] The only major difference is that the transpulmonary curve appears later and has a lower peak temperature than that observed with pulmonary artery thermodilution. Research indicates that TDCO and PiCCO may be used interchangeably for CO measurement even under acute hemodynamic changes.[15,16]

LiDCO. The LiDCO (lithium dilution cardiac output) method consists of injecting a small dose of lithium chloride (LiCl) through a peripheral venous line.[17] The resulting lithium concentration-time curve is recorded by withdrawing blood past a lithium sensor attached to the patient's existing arterial line (Fig. 16-7). Primary and secondary indicator dilution curves for lithium dilution CO are obtained, and CO is calculated using a variation of the Steward-Hamilton formula that accounts for packed cell volume (needed because lithium is distributed only in the plasma). Research evidence indicates that this method correlates well with TDCO in a variety of clinical settings.[18]

Although less risky and generally as accurate and repeatable as pulmonary artery thermodilution, transpulmonary indicator-dilution methods still provide only intermittent measures of CO.

Continuous Cardiac Output Monitoring

Continuous cardiac output (CCO) monitoring is preferable to intermittent measurement, especially during rapid changes in hemodynamic function of critically ill patients. CCO is considered the ideal method for monitoring the response to a fluid challenge because it has been shown to reduce hospital stay and postoperative complications.[19] Two CCO methods are in current use: (1) continuous PA thermal dilution, and (2) arterial pulse contour analysis.

Continuous PA Thermal Dilution Cardiac Output Monitoring. PA-based continuous thermodilution methods use a modified PA catheter that includes a thermal filament located between 14 and 25 cm from the distal tip of the catheter. Every 30 to 60 seconds, the thermal filament heats the surface of the catheter to about 5° C above body temperature. As with intermittent bolus injections, the subsequent change in blood temperature (in this case warming) is measured by a thermistor near the PA catheter tip, with CO calculated using the same basic Steward-Hamilton equation.

Invasive Arterial Pulse Contour Analysis. In recent years, several techniques that estimate CO by analysis of the arterial line waveform have been developed and applied at the bedside. Collectively, these techniques, known as *arterial pulse contour (APC) analysis*, have become the most frequently described method for continuous CO monitoring in the literature.[20] APC analysis is considered a minimally invasive and indirect method used to assess CO. CO is computed from a pressure pulsation on the basis of a criterion or a model.[21] APC provides beat-to-beat CO measurement and permits preload assessment using volumetric parameters, an assessment tool critically important to guide fluid therapy.[22] The origin of the APC method for estimation of beat-to-beat SV goes back to the classic model described by Otto Frank in 1899. In its most simple conceptual formulation, SV is proportional to the area under the arterial pulse-pressure waveform.

As of this writing, three invasive APC methods are in common clinical use: (1) PulseCO (LiDCO Group), (2) PiCCO (Pulsion), and (3) FloTrac (Edwards Lifesciences). All three methods use arterial blood pressure measured invasively

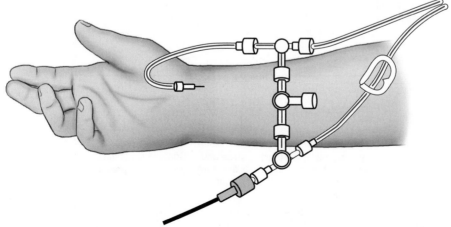

FIGURE 16-7 LiDCO system. The sensor consists of a disposable lithium-selective electrode in a flow-through cell. The sensor is connected to a three-way tap on the arterial line, and a small peristaltic pump restricts the flow through it to 4.5 mL/minute.

through an arterial line (see Chapter 15). The PulseCO and PiCCO methods require calibration through one of the indicator-dilution methods previously described. The Flo-Trac system requires no external calibration.

The PulseCO and PiCCO systems both calculate continuous beat-to-beat SV and CO through complex analysis of the arterial blood pressure waveform (Fig. 16-8). The PulseCO system requires calibration by a transpulmonary lithium dilution CO measurement using the LiDCO technology previously described,[23] whereas the PiCCO system calibration is by transpulmonary thermodilution.[14] Both systems have proved accurate and reliable in the perioperative and ICU settings. In a recent evaluation of this method in patients undergoing off-pump coronary artery bypass grafting, calibrated PulseCO values were interchangeable with the those obtained by intermittent PA TDCO.[24] However, other studies have indicated that the values of cardiac function measured by calibrated PulseCO may not always be consistent with those measured by the gold standard of PA TDCO.[25,26] A check on the calibration is required only every 8 hours, and the software can track changes in CO even in the presence of moderately dampened arterial lines.[26]

In combination with the Vigileo monitor, the Flo-Trac sensor only requires access to the radial or femoral artery using a standard arterial catheter and does not need an external calibration.[21] This technique has been recently validated in critically ill patients and has been found to correlate well with values obtained by TDCO and PulseCO.[17,22,26-33] CO measurement based on uncalibrated pulse contour analysis correlates well with CO measured with the continuous thermodilution method in patients undergoing uncomplicated coronary artery surgery. However, in situations in which the arterial pressure waveform is changed, agreement between techniques may be altered,

and data obtained with uncalibrated pulse contour analysis may become less reliable.[34-37]

> ### SIMPLY STATED
>
> CCO monitoring is preferable to intermittent cardiac output measurement, especially during the rapid changes in hemodynamic function that commonly occur in critically ill patients

Transesophageal, Transtracheal, and Intravascular Doppler Monitoring

Technologic advances have led to new miniature Doppler ultrasonic probes that can be positioned on tubes or catheters inserted into different body locations to obtain CO measurements. The technique measures the velocity of blood flow and vessel diameter in a nearby artery. With blood velocity and vessel diameter known, volumetric blood flow in liters per minute can be calculated.

The transesophageal probe is positioned in the esophagus at the level of the fifth and sixth vertebrae (approximately 35 to 45 cm from the nose) and pointed posteriorly to assess descending thoracic aortic blood flow. It can be used to derive CO from measurement of blood flow velocity by recording the Doppler shift of ultrasound reflected from the red blood cells. The time velocity integral, which is the integral of instantaneous blood flow velocities during one cardiac cycle, is obtained for the blood flow in the left ventricular outflow tract. This is multiplied by the cross-sectional area and the HR to give CO. Signals can be obtained every 2 to 10 minutes.

Transesophageal probes have been left in place for up to 4 days without significant complications. Esophageal Doppler has been considered clinically acceptable and has

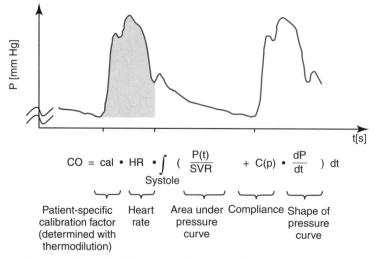

FIGURE 16-8 Computation of cardiac output from arterial pulse contour (APC) analysis (PiCCO system as an example). The calibration factor is determined by intermittent transpulmonary indicator dilution measurement of CO (thermodilution for the PiCCO system). SV is computed as a complex integral that includes three factors: the area and shape of the pressure curve and the compliance of the arterial system. (From PULSION Medical Systems)

shown good agreement with values obtained by CCO and PulseCO.[38,39] The main disadvantages of the method are that a skilled operator is needed, the probe is large and therefore heavy sedation or anesthesia is needed, the equipment is very expensive, and the probe cannot be fixed to give continuous CO readings without an expert user being present.[40]

Transtracheal Doppler ultrasound is accomplished by a transducer attached to the end of an endotracheal tube so that it can be in continuous contact with the tracheal wall. Because these devices look at flow in the descending aorta, which does not reflect total CO, they cannot provide an actual CO measurement. However, they can provide measures of flow—including flow time, peak velocity, and stroke distance—that correlate with SV. One-time calibration using transcutaneous Doppler ultrasound CO measurements has been used to convert the descending aorta flow measurements to total CO measurement. This technique has not proved reliable. However, these devices may find more use in situations in which it is important to identify hemodynamic changes but not necessary to know the actual CO.

Continuous intravenous Doppler ultrasound CO measurements are obtained by a transducer mounted on the distal section of a PA catheter and positioned in the main pulmonary artery proximal to the bifurcation. CO measurements obtained by this method have a moderate correlation to the bolus PA thermodilution technique.

Noninvasive Methods

Early assessment of SV or CO is important for the management of critically ill patients in the ICU or high-risk surgical patients in the operating room, as well as for assisting in the triage of patients with hemodynamic compromise in the emergency department. However, the invasiveness and complexity of the established CO monitoring techniques often preclude this early evaluation. To that end, newer, noninvasive methods are gaining acceptance among clinicians.[41,42] An ideal noninvasive monitoring is one that is accurate and cost-effective, is easy to set up and use, and, provides readily interpretable data, and presents minimal hazards and complications.[43]

Continuous Measurement of Cardiac Performance Using Transthoracic Electrical Bioimpedance

Transthoracic electrical bioimpedance was first described by Kubicek and associates in 1966 and reviewed by Critchley in 1998. It allows the intrabeat measurement of changes in transthoracic voltage amplitude in response to an injected high-frequency current.[44] Contraction of the heart produces a cyclical change in transthoracic impedance of about 0.5%, unfortunately giving a rather low signal-to-noise ratio. It provides continuous, real-time, noninvasive measurement of variables that describe global blood flow, left ventricular performance, pumping efficiency, and volume status. Because blood is the most electrically conductive substance in the body and because the thorax can act like a transducer, the electrical

conductivity in the thorax can be translated into blood flow data. Eight electrocardiogram-type electrodes, two on each side of the neck and two on each side of the chest, form the interface between the patient and the computer terminal. Digitally displayed variables include CO, SV, HR, ejection velocity, ejection time, and thoracic fluid index. Additional variables include end-diastolic volume, peak flow, index of contractility, acceleration index, ejection ratio, and systolic time ratio.

This technique is promising because continuous real-time hemodynamic data can be obtained noninvasively at no risk to the patient. Changes in fluid content also induce changes in thoracic capacitive and inductive properties; thus, bioimpedance is limited in some clinical settings such as sepsis, intracardiac shunts, cardiac dysrhythmias, and hypertension because of inherently low signal-to-noise ratio. Preclinical and clinical data demonstrate the feasibility of using transthoracic electric signals to perform noninvasive CCO monitoring that closely correlates with TDCO.[44]

A new endotracheally sourced impedance cardiography-based CO monitor (ECOM, ConMed Corporation) potentially increases accuracy of SV measurement by placing the monitoring electrodes on an endotracheal tube, resulting in close proximity to the ascending aorta. Once the ECOM endotracheal tube is placed, two cables connect the endotracheal tube and arterial catheter transducer to the ECOM monitor. The system reports CO, CI, SV, and SVR. A recent evaluation showed that ECOM has poor correlation with measurements obtained with the gold standard, TDCO, as well as other transesophageal echocardiographic monitoring.[45] However, because the method does provide clinically acceptable trending of CO, it retains potential utility for monitoring changes in whole body perfusion of critically ill patients.

Periodic Noninvasive Measurement of Cardiac Performance

Transthoracic Echocardiography. Transthoracic echocardiography (TTE) provides a noninvasive method of obtaining periodic data on cardiac performance. The use of Doppler color-flow mapping with two-dimensional and M-mode echocardiography allows assessment of global ventricular function, including left ventricular volume, EF, fractional shortening, and circumferential fiber shortening. Additionally, echocardiography can be used to describe intracardiac blood flow and the origin of intracardiac shunts, diagnose pathologic lesions in and around the heart, evaluate regional wall motion and its relationship to coronary artery insufficiency, and suggest the possibility of rejection in the infant with a transplanted heart. Although echocardiography does not provide continuous assessment of cardiac function, the portability of the current machines allows quality studies to be performed at the patient's bedside in the ICU or ED. However, bandages, obesity, inability to turn or maintain a desired position, and air trapping in the lungs (as occurs in patients with emphysema) may make it difficult to obtain an adequate study using transthoracic imaging.

This technique has been shown to accurately predict fluid responsiveness in critically ill patients because it measures the dynamic markers of preload that affect SV or CO.[46,47]

Real-time three-dimensional echocardiography (RT-3DE), unlike two-dimensional echocardiography, can measure SV without inaccurate geometric assumptions. Recent research has indicated a close correlation between RT-3DE and TDCO under the same hemodynamic conditions.[48]

When a quality image cannot be obtained using a chest transducer, transesophageal imaging can be performed. Esophageal imaging provides especially good images of the chambers and the mitral valve because the transducer is positioned immediately behind the left ventricle or left atrium.

Although TTE has the potential of becoming a valuable method for rapid assessment of CO, especially in the emergency setting, further studies are still warranted. Given the currently moderate level of evidence, the use of TTE should be restricted to well-defined clinical studies until more evidence has emerged.[49]

Radionuclide Cardiac Imaging. Radionuclide cardiac imaging techniques can be used to provide periodic information about cardiac performance.[50,51] Thallium-201 can be injected, and myocardial perfusion scanning can be done with a gamma camera or single-photon emission computed tomography. Areas of decreased perfusion or scars pick up reduced amounts of thallium, creating "cold" spots on the image. Radionuclide angiography can be done by two techniques: first pass and gated blood pool (multiple-gated acquisition). Technetium-99m is the radioisotope injected in both cases. The images obtained permit visualization of wall motion and calculation of EF.

Blood Pressure. Obtaining CO measurements noninvasively during routine blood pressure recording can improve management of hypertension. A new method has been developed that estimates CO using pulse waveform analysis from a brachial cuff sphygmomanometer. The method correlates well with CO values derived by Doppler ultrasound during dobutamine stimulation.[52]

Pulse pressure (the difference between the systolic and diastolic arterial pressure) can be used as a rough estimate of stroke index (1 mm Hg = 1 mL/m²) because SV is the major determinant of pulse pressure. This estimate does not take into account the effects of peripheral vascular resistance on CO but may be useful for trending when perfusion parameters are changing rapidly and no other methods are available for measuring CO.

Elevation of the lower limbs or passive leg raising induces an autotransfusion hemodynamically equivalent to an exogenous fluid challenge. For this reason, changes in CO and pulse pressure in response to passive leg raising are considered good predictors of fluid responsiveness, even in patients receiving positive-pressure ventilation.[53]

Finger Arterial Pressure Waveform. Two technologies currently are used to provide cardiac performance data noninvasively by measurement of a finger arterial pressure waveform: (1) the Finometer (Finapres Medical Systems) and the (2) Nexfin monitor (BMEYE).

The Finometer measures arterial pressure using a finger cuff and an inflatable bladder in combination with an infrared plethysmograph. As with a pulse oximeter, the infrared light is absorbed by the blood, and the arterial pulsations are measured by a light detector. To correct for distortions in finger pressure relative to brachial artery pressure, electronic filtering and computer reconstruction techniques are applied. Then a proprietary algorithm (Modelflow) is used to model aortic flow from the reconstructed brachial artery waveform. Calibration is via pressure measurements during automated brachial arm cuff inflation/deflation. Although the technology appears to provide useful beat-to-beat information on arterial pressure trends, marked variability in pressure and flow (CO) accuracy limits its utility in the critical care setting.[54,55]

The Nexfin monitor also employs analysis of the blood pressure waveform produced by a finger cuff to measure blood pressure, HR, SV, and CO.[56] Because of its ease of use, this method may be best suited for clinical areas where blood pressure measurement is necessary but blood sampling is not. Although a recent evaluation of this method demonstrated a good correlation with thermodilution measurements of CO during and after cardiac surgery,[57] it was determined to be less reliable than invasive blood pressure monitoring.[58] Although an invasively derived calibration is still needed to obtain absolute data on CO, relative changes in CO can be accurately monitored using this method.[59]

Partial CO₂ Rebreathing. Partial CO_2 rebreathing is a method of CO monitoring based on a modification of the Fick principle. This "indirect Fick" method uses the Fick method applied to CO_2 produced by the body and eliminated through gas exchange by the lungs. The equation for differential Fick partial rebreathing CO_2 is as follows:

$$CO = \frac{(V_{CO_2}N - V_{CO_2}R)}{(Ca_{CO_2}R - Ca_{CO_2}N)} = \frac{\Delta V_{CO_2}}{\Delta Ca_{CO_2}} = \frac{\Delta V_{CO_2}}{S\Delta etc_{O_2}}$$

where $V_{CO_2}N$ and $V_{CO_2}R$ are the arterial CO_2 concentrations during normal and rebreathing periods, respectively; ΔV_{CO_2} and ΔCa_{CO_2} represent the changes in CO_2 and arterial content of CO_2 (Ca_{CO_2}) between normal and rebreathing periods, respectively; changes in arterial CO_2 concentration are reflected in end-tidal CO_2 (etc_{O_2}) value; and S represents CO_2 dissociation curve.

Although this method has been found to be accurate and precise compared with thermodilution and TTE in some evaluations,[60,61] a lack of agreement with TDCO also has been reported.[62]

A noninvasive CO monitor that uses the partial CO_2 rebreathing method is available for mechanically ventilated patients (NICO, Philips Respironics; Fig. 16-9). The NICO monitor measures CO based on changes in respiratory CO_2 concentration during a brief period

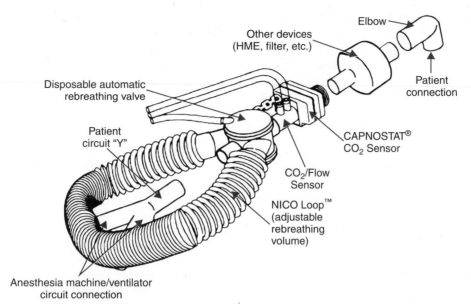

Other devices
(HME, filter, etc.)

Elbow

Patient
connection

Disposable automatic
rebreathing valve

Patient
circuit "Y"

CAPNOSTAT®
CO_2 Sensor

CO_2/Flow
Sensor

NICO Loop™
(adjustable
rebreathing
volume)

Anesthesia machine/ventilator
circuit connection

FIGURE 16-9 NICO Sensor, consisting of a rebreathing valve and a combined CO_2/flow sensor. The sensor is placed into the ventilator circuit between the patient elbow and ventilator wye. The rebreathing valve is automatically controlled by the monitor. When the valve is activated, the flow of the inspired and expired gas is diverted through a rebreathing loop. When the valve is deactivated, this additional rebreathing volume is bypassed, and normal ventilation resumes. Every 3 minutes, a baseline, rebreathing, and stabilization phase occurs. A noninvasive cardiac output calculation is made after the end of each 3-minute cycle. The calculation is based on the changes induced in CO_2 elimination and end-tidal CO_2 in response to the rebreathing volume. The increase in end-tidal CO_2, which reflects the increase in $Paco_2$, is usually 3 to 5 mm Hg. HME, heat and moisture exchanger. (From User's Manual. Non-Invasive Cardiac Output Monitor Model 7300 [Catalog No. 9226-23-05]. © 2001. Novametrix Medical Systems Inc. [now Phillips Respironics].)

of partial rebreathing. Every 3 minutes, the patient's inhaled and exhaled gases are diverted through a tubing loop for 50 seconds by the rebreathing valve; this prevents normal volumes of CO_2 from being eliminated, and as a result, the CO_2 elimination decreases and concentration of CO_2 in the pulmonary artery increases. Although a recent evaluation of the NICO showed a tendency to underestimate CO compared with TDCO at all measurement times in patients undergoing thoracic surgery, the CO readings were comparable.[63] NICO remains one of the least expensive and easiest to use methods for measuring CO.[64]

The use of noninvasive methods, although attractive, has to be validated against the gold standard thermodilution method. A recent meta-analysis of accuracy and precision of four minimally invasive methods (transthoracic electric bioimpedance, pulse contour, esophageal Doppler, and partial CO_2 rebreathing) found that they did not achieve agreement[65] with bolus thermodilution in patients during surgery and in the critical care setting. The correlations between these methods and the thermodilution were 0.79, 0.75, 0.69, and 0.57, respectively.[66]

An overview written by Hofer and colleagues based on recent validation studies demonstrated that pulse wave analysis may be used reliably as an alternative to the PA catheter in a variety of clinical settings.[67] The use of

transesophageal echography and Doppler monitoring is limited because it requires high operator dependency, the partial CO_2 rebreathing technique should be applied in a precisely defined clinical setting to mechanically ventilated patients only, and pulsed dye densitometry as well as the bioimpedance technique are currently primarily applied in an investigational setting. Although minimally-invasive and noninvasive CO monitoring may replace measures obtained from the PA catheter in some settings, the traditional invasive approach may still be recommended for CO measurement when PA pressure monitoring is needed.[65]

KEY POINTS

▶ The amount of blood pumped out of the left ventricle in a minute is known as CO. It is the product of HR and SV, which is the volume of blood ejected by the ventricle by a single heartbeat.

▶ CI is CO divided by BSA and is reported as liters per minute per square meter ($L/minute/m^2$) so that comparisons can be made among patients of different heights and weights.

▶ Cardiac work is a measurement of the energy the heart uses to eject blood against the aortic or pulmonary pressures (resistance) and increases as the end-diastolic ventricular size increases. Cardiac work correlates well with the oxygen requirements of the heart.

KEY POINTS—cont'd

▶ End-diastolic ventricular size can be assessed by the EDV, defined as the amount of blood in the ventricle at the end of filling (diastole). The most common indirect method of measuring the end-diastolic ventricular size is the measurement of the EDP.

▶ EF represents the percentage of the EDV ejected with each beat. Normal EF is 65% to 70%.

▶ The performance ability of the heart (CO) is determined by both HR and SV. SV is determined by three factors: preload, afterload, and contractility.

▶ Preload is the stretch on the ventricular muscle fibers before contraction. Preload is created by the end-diastolic volume.

▶ The filling pressure for the right heart is right atrial pressure, commonly measured as CVP.

▶ The filling pressure for the left heart is left atrial pressure, commonly measured as PAWP.

▶ Afterload, the resistance or sum of the external factors that oppose ventricular ejection, has two components: tension in the ventricular wall and peripheral resistance (sometimes called *impedance*).

▶ Contractility is a measure of myocardial contraction strength.

▶ Inotropic drugs are medications that affect the force or energy of muscular contraction, typically by increasing cellular levels of calcium. A drug with a positive inotropic effect increases the strength of contraction but also may increase myocardial oxygen consumption as cells are stimulated to work beyond their metabolic capacity.

▶ Drugs with a negative inotropic effect decrease the strength of contraction but may also decrease the myocardial oxygen demand.

▶ The ideal characteristics for CO monitoring techniques are accuracy, reproducibility or precision, fast response time, operator independence, ease of use, noninvasive access, continuous use, cost-effectiveness, and no increased mortality and morbidity.

▶ Despite the introduction of various less-invasive concepts of CO measurement, pulmonary artery thermodilution is still considered the gold standard technique for measuring CO.

▶ APC analysis is an indirect method to assess CO. CO is computed from a pressure pulsation on the basis of a criterion or model.

▶ Continuous intravenous Doppler ultrasound CO measurements are obtained through a transducer mounted on the distal section of a PA catheter and positioned in the main pulmonary artery proximal to the bifurcation.

▶ Echocardiography provides a noninvasive method of obtaining periodic data on cardiac performance. Near-continuous invasive measurement of cardiac performance can be provided by a special thermodilution PA catheter that heats the blood, by arterial line pulse contour analysis, or Doppler ultrasound using an esophageal, tracheal or PA transducer.

▶ True noninvasive methods for assessing cardiac performance include transthoracic electrical bioimpedance, transthoracic echocardiography, finger arterial pressure waveform analysis, and partial CO_2 rebreathing.

ASSESSMENT QUESTIONS

See Appendix for answers.

1. Given a stroke volume of 62 mL and an HR of 88 beats/minute, what is the CO?
   a. 5.5 L/min
   b. 6.2 L/min
   c. 7.0 L/min
   d. 11.0 L/min

2. What is the normal range for CO in an adult?
   a. 2 to 4 L/min
   b. 4 to 8 L/min
   c. 6 to 10 L/min
   d. 10 to 13 L/min

3. A 75-year-old man is admitted to the ICU after aortic valve surgery. A pulmonary artery catheter yields the following data: central venous pressure (CVP): 5 mm Hg; cardiac output (CO): 4.0 L/min; mean arterial pressure (MAP): 80 mm Hg; mean pulmonary artery pressure (MPAP): 26 mm Hg; pulmonary artery wedge pressure (PAWP): 10 mm Hg; and heart rate (HR): 80 beats/min. Calculate the patient's pulmonary vascular resistance (PVR):
   a. 40 dynes-sec/cm^5
   b. 320 dynes-sec/cm^5
   c. 160 dynes-sec/cm^5
   d. 220 dynes-sec/cm^5

4. What happens to CO in the presence of sympathetic nervous stimulation?
   a. Increases significantly
   b. Decreases significantly
   c. Remains unchanged
   d. Decreases by only 20%

5. Which of the following statements are true regarding the distribution of blood flow and venous return?
   1. 60% to 70% of the total blood volume is in the venous system.
   2. Blood is shunted to vital organs during cardiac failure.
   3. Circulatory function and pressures can be maintained with a loss of 20% of the blood volume.
   4. 50% of the total blood volume is in the venous system.
      a. 1, 2, and 3
      b. 2 and 3
      c. 1 and 2
      d. 2, 3, and 4

6. What is the normal range for CI?
   a. 0.2 to 1.3 L/min/m^2
   b. 1.5 to 2.6 L/min/m^2
   c. 2.5 to 4.0 L/min/m^2
   d. 4 to 8 L/min/m^2

7. Which of the following correlates best with the oxygen requirements of the heart?
   a. SV
   b. EF

c. EDV

d. Cardiac work

8. What is the normal range for ejection fraction?

a. 25% to 40%

b. 40% to 55%

c. 65% to 70%

d. 75% to 85%

9. The amount of precontraction stretch applied to the ventricles is called:

a. Preload

b. Afterload

c. Contractility

d. EF

10. Preload of the left ventricle is assessed by which of the following parameters?

a. Arterial diastolic blood pressure

b. MAP

c. CVP

d. PAWP

11. Which of the following conditions would cause a reduction in ventricular preload?

a. Decreased ventricular compliance

b. Increased venous return

c. Cardiac tamponade

d. Hypovolemia

12. Which of the following are possible hemodynamic effects of using mechanical ventilation?

1. Reduced preload

2. Reduced CO

3. Increased PVR

4. Increased preload

a. 1, 2, and 3

b. 2, 3, and 4

c. 1 and 2

d. 3 and 4

13. Which of the following conditions would increase left ventricular afterload?

a. Pulmonic valve stenosis

b. Decreased blood viscosity

c. Positive end-expiratory pressure

d. Systemic hypertension

14. Which of the following is most closely related to systemic vascular resistance?

a. Right ventricular afterload

b. Left ventricular afterload

c. CO

d. Left ventricular preload

15. Which of the following abnormalities would increase PVR?

1. Hypoxemia

2. Acidosis

3. Pulmonary emboli

4. Hypervolemia

a. 1, 3, and 4

b. 1, 2, and 3

c. 2 and 4

d. 1, 2, 3, and 4

16. Which of the following is TRUE regarding cardiac contractility?

a. It cannot be measured directly.

b. It is increased by β-blocking drugs.

c. It is increased by hypercapnia.

d. It is increased by parasympathetic neural stimulation.

17. Which of the following invasive CO techniques requires the measurement of inhaled and exhaled gas concentrations?

a. Thermodilution

b. Fick

c. Pulse contour

d. Transtracheal Doppler

18. Which of the following techniques can provide beat-by-beat measurement of stroke volume and cardiac output?

a. Thermodilution

b. Fick

c. Pulse contour

d. NICO

19. Which of the following are noninvasive techniques for determining cardiac performance?

1. Echocardiography

2. Transthoracic electrical bioimpedance

3. Partial CO_2 rebreathing

4. Thermodilution

a. 1, 2, and 3

b. 1, 2, and 4

c. 2, 3, and 4

d. 2 and 4

References

1. Jhanji S, Dawson J, Pearse RM. Cardiac output monitoring: basic science and clinical application. *Anaesthesia* 2008;**63**:172–81.

2. Guyton AC. *Human physiology and mechanisms of disease*. 4th ed. Philadelphia: WB Saunders; 1987.

3. Pollard E, Seliger E. *An implementation of bedside physiological calculations*. Waltham, MA: Hewlett-Packard; 1985.

4. Shoemaker WC. Monitoring of the critically ill patient. In: Shoemaker WC, editor. *Textbook of critical care medicine*. 2nd ed. Philadelphia: WB Saunders; 1989.

5. Margulies DM, Thaler MS. *The physician's book of lists*. New York: Churchill Livingstone; 1983.

6. Middleton PM, Davies SR. Noninvasive hemodynamic monitoring in the emergency department. *Curr Opin Crit Care* 2011;**17**:342–50.

7. Geerts BF, Aarts LP, Jansen JR. Methods in pharmacology: measurement of cardiac output. *Br J Clin Pharmacol* 2011;**71**:316–30.

8. Reuter DA, Huang C, Edrich T, et al. Cardiac output monitoring using indicator-dilution techniques: basics, limits, and perspectives. *Anesth Analg* 2010;**110**:799–811.

9. Hathaway R. The Swan-Ganz catheter: a review. *Nurs Clin North Am* 1978;**13**:389–407.

10. Wiener RS, Welch HG. Trends in the use of the pulmonary artery catheter in the United States, 1993-2004. *JAMA* 2007;**298**:423–9.

11. Alhashemi JA, Cecconi M, della Rocca G, et al. Minimally invasive monitoring of cardiac output in the cardiac surgery intensive care unit. *Curr Heart Fail Rep* 2010;**7**:116–24.

12. Pugsley J, Lerner AB. Cardiac output monitoring: is there a gold standard and how do the newer technologies compare? *Semin Cardiothorac Vasc Anesth* 2010;**14**:274–82.

13. Richard C, Monnet X, Teboul JL. Pulmonary artery catheter monitoring in 2011. *Curr Opin Crit Care* 2011;**17**: 296–302.

14. Martin Vivas A, Saboya Sanchez S, Patino Rodriguez M, et al. Hemodynamic monitoring: PiCCO system. *Enferm Intensiva* 2008;**19**:132–40.

15. Bajorat J, Hofmockel R, Vagts DA, et al. Comparison of invasive and less-invasive techniques of cardiac output measurement under different hemodynamic conditions in a pig model. *Eur J Anaesthesiol* 2006;**23**:710.

16. Nusmeier A, van der Hoeven JG, Lemson J. Cardiac output monitoring in pediatric patients. *Expert Rev Med Devices* 2010;**7**:503–17.

17. Reuter DA, Huang C, Edrich T, et al. Cardiac output monitoring using indicator-dilution techniques: basics, limits, and perspectives. *Anesth Analg* 2010;**110**:799–811.

18. Costa MG, Della Rocca G, Chiarandini P, et al. Continuous and intermittent cardiac output measurement in hyperdynamic conditions: pulmonary artery catheter vs. lithium dilution technique. *Intensive Care Med* 2008;**34**:257–63.

19. Cecconi M, Parsons AK, Rhodes A. What is a fluid challenge?. *Curr Opin Crit Care* 2011;**17**:290–5.

20. Critchley LA, Lee A, Ho AM. A critical review of the ability of continuous cardiac output monitors to measure trends in cardiac output. *Anesth Analg* 2010;**111**:1180–92.

21. Morgan P, Al-Subaie N, Rhodes A. Minimally invasive cardiac output monitoring. *Curr Opin Crit Care* 2008;**14**:322–6.

22. Lavrentieva A, Palmieri T. Determination of cardiovascular parameters in burn patients using arterial waveform analysis: a review. *Burns* 2011;**37**:196–202.

23. Sundar S, Panzica P. LiDCO systems. *Int Anesthesiol Clin* 2010;**48**:87–100.

24. Chakravarthy M, Patil TA, Jayaprakash K, et al. Comparison of simultaneous estimation of cardiac output by four techniques in patients undergoing off-pump coronary artery bypass surgery-a prospective observational study. *Ann Card Anaesth* 2007;**10**:121–6.

25. Cecconi M, Dawson D, Casaretti R, et al. A prospective study of the accuracy and precision of continuous cardiac output monitoring devices as compared to intermittent thermodilution. *Minerva Anestesiol* 2010;**76**:1010–7.

26. Pittman J, Bar Yosef S, SumPing J, et al. Continuous cardiac output monitoring with pulse contour analysis: a comparison with lithium indicator dilution cardiac output measurement. *Crit Care Med* 2005;**33**:2015–21.

27. Button D, Weibel L, Reuthebuch O, et al. Clinical evaluation of the FloTrac/Vigileo system and two established continuous cardiac output monitoring devices in patients undergoing cardiac surgery. *Br J Anaesth* 2007;**99**:329–36.

28. Compton FD, Zukunft B, Hoffmann C, et al. Performance of a minimally invasive uncalibrated cardiac output monitoring system (Flotrac/Vigileo) in haemodynamically unstable patients. *Br J Anaesth* 2008;**100**:451–6.

29. Cannesson M, Attof Y, Rosamel P, et al. Comparison of FloTrac cardiac output monitoring system in patients undergoing coronary artery bypass grafting with pulmonary artery cardiac output measurements. *Eur J Anaesthesiol* 2007;**24**:832–9.

30. Manecke Jr GR, Auger WR. Cardiac output determination from the arterial pressure wave: clinical testing of a novel algorithm that does not require calibration. *J Cardiothorac Vasc Anesth* 2007;**21**:3–7.

31. Vasdev S, Chauhan S, Choudhury M, et al. Arterial pressure waveform derived cardiac output FloTrac/Vigileo system (third generation software): comparison of two monitoring sites with the thermodilution cardiac output. *J Clin Monit Comput* 2012;**26**:115–20.

32. Hofer CK, Button D, Weibel L, et al. Uncalibrated radial and femoral arterial pressure waveform analysis for continuous cardiac output measurement: an evaluation in cardiac surgery patients. *J Cardiothorac Vasc Anesth* 2010;**24**:257–64.

33. Scheeren TW, Wiesenack C, Compton FD, et al. Performance of a minimally invasive cardiac output monitoring system (Flotrac/Vigileo). *Br J Anaesth* 2008;**101**:279–80.

34. Lorsomradee S, Lorsomradee S, Cromheecke S, et al. Uncalibrated arterial pulse contour analysis versus continuous thermodilution technique: effects of alterations in arterial waveform. *J Cardiothorac Vasc Anesth* 2007;**21**:636–43.

35. Lorsomradee S, Lorsomradee SR, Cromheecke S, et al. Continuous cardiac output measurement: arterial pressure analysis versus thermodilution technique during cardiac surgery with cardiopulmonary bypass. *Anaesthesia* 2007;**62**:979–83.

36. McGee WT, Horswell JL, Calderon J, et al. Validation of a continuous, arterial pressure-based cardiac output measurement: a multicenter, prospective clinical trial. *Crit Care* 2007;**11**:R105.

37. Prasser C, Bele S, Keyl C, et al. Evaluation of a new arterial pressure-based cardiac output device requiring no external calibration. *BMC Anesthesiol* 2007;**7**:9.

38. Mowatt G, Houston G, Hernández R, et al. Systematic review of the clinical effectiveness and cost-effectiveness of oesophageal Doppler monitoring in critically ill and high-risk surgical patients. *Health Technol Assess* 2009;**13**:1–95.

39. Ferreira RM, do Amaral JL, Valiatti JL. Comparison between two methods for hemodynamic measurement: thermodilution and oesophageal Doppler. *Rev Assoc Med Bras* 2007;**53**:349–54.

40. Nusmeier A, van der Hoeven JG, Lemson J. Cardiac output monitoring in pediatric patients. *Expert Rev Med Devices* 2010;**7**:503–17.

41. Cholley BP, Payen D. Noninvasive techniques for measurements of cardiac output. *Curr Opin Crit Care* 2005;**11**:424–9.

42. Marik PE, Baram M. Noninvasive hemodynamic monitoring in the intensive care unit. *Crit Care Clin* 2007;**23**:383–400.

43. Absi MA, Lutterman J, Wetzel GT. Noninvasive cardiac output monitoring in the pediatric cardiac intensive care unit. *Curr Opin Cardiol* 2010;**25**:77–9.

44. Keren H, Burkhoff D, Squara P. Evaluation of a noninvasive continuous cardiac output monitoring system based on thoracic bioreactance. *Am J Physiol Heart Circ Physiol* 2007;**293**:H583–9.

45. Maus TM, Reber B, Banks DA, et al. Cardiac output determination from endotracheally measured impedance cardiography: clinical evaluation of endotracheal cardiac output monitor. *J Cardiothorac Vasc Anesth* 2011;**25**:770–5.

46. Mandeville JC, Colebourn CL. Can transthoracic echocardiography be used to predict fluid responsiveness in the critically ill patient? A systematic review. *Crit Care Res Pract* 2012;**513480**:2012.

47. Biais M, Vidil L, Sarrabay P, et al. Changes in stroke volume induced by passive leg raising in spontaneously breathing patients: comparison between echocardiography and Vigileo/FloTrac device. *Crit Care* 2009;**13**:R195.

48. Hoole SP, Boyd J, Ninios V, et al. Measurement of cardiac output by real-time 3-D echocardiography in patients undergoing assessment for cardiac transplantation. *Eur J Echocardiogr* 2008;**9**:334–7.

49. Meyer S, Todd D, Wright I, et al. Review article: non-invasive assessment of cardiac output with portable continuous-wave Doppler ultrasound. *Emerg Med Australas* 2008;**20**:201–8.

50. Petri S, Esko V, Esa J, et al. A prospective comparison of cardiac magnetic resonance imaging and radionuclide ventriculography in the assessment of cardiac function in patients treated with anthracycline-based chemotherapy. *Nucl Med Commun* 2012;**33**:51–9.

51. Friehling M, Chen J, Saba S, et al. A prospective pilot study to evaluate the relationship between acute change in left ventricular synchrony after cardiac resynchronization therapy and patient outcome using a single-injection gated SPECT protocol. *Circ Cardiovasc Imaging* 2011;**4**:532–9.

52. Chio SS, Tsai JT, Hsu YM, et al. Development and validation of a noninvasive method to estimate cardiac output using cuff sphygmomanometry. *Clin Cardiol* 2007;**30**:615–20.

53. Cavallaro F, Sandroni C, Marano C, et al. Diagnostic accuracy of passive leg raising for prediction of fluid responsiveness in adults: systematic review and meta-analysis of clinical studies. *Intensive Care Med* 2010;**36**:1475–83.

54. Stokes DN, Clutton-Brock T, Patil C, et al. Comparison of invasive and non-invasive measurement of continuous arterial pressure using the Finapres. *Br J Anaesth* 1991;**67**:26–35.

55. Remmen JJ, Aengevaeren WR, Verheugt FW, et al. Finapres arterial pulse wave analysis with Modelflow is not a reliable non-invasive method for assessment of cardiac output. *Clin Sci (Lond)* 2002;**103**:143–9.

56. Martina JR, Westerhof BE, Van Goudoever J, et al. Noninvasive blood pressure measurement by the Nexfin monitor during reduced arterial pulsatility: a feasibility study. *ASAIO J* 2010;**56**:221–7.

57. Broch O, Renner J, Gruenewald M, et al. A comparison of the Nexfin and transcardiopulmonary thermodilution to estimate cardiac output during coronary artery surgery. *Anaesthesia* 2012;**67**:377–83.

58. Stover JF, Stocker R, Lenherr R, et al. Noninvasive cardiac output and blood pressure monitoring cannot replace an invasive monitoring system in critically ill patients. *BMC Anesthes* 2009;**9**:6.

59. de Jong RM, Westerhof BE, Voors AA, van Veldhuisen DJ. Noninvasive haemodynamic monitoring using finger arterial pressure waveforms. *Netherlands J Med* 2009;**67**:372–5.

60. Peyton PJ. Continuous minimally invasive peri-operative monitoring of cardiac output by pulmonary capnotracking: comparison with thermodilution and transesophageal echocardiography. *J Clin Monit Comput* 2012;**26**:121–32.

61. Peyton PJ, Thompson D, Junor P. Non-invasive automated measurement of cardiac output during stable cardiac surgery using a fully integrated differential CO_2 Fick method. *J Clin Monit Comput* 2008;**22**:285–92.

62. Møller-Sørensen H, Hansen KL, Ostergaard M, et al. Lack of agreement and trending ability of the endotracheal cardiac output monitor compared with thermodilution. *Acta Anaesthesiol Scand* 2012;**56**:433–40.

63. Ng JM, Chow MY, Ip-Yam PC, et al. Evaluation of partial carbon dioxide rebreathing cardiac output measurement during thoracic surgery. *J Cardiothorac Vasc Anesth* 2007;**21**:655–8.

64. Young BP, Low LL. Noninvasive monitoring cardiac output using partial CO_2 rebreathing. *Crit Care Clin* 2010;**26**:383–92.

65. Cecconi M, Rhodes A, Poloniecki J, et al. Bench-to-bedside review: the importance of the precision of the reference technique in method comparison studies—with specific reference to the measurement of cardiac output. *Crit Care* 2009;**13**:201.

66. Peyton PJ, Chong SW. Minimally invasive measurement of cardiac output during surgery and critical care: a meta-analysis of accuracy and precision. *Anesthesiology* 2010;**113**:1220–35.

67. Hofer CK, Ganter MT, Zollinger A. What technique should I use to measure cardiac output? *Curr Opin Crit Care* 2007;**13**:308–17.

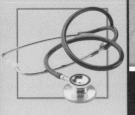

Chapter 17

Bronchoscopy

ZAZA COHEN*

CHAPTER OUTLINE

LEARNING OBJECTIVES

After reading this chapter, you will be able to:
1. Define the basic terms used with endoscopy.
2. Describe the characteristics and capabilities of the flexible bronchoscope.
3. Identify common indications for bronchoscopy.
4. Distinguish diagnostic and therapeutic indications for bronchoscopy.
5. Explain the uses of bronchoalveolar lavage, brushings (both sterile and nonsterile), and forceps and needle biopsies.
6. Discuss the major concepts of interventional bronchoscopy.
7. Discuss the complications of flexible bronchoscopy and the relative risks involved in the procedure.
8. Identify the contraindications to performing a bronchoscopy.
9. List the essential equipment needed to perform a bronchoscopy safely.
10. Review the role of the respiratory therapist in bronchoscopy.
11. Discuss step-by-step preparation of the patient and the equipment for the bronchoscopy.

KEY TERMS

bronchoalveolar lavage (BAL)	**endoscopy**	**transbronchial biopsy (TBB)**
bronchoscope	**fiberoptic bronchoscope**	
bronchoscopy	**fluoroscopy**	
electromagnetic navigation bronchoscopy	**interventional bronchoscopy**	
	moderate sedation	

*Dr. James Dexter contributed some of the content for this chapter as coeditor of the prior edition of this text.

The word **endoscopy** (from Greek words *endo*, meaning "inside," and *skopeo*, "to examine") describes examination of the interior of a canal or a hollow viscus by means of a special instrument, such as an endoscope. Endoscopy is a somewhat general term that includes procedures, such as *laryngoscopy*, examination of the larynx; **bronchoscopy**, examination of the bronchi; *gastroscopy*, examination of the stomach; and *colonoscopy*, examination of the colon, among many others. Gustav Killian, widely regarded as the "father" of bronchoscopy, was first to visualize the bronchial tree through a hollow tube (**bronchoscope**) inserted in the patient's larynx in 1897. Two major advances of the 20th century in the field of bronchoscopy were the addition of the suction channel by Chevalier Jackson and the use of fiberoptics for the light source by Shigeto Ikeda.

The early versions of bronchoscopy used straight pieces of open pipe, beveled on the end to prevent tearing the trachea while being forced into the anesthetized patient with the head tipped back as far as possible. A simple light shining down the tube allowed limited viewing of the trachea and mainstem bronchi. Although these rigid devices provided a limited view of the larger airways, they allowed removal of large volumes of blood, mucus, or foreign objects and biopsy of tumors in the upper airway. At the same time, mechanical ventilation was provided to ensure better gas exchange during the procedure. Those early rigid bronchoscopes have been replaced by more sophisticated rigid instruments with lights at the tips and valves to allow general anesthesia, oxygenation, suctioning, and biopsy. The new rigid bronchoscopes remain useful for a few problems, such as removal of difficult foreign bodies and management of severe bleeding, but well more than 90% of bronchoscopy procedures now are done with flexible fiberoptic bronchoscopes. Given that the emphasis of this text is on patient assessment, and that rigid bronchoscopy is relatively infrequently performed, the focus of this chapter is on flexible fiberoptic bronchoscopy.

The first application of flexible fiberoptics to the field of endoscopy was in 1957 and was initially applied to gastroscopes. As experience grew and the techniques improved, it was applied to the other disciplines within the field of endoscopy. In the 1960s, Shigeto Ikeda of Japan designed the first **fiberoptic bronchoscope**, which incorporated fiberoptics into a flexible tube suitable in size and length to enter the trachea and visualize the lower airway. The first bronchoscopy in the United States using flexible fiberoptic technique was done in the Mayo Clinic in 1969. The flexible fiberoptic bronchoscope has greatly expanded the practice of pulmonary medicine by allowing inspection of the airways, removal of many different foreign bodies, and biopsy of airway and peripheral lung tissue. Most of these activities can be performed in the outpatient setting with **moderate sedation**.

In most institutions, flexible bronchoscopy is performed by a properly trained and licensed physician (usually a pulmonologist, but sometimes a surgeon or a critical care physician) and one or two assistants, usually a respiratory therapist (RT) or a registered nurse (RN). For the remainder of this chapter, we refer to the physician performing the procedure as "the bronchoscopist" and the RN or the RT assisting as "the assistant." In many teaching institutions, students, medical residents, or other trainees may also be present and participate in various parts of the procedure under the supervision of a licensed health care provider. Sometimes, a radiology technician is available to perform fluoroscopy (see the discussion on fluoroscopy later in this chapter or in Chapter 10), as well as a histology technician to evaluate the quality of the specimen from biopsy or brushings. RTs are educated and trained about flexible fiberoptic bronchoscopes because they often maintain the equipment and the materials needed for the procedure. The RT has become indispensable in helping the physician perform the procedure both in hospitals and outpatient clinics.

> ### SIMPLY STATED
>
> Endoscopy is a field of medicine that uses instruments to look into different parts of the body to diagnose various diseases and explain certain conditions. Bronchoscopy is the process of visualizing the airways below the larynx with a bronchoscope.

Characteristics and Capabilities of the Bronchoscope

The bronchoscopes available today serve a wide range of applications, from small-diameter scopes used for viewing the airways of infants and children to larger-diameter scopes with suction channels used to remove thick secretions from patients on ventilators in the intensive care unit (ICU), to scopes that incorporate ultrasound equipment for better visualization of the structures. Many bronchoscopes are now digital. Light is produced in an external light source and carried into the airways through a fiberoptic bundle. A digital video camera on the end of the bronchoscope acquires the images of the lighted airways, and the real-time images are displayed on a large video monitor. This allows easier and more hygienic manipulation of the bronchoscope and allows both still and video photographs of the procedure for documenting and teaching purposes.

The standard flexible bronchoscope has an external diameter of 5.3 mm and a total length of 605 mm (Fig. 17-1). It can pass easily down the trachea (first-order bronchus) and into the right or left mainstem bronchus. From there, it can be advanced through most fourth-order bronchi and one third of all fifth-order bronchi (Fig. 17-2). Visualization of half of the lung's sixth-order bronchi is possible. Ultrathin scopes with a 2.7-mm external diameter and 0.8-mm biopsy channels will pass down 3.5-mm or larger endotracheal tubes, making it easier to study and perform

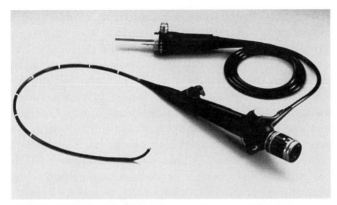

FIGURE 17-1 Flexible fiberoptic bronchoscope (Courtesy Olympus America, Inc. Melville NY).

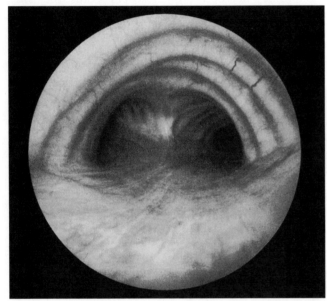

FIGURE 17-2 Normal main carina showing left (L) and right (R) mainstem bronchi.

biopsies on infants and children who are intubated. One must keep in mind that even with such depth of visualization, bronchoscopy still allows examination of only a small percentage of all airways. For comparison, colonoscopy allows the entire length of the colon to be examined during the procedure.

SIMPLY STATED

The standard adult bronchoscope is an instrument about 60 cm long and 5 mm thick, with hand controls for directing the tip. There are two ports near the hand controls: one for suctioning and the other for inserting biopsy tools and flushing fluids into distal airways.

The amount of tip angulation, which makes the scope directional, is crucial to the scope's utility and ability to visualize hard-to-reach but important airways. Most bronchoscope tips can bend from the axial plane at least 130 degrees in one direction and 160 degrees in the other. Bronchoscopes flex less with a brush, forceps, or needle in

place, and all bronchoscopes lose flexibility at the tip over time and with use.

A light source is the foundation for fiberoptic bronchoscopy. Light sources range in size from 2-inch battery cases that attach to the head of the bronchoscope to large units that deliver light at varied intensities, in different wavelengths, and in pulses for photography or other specialized jobs.

Biopsy devices can be passed down the scope and greatly extend the scope's use. The devices include biting and grasping forceps, brushes (shielded and unshielded), sheathed needles, and sampling catheters. The biting forceps come in various types (biting cusps with smooth edges or serrated edges). Smooth-cusped flexible forceps can be used if the physician needs to obtain a piece of lung parenchyma during the procedure. If a large, dense (tough) lesion is seen in the larger airways, a serrated forceps capable of cutting tissue is preferred. Forceps are metallic, are easily visualized by radiographs, and can be directed to the desired area for biopsy of peripheral lung lesions using real-time radiography (**fluoroscopy**).

A hollow needle fixed to a long, small-lumen plastic tube can be passed down the scope to perform biopsy on lesions under the mucosa. Specimens usually contain a few cells, rather than a larger piece of actual tissue sample with preserved lung architecture that is obtained during forceps biopsy. Positive yields (obtaining diagnostic tissue samples) from submucosal lesions are less than those for large cancers growing in the larger airways.

Unshielded brushes are used to harvest cells from tumor masses, located both centrally and in the periphery. The double-shielded sterile brush is used to gather microbiologically important material to diagnose infections in the lung. Because the bronchoscope is passed into the lung by way of the nose or mouth, the entire scope immediately becomes contaminated with the patient's upper-tract bacterial mix (normal flora). Thus, unshielded sampling may misrepresent the specific bacteria present in the lower lung and causing the lung infection. Sterile double-shielded brushes are passed through the entire length of the scope until the bronchoscopist sees that the tip is well in view into the airway of concern. The inner sheath is then advanced, followed by the wire brush that comes out of the sterile inner sheath. The sampling is done by gently brushing the airway. The wire is then drawn back into its sheath and pulled from the bronchoscope. The wire tip is cut off with sterile scissors, placed in a sterile container with sterile normal saline, and sent for microbiologic studies.

During the **bronchoalveolar lavage (BAL)**, the bronchoscope is passed to the affected part of the lung, and the tip of the scope is positioned into a fourth-generation bronchus. A total of about 100 mL of normal saline is flushed through the scope's suction channel in four or five increments of 20 to 30 mL to distend the distal bronchioles and fill the alveoli, thereby washing out samples of any microorganisms. A little more than half of the BAL fluid is usually suctioned back into a collection chamber, and the balance is absorbed by the lymphatic system. The lavage is typically done for diagnostic purposes: to look for infection (smears and cultures) or certain types of interstitial diseases (cell count and differential). In rare situations, such as patients with pulmonary alveolar proteinosis and highly selected patients with severe asthma, the lavage can be done for therapeutic purposes. The fluid is collected very carefully to avoid contamination from oral or upper airway secretions. In normal patients, the fluid is sterile and contains predominantly macrophages.

> ### SIMPLY STATED
>
> Because the mouth harbors bacteria, shielded brushes must be used to get uncontaminated material from the area of the lung where pneumonias are located to accurately determine which organism is causing the pneumonia. When the offending organism is determined, the appropriate antibiotic can be selected.

Patients accidentally inhale a remarkable variety of objects, including corn, peas, beans, peanuts, garlic cloves, teeth, dental crowns, dental fillings, dental drill bits, pills, coins and, beads. These objects, as well as mucous plugs or clots, can be retrieved with a bronchoscope. In some cases, these items or conditions do not show up on the chest radiograph, and their discovery by bronchoscopy is based on the patient's history or is an unexpected discovery during an evaluation for chronic cough. Grasping forceps and snares can be used with the bronchoscope to retrieve foreign objects (Figs. 17-3 and 17-4). Grasping forceps are available with rubber tips for needle and nail removal; basket types for removal of marbles, seeds, and nuts; "pelican" types for removal of food particles; and W-shaped forceps for the removal of coins.

Lasers can be used to obliterate tumors obstructing large airways. Flexible quartz monofilaments pass through the bronchoscope and conduct a laser beam beyond the end of the scope. The bronchoscopist can direct the red "aiming dot" with precision, step on the foot pedal to activate the laser beam, and send a pulsed beam of tissue-vaporizing laser energy into the tumor. Safety is a major issue because lasers are more likely to ignite airway fires if the oxygen concentration is above 30%. Other specialty catheters available for use through a bronchoscope include suture cutters, magnetic extractors, and injector catheters to direct medications into an area of the lung. Coagulation electrodes and hot biopsy forceps are also available.

Interventional Bronchoscopy

The past two decades of the 20th century saw a great expansion in the types of secondary procedures performed during bronchoscopy, leading to the development of a new

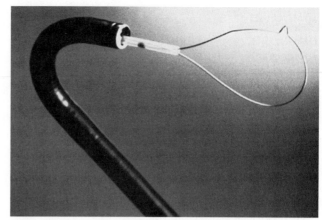

FIGURE 17-3 Electrosurgical snare. (Courtesy Olympus America Inc., Melville, NY.)

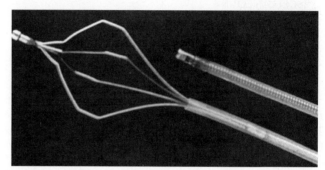

FIGURE 17-4 Retrieval snare. (Courtesy Olympus America Inc., Melville, NY.)

discipline interventional bronchoscopy, within the field of bronchoscopy. In a combined European Respiratory Society and American Thoracic Society (ERS/ATS) statement, **interventional bronchoscopy** was defined as "the art and science of medicine as related to the performance of diagnostic and invasive therapeutic procedures that require additional training and expertize beyond that required in a standard pulmonary medicine training programme." The field of interventional bronchoscopy includes procedures such as autofluorescent bronchoscopy, endobronchial ultrasound (EBUS), laser bronchoscopy, endobronchial electrosurgery, **electromagnetic navigation bronchoscopy (ENB),** argon-plasma coagulation, bronchial thermoplasty, endobronchial cryotherapy, airway stent placement, endobronchial brachytherapy, photodynamic therapy, percutaneous tracheostomy placement, and endobronchial valve placement, and it is constantly expanding. A detailed description of these procedures is outside the scope of this chapter. A review of the aforementioned ERS/ATS statement is highly recommended for a better understanding of these procedures.

> ### SIMPLY STATED
>
> The field of interventional bronchoscopy is rapidly expanding and permits many secondary therapeutic procedures to be performed during bronchoscopy.

DIAGNOSTIC
- Radiographic finding suggestive of neoplasia
- Pneumonia
- Hemoptysis
- Persistent atelectasis
- Unexplained and persistent pleural effusion
- Unexplained and persistent paralysis of a hemidiaphragm
- Interstitial lung disease
- Unexplained hoarseness

THERAPEUTIC
- Atelectasis (to remove mucous plugs and secretions)
- Removal of foreign bodies
- Tamponade of a bleeding source
- Advanced procedures (see section on interventional bronchoscopy)

MISCELLANEOUS
- Difficult intubations
- Research

Indications for Bronchoscopy

There are two basic categories of indications for flexible fiberoptic bronchoscopy: diagnostic and therapeutic (Box 17-1). The flexible fiberoptic bronchoscope is used most often for diagnostic purposes, with therapeutic indications being less common. The most common indication for flexible bronchoscopy is to diagnose the cause of an abnormality seen on a chest radiograph. These abnormalities include infiltrates of any size or location, atelectasis, or mass lesions. These lesions are of particular concern if recently they have appeared on the chest radiograph, or if the patient has risk factors for malignancy, such as history of previous cancer diagnosis or history of smoking. Bronchoscopy may be indicated in the patient with a normal chest radiograph if the patient has symptoms of chronic cough, stridor, hoarseness, or history of choking.

Nodules and Masses

Radiologists and pulmonologists often distinguish between pulmonary nodules and masses. An abnormal solid structure in the pulmonary parenchyma that is smaller than 3 cm on a chest radiograph or computed tomography (CT) scan is typically called a *nodule*. Structures larger than 3 cm are referred to as *masses*. Rounded small lesions are often called *coin lesions* because their shadows resemble coins. The malignant potential of these lesions depends on their size, location, shape, rate of growth, and the patient's history (smoking, weight loss, hemoptysis, history of cancer, or other risk factors for malignancy). Although most nodules and some masses turn out to be benign, a biopsy is often necessary for accurate diagnosis. The possibility of obtaining adequate tissue for diagnosis depends on the lesion size, its location (endobronchial or not, central vs. peripheral), and the expertise of the bronchoscopist.

Naturally, large lesions that are in the central airways are easy to find and excise for biopsy. However, coin lesions are often in the lung periphery and cannot be seen through a flexible bronchoscope. Fluoroscopy is used to aim the tip of the bronchoscope toward the lesion (see Chapter 10 on chest imaging for the utility and limitations of the fluoroscopy). Biopsy forceps can then be advanced into the appropriate subsegmental bronchus to reach the lesion and snip off pieces to be sent for analysis. New advanced bronchoscopy techniques such as ENB and EBUS increase the likelihood of obtaining adequate tissue sample. During ENB, the patient's lungs and the lesion are mapped out using conventional CT scan, and then the software guides the bronchoscope toward the lesion even when the lesion cannot be directly visualized. During EBUS, the ultrasound probe that is mounted on a special bronchoscope guides the biopsy needle into the submucosal lymph nodes that cannot otherwise be seen.

> **SIMPLY STATED**
>
> The larger the lung tumor and the closer to the hilar area it is growing inside a large airway, the easier it is to make a tissue (adenocarcinoma or squamous cell, small cell, or large cell cancer) diagnosis. If the cancer is outside an airway and in the periphery of the lung, it is less likely that flexible bronchoscopy will be able to get adequate tissue to make a diagnosis.

Hemoptysis

Hemoptysis is commonly caused by infection of the lower respiratory tract, and milder cases frequently can be treated with antibiotics. Lung tumors can also cause moderate to severe hemoptysis. As a result, bronchoscopy is usually indicated for the evaluation of more severe cases of hemoptysis, particularly in patients with risk factors for lung cancer.

Usually, the patient with hemoptysis coughs up small amounts of blood and then stops. Occasionally, massive hemoptysis (>200 mL/24 hours) occurs, making intervention more urgent. Large-bore rigid bronchoscopes (Figs. 17-5 and 17-6) are often used in this setting because they allow more rapid removal of blood than do flexible fiberoptic bronchoscopes, but they generally require an operating room, which takes more preparation time than a flexible fiberoptic bronchoscopy performed at the bedside. Fiberoptic bronchoscopy provides a more detailed and distal examination of the airways, making it a good alternative in most instances of hemoptysis. Sometimes, flexible bronchoscopy is performed at bedside urgently to localize the site of bleeding, without attempts to stop it. Once the site has been identified, the patient is then taken to a special suite in radiology, where a corresponding bronchial vessel is cannulated and then special material injected into it, leading to obstruction of the blood flow through the vessel (a procedure called *bronchial artery embolization*) in hope of stopping the bleeding.

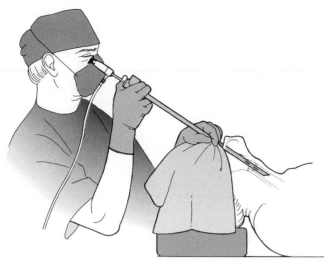

FIGURE 17-5 Placement of a rigid bronchoscope in the trachea of an anesthetized patient. (From Stradling P: *Diagnostic bronchoscopy,* ed 6, New York, 1991, Churchill Livingstone.)

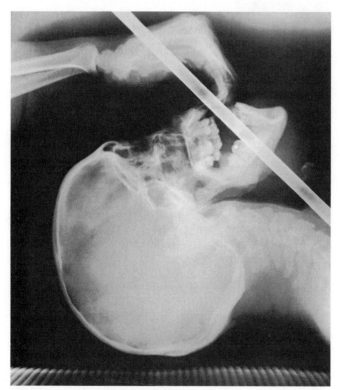

FIGURE 17-6 Lateral neck radiograph of a rigid bronchoscope in place. (From Stradling P: *Diagnostic bronchoscopy,* ed 6, New York, 1991, Churchill Livingstone.)

Pneumonia

Most patients with pneumonia do not require bronchoscopy. The diagnosis is usually made based on clinical information (history and physical examination), routine laboratory tests, and chest imaging. The treatment is often started empirically, without the knowledge of sputum or blood culture results. A more accurate microbiologic

diagnosis—microorganism species and antibiotic sensitivity—may be necessary in certain situations, such as in a patient with persistent pneumonia, on mechanical ventilation, or with severe immunosuppression (human immunodeficiency virus infection or acquired immunodeficiency syndrome, chronic steroid use, organ transplantation, or cancer therapy). In such patients, BAL fluid and sometimes biopsy samples are obtained and sent to the laboratory for smears and cultures. If biopsy samples are obtained for culture purposes, the specimens must be placed in sterile saline solution, rather than formalin, to avoid suppression of bacterial growth by formalin.

For patients on ventilators who are receiving antibiotics, diagnosis of the organisms responsible for persistent and severe pneumonias is a serious issue. In these cases, the double-sheathed sterile brush is used to distinguish the pathogenic organism from organisms that have merely colonized the lower respiratory tract. It is assumed that some bacteria will grow from a respiratory sample of nearly every intubated patient, so the cultures are often done in a quantitative fashion, and a certain threshold of bacterial load must be reached for the cultures to be considered positive. This approach is the best available, but even with careful attention to technique, the results of sterile brushing directly into an infiltrate may not establish the identity of the offending pathogen. Biopsies are typically not performed while the patient is on a ventilator because positive-pressure ventilation increases the risk for pneumothorax.

Interstitial Lung Diseases

Interstitial lung disease is a loosely defined term that encompasses about 200 clinical syndromes and diagnoses. Many of these diseases affect not only the lung interstitium but also the parenchyma, the airways, and the pleural space, leading to a certain degree of confusion. In addition, many other diseases that do not affect the interstitial space give a pattern of infiltrates on a chest radiograph that is often described as "interstitial infiltrates," leading to further confusion. Flexible bronchoscopy has a limited role in evaluation of patients with interstitial lung disease, or the interstitial pattern of infiltrates. With the exception of sarcoidosis, some cancers, and most infections, fiberoptic bronchoscopy provides insufficient material to make a definitive diagnosis of interstitial lung disease. The lavage analysis for cell count and differential is often nonspecific (Table 17-1). **Transbronchial biopsy (TBB)** gives a poor diagnostic specimen because of small sample size (absence of the detailed lung architecture needed for a definitive diagnosis), sampling error (excising an area with minimal involvement), and crushing artifact (distortion of the lung architecture from the shearing forces of the biopsy forceps). This usually creates a dilemma for the patient care team regarding whether to perform a bronchoscopy first (easy, safe, outpatient procedure, but less likely to lead to a definitive

TABLE 17-1

Interstitial Lung Diseases and Fiberoptic Bronchoscopy

Disease	Technique	Findings
Sarcoidosis	TBB	Noncaseating granulomas
	BAL	Altered T-lymphocyte helper-to-suppressor ratio
Pulmonary alveolar proteinosis	TBB	PAS stain and alveolar exudates
Lymphangitic spread of cancer	TBB	Tumor cells in interstitial areas
Alveolar cell cancer	TBB	Tumor cells in alveolar space
Idiopathic interstitial fibrosis	BAL	Increased PMNs
Collagen vascular diseases	BAL	Increased PMNs
Pneumoconiosis	BAL	Increased PMNs
Bronchiolitis obliterans	BAL	Increased PMNs
Amiodarone toxicity	BAL	Lipid-laden macrophages
Goodpasture syndrome	BAL	Hemosiderin-laden macrophages
Eosinophilic pneumonia	BAL	High eosinophil concentration
Hypersensitivity pneumonitis	BAL	Altered T-lymphocyte helper-to-suppressor ratio

BAL, bronchoalveolar lavage; PAS, periodic acid–Schiff; PMN, polymorphonuclear cells (neutrophils); TBB, transbronchial biopsy.

diagnosis) or an open lung biopsy, which requires general anesthesia, opening the chest in an operating room, and allowing postoperative time in the hospital. Ultimately, the decision is based on the likelihood that the patient has sarcoidosis, cancer, or infection—diseases that can be reliably diagnosed by the specimens obtained during bronchoscopy.

SIMPLY STATED

Interstitial lung diseases may necessitate several methods (transbronchial biopsy, bronchoalveolar lavage) to obtain diagnostic material through a flexible bronchoscope, or an open lung biopsy.

Foreign Bodies

As described earlier, various objects have been reported to have been aspirated and then retrieved from the airways. The bronchoscopy (rigid vs. flexible) method for retrieval often depends on the size of the object and the expertise of the bronchoscopist. If a large foreign body has been inhaled into the airway, a large-bore rigid bronchoscope inserted during general anesthesia is most useful to remove the object. Sometimes, the aspirated object is small and passes beyond the reach of a rigid scope. In these cases, the flexible fiberoptic bronchoscope is used. Regardless of the type of scope used, control of the airway is of the greatest concern. If the object is dislodged, it can move to a new location where obstruction of the airway can endanger the patient.

Of special concern is the ability to apply suction while removing foreign bodies. Prolonged suctioning while performing bronchoscopy may significantly reduce the inspired air, thereby creating a risk for intraoperative atelectasis and hypoxemia. Careful attention to suctioning technique and grasping of the foreign body to avoid

Box 17-2	**Complications of Flexible Bronchoscopy**

1. Adverse effects of associated medications (i.e., Lidocaine)
2. Hypoxemia
3. Hypercarbia
4. Bronchospasm
5. Hypotension
6. Laryngospasm, bradycardia, or other vagal responses
7. Mechanical complications such as epistaxis, pneumothorax, and hemoptysis
8. Increased airway resistance
9. Death
11. Cross-contaimination of specimens or bronchoscopes
12. Nausea, vomiting, fever, and chills
13. Cardiac dysrhythmias

(Adapted from AARC Clinical Practice Guidelines, Bronchoscopy Assisting - 2007 Revision and Update, Respiratory Care, Jan. 52:1, 2007)

damaging the airway requires proficiency by the medical staff.

Complications

Few complications are associated with fiberoptic bronchoscopy (Box 17-2). When they do occur, they are most often associated with medications used in the procedure, not the procedure itself. The overall mortality rate from flexible bronchoscopy is less than 0.01%. A careful preprocedure history and physical will identify high-risk patients, and questions about previous bleeding problems to screen for clotting abnormalities will alert the bronchoscopist that biopsy may be risky.

Respiratory failure is more common in patients with advanced lung disease. There are typically multiple factors that lead to the development of respiratory failure in a given patient undergoing bronchoscopy. These factors are asterisked in Box 17-2.

Bleeding and pneumothorax are potential serious complications associated with transbronchial biopsies. The risk for both problems can be reduced with careful attention to technique. In some studies, bronchial brushings were reported to cause rates of bleeding similar to those from TBB. Bilateral TBB is usually avoided because bilateral post-procedure pneumothorax could be life threatening.

After bronchoscopy, patients may develop a transient low-grade fever. It occurs in about 5% of bronchoscopy patients, usually starting 6 to 8 hours after the procedure but lasting only 12 to 24 hours. The exact cause of the fever is unknown, but it is not believed to be a sign of a new infection.

The longer the procedure duration, the greater is the risk for hypoxemia and hypercapnia. When these conditions occur, side effects of the anesthetic agents and arrhythmias become more likely.

SIMPLY STATED

Flexible fiberoptic bronchoscopy is safe. Careful patient selection and attention to detail during and after the bronchoscopy make the risk-to-benefit ratio excellent for this procedure.

Outpatient Bronchoscopy

With the increasing demand for more cost-effective ways to render care, the outpatient clinic has been shown to be a safe and inexpensive site for routine flexible bronchoscopy.

The outpatient bronchoscopy room should be equipped with adequate suction capability; electrocardiographic, arterial oxygen saturation (SpO_2), and blood pressure monitoring; an oxygen source; a bag-valve-mask system; and a crash cart with defibrillator and appropriate drugs, in the event that cardiopulmonary resuscitation is needed. Specifically, naloxone and flumazenil (direct antagonists to opiates and benzodiazepines, respectively) should be immediately available.

A complete history and physical examination are performed to assess the patient and the appropriateness of the bronchoscopy. Box 17-3 lists contraindications to performing the bronchoscopy in the outpatient setting.

SIMPLY STATED

There are specific contraindications to performing flexible bronchoscopy in the outpatient setting as opposed to the hospital. Because there is less support in an outpatient clinic if complications occur, these guidelines must be applied carefully to patient selection to ensure patient safety.

Box 17-3	Contraindications for Outpatient Flexible Bronchoscopy

- Recent myocardial infarction
- Lack of patient cooperation
- Unstable severe asthma
- Severe hypoxemia and/or severe hypercapnia
- Bleeding disorders
- Potentially lethal cardiac arrhythmias
- Lung abscess
- Renal failure
- Immunosuppression
- Obstruction of the superior vena cava

Preparation

As previously described, bronchoscopies are typically performed by an experienced team consisting of the bronchoscopist (physician) and two assistants, often an RT and a RN; one monitors the patient's clinical status and records vital signs every 5 minutes, and the other prepares the equipment and directly assists the bronchoscopist in performing the procedure. It is extremely important that the roles of each team member are clearly defined in advance and that all members of the team communicate clearly with one another before, during, and after the procedure.

Given that bronchoscopy is an invasive procedure with hazards and side effects, safety protocols must be in place for such procedures. Infection control protocols require that the bronchoscopist and the assistants wear gowns, masks, goggles, and gloves. Additional protective equipment, such as lead aprons, may be necessary if fluoroscopy, which involves ionizing radiation, is performed. Another protocol that is typically in place is to take a preprocedure "time-out" to confirm that the correct procedure is being performed on the right patient.

Appropriate preparation of the patient for bronchoscopy is crucial to the success of the procedure. The preparation should start the night before so that when the patient arrives for the procedure, he or she has been fasting for a minimum of 6 hours.

Before the procedure can be performed, an informed consent must be obtained from the patient (or a surrogate, such as close relative, if the patient is heavily sedated or comatose). The patient must understand the reason for the bronchoscopy (diagnostic or therapeutic) and other alternatives available to obtain similar results. The patient also must understand the potential risks and complications of both the procedure and the anesthesia to be used. He or she must also be aware of what to expect after the procedure.

The patient is encouraged to ask questions about the bronchoscopy before signing the consent form. The bronchoscopist should already have explained the procedure in detail and should be available to answer any new questions. Risks and benefits are again discussed. Issues, such as the patient's inability to speak during the procedure, supplemental oxygen, and local anesthetic medicines, are covered. The concept of intravenous (IV) moderate sedation is explained to the patient, and possible medication allergies are reviewed again. The effects and side effects of the anesthetic drugs must be explained. Because of the use of moderate sedation, the patient must also be told to have an adult accompany him or her to and from the procedure because the sedative effects of the medications may linger long after the procedure. The patient is then informed of the process necessary for adequate preparation. It is explained to the patient that during the procedure the assistant will monitor and record the patient's vital signs, including blood pressure, heart rate, respiratory rate, temperature, and initial room air oxygen saturation measured by pulse oximetry (SpO_2). Cardiac status and SpO_2 are monitored continuously while supplemental oxygenation through nasal cannula is supplied at a rate adequate to keep the patient in a safe range of oxygenation during all phases of the bronchoscopy.

After all issues are covered to the patient's satisfaction, the consent is signed and witnessed. It is important to steer clear of medical terminology and use simple language to avoid patient confusion.

It is also important that the assistant carefully review the chart to ensure that there is appropriate documentation for the procedure and that no contraindications exist (see Chapter 21). This involves ensuring that the informed consent has been properly signed, the time-out procedure has been completed, there is a valid physician's order, and there are no absolute contraindications.

> **SIMPLY STATED**
>
> Patient preparation should include answering all the patient's questions. The RT usually has this responsibility and must understand all aspects of the procedure.

For the bronchoscopy to be successful, the patient will need moderate sedation with IV agents, as well as local anesthesia. There are numerous ways to achieve local anesthesia, and the chosen method for a given procedure usually depends on the clinician's experience and the patient's characteristics (e.g., anatomy, personal choices). The patient is usually positioned upright, and 10 to 20 mg of lidocaine is delivered topically to the nasopharynx and oropharynx. The delivery methods include instillation of liquid or viscous lidocaine, inhalation through nebulizer or atomizer, or combination thereof. It is common to ask the patient whether he or she feels the throat getting numb throughout this process to gauge the results. Some bronchoscopists choose to administer recurrent laryngeal nerve block, which involves injection of 1 to 2 mg of lidocaine in the area of the recurrent laryngeal nerve bilaterally. This often leads to numbing up the entire throat, much like the injection of lidocaine in the back of the jaw leads to numbing of the entire jaw during a dental procedure. Once it is

believed that the patient is adequately anesthetized, some bronchoscopists administer a "road test." During such a test, two long cotton swabs are dipped in viscous lidocaine and then carefully placed inside the patient's nostril. The collective diameter of the two swabs is about that of a standard bronchoscope, and if the swabs can be fully passed down the nostril, so can the bronchoscope. If the patient experiences discomfort during the swab insertion, it is likely due to inadequate anesthesia, and more lidocaine is given. Otherwise, the swabs are left in for another minute or so. Similarly, a curved clamp is wrapped in gauze or cotton and then dipped in liquid lidocaine. Then, the clamp is placed behind the tongue. Gagging, choking, or discomfort is again indicative of incomplete anesthesia, and more lidocaine is given. If the patient tolerates both swabs and clamp insertion without discomfort, IV sedation can be given, and the procedure can be started.

It is assumed that even patients with normal gas exchange before the procedure will require supplemental oxygen. The need for the oxygen comes from decreased alveolar ventilation due to anesthesia, loss of tidal volume due to suctioning, airway obstruction from the bronchoscope, additional airway edema from the mechanical trauma, local pulmonary edema after instillation of saline for the lavage, or combination thereof. Almost all patients should receive supplemental oxygen during bronchoscopy. This is usually achieved by giving oxygen by nasal cannula at 2 to 6 L/minute. Some patients will require higher flow that cannot be delivered by nasal cannula. In such situations, a small hole is cut out of the mask that is used for oxygen delivery to allow passage of the bronchoscope. Yet other patients will have such a degree of gas exchange abnormalities that the procedure may need to be performed in the ICU, or even after the intubation, to ensure the availability of proper support staff in case of patient deterioration. The decision about the need for supplemental oxygen, or the need for mechanical ventilation before bronchoscopy, is often made by the bronchoscopist and the assistant in collaboration.

Suctioning through the bronchoscope is critical to keep the airway clear of mucus and blood and to help keep the bronchoscope lens clear. The suction is connected to a sterile 80-mL specimen trap, which must be secured so that it will not tip and thereby lose the washing from the patient's airway. Several of these traps are needed. Because the first one is usually contaminated with mouth flora, it is usually discarded, along with its contents. If heavy bleeding occurs during biopsy, the trap may become clogged with blood and thus inappropriate for cytologic analysis or cultures and may need to be discarded. A separate suction channel is set up for oropharyngeal suctioning to avoid cross-contamination with lower airway specimens.

The final stage of preparation is to administer IV moderate sedation. Moderate sedation is a state of consciousness that may be described as a "twilight sleep," whereby the patient may be aroused if necessary through stimulation or by administering a chemical agent to reverse the effects of sedation. Commonly, a combination of a sedative benzodiazepine like midazolam (Versed) and opioid narcotic like fentanyl is used. Although midazolam relaxes the patient and eases him or her to sleep, fentanyl provides pain control as well as cough suppression. These drugs are chosen for their quick on-and-off action. Benzodiazepines are a good amnestic agent as well, so even when the patient is uncomfortable during the procedure, he or she often does not remember it afterward. Some bronchoscopists also give codeine to further suppress the cough and atropine to decrease the secretions about 30 minutes before the procedure. As soon as the patient relaxes and appears to be asleep and all preparation is done, the bronchoscopy can begin.

Procedure

For spontaneously breathing patients, the bronchoscope is passed through the nares. This allows for more stable scope position and less likelihood of patient biting and damaging the optical fibers. In some patients, the nasopharynx is too small for the bronchoscope, or previous trauma or surgery does not allow the scope to be passed. In this case, an oral airway or "bite block" is inserted into the mouth and the bronchoscope advanced through it.

Once the bronchoscope passes through the pharynx (nasopharynx, oropharynx, or artificial airway, as the case may be), the epiglottis and then the vocal cords come into view. A small amount of lidocaine is injected to numb the cords and allow easy passage of the bronchoscope through them. Sometimes, especially in patients with suspected cancer, the bronchoscopist will ask the patient to say "eeeee" to see the vocal cords adduct. Patients with cancer infiltrating the recurrent laryngeal nerve may be unable to fully adduct (close) their vocal cords.

Once the cords have been anesthetized, the patient is asked to take deep breaths. This will allow a full abduction (opening) of the vocal cords and passage of the bronchoscopy through them. It is common for the cough reflex to close the vocal cords and not allow the advancement of the scope.

Once in the trachea, the scope is advanced firmly to avoid being bounced back by the strong cough. Nearly all spontaneously breathing patients will start coughing at this point, requiring large, sometimes repeated doses of lidocaine or fentanyl.

During the passage of the scope through the pharynx and the vocal cords, it is possible to rotate it 180 degrees, resulting in an upside-down appearance of the trachea. How can one be sure that the airway on the right is leading to the right, not the left, lung (see Fig. 17-2)?

There are a few ways to orient the bronchoscopist. First, and most reliable, the tracheal rings have cartilage in front and muscle in back. So, if the cartilaginous part appears to be on the top of the image, the orientation is proper, and the right lung will be on the right side of the image. Second,

the angle of the right mainstem bronchus is straighter (this is also good to remember when discussing why aspirated objects often settle on the right side and why blindly advanced devices, such as suction catheters and endotracheal (ET) tubes, tend to be in the right mainstem bronchus). However, this angle is not as reliable because tumors may push on the bronchi and distort anatomy. The third, and probably least important sign is the length of the right mainstem bronchus. Shortly after its takeoff from the main carina, the right mainstem bronchus divides into the bronchus intermedius and the right upper lobe bronchus. This makes the right mainstem bronchus very short (a few millimeters), as opposed to the left mainstem bronchus (2 to 3 cm).

Once the mainstem bronchi are identified and examined, the plan of action is devised. If the disease is unilateral, the normal side is examined first, to avoid cross-contamination (e.g., infection, tumor material). In general, the extent and the order of the procedures performed will vary depending on the nature and etiology of the disease being evaluated during bronchoscopy.

> ### SIMPLY STATED
>
> *Moderate sedation* is a term used to denote a state of anesthesia in which the patient is in a "twilight sleep" for approximately 15 to 30 minutes. The medications used to achieve this state are given intravenously and can be reversed in seconds by specific antagonists, also given intravenously.

Samples are usually obtained quickly, so the assistant must have an organized working surface with easily accessible supplies. The exact list of supplies requested for bronchoscopy varies from hospital to hospital and bronchoscopist to bronchoscopist. These supplies are placed in medication cups and are clearly labeled. A labeled syringe is placed with each labeled medication cup to match each medication. Below is the list of commonly used materials:

- 2% topical lidocaine to be used if needed above the vocal cords
- 1% topical lidocaine to be used if needed below the vocal cords
- 0.9% sodium chloride (NaCl) for irrigation (a larger container may be necessary if BAL is needed)
- 1:19 solution of epinephrine (1 mL 1:1000 epinephrine diluted with 19 mL 0.9% NaCl)
- Syringes of various size, with the proper tip to adapt to the working channel of the bronchoscope

It is important that when the syringes with lidocaine are handed to the bronchoscopist during the procedure, they contain a known amount of lidocaine, with plenty of air in the syringe barrel. This allows the bronchoscopist to push the lidocaine all the way down the approximately 2 feet of the scope's channel. Because it is possible to administer an overdose of lidocaine, having a small amount

(1 to 2 mL) in each syringe helps limit the lidocaine given. It is impossible to know how much lidocaine the patient absorbs as a total dosage because suctioning during the procedure removes some of the lidocaine before it is absorbed. Nevertheless, it is important to keep the total dosage of lidocaine below 300 mg. Seizures are the most common sign of acute lidocaine overdose.

Some pathologists prefer cytology specimens fixed on slides. There should be four sets of frosted slides placed back to back and labeled legibly with the patient's name, history number, physician number (if applicable), and date. Two slide bottles with 90% alcohol and one biopsy specimen bottle containing 10% formalin should be available. Other pathologists prefer cytology specimens preserved in Saccomanno solution.

An 80-mL mucus specimen trap is placed in-line between the suction source and the bronchoscope. Standard biopsy forceps, a brush holder loaded with a disposable wire brush, and an aspiration needle accompanied by a 10-mL syringe filled with 5 mL 0.9% NaCl should be available, depending on the specimens the bronchoscopist needs to collect.

To obtain a lung brushing, the bronchoscopist gently brushes the abnormal-appearing area, then withdraws the brush from the scope. The assistant rubs the brush lightly on the frosted side of a slide, making a smear about the size of a dime. This slide is then placed in the slide bottle containing 90% alcohol (or the brush is agitated in the Saccomanno solution). This procedure should take no longer than 10 seconds.

Lung biopsy specimens are placed into a labeled specimen bottle filled with formalin. Usually, four to six samples are obtained. Formalin is an airway irritant, so if any amount of it ends up on the forceps, it is usually removed by rinsing the forceps in saline. It is often necessary for the assistant to tease the small piece of tissue out of the biopsy cusps with a needle. Some bronchoscopists prefer to "evaluate" the quality of biopsy specimens by visually inspecting the specimens in formalin and observing whether they float. Although commonly practiced, the clinical value and accuracy of such evaluation is hard to ascertain.

Obtaining a needle aspiration sample requires the bronchoscopist to place two or three drops of specimen on the frosted side of a slide (or into Saccomanno solution). The assistant then places a second slide, frosted side down, on top of the original slide containing the specimen and slowly slides it across this slide. Both slides should be placed into a slide bottle containing 90% alcohol. This procedure is repeated with each new specimen collected.

BAL is performed with repeated instillations of 20 mL of preservative-free 0.9% NaCl. The instillations are followed by suctioning into an 80-mL mucus specimen trap. It is usually sent for smears and cultures (e.g.,

routine, acid-fast bacilli, fungal) when infection is suspected, cell count and differential when interstitial lung disease is suspected, or cytology when malignancy is suspected. The sample is usually split into different cups (all need to be appropriately labeled) to be sent to the different parts of the laboratory. Contamination should be avoided, especially for the sample sent to the microbiology laboratory.

> ### SIMPLY STATED
>
> After patient safety, collection of samples and their careful management is the most important job of the RT or other clinician assisting with the procedure.

Post-Procedure Considerations

On completion of the bronchoscopy, the patient is monitored closely while recovering. Vital signs, including blood pressure, heart rate, respiratory rate, and SpO_2, are monitored and recorded by the RT or RN every 5 to 15 minutes. The bronchoscopist must be notified of significant changes in any of these parameters. It is essential to recognize signs of increased discomfort, bleeding, or respiratory distress. The IV site should be examined periodically for signs of infiltration or blockage until its discontinuation.

Once the patient is alert and oriented, usually within an hour of the procedure's completion, the patient is given a small sip of water to see whether his or her gag reflex and sensation in the throat have returned to normal. If these parameters are normal, the IV is removed, and a final set of vital signs is obtained. The following criteria should be met before discharge:

- The patient is alert and oriented.
- Gag reflex is present.
- Sensation in the throat has returned to normal.
- Vital signs are stable.
- No significant bleeding is present.

At this time, the bronchoscopist can explain the findings to the patient and patient's family and tell the patient that he or she might cough up small amounts of blood or develop mild fever for up to 24 hours after the procedure. Larger amounts of blood, sudden shortness of breath, pain, or high-grade fever should prompt a call to seek medical attention. Arrangements are made for a return visit in 5 to 7 days to review the findings from the patient's specimens and to make recommendations.

The patient can then be liberated from all monitors and assisted in dressing. A wheelchair should be available to transport the patient out to his or her attendant. It is imperative to remind the patient not to drive for several hours. The patient and attendant are reminded that if any unusual bleeding, shortness of breath, fever, or pain occurs, they are to seek medical attention immediately.

All specimens must be handled appropriately for transport to the laboratory. Biopsies, brushings, needle aspirations, and lung washings should be labeled with the patient's name, history number, physician number, date, and site of origin. Necessary pathology or laboratory slips should also contain similar data, including what tests should be performed.

Finally, any additional charting should be completed, signed by the bronchoscopist, and filed in the patient's chart. The bronchoscopist must also make his or her own notes of the entire procedure, including indications, medications given, specimens collected, tests requested on the specimens, any intraoperative complications, and postoperative impression.

Inpatient Bronchoscopy

It should also be noted that bronchoscopy can be performed on hospitalized patients with an artificial airway such as an ET or a tracheostomy (T) tube. Although much of the steps described earlier apply to both spontaneously breathing outpatients and those in the hospital with artificial airways on mechanical ventilation, there are several modifications to remember. In such patients, the procedure is often done at the bedside because the patient is often too unstable to travel to the endoscopy suite. A special adaptor is placed between the ET tube and the ventilator circuit to allow passage of the bronchoscope without interrupting ventilation, and a bite block is placed in the patient's mouth to prevent biting down on the bronchoscope. A special consideration must be given to the size of the ET tube in relation to the size of the bronchoscope. Most standard bronchoscopes can easily pass through the size 8 ET tube. A smaller bronchoscope will need to be used in a patient with smaller ET tubes. Using an inappropriately large bronchoscope may be dangerous not only for the obvious reason of being wedged inside the tube but also by obstructing a large percentage of the airway lumen and making mechanical ventilation difficult. Once the right-sized bronchoscope is chosen for a given ET tube, it can be advanced through the artificial airway and into the trachea without much difficulty. In addition, many patients (especially those in the ICU) may already be adequately sedated for the purposes of the bronchoscopy.

Role of the Respiratory Therapist

As suggested previously, it is common for the RT to be involved in assisting the physician with many aspects of the preparation, performance, and post-procedure considerations associated with bronchoscopy. These may include reviewing the medical record for proper documentation, preparing the equipment, assisting with the procedure, and monitoring the patient's clinical status before, during, and after the procedure (Fig. 17-7). Table 17-2 summarizes the common functions of the RT before, during, and after the bronchoscopy.

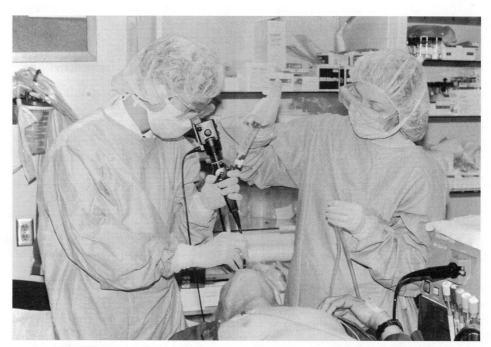

FIGURE 17-7 Typical outpatient set-up for performing flexible bronchoscopy.

TABLE 17-2

Respiratory Therapist's Role When Assisting with Bronchoscopy

Therapist's Function	Purpose
Before the Procedure	
Help identify potential need for a bronchoscopy	Determine which patients may benefit from the procedure
Review chart to confirm: physician order, signed consent form, no contraindications	Confirm physician's order, that the patient has agreed to it, and that it isn't contraindicated, and any special considerations
Prepare/ensure proper function of equipment, including bronchoscope, light source, monitor, video recorder, medications, specimen traps	Minimize unnecessary delay and likelihood of patient harm from procedure
Prepare patient, providing patient education and premedication	Minimize untoward delays and patient's well-being
Ensure "time out" to confirm correct patient and procedure	Minimize patient harm and medical errors
During the Procedure	
Ensure proper functioning of all equipment (bronchoscope, light source, TV monitor) needed during procedure	Minimize unnecessary delay from equipment failure
Assist physician in obtaining specimens; help with medication preparation	Minimize unnecessary delay and likelihood of patient harm from procedure
Monitor patient vital signs and overall clinical status; respond to adverse reactions	Minimize patient harm from adverse reactions
After the Procedure	
Monitor patient's vital signs and clinical status	Ensure the patient has tolerated procedure and detect adverse reactions
Ensure specimens are properly labeled and sent to laboratory	Help obtain accurate diagnosis and treatment
Clean, disinfect/sterilize equipment, then ensure it is properly stored	Minimize nosocomial infection risk and potential damage to equipment
Record results in chart and other pertinent records	Maintain medical and legal record of procedure and patient response

KEY POINTS

▶ Rigid bronchoscopes allow good access to large airways and allow ventilation during the procedure. However, rigid bronchoscopy requires general anesthesia for patient comfort.

▶ In 1969, Shigeto Ikeda of Japan brought the first bronchoscope to the Mayo Clinic, which incorporated fiberoptics into a flexible tube suitable in size and length to enter the trachea and visualize the lower airway.

▶ Today, flexible fiberoptic bronchoscopes allow better access to small airways and are comfortable enough that only light to moderate sedation is needed. The patient can breathe spontaneously during the procedure.

▶ The standard flexible bronchoscope has an external diameter of 5.3 mm and a total length of 605 mm.

▶ The flexible fiberoptic bronchoscope has greatly expanded the practice of pulmonary medicine, allowing inspection of the airways, removal of many different foreign bodies, and biopsy of airway and peripheral lung tissue.

▶ The most common indication for flexible bronchoscopy is to diagnose the cause of an abnormality seen on a chest radiograph. These abnormalities include infiltrates of any size or location, atelectasis, or mass lesions.

▶ The flexible fiberoptic bronchoscope can be used to reach to the periphery of the lung and remove a small piece of lung biopsy for submission to the pathologist. In certain clinical scenarios, this is helpful in the diagnosis of interstitial lung disease.

▶ If a large foreign body has been inhaled into the airway, a large-bore rigid bronchoscope inserted during general anesthesia is most useful to remove the object.

KEY POINTS—cont'd

▶ Sometimes the aspirated object is small and passes beyond the reach of a rigid scope. In these cases, the flexible fiberoptic bronchoscope is used.

▶ Few complications are associated with fiberoptic bronchoscopy. When they do occur, they are most often associated with medications used in the procedure, not the procedure itself.

▶ Bleeding, pneumothorax, and respiratory failure are the potential major complications associated with bronchoscopy, especially when tissue biopsy is performed.

▶ RTs commonly provide technical support for bronchoscopy procedures.

▶ RT activities include setting up the bronchoscopy suite, providing medications for the physician, operating biopsy forceps, collecting specimens and preparing them for presentation to the pathologist, cleaning the bronchoscope and biopsy equipment, and preparing the suite for the next procedure.

ASSESSMENT QUESTIONS

See Appendix for answers.

1. In most patients, the standard adult bronchoscope can visualize:
   a. Third-level bronchi
   b. Fourth-level bronchi
   c. Fifth-level bronchi
   d. Sixth-level bronchi

2. Double-sided brushes are used during bronchoscopy to:
   a. Clean the fiberoptics
   b. Obtain microbiologic samples
   c. Assist in cleaning the smaller airways of mucous plugs
   d. Assist in diagnosing malignancies
3. The purpose of using lasers during bronchoscopy is to:
   a. Obliterate obstructing tumors
   b. Stop excessive bleeding
   c. Open mucous-plugged airways
   d. Improve visualization of smaller airways
4. The most common indication for the use of a bronchoscope is:
   a. To retrieve inhaled foreign objects
   b. To obtain microbiologic samples
   c. To help diagnose abnormalities seen on chest radiograph
   d. To treat hemoptysis
5. The rigid bronchoscope most likely is used for:
   a. Pneumonia
   b. Massive hemoptysis
   c. Tumors
   d. Interstitial lung disease
6. The most common complication associated with bronchoscopy is:
   a. Side effects of the medications used in the procedure
   b. Pneumothorax
   c. Secondary infection
   d. Excessive bleeding
7. A patient who develops hypoxemia during a bronchoscopy procedure is less likely to demonstrate arrhythmias due to:
   a. Use of sedative medications
   b. Use of lidocaine before the procedure
   c. Lack of heart problems in most patients undergoing bronchoscopy
   d. Hypoxia being rare cause of arrhythmias

8. In addition to lidocaine and normal saline, the most commonly used medication to be delivered into the airways during bronchoscopy is:
   a. Acetylcysteine (Mucomyst)
   b. Epinephrine
   c. Sterile water
   d. Midazolam (Versed)
9. The most common sign of lidocaine overdose during bronchoscopy is:
   a. Tachycardia
   b. Bradycardia
   c. Seizures
   d. Apnea
10. This clinical observation may be present in a post-bronchoscopy patient before discharge:
    a. Poor gag reflex
    b. Sputum with small flecks of blood
    c. Respiratory distress
    d. Confusion and disorientation

Bibliography

American Thoracic Society. *Patient Information Series. Fiberoptic bronchoscopy.* Available at http://patients.thoracic.org/information-series/en/resources/fiberoptic-bronchoscopy.pdf.

Flexible bronchoscopy update. In: Mehta Atul, guest, editors. *Clin Chest Med.* 2001;**22**:2.

Bolliger CT, Mathur PN, Beamis JF, et al. ERS/ATS statement on interventional pulmonology. *Eur Respir J* 2002;**19**:356.

Kacmarek RM, Stoller JK, Heuer AJ. *Egan's fundamentals of respiratory care.* 10th ed. St. Louis: Mosby-Elsevier; 2013.

Silus MHU, Bolliger CT. *Educational Resources for Bronchoscopy.* Retrieved March 12, 2012, from http://www.thoracic.org/clinical/best-of-the-web/pages/patient-education/educational-resources-for-bronchoscopy.php.

Sokolowski JW, Burgher LW, Jones FL, et al. Guidelines for fiberoptic bronchoscopy in adults. *Am J Respir Crit Care Med* 1987;**136**:1066.

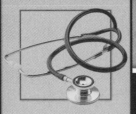

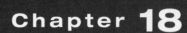

Chapter 18

Nutrition Assessment

JANE E. ZIEGLER*

LEARNING OBJECTIVES

After reading this chapter, you will be able to:
1. Recognize how nutrition and respiration and pulmonary status are interrelated.
2. Recognize the functional importance of oxygen in nutrition.
3. Identify the nutritional significance of measuring oxygen uptake.
4. Identify the value of determining the resting energy expenditure.
5. Recognize how starvation affects the following:
    a. Body weight
    b. Muscle mass (diaphragm and other respiratory musculature)
    c. Forced vital capacity, forced expiratory volume in 1 second, and diffusing capacity of the lung for carbon dioxide
    d. Surfactant production
6. Recognize how some respiratory treatment modalities may inhibit the nutritional status of patients.
7. Identify the by-products of anaerobic (without oxygen) metabolism.
8. Identify oxygen's importance in terms of adenosine triphosphate production.
9. Recognize how fat, carbohydrate, and protein metabolism affect the respiratory quotient.
10. Recognize the daily nutritional requirements for carbohydrate, protein, and fat.
11. Identify the protein requirements for normal and severely catabolic patients.
12. Recognize the significance of measuring nitrogen balance.
13. Recognize the problems associated with a low-protein diet.

*James A. Peters and Cheryl D. Thomas-Peters contributed some of the content of this chapter as contributors to the prior edition of this text.

LEARNING OBJECTIVES—cont'd

14. Recognize the advantages and disadvantages of a high-carbohydrate diet in regard to the pulmonary system.
15. Identify the importance of vitamins and minerals in respiratory function.
16. Recognize the methods available for meeting nutritional requirements and their advantages and disadvantages.
17. Recognize the methods for assessing nutritional status.
18. Identify the role of the respiratory therapist in nutritional assessment in relation to inspection, auscultation, and laboratory and pulmonary function findings.

KEY TERMS

adenosine triphosphate (ATP)	direct calorimetry	oxygen uptake
anabolism	gluconeogenesis	parenteral
anemia	glycolysis	parenteral nutrition (PN)
basal energy expenditure (BEE)	ideal body weight	phytochemicals
basal metabolic rate (BMR)	indirect calorimetry	protein-energy malnutrition
body mass index (BMI)	kilocalories	(PEM)
cachectic	lactic acid	respiratory quotient (RQ)
catabolism	metabolic cart	resting energy expenditure
creatine phosphate	metabolism	(REE)
creatinine	nitric oxide	serum albumin
creatinine-height index (CHI)	nitrogen balance	serum transferrin
diet-induced thermogenesis	oncotic pressure	skinfold measurement

The pulmonary system has a synergistic relationship with nutrition throughout life, beginning with the fetus and extending through adulthood. Although nutritional status and pulmonary function are interdependent, a healthy pulmonary system supports the body through its ability to obtain oxygen needed for cellular demands of the metabolism of the three macronutrients: carbohydrates, proteins, and lipids. Provision of adequate nutrition to maintain optimal nutritional status assists in ensuring growth and development of the pulmonary system, including its supporting structures. The skeletal and respiratory muscles, as well as the nervous system and immune system, are supported and maintained through optimal nutrition. A person's nutritional status and ability to metabolize carbohydrates, proteins, and fats is directly related to a healthy pulmonary system.[1]

Pulmonary dysfunction or changes in pulmonary status can occur throughout life, from the premature infant with bronchopulmonary dysplasia, to the child with asthma or the adolescent with an eating disorder, to adulthood and the senior years. Significant pulmonary disorders with nutrition concerns include asthma, cystic fibrosis, bronchopulmonary dysplasia, chronic obstructive pulmonary disease (COPD), and emphysema, as well as acute respiratory distress syndrome. The nutritional needs and nutritional status of patients with pulmonary disease have emerged as major factors influencing acute and long-term patient outcomes. The major function of the pulmonary system is gas exchange, with the lungs providing oxygen for cellular metabolic demands and allowing for removal of carbon dioxide from these metabolic processes. Lungs also assist in the regulation of acid-base balance, synthesize surfactant and arachidonic acid, and convert angiotensin I to angiotensin II.

Breathing provides the oxygen necessary for metabolism of nutrients to meet the energy needs of individuals. Nutrition affects the efficiency of the metabolic processes and influences the amount of oxygen needed and the amount of carbon dioxide exhaled. Nutrition influences the immune defense mechanisms, thereby affecting the patient's susceptibility to infection and ability to deal with physiologic stress. The ability to assess and interpret the role of and need for nutrition in maintaining normal respiratory function and in combating pulmonary disease is important for today's respiratory therapist (RT).

Malnutrition and the Pulmonary System

Malnutrition adversely affects the structure, elasticity, and function of the lungs as well as the mass, strength, and endurance of muscles involved in the respiration process.[2-4] Malnutrition-altered lung function includes decreased strength, power, and endurance of respiratory muscles and increased respiratory muscle fatigue. In addition, skeletal muscle relaxation slows, and muscle mass is diminished due to specific reduction in muscle fiber size and type. During starvation or malnutrition, respiratory muscles and skeletal muscles are subject to **catabolism**, providing energy to the body. The resultant reduction in the mass of the diaphragm, diminished inspiratory and expiratory muscle strength, and decreased vital capacity and endurance result in impaired pulmonary function.[4-9] Inadequate nutrition or an increase in energy needs can result in malnutrition, leading to alterations in pulmonary muscle function.

Within days, protein deficits in the diet result in a decline in respiratory muscle function.[7] Low levels of proteins in the blood (hypoalbuminemia) contribute to pulmonary edema as colloid osmotic pressure is decreased, allowing a fluid shift into the interstitial space. Extravascular lung water increases, resulting in a decrease in functional residual capacity and pulmonary reserve. Low serum albumin levels can result in an increase in extracellular fluid volume and a reduction in the intracellular space.[7,9] Surfactant provides the low surface tension at the air-liquid interface, preventing the atelectasis, alveolar collapse, alveolar flooding, and severe hypoxia that result in respiratory distress. Even short periods of starvation result in a decreased synthesis and secretion of surfactant.[10] Reduced surfactant, which is synthesized from proteins and phospholipids, contributes to the collapse of alveoli, resulting in an increased effort of breathing. Airway mucus is composed of glycoproteins, water, and electrolytes. Malnutrition results in depletion of liver and muscle glycogen and energy-rich compounds used to provide cellular energy, resulting in metabolic and muscular endurance dysfunction. This reduction in respiratory muscle function often coexists with increased energy requirements, resulting in a deterioration of gas exchange and an increased work of breathing, which can lead to pulmonary failure.[7,9]

Micronutrients consistent of vitamins and minerals. Micronutrient imbalances and deficiencies can affect pulmonary function in several ways. Iron deficiency can result in low hemoglobin levels, thus reducing the oxygen-carrying capacity of the blood. Low levels of other micronutrients, such as potassium, phosphorus, calcium, and magnesium, affect cellular processes. Collagen, composing the supporting connective tissue of the lungs, requires vitamin C for synthesis. Low levels of phosphorus result in neuromuscular dysfunction and can exacerbate pulmonary failure. A reduction in 2,3-diphosphoglycerate (2,3-DPG) in the red blood cells due to reduced phosphorus levels decreases oxygen delivery to tissues and decreases the contractibility of respiratory muscles. Muscle strength is reduced in the presence of magnesium deficiency.[7] Deficiencies in vitamin A, pyridoxine, and zinc may impair immune status and increase risk for pulmonary infections.[5,11] Antioxidant nutrients, including vitamins A, C, and E and flavonoids, have been reviewed for their relationship to the pathogenesis or exacerbations in patients with COPD. Reduced serum or tissue levels of antioxidant vitamins were found in people with COPD; however, other studies did not show significant effects.[12] Malnutrition has been found to be an independent predictor of higher morbidity and mortality in respiratory disease.[4]

Effect of Pulmonary Disease on Nutritional Status

Diseases of the pulmonary system can increase energy requirements. In addition, complications and treatment of pulmonary disease affect the ability to ingest and digest adequate food and affect the circulation, cellular use, storage, and excretion of most nutrients. The increased work of breathing, chronic infection, and medical treatments used to treat pulmonary diseases, such as chest physical therapy and some medications, increase energy requirements. Medications such as bronchodilators, steroids, and antibiotics used to treat disease may have other nutritional implications and need to be considered in the nutritional evaluation. Patients with pulmonary disease usually present with a reduced nutritional intake attributed to fluid restrictions, gastrointestinal discomfort, vomiting, anorexia, shortness of breath, and decreased oxygen saturation when eating. A reduced ability to prepare foods because of fatigue and shortness of breath, impaired feeding skills, altered metabolism, and financial limitations all result in additional limitations in achieving adequate nutritional intake. Also, some diseases, such as cystic fibrosis, affect not only the lungs but also the pancreas, resulting in inadequate production of certain enzymes necessary in the digestion of fats. This exposes cystic fibrosis patients to certain types of malnutrition, unless certain dietary supplements are taken to compensate.

Interdependence of Respiration and Nutrition

Respiration and nutrition are interdependent (Fig. 18-1). Air and food share common pathways during ingestion and then separate only briefly during "digestion," with air going to the lungs for distribution and food to the stomach and intestinal tract for digestion and absorption. Oxygen and nutrients then combine in the blood and are distributed to the tissues of the body. The use of food for energy at the cellular level requires oxygen to support a controlled combustion process that produces energy molecules of **adenosine triphosphate (ATP)**, which are used in all of the body processes for energy (Fig. 18-2).

Body heat is a result of a combustion process called **metabolism**. Metabolism requires fuel in the form of food. For combustion to occur, oxygen must be present, provided through the process of breathing. Unless oxygen is delivered to the cells, the food eaten cannot be used. Nutrition and respiration are truly interdependent because breathing and oxygenation are considered part of the process of providing nutrition to the body's tissues.

Titrating the proper amount of oxygen and eliminating carbon dioxide (the metabolic "smoke" of the combustion process) is the job of the respiratory system, coupled closely with the cardiovascular system. The respiratory system must be sensitive to the metabolic needs of the entire body. This process requires the integration of several organ systems. The respiratory system consists of neurologic components, cardiovascular components, respiratory muscles, and lungs (Fig. 18-3).

The metabolic rates of the tissues dictate the amount of oxygen needing to be picked up in the lungs. **Oxygen** uptake ($\dot{V}_{O_2}$) is a respiratory factor that can be measured in the laboratory or at the bedside using specialized equipment. Nutritionally speaking, it is this measure that indicates the patient's energy requirement. If $\dot{V}_{O_2}$ is measured while a person is in a resting, nonstressed state, the **basal metabolic rate (BMR)** or **basal energy expenditure (BEE)**

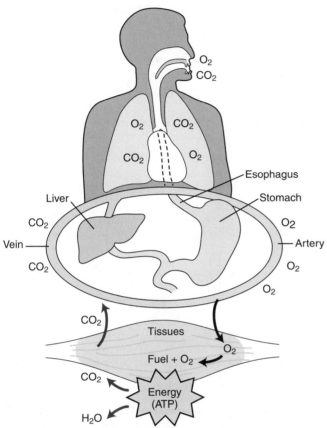

FIGURE 18-1 Nutrition and breathing are interrelated. Air and food share common pathways of entry during ingestion and then separate only briefly during "digestion," with air going to the lungs for distribution and food to the stomach and intestinal tract for digestion and absorption. Oxygen and nutrients then combine in the blood and are distributed to the tissues of the body. The use of food for energy at the cellular level requires oxygen to support a controlled combustion process that produces energy molecules of adenosine triphosphate (ATP), which is used in all of the body processes for energy, carbon dioxide, and water.

can be calculated. The BEE is the measure obtained when a person is at absolute rest with no physical movement, which is not clinically possible in the hospitalized patient. The term **resting energy expenditure (REE)** is used when a person is at rest upon waking. REE is the measurement used in hospitalized patients and is about 10% higher than BEE[13] because measurements are done when the patient is awake and at rest but not at basal conditions. A variety of predictive equations have been developed for use in estimating REE. For the purposes of predicting energy needs through predictive equations in nonobese critically ill patients when indirect calorimetry is not available, four equations were considered precise and unbiased in this population. In patients younger than 60 years and in those older than 60 years, respectively, the equations and their accuracy are as follows: Penn State Equation (69%, 77%), Brandi equation (61%, 61%), Mifflin-St. Jeor equation × 1.25 (54%, 54%), and Faisy equation (65%, 37%). The Penn State equation was validated in 2009 and is calculated as follows[14]:

$$\text{Resting metabolic rate (RMR)} = \text{Mifflin } (0.96) + V_E (31) + T_{max} (167) - 6212$$

Because calculating the REE produces only an estimate, it is preferable to measure the actual metabolic rate by indirect calorimetry in order to know the patient's true energy needs. This eliminates some of the guesswork, especially when treating critically ill or metabolically challenged patients.

Adequate nutrition support depends on the ability to determine a patient's energy needs. There are several ways to determine energy needs, including direct and indirect calorimetry and whole-body potassium measurement. Total daily energy expenditure is usually divided into three components:
1. REE, which includes metabolic rate at rest while the patient is awake
2. **Diet-induced thermogenesis**
3. Energy cost of physical activity[15]

Energy production generates heat, and heat is measured in calories. **Direct calorimetry** directly measures the heat given off by the body in a carefully designed room. This measurement is not practical in clinical settings and cannot be used with compromised patient populations. **Indirect**

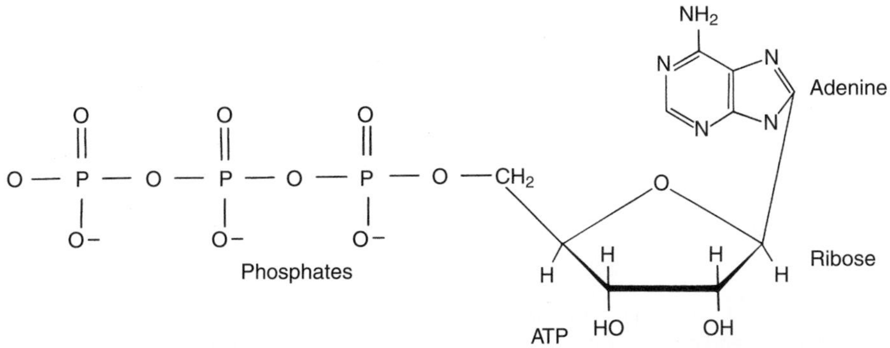

FIGURE 18-2 Functions of adenosine triphosphate (ATP) are as follows: muscle contraction and relaxation, active transport of substances across membranes, substrate for cyclic adenosine monophosphate, energy for synthesis of various chemical compounds, and energy storage.

calorimetry is the method most commonly used in clinical environments. Indirect calorimetry is the calculation of energy expenditure using measured respiratory parameters of oxygen consumption ($\dot{V}o_2$) and carbon dioxide production ($\dot{V}co_2$). $\dot{V}o_2$ and $\dot{V}co_2$ require precise measurements of inspired and expired gas concentrations and volume. $\dot{V}o_2$ and $\dot{V}co_2$ are converted to energy expenditure through the application of the abbreviated Weir equation[13,16,17]:

$$\text{Energy expenditure (kcal)} = [(\dot{V}o_2 \text{ L/min}) (3.941) + (\dot{V}co_2 \text{ L/min})(1.11)]1400 \text{ minutes}$$

where $\dot{V}o_2$ and $\dot{V}co_2$ are expressed in liters per minute, and 1440 is the number of minutes in a day.

Because oxygen is not stored in the body, measuring oxygen uptake ($\dot{V}o_2$) correlates directly with energy (ATP) creation and use. Metabolism (REE) then can be measured by oxygen consumption and is directly related to the energy (calories) used. Indirect calorimetry may be clinically beneficial in the identification of patients who will not be able to sustain spontaneous ventilation because of excessive pulmonary work.[18] The work of breathing is attributable to about 2% to 3% of the REE in the normal adult; however, in the pulmonary-compromised patient, as much as 25% of the REE can be attributed to the work of breathing.[19] The **respiratory quotient (RQ)** ($\dot{V}co_2/\dot{V}o_2$) is also obtained from indirect calorimetry, which is used in the interpretation of net substrate use and as an indicator of test validity. The normal RQ range in humans is 0.67 to 1.2.[17] Because energy measurements by indirect calorimetry are respiratory measurements, the RT is one of the members of the patient care team who commonly performs these measures in clinical settings. The RT who is trained to perform indirect calorimetry measurements is an important contributor to the assessment of nutritional needs of patients.

Indirect calorimetry measurements are usually performed using a metabolic cart, although different types of calorimeters exist. A **metabolic cart** is a computer-controlled unit composed of oxygen and carbon dioxide gas analyzers and flow transducers. The cart automatically measures patients' airflow and expiratory volumes, applies correction factors, and prints out and graphs the results. Different types of gas collection devices, such as a facemask, mouthpiece with nose clip, or canopy, can be used as long as rigorous control is used and no air leaks occur.[14]

Having an understanding of this procedure will help the RT better understand what is automatically calculated by a metabolic cart. The following is a summary of the traditional energy measurement procedure:

1. Collect expired gas in a bag or Tissot spirometer for several minutes.
2. Analyze for carbon dioxide and oxygen (or oxygen and nitrogen).
3. Measure the volume of the gas collected in the bag.
4. Calculate:
   a. If oxygen and carbon dioxide are measured:

$$\dot{V}o_{2(STPD)} = \frac{\dot{V}_{E(ATPS)} \times (P_B - H_2O) \times 21.55}{\text{Collection time} \times (273 + \text{temp in} ^{\circ}C)}$$
$$\times \left[\frac{1 - F_EO_2 - F_ECO_2 \left(\frac{PH_2O}{P_B} \right)}{1 - \frac{F_IO_2}{F_IO_2}} \right] - F_EO_2$$

$$\text{Note:} \frac{(273^{\circ} \text{ K} \times 60 \text{ sec})}{760 \text{ mm Hg}} = 21.55$$

If gas is analyzed with desiccant (a drying agent) in line, then

$$PH_2O/P_B = 0$$

where $\dot{V}o_{2(STPD)}$ = oxygen uptake, standard conditions
$\dot{V}_{E(ATPS)}$ = minute volume; ambient temperature and pressure, saturated
P_B = barometric pressure
F_EO_2 = fraction of expired oxygen

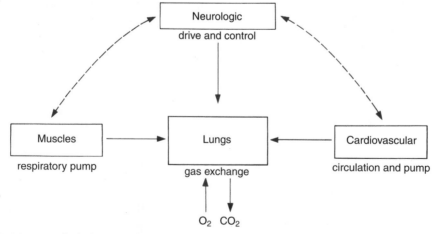

FIGURE 18-3 Block diagram illustrating components of the respiratory system. The neurologic component drives and controls respiration at the lungs by the respiratory muscles. It also affects the cardiovascular system by altering heart function and circulatory resistance. All components are necessary to achieve respiration. Nutritional quality and quantity directly affect the functioning of each system.

F_ECO_2 = fraction of expired carbon dioxide
PH_2O = water vapor pressure
F_IO_2 = fraction of inspired oxygen

    b.

$$\dot{V}co_2 = \dot{V}_E \times (F_ECO_2 - 0.0003)$$

where $\dot{V}co_2$ = carbon dioxide production

    c.

$$RQ = \dot{V}co_2 / \dot{V}o_2$$

where RQ = respiratory quotient

    d.   If only oxygen and nitrogen are measured,

$$\dot{V}o_2 = \dot{V}_E \times (F_EN_2/F_IN_2) \times F_IO_2 - \dot{V}_E \times F_EO_2)$$

where F_EN_2 = fraction of expired nitrogen
F_IN_2 = fraction of inspired nitrogen

For patients confined to a hospital bed, portable equipment is used. For patients who are not intubated and whose condition does not allow them to cooperate with the procedure using a nose clip and mouthpiece, a special hood or canopy apparatus becomes necessary. The RT's interactions with the nutritional support team for metabolic measurements is most helpful because respiratory therapy departments are usually equipped and therapists are trained for such measurements.

In nutrition, energy is quantified in terms of **kilocalories** (kcal); 1 kcal is the amount of energy it takes to raise the temperature of 1 kg of water 1° C. (Although kilocalories have been used most frequently in clinical nutrition, the kilojoule [kJ] is often used in research because kJ is the international unit for energy. To convert kcal to kJ, multiply kcal by 4.184.) For approximately every 5 kcal burned, 1 L of oxygen is used by the tissues. Therefore, if a patient's $\dot{V}o_2$ is measured as 300 mL oxygen/minute, then 300 mL oxygen × 60 minutes × 24 hours equals 432 L of oxygen required per day and 5 kcal × 432 L oxygen/day equals 2160 kcal/day that should be given to the patient. If less than this amount of energy is given, the patient must use body energy stores (glycogen, adipose tissue, and lean muscle mass), which are often already depleted in chronically ill patients. The abbreviated Weir equation is used for more precise conversion of $\dot{V}o_2$ to kilocalories,[16] as follows:

$$kcal/min = (3.94 \times \dot{V}o_2 \text{ L/min}) + (1.11 \times \dot{V}co_2 \text{ L/min})$$

$$\text{Energy expenditure} = kcal/min \times 1440 \text{ min (per day)}$$

Nutritional Depletion and Respiration

A patient who is not ingesting food enterally (through the gastrointestinal tract) probably will be placed on intravenous (IV) therapy. An IV solution of 5% dextrose running at 3 L/day will provide the patient with only 600 kcal/day (0.05 × 3000 mL × 3.41 kcal/g of glucose). (Note: glucose, when given in hydrated form [IV D_5/W and so on], yields 3.41 kcal/g; otherwise the yield is about 4 kcal/g of carbohydrate.) This is far from what is needed to meet a person's energy needs and does not include requirements for protein, vitamins, and minerals.

Blood sugar levels are maintained from liver glycogen (carbohydrate) stores between meals and during fasting. The liver's glycogen stores come from the carbohydrates (starches and sugars) that are eaten in the diet and converted to glucose and stored as glycogen. However, liver glycogen will be depleted within 12 to 16 hours unless sufficient carbohydrate is provided again. When the liver glycogen is depleted, the body obtains sugar by converting protein (amino acids) to sugar. This process is called **gluconeogenesis** (*gluco,* meaning "glucose sugar"; *neo,* meaning "new"; and *genesis,* meaning "to create"). The protein used for gluconeogenesis is obtained from functional proteins (muscles and enzyme systems) because protein is never stored like fat in the body. Protein in the body is always a part of structural or functional tissue, organ, enzyme, or other biochemical action molecule, or is in an "amino acid pool" in circulation while waiting to be incorporated into body systems. Therefore, in patients who have a consistently inadequate nutritional intake, protein, instead of serving a functional role, must be used for more and more of the body's energy needs. This leads to a loss of functional tissue. Skeletal muscle tissues, including the diaphragm and other respiratory muscles, lose muscle mass, with a resultant decrease in endurance and strength. The depletion of protein from the body is also reflected in lowered blood albumin levels; however, low albumin levels may be a result of other metabolic conditions, such as stress and inflammation. In starvation or semistarvation states, respiratory muscle strength can diminish, producing a decrease in forced vital capacity (FVC) and forced expiratory volume in 1 second (FEV_1) because the muscles of respiration, as well as other skeletal muscles, are being catabolized for energy. In starvation, a decrease in carbon monoxide diffusing capacity (D_{LCO}) also occurs, which reflects a diminished gas exchange capacity of the lungs. The decline in FEV_1 also correlates with a decreased **creatinine-height index (CHI)**, indicative of loss of muscle mass. Because immune antibodies are composed of proteins, persistent inadequate calorie and protein intake will also compromise the immune system, thereby limiting the body's ability to fight pneumonia or other infections.

If the calorie intake is less than needed, there will be a decrease in weight, as is commonly seen in patients with COPD. Patients with emphysema are more commonly underweight, appearing thin and often **cachectic** (nutritionally depleted) compared with those with chronic bronchitis, who may be of normal weight and often are overweight. Emphysema produces a catabolic state that usually results in weight loss and mild hypoxemia. Nutritional depletion is evidenced by low body weight or **body mass index (BMI)** and a reduced triceps skinfold thickness measurement. Lean body mass may be decreased, although weight may be stable. BMI alone may not be indicative of a patient's nutritional status, and body composition measurement is preferred in this population to detect alterations in body compartments. Body composition can help differentiate lean body mass from adipose tissue and overhydration from dehydration because changes in hydration status can hide actual body wasting. In patients who retain fluids, it is important to carefully assess anthropometric measurements and biochemical measurements in light of fluid status.

Measures of REE are consistently higher in malnourished emphysematous patients.[20] This increased REE leads to nutritional depletion and eventually malnutrition. Malnutrition can exacerbate symptoms of COPD by decreasing respiratory muscle strength and exercise tolerance and can compromise immune function, leading to increased respiratory infections. Energy expenditure is usually elevated related to pulmonary complications, including the degree of airway obstruction and resultant increased work of breathing.[21] Respiratory inflammation, carbon dioxide retention, gas diffusing capacity, and other mediators, including hormones and cytokines, affect energy expenditure. In addition, insufficient absorption of some nutrients may lead to muscle wasting and malnutrition. Adequate protein intake is needed to maintain or restore lung and muscle strength in these patients.[21] COPD presenting with chronic hypoxia and oxidative stress could be responsible for the catabolic state seen in these patients. Systemic inflammation, anorexia, and muscle dysfunction may all relate to the hypoxia. Correction of the hypoxia by oxygen supplementation seems to allow weight gain and in the short term improve exercise tolerance.[22,23] This improvement is usually not sustained because the underlying metabolic increase is not reversed, and the patient's appetite is not improved.

> **SIMPLY STATED**
>
> Chronic nutritional depletion eventually weakens the muscles of breathing and can contribute to the onset of respiratory failure, especially in patients with chronic lung disease.

If an increased amount of food is consumed, weight can begin to normalize, but emphysematous patients are not comfortable eating larger quantities of foods. In one study, it was necessary to increase intake above 140% of the BMR before improvement of the nutritional status of COPD patients was achieved.[24] If not continuously encouraged to do so, patients typically return to eating their normal amount, which is insufficient to maintain a normal weight. In addition, patients with chronic **protein energy malnutrition (PEM)**, also known as *protein-calorie malnutrition (PCM)*, experience higher morbidity and mortality rates. With loss of body protein, there is a subsequent loss not only of muscle and various enzyme systems but also of immunoglobulins (IgA, IgG, and IgM). Thus, susceptibility to respiratory infections is increased because of decreased immunocompetence.

Therapeutic Interactions of Respiration and Nutrition

Nutritional repletion in respiratory patients is often hindered by some of the necessary therapeutic actions.

Bronchodilators may produce nausea; oxygen by nasal cannula disturbs the sense of smell and therefore taste because 70% of the taste of food is contributed from the sense of smell. Medications the patients are taking may also interact with nutrients and render them less available for absorption or even inhibit specific metabolic enzymes. An intubated patient really complicates the process of eating, requiring specialized feeding approaches. Furthermore, eating large meals expands the stomach, thereby limiting the movement of the diaphragm, the main muscle of respiration. Because of this, frequent small meals may be necessary, requiring greater effort in food preparation. Eating more frequently is also shown to burn more calories than fewer, larger meals eaten each day. These factors, along with shortness of breath, fatigue, increased work of breathing, and a greater prevalence of peptic ulcers, increase the risk for malnutrition. Being knowledgeable about these factors can help the patient to improve both nutritional status and respiratory function.

The respiratory response to the body's need for oxygen and carbon dioxide elimination is usually regulated by the carbon dioxide produced ($\dot{V}co_2$). At the oxygen sensor level, increased hydrogen ion (H^+) concentration in addition to carbon dioxide drives ventilation; this occurs when the amount of oxygen present is insufficient with respect to metabolic need, resulting in lactic acidosis. Oxygen levels, when low enough, become an important stimulus for breathing. A semistarved state can decrease hypoxic drive,[25] compromising a patient even further.

Oxygen uptake and carbon dioxide excretion are as much a part of nutrition as are eating and the elimination of food by-products through the gastrointestinal tract and kidneys. Usually, respiration is not thought of in this way because of the abundance of air and the minimal effort involved in its continuous "ingestion" (breathing). However, patients with respiratory disease often find themselves needing higher levels of the "nutrient" oxygen or assistance in getting rid of the metabolic waste, carbon dioxide. Under these conditions, breathing becomes a more conscious and deliberate effort. In critical care patients, both feeding and breathing often require continuous assistance. Just as patients require intubation when the ventilatory status is compromised sufficiently, they may also require nasogastric or enteral feeding tubes or **parenteral** (into a vein) IV feeding. Matching a patient's energy and nutritional needs with ventilatory needs can become a challenge. Meeting this challenge is necessary to achieve better survival for the patient.

Respiratory System and Nutritional Needs

For optimal ventilatory function, proper nutrition is needed for all components of the respiratory system (see Fig. 18-3).

Neurologic Component

The neurologic component drives and controls ventilation. The higher the $\dot{V}co_2$ level, the greater the blood carbon dioxide concentration and therefore the greater the stimulus to the chemoreceptors. $\dot{V}co_2$ is increased in the body by metabolism, buffering of fixed acids, or both. This in turn increases the electrical activity in the respiratory centers of the central nervous system (CNS), resulting in increased minute ventilation. The nervous system's fundamental requirement is for glucose. The energy derived from glucose is used to maintain an electrical charge across the nerve cell membrane, allowing for depolarization (action potential) and subsequent repolarization. The neurotransmitters at the synaptic ends are amino acids or derivatives of them, and their presence is necessary for the relay of information from one neuron to another and from nerve to muscle. Apparently, the sensitivity of the respiratory centers (either peripheral or central chemoreceptors) is affected by the amount and quality of protein ingested. The respiratory response to carbon dioxide or low levels of oxygen is increased with high protein intake.[26] However, too much protein may make some patients too sensitive to gas partial pressure changes, thus increasing the work of breathing. Giving the optimal amount of protein is the task of the nutritional support team.

Respiratory Muscle Component

The respiratory muscles make up the pump that drives the lungs. They receive the final stimulus from the CNS and produce the appropriate breathing rate and tidal volume as dictated by the CNS and local feedback pathways. The muscles require energy for contraction and relaxation. This energy is derived from blood glucose, free fatty acids from fat stores, muscle glycogen, and at times, branched-chain amino acids. The muscle glycogen stores are the most readily available source of energy for the muscles; however, the amount of glycogen stored depends on the level of carbohydrate in the diet as well as the exercise history of the muscle. A muscle that has been exercised has a greater ability to store glycogen (muscle carbohydrate) after a meal than when one eats without having exercised first. In any case, for the body to store muscle glycogen, there must be an adequate amount of carbohydrate in the diet. The diaphragm, being the main muscle of respiration, needs adequate glycogen stores to be able to meet the metabolic demand of breathing.

Cardiovascular Component

The heart and the circulatory system are vital for pumping the blood through the lungs and throughout the body carrying both nutrients and oxygen to all the tissues. The requirements of the cardiovascular system for food energy for the heart muscle are similar to those of the respiratory muscles.

Protein is needed to maintain and build up the heart muscle and other structural components of tissue. Protein is also a part of buffering actions, clotting factors in the blood, and transport of lipids and iron. **Oncotic pressure** (a form of osmotic pressure that tends to pull water into the blood vessels from the tissue) in the blood is maintained primarily through albumin, the major blood protein produced by the liver. Arginine, one of the amino acids that make up proteins in the body, is the main contributor of nitrogen for the crucial vasodilating molecule **nitric oxide** (NO). NO plays the key role in relaxing the smooth muscles around the artery walls, resulting in vasodilation and thereby regulating blood flow throughout the body. NO is also involved in some end processes of the immune system. Arginine is found in highest concentrations in plant-based proteins.

Carbohydrate is the major fuel for heart muscle. Carbohydrate metabolism is also the source of 2,3-DPG that facilitates oxygen release in the tissue. 2,3-DPG, synthesized by the red blood cells, is an important regulator for the affinity of hemoglobin for oxygen. Phosphorus is also a crucial nutrient in the synthesis of this compound. Blood sugar levels come primarily from dietary carbohydrate and release of stored liver glycogen between meals. Regulation of blood sugar (glucose) is key to normal metabolic function.

Fat is an important component of all cell membranes and is a part of packaging of molecules that are produced by cells. Fat is also a source of fuel for heart muscle, especially when blood glucose levels or muscle glycogen runs low. Essential fatty acids are the backbone of prostaglandins and help regulate blood lipid levels, blood glucose levels, and blood pressure. The fat in nuts also appears to have antiarrhythmic properties and contains omega-3 fatty acids as found in flaxseed and fish oils.

Vitamins and minerals are needed to maintain the metabolic pathways, integrity of cell membranes, and antioxidant activity of cells. They are major players in all body enzyme and metabolic systems. Iron is a major mineral that is a structural part of the heme of hemoglobin and is where oxygen attaches and is carried by the blood. Phosphate stores are commonly depleted in patients with COPD,[27] and medications used in the treatment of COPD, such as corticosteroids, diuretics, and bronchodilators, are associated with phosphate depletion and may contribute to these low stores. Serum phosphate levels should be closely monitored.

Water is the major constituent of the blood and body cells. Sufficient water intake is necessary for proper circulation, clearing of waste from the body, and maintenance of blood pressure. What is eaten or drunk has a vital effect on the cardiovascular system.

Gas Exchange Component (Lungs)

The lungs, which introduce air from the atmosphere into the circulatory system, require a delicate balance of various systems to achieve efficient gas exchange. Alveolar ventilation must be matched with alveolar circulation to allow the efficient transfer of gases between blood and air. To prevent alveolar collapse, surfactant is needed to lessen the surface-active forces that promote collapse of the lung. Starvation leads to decreased surfactant synthesis as well as emphysematous changes in the lung.[28] Humidity and mucociliary performance in the lung require adequate hydration. Smooth muscle function, macrophage activity, and secretion of immunoglobulins (e.g., IgA) into mucus all depend on good nutrition. Obesity changes the physiology of several organ systems. Decreased compliance of the lungs is caused by accumulation of fat tissue around the chest wall, ribs, diaphragm, and abdomen, resulting in impaired lung expansion. Compliance of the pulmonary system declines with increasing BMI. Results of decreased compliance include shallow and rapid breathing and an increased work of breathing. Functional residual capacity declines with increasing BMI, resulting in a small airway closure, right-to-left shunting, and arterial hypoxemia. High levels of adipose tissues result in increased metabolic activity of the fat cell resulting in increased oxygen consumption and CO_2 production. Gas exchange is severely impaired postoperatively and when in a supine position. Obstructive sleep apnea leads to hypoxemia and hypercapnia.[29]

Metabolism

Because basic requirements for both oxygen and nutrients are determined by the cellular metabolic rate, an understanding of metabolism is essential for both respiratory and nutritional assessment.

Metabolism is the body's way of transferring energy from food to the body's energy currency molecules: ATP. The metabolic process can be divided into two pathways: those that break down molecules as energy is released (catabolism) and those that build up new molecules (**anabolism**) to be used in a structural or a functional role. The catabolic pathways produce ATP, which is used for energy to drive the anabolic pathways for growth and maintenance of the organism or simply for the organism's movement in the environment. Therefore, energy is the fundamental need of the body. If sufficient food is eaten, the body can maintain its equilibrium and satisfy the demands placed on it by changes in the environment. However, if too little food is ingested, the body must rely on energy previously stored. If the stored energy—fat and carbohydrate (glycogen)—is not sufficient, the body will break down protein to produce ATP. As mentioned previously, this condition is undesirable because the protein comes from functioning tissue and therefore lessens the functional capability of the organism.

If too much food energy is taken in, the body must use some of its energy to convert the excess carbohydrate or protein so that it can store the excess in the form of fat. As the level of body fat increases, the metabolic cost of moving and breathing increases along with the risk for various diseases. Again, the functional capability of the organism is decreased.

A basic understanding of the metabolic pathways is essential when planning nutritional and ventilatory support. Figure 18-4 illustrates schematically the major energy-producing pathways used by almost every cell of the body.

The reader is encouraged to refer to biochemistry or physiology texts for a more complete discussion of metabolism.

The metabolic process can be viewed as having four major phases (see Fig. 18-4). The first is the digestive phase, in which the food substrates are broken down to the basic components: fat (fatty acids and glycerol), carbohydrates (sugars), and protein (amino acids). The food components are then absorbed from the gastrointestinal tract into the blood, to the liver from which they eventually travel to every cell in the body.

The second phase involves the catabolism of the food components within the cell down to a common molecule, acetylcoenzyme A (acetyl CoA). A small amount of the food energy is used directly to produce a few ATP molecules or transferred to molecular energy shuttles (energy intermediates) in this phase, but acetyl CoA still contains the bulk of the food energy. It is also possible for the metabolic pathways in this phase to go in the opposite direction, from acetyl CoA to form the basic food components again. However, molecules move in this anabolic direction only when the cell has plenty of energy currency (ATP) available. Also note that anaerobic metabolism (energy—ATP—being formed without the presence of oxygen) can occur only in this second phase of metabolism, in the pathway labeled **glycolysis**. In anaerobic metabolism, pyruvate produces lactate (**lactic acid**) rather than acetyl CoA. The greater the energy production without sufficient oxygen, the more lactic acid produced. This can result in lactic acidosis. If this occurs, the acid must be buffered with bicarbonate (HCO_3^-), and carbon dioxide is produced in the process. This requires increased minute ventilation to eliminate the carbon dioxide generated.

Whereas the phases just described have different pathways for each of the food components, the third phase uses the same tricarboxylic acid (TCA) pathway (also called the *Krebs* or *citric acid cycle*), regardless of the origin of the acetyl CoA. The rest of the food energy is removed in the TCA phase, again transferring the energy to molecular energy shuttles. It is here that most of the energy-depleted carbon "skeletons" are discarded as carbon dioxide. For the TCA cycle to be active, the energy shuttles, nicotinamide adenine dinucleotide (NAD) and flavoprotein adenine dinucleotide (FAD), must be able to unload their energy-rich hydrogen and electrons into the respiratory transport chain (oxidative phosphorylation). This requires the presence of oxygen. Without it, the TCA cycle grinds to a halt.

The fourth phase occurs in the cell's mitochondria and is the final destination of the molecular energy shuttles, in which they "dump" their energy-rich loads of hydrogen and electrons into the oxidative phosphorylation system where ATP molecules are mass produced. This is also the final destination of the oxygen that was inhaled. Here, the energy is extracted from the hydrogen and electrons; in the energy-depleted form, the hydrogen and electrons combine with oxygen to form water.

It is in the metabolic pathways just outlined where the body's oxygen is used and carbon dioxide is produced. The

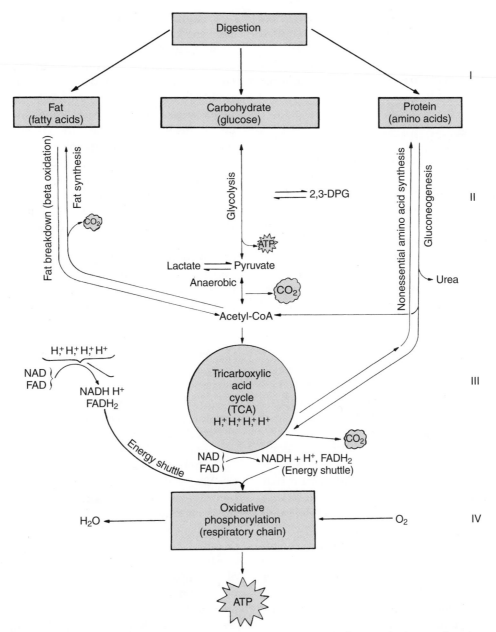

FIGURE 18-4 Four major phases of metabolism are schematically illustrated. Phase I: digestion and nutrient absorption of fat, carbohydrate, and protein. Phase II: breakdown of fatty acids, glucose, and amino acids to acetyl CoA, which either can go on to synthesize (directly or indirectly) fat, carbohydrate, or amino acids, as need be, or can have more energy extracted from it in phases III and IV. Phase III: tricarboxylic acid cycle, where most of the body's carbon dioxide is produced and where most of the molecular energy shuttles (nicotinamide adenine dinucleotide [NAD] and flavoprotein adenosine dinucleotide [FAD]) receive their energy supply in the form of hydrogen atoms. Shuttles transport energy to the respiratory chain. Phase IV: inner mitochondrial membrane where oxidative phosphorylation (production of adenosine triphosphate [ATP] in the presence of oxygen) occurs. Oxygen is the final acceptor of the now energy-depleted electrons and hydrogen ions. 2,3-DPG, 2,3-diphosphoglycerate; FADH, flavoprotein adenine dinucleotide dehydrogenase; NADH, nicotine adenine dinucleotide dehydrogenase.

oxygen used can be measured and is expressed as the oxygen uptake per minute ($\dot{V}_{O_2}$). The measured carbon dioxide produced per minute is expressed as the $\dot{V}_{CO_2}$. The ratio of $\dot{V}_{CO_2}$ to $\dot{V}_{O_2}$ is the RQ. The RQ is determined simply by the amount of fat, carbohydrate, or protein one has eaten or is metabolizing. Pure fat metabolism has an RQ of 0.7 (more oxygen used than carbon dioxide produced), protein has a value of 0.85, and carbohydrate has a value of 1.0 (an even ratio, where one carbon dioxide molecule is produced for each molecule of oxygen used). A mixture of the three different types of foods used for energy at the same time results in an RQ of about 0.8. (This is the R value used most often in the alveolar air equation.) In indirect calorimetry, the RQ should be used as a measure of test validity; measures in the range of 0.6 to 1.2 are within normal physiologic range.[17]

Nutritional Requirements

The basic nutritional requirements include carbohydrate, protein, fat, vitamins, minerals, and water. In light of the present discussion, it would not be wrong to include oxygen as a nutrient because food is of no value unless oxygen is present, although traditionally it is not included in discussions of nutritional requirements. Carbohydrate, protein, and fat provide the energy the body needs as well as the basic chemical skeletons on which structural and functional body systems are built. Vitamins, being part of coenzymes, work along with enzymes in various metabolic pathways and allow specific reactions to occur. Minerals often are elements of specific molecules such as hemoglobin, cytochromes, and thyroxin and may function as cofactors in enzyme systems. Water is the medium in which the various chemical reactions take place within cells. It is also responsible for the fluidity of the blood, which allows blood to circulate. It is not surprising that 50% to 70% of the body's weight is made up of water.

The optimal amount of each of the nutritional components has not been determined precisely, especially for those required in trace amounts. There is agreement that a minimum nutrient level should be high enough so that deficiency symptoms cannot be detected and low enough to prevent toxicity. Within this range, there is much discussion as to what is the right amount because nutritional requirements vary from person to person. Greater or lesser amounts of specific nutrients may be needed because of genetically induced enzyme defects, various disease states, varying amounts of energy expenditure, and various drug-nutrient interactions. Because of the complexity of nurturing the body, a careful nutritional assessment by a nutritional support team, composed of at least a physician and dietitian, is essential. A clinical pharmacologist, for nutrition given parenterally, and an RT, for assessing $\dot{V}co_2$ and $\dot{V}o_2$, are important additions to the team.

Energy

Energy requirements of people with COPD are variable owing to differences in REE and levels of physical activity. COPD, whether stable or in exacerbation, results in an increase in inflammation resulting in an increase in REE. Other influences on energy needs include the efficiency of breathing, thermic effect of food and medications, and others that are beyond the scope of this text.[12] To meet these energy needs and the overall nutritional requirements of the body, a proper balance of macronutrients (carbohydrates, protein, and fat) and micronutrients (vitamins and minerals) is required.

The macronutrient food component that should compose the largest amount of the dietary intake is carbohydrate. Carbohydrates are sometimes broadly classified as complex or simple. The complex carbohydrates are starches (sugar molecules linked together in long branching chains) readily found in a variety of foods; the best sources are grains, vegetables, and fruits. Foods high in complex carbohydrates usually contain the vitamins required in the metabolic pathways for catabolism. In addition, these foods provide water, fiber, protein, and chemical components that are associated with a decrease in chronic disease processes. Simple carbohydrates are free sugars; in natural foods, the largest amounts of simple carbohydrates are found in fruits. However, the majority of sugar consumed comes from processed, refined foods. Ingestion of simple carbohydrates (not including fruits) should be at a minimum because their nutritional value is quite low, but their metabolic demand is quite high (i.e., they travel down the glucose metabolic pathway or go to fat synthesis, but do not "pay any taxes" in the form of vitamins or minerals for the maintenance of the metabolic machinery). They can provide a quick form of energy, but when ingested alone, they can stimulate an exaggerated insulin response because of their rapid absorption from the intestinal tract. Complex carbohydrates tend not to trigger this response because they have to be broken down to free sugars, which takes time, before they are absorbed. Various complex carbohydrate foods differ from one another in their effects on blood sugar levels.

Carbohydrate has often been contrasted with fat. Because the $\dot{V}co_2$ with fat metabolism is lower than that with carbohydrate, it has been suggested by some that minimizing the dietary intake of carbohydrate is to the advantage of the patient with respiratory disease. A patient's response to carbohydrate should be evaluated so that adverse effects can be avoided. It appears, however, that when high levels of carbohydrate are given enterally to patients with COPD who retain carbon dioxide, elevated arterial carbon dioxide tension ($Paco_2$) levels do not always occur.[30-32] In fact, there are even some advantages. A load of ingested carbohydrate can elevate the arterial blood oxygen level (Pao_2) by a modest amount of 7 to 9 mm Hg.[30,33] This is of definite benefit to patients with low oxygen saturations. When the oxygen saturation is low, small increases in Pao_2 can produce significant increases in oxygen content. In addition, a high-carbohydrate diet can significantly increase endurance[34] and allow a given amount of work to be performed with less oxygen than with low-carbohydrate diets. The low $\dot{V}co_2$ advantages of a high-fat diet may be offset in some patients by the increased oxygen requirement for a given work rate. The major problem that has arisen with carbohydrate intake in patients with respiratory disorders occurs when glucose has been given in excess. The increased $\dot{V}co_2$ (a result of both the high RQ of glucose metabolism and its conversion to fat) has induced respiratory difficulty in patients being weaned from mechanical ventilators.[35] This has been observed primarily when glucose has been administered by the parenteral (IV) route.

SIMPLY STATED

Excessive glucose intake leads to an increase in carbon dioxide production, and the respiratory system must work harder to rid the body of this extra carbon dioxide.

Clearly, the problem with glucose lies not in its use, but in its "abuse" or overuse. It is recommended that with the use of parenteral nutrition in critically ill patients, fat should be infused along with the glucose. The infused fat not only helps provide energy but also inhibits the fat synthesis pathway, thereby preventing excessive carbon dioxide production.

Despite the advantages of carbohydrates, diets must be individualized for each patient. Identification of the causes of reduced or inadequate intake is required to develop a nutrition plan that will be effective. Patients with more severe COPD often do better with a higher fat content in the diet and less carbohydrate because there is less carbon dioxide production. But this does not lessen the importance of carbohydrates. Various carbohydrate and dietary fat percentages should be tried until the best combination is found for each patient. This point is stressed because there is a tendency to simply put patients with COPD on a high-fat diet without determining how much carbohydrate they can handle before their condition becomes compromised. Generally, carbohydrates should make up about 55% to 60% of the caloric intake of enterally fed patients. If a patient is having difficulty weaning from mechanical ventilation, a higher fat diet may be useful during the weaning process, in particular those with high P_{CO_2} and CO_2 levels. Follow-up assessment of patients by a registered dietitian familiar with COPD allows proper dietary adjustments.

Protein

Protein should make up 12% to 15% of the caloric intake. The recommended dietary allowance (RDA) of protein for a healthy person has been set at 0.8 g/kg of body weight each day. Thus, a 70-kg person should obtain about 56 g of protein each day. Typically, a person who ingests an adequate number of calories each day, from a variety of foods, will get sufficient protein. In general, protein intake should be sufficient to establish positive nitrogen balance in patients who are nutritionally compromised. A nitrogen balance of +2 g/24 hours is desirable for repletion (ASPEN 4).

Protein is determined by calculating grams of protein per kilogram of body weight (actual or ideal, whichever is lower):
- 0.8 g/kg for the normal healthy adult
- 1.2 to 1.5 g/kg for the initial provision of protein in the pulmonary compromised patient. If protein depletion is present, assessing nitrogen balance and reassessing protein needs is critical.
- 2.0 to 2.5 g/kg for severe catabolic conditions

Nitrogen values are often referred to in discussion of protein requirements because nitrogen is only found in the amino acids that make up proteins. Thus, measuring nitrogen, which is a simple laboratory measure, is the easiest way to measure protein intake or excretion. Amino acids make up all the proteins. Amino acids contain an acid group, COOH, and an amino group, NH_2. The amino group is the nitrogen-containing portion of the amino acid. Specific laboratory methods are used to measure nitrogen in the blood (blood urea nitrogen [BUN]) or in the urine (urinary urea nitrogen [UUN]). Because every 100 g of proteins contains approximately 6.25 g of nitrogen, grams of nitrogen can readily be converted to grams of protein by multiplying by 6.25. Conversely, to find how much nitrogen there is in a given amount of protein, in grams, divide by 6.25 (or the appropriate factor for the specific protein).

When considering adequacy of protein intake, both quantity and quality of the protein must be considered. The quality of a protein is determined by the amount of each essential amino acid it contains. Essential amino acids cannot be synthesized by the body in sufficient quantities to meet body needs or cannot be synthesized at all. Of the 20 amino acids, 9 are considered essential for the healthy adult: histidine, isoleucine, leucine, lysine, methionine, phenylalanine, threonine, tryptophan, and valine. By definition, the greater the number of essential amino acids contained in a protein, the higher its quality. The ratio of various key amino acids is emerging as an important factor in nutritional health. Soy protein is considered a high-quality protein, along with milk or egg protein; however, soy protein has an additional benefit of lower insulin stimulation and a lowering of cholesterol. With milk or egg protein, there is an opposite effect. Plant-based proteins lower many of the risk factors for many chronic diseases. Most of the plant proteins have lower essential amino acid profiles than do animal proteins, but when combined with other complementary plant protein, complete essential amino acid profiles can be obtained.

As with anything else, the extremes of protein intake, either too little or too much, can have detrimental effects. Too little protein compromises the immune system, contributes to edema and ascites, produces generalized wasting of muscle tissue, and retards growth and proper development in children. Too much protein, although not as harmful, increases the requirements for some other nutrients, notably calcium and water. In addition, there may be an increase in the work of breathing, as noted previously, and increased stress on the liver and kidneys (of concern mostly in patients with liver or renal insufficiency). The final consideration involves the body's acid-base balance. Protein is the major source of fixed acids that are ingested (fixed acids must be cleared by the kidney; volatile acids, like carbon dioxide, can be cleared by the lungs). Patients with COPD who are in a state of respiratory acidosis may experience more difficulty if an increased fixed acid load (large quantity of protein) is ingested. Protein from plant-based sources is more alkaline in nature. In fact, fruits and vegetables leave an alkaline residue in the body after metabolism, and they help buffer the acids from the proteins. Without sufficient fruits and vegetables, more calcium must be pulled from the bones, forming calcium carbonate, which is then used to buffer the fixed acids from the proteins. So, in patients who have respiratory acidosis and are in need of more protein intake, the acid-base balance is better regulated by adding more plant-based foods in the diet.

To establish the optimal amount of protein, a patient needs the measurement of protein intake (nitrogen intake) and nitrogen excretion. A patient whose intake of nitrogen equals excretion of nitrogen is said to be in **nitrogen balance**. If more nitrogen is excreted than ingested, negative nitrogen balance exists. Conversely, positive nitrogen balance exists when the nitrogen intake is greater than the nitrogen excretion. Patients who are severely ill or who are simply not getting enough calories are often in negative nitrogen balance. This is undesirable because it indicates that body protein is being used for energy. Patients who are nutritionally depleted need to be in positive nitrogen balance to build up body tissues. In the well-nourished patient, the clinical goal is to maintain nitrogen balance.

SIMPLY STATED

A negative nitrogen balance is common in critically ill patients who are not able to eat and indicates that more nitrogen is excreted than ingested. Body protein stores are being consumed in such cases, and muscle wasting is occurring.

Fat

Dietary fat plays a number of important roles in the body. The fat-soluble vitamins, A, D, E, and K, are carried in fats and oils. These vitamins are involved in immunity, antioxidant activity, blood clotting, and bone and arterial health. Fat is energy dense and contains twice as many calories per gram weight as carbohydrate or protein. Because of this, fat is the best storage form of energy, and this is why the body stores excess calories in the form of fat or triglycerides in the adipose tissue. Fat is also the most efficient way to provide more calories to hospitalized patients when they are fluid restricted or cannot tolerate large volumes of food. Fat provides a feeling of fullness (satiety), improves palatability of food, and is digested more slowly than proteins and starches. There are two essential fats, linolenic (omega-3) and linoleic (omega-6), that the body must obtain from the diet. These fats are needed for modulation of inflammatory processes, nerve function, and other essential chemical activities.

Within the body, fat is involved in many different functions. Notably, fat is a component of all cell membranes, provides energy storage and organ protection, and is the major component of surfactant (dipalmitoyl lecithin). However, these tasks do not require much fat to be eaten. The typical American diet is composed of more than 30% of calories from fat. This is more than necessary. With excess

dietary fat comes increased risk for heart disease, breast cancer, colon cancer, and lung cancer in women. Increased fat also decreases oxygenation of the tissues,[36,37] impairs pulmonary gas diffusion (D_{LCO}), and hinders capillary circulation by promoting the clumping of red blood cells.[38] However, these outcomes do not always occur because the effects seen depend on the amount of fat that is circulating, the rate of clearance of fat, and possibly the type of fat. As the fat content of the diet increases, there is a measurable decrease in $\dot{V}CO_2$. For many patients with COPD, this results in less dyspnea and improved function.[39,40]

SIMPLY STATED

Excessive fat intake can decrease tissue oxygenation. Strive for a balance between fat and carbohydrate intake so that oxygenation is maximized and carbon dioxide production is minimized.

The main concern of nutritionists is to determine the optimal percentage of calories that should come from carbohydrate and protein. With that established, the remaining amount of calories required can come from fat.

With the quantity of fat determined, one must be concerned with the quality of fat. Fat can be either saturated (no double bonds present in the fatty acid chain) or unsaturated (some of the fatty acid carbons contain double bonds). The two types of unsaturated fat are polyunsaturated (more than two double bonds in the fatty acid chain) and monounsaturated (only one double bond present). Most diets are too high in saturated fat, and a higher intake of monounsaturated fat is recommended. Monounsaturated fat, found in olives, nuts, and avocados, has numerous health benefits. This type of fat lowers total and low-density lipoprotein (LDL) cholesterol with no adverse effect on the high-density lipoprotein (HDL) cholesterol, thereby lowering the risk for heart disease. Monounsaturated fat also helps regulate both blood sugar and blood pressure. Olive oil and canola oil are the recommended choices. Despite all the information available about the advantages and disadvantages of given foods and optimal combinations of carbohydrate, fat, and protein, dietary patterns established early in life are difficult to change in later years. Patients should be encouraged to eat foods that provide good nutrition and do not aggravate a compromised respiratory condition. However, some patients will not adapt to a change in diet, and in these cases, any nutrition is better than no nutrition.

Vitamins, Minerals, Phytochemicals, and Other Nutrients

Vitamins can be classified into two main categories: water soluble and fat soluble. Water-soluble vitamins are those of the B group and vitamin C. The fat-soluble vitamins are A, D, E, and K. Vitamins are cofactors in the enzyme systems needed for various metabolic pathways and body processes. The minerals can be divided into either macronutrient elements or micronutrient (trace) elements. Minerals are used in all of the body chemical reactions and are part of numerous enzyme systems serving as cofactors. It is just as important to supplement with minerals as it is with vitamins when there appears to be a deficient food intake.

For most people who eat a variety of foods each day, ingesting the recommended amounts of vitamins and minerals is not difficult. But when physiologic functioning has been altered by a disease process, an increased need for specific nutrients may arise. Vitamin and mineral supplementation will also be more necessary when there is a decreased consumption of food because of, for example, loss of appetite. The less food eaten, the more difficulty there will be in obtaining all the different nutrients. Furthermore, various medications can interact with the absorption, function, or excretion of some nutrients, thereby altering the required amount. Studies show that in older people, supplementation with a basic vitamin and mineral results in fewer infections and more days of wellness each year.[41-43] However, not all studies confirm these findings. The differing results might be due to different levels or combinations of supplementations. There appears to be a consistent finding that higher antioxidant levels in the blood correlate with improved lung function, but this may be more likely from the diet rather than the supplements.[44] Subjects with higher plasma β-carotene are shown to have higher FVC levels, and vitamin D is linked to improved lung function.[45,46] Higher intakes of vitamin C or β-carotene are protective for FEV_1 and FVC.[47] These observations are important for COPD patients because there is a decrease in plasma antioxidants in people who smoke; this is associated not only with decreased lung function but also with greater mortality.[48,49] It has also been found that a deficiency of vitamins C and E is associated with more wheezing symptoms.[50] Higher levels of dietary intakes of antioxidants appear to be associated with higher skeletal muscular strength in elderly persons.[51] This relationship would apply to the respiratory muscles, which are skeletal muscles.

A few nutrients deserve special mention because of their importance in patients with lung disease. Iron's role in oxygen transport and use in hemoglobin and myoglobin and within the respiratory transport chain makes it necessary to maintain iron at normal levels. It has also been found that **anemia** is associated with decreases in muscular strength.[52] Vitamin A promotes optimal functioning of mucous membranes and helps promote resistance to respiratory tract infections.[53] Vitamin A depletion induced by cigarette smoking has been associated with development of emphysema in rats.[54] Carotene, a vitamin A precursor, and vitamin C have been found to be associated with a decreased risk for certain types of lung cancers.[55] A number of studies show that the benefits from these nutrients are better realized from eating the fruits and vegetables that contain them than from simply supplementing the isolated vitamin.[56] Vitamins

E and C and selenium, which are antioxidants, appear to help lessen the effects of oxygen toxicity and ozone on lung tissue.[57-60] Vitamin D in the form of D_3 (also known as cholecalciferol) has come to the forefront in recent years because of numerous benefits: improved lung function, immunity and resistance against some cancers and viruses, bone density, calcium uptake, muscle strength, and relief of aches and pains. Vitamin D is the "sunshine" vitamin, and proper exposure to the sun can help a person achieve sufficient levels; however, in many areas, sufficient exposure to the sun is not readily available, and oral supplementation should be used to optimize the amount of vitamin D received. Monitoring blood levels of vitamin D is recommended so that proper dosing adjustments can be made as needed.

Any chronically ill patient may have altered eating habits that are insufficient to meet nutrient requirements. The severity of nutritional depletion appears to be related to the severity of COPD despite an adequate caloric intake.[61,62] This may result in a need for supplementation of some or all of the vitamins and minerals.

Phytochemicals are plant components that make up plant colors and other active components of plants. Intake of plant **phytochemicals**, as would be obtained from eating whole plant foods, lowers risk for chronic diseases, including asthma.[63] Flavonoids and other phytochemicals, which are only found in plant foods, especially fruits, vegetables, and berries, have potent antioxidant tissue-protective effects that are vital to health and disease prevention. Diets need to ensure generous amounts of these types of foods.

COPD patients, as with other patients with chronic diseases, are often found to have an underlying inflammatory component. Skeletal muscle loss in COPD appears to be linked with systemic inflammation.[64] It is also known that the underlying problem with asthma is airway inflammation, which leads to bronchoconstriction. Dietary omega-3 polyunsaturated fatty acids, which are found in flaxseeds and fish oils, have important anti-inflammatory effects in the body and may benefit patients with lung disease.[65]

Fluids and Electrolytes

Adequate fluid intake is extremely important for patients with respiratory disorders. Proper function of the lung's mucociliary clearance mechanism requires good hydration. Although the body is composed of about 60% water by weight, it is constantly losing water through urine, feces, sweat, breathing, and, in patients with respiratory problems, expectoration. This requires continual fluid replacement.

Patients with respiratory problems often develop heart failure (right or left, or eventually both), which complicates the fluid replacement process. The need for fluids must be carefully balanced with the need to restrict fluids because of the fluid retention resulting from the heart problem. In a patient who has a heart problem, both fluid and sodium intake must be monitored. Sodium levels determine how much water the body will retain; therefore, dietary sodium often must be limited.

Water is the best fluid to provide hydration. However, fruit or vegetable juices add some variety as well as some nutrition and more calories for those who need additional caloric intake. Low-sodium juices can be obtained. Drinks containing caffeine promote bronchodilation to some extent because caffeine is in the same family as theophylline; both are xanthines.[66] If a patient is using theophylline-type bronchodilators and is also a heavy user of drinks containing caffeine, there is a greater chance of side effects. Because the ingestion of alcohol has been correlated with decreased FVC and FEV_1,[67] bronchoconstriction,[68] impairment of lung defenses,[69] and increased likelihood of sleep apnea,[70] its use is contraindicated. Good nutrition for the respiratory system involves not only getting enough of that which is essential but also avoiding that which is harmful.

Patients receiving IV fluids must have the input and output amounts monitored continually so that neither too much nor too little is given. Fluid overload often results in pulmonary congestion or edema, further complicating a poorly functioning lung.

In addition to serum sodium levels, potassium and chloride values should be checked. All of these electrolytes play an important role in acid-base balance and nerve function. Potassium also plays an important role in heart, muscle, and nerve function as well as in stimulation of aldosterone secretion (along with angiotensin II) from the adrenal cortex.

One must not forget that fluid and sodium intake can occur with medication and normal saline nebulization. Nebulized fluid retention is most critical when dealing with small children and infants, especially when an ultrasonic nebulizer is used.

SIMPLY STATED

Excessive intake of sodium can lead to fluid retention, especially in the patient with heart failure.

Methods of Meeting Nutritional Requirements

Nutritional requirements are not always achieved easily. Dietitians often work against patient factors such as loss of appetite, dyspnea that is increased with eating, inability to eat normal amounts of solid food, fluid restrictions, inability to take food by mouth, and a comatose state. Careful evaluation of a patient's nutritional needs, food preferences, educational and economic status, cooking facilities, and self-help level is necessary. All factors influence a patient's ability to reach the nutritional goals set.

The routes of nutritional administration can be either enteral or parenteral. The preferred route is enteral. If a patient is intubated and cannot take food by mouth, enteral tube feeding is instituted. The last resort, when all other attempts at feeding are unsuccessful or not recommended, is **parenteral nutrition (PN)**. PN is the feeding of patients by direct infusion of nutrients into either a peripheral or a central vein. There is a reluctance to feed patients by PN because it is not as efficient as the enteral route, it is expensive, and there are increased risks for complications such as infection. However, because nutrition is so important, it is used. Nutritionally depleted or catabolic patients should never go without nutritional support for more than a day.

Patients with emphysema are often underweight and need to gain weight, whereas those with chronic bronchitis are likely to be overweight and need to lose weight. Patients with COPD may find it uncomfortable to eat a large meal because a flattened diaphragm along with a full stomach makes it even more difficult to function. To avoid this problem, frequent small meals may be helpful. The goal for a patient with emphysema is a positive nitrogen balance and an increase in caloric intake because respiratory muscle function improves with an increase in weight (muscle mass). The goal for an overweight patient with bronchitis is maintenance of nitrogen balance with decreased caloric intake because respiratory muscle function improves with a loss of weight due to fat.

Patients being assisted by continuous mechanical ventilation provide an additional nutritional challenge. Positive-pressure breathing can affect splanchnic (internal organs of the abdomen) circulation and can cause increased resistance to portal blood flow to the liver, increased resistance to bile flow down the bile duct, and decreased blood flow to the kidneys. These effects are increased as the pressure is increased and are most pronounced with the use of continuous positive airway pressure (CPAP) or positive end-expiratory pressure (PEEP). However, these effects may reach significance only for a minority of patients. Yet any alteration in blood flow in the gastrointestinal tract, liver, or kidneys can have an effect on the nutritional status of the patient, thus making it more difficult to meet his or her nutritional requirements.

In addition and as previously indicated, a disease such as cystic fibrosis affects not only the lungs but also other organ systems, including the pancreas. As a result, patients with cystic fibrosis tend to have a deficiency of certain digestive enzymes produced in the pancreas and needed for digesting fats. To address this and enable the body to better digest and absorb fats, such patients generally need to take digestive enzyme supplements.

SIMPLY STATED

Patients with cystic fibrosis tend to have a deficiency of enzymes produced in the pancreas and need for the digestion of fats. As a result, most patients with cystic fibrosis need to take digestive enzyme supplements to minimize the likelihood of a certain type of malnutrition.

Nutritional Assessment

The RT is not responsible for the nutritional assessment of the patient but should be familiar with the process and may actually participate in it. Because the RT and the nurse usually spend the most time with a patient, their observations are valuable. A complete nutritional assessment is performed by the registered dietitian and may include some factors assessed by other members of the health care team. The components of nutritional assessment consist of medical and diet histories, including medications with nutritional considerations, anthropometric measurements (weight, body composition, skinfold, and waist and limb circumferences), biochemical evaluations, energy and macronutrient and micronutrient evaluations, and immunologic evaluations. The areas to be assessed in determining the patient's nutritional profile are summarized in Box 18-1.

Data Gathering and Interpretation
History
Conditions that should be discovered in the medical history are as follows:
- Multiple surgical or nonsurgical trauma
- Fever
- Infection acute and chronic
- Burns
- Long bone fractures
- Hyperthyroidism
- Prolonged corticosteroid therapy

These conditions increase a patient's metabolic rate or caloric and other nutrient requirements. Such metabolic challenges pose a serious threat to the homeostatic maintenance of a marginally nourished patient with COPD. A patient with one of these conditions should be evaluated further with an REE using indirect calorimetry.

During the patient interview, the following information is collected:
- Smoking or other tobacco habits
- Occupation and usual daily activity
- Use of supplemental oxygen
- Usual energy and nutrient intake through 24-hour recall, usual daily intake or food frequency pattern
- Special diet restrictions at home
- Food aversions, intolerances, and allergies
- Medications (prescription and over the counter), nutritional, botanical and herbal supplements
- Mechanical feeding problems (e.g., biting, chewing or swallowing, mouth sores)
- Changes in appetite
- Changes in food intake or food patterns
- Gastrointestinal problems (e.g., anorexia, nausea, vomiting, or heartburn)
- Elimination pattern and consistency of stool
- Maximal weight attained and how long ago it was attained

Box 18-1	Areas Requiring Assessment to Determine a Patient's Nutritional Profile

PHYSIOLOGIC
- Types of diseases present
- Severity of illness
- Metabolic stress of disease
- Medications being used (both prescription and over the counter)
- Botanical and/or herbal therapies
- Genetic deficiencies
- Activity level
- Resting energy expenditure (REE)
- Food allergies and intolerances
- Current nutritional status
  - Anthropometric
  - Biochemical
  - Immunologic

PSYCHOSOCIAL
- Mental state (mood, alertness)
- Culture
- Food preparation skills
- Appetite
- Learned eating behaviors/habits (food preferences)
- Motivation
- Habits: alcohol, smoking
- Education
- Income
- Support system

ENVIRONMENTAL
- Mechanical hindrances to eating (continuous mechanical ventilation and tracheostomy)
- Food availability
- Temperature
- Humidity

SUGGESTED MEASUREMENTS
- Skinfold thickness
- Skinfold + arm circumference = arm, muscle circumference, muscle and fat area
- Body mass index (BMI)
- Percent body fat
- Percent lean body mass—body protein reserves (an indicator of protein energy nutrition)
- Body fat stores (an indicator of energy reserves)
- Result of long-term nutritional status

- Usual weight, recent weight changes
- Alcohol intake

This information is usually obtained from the patient or family members during the initial evaluation.

Physical Examination
The physical examination often yields clues to the patient's nutritional status; however, many signs of nutritional deficiency can be missed by the inexperienced RT or other member of the patient care team. Look at the health of

the patient's hair and check for sparseness, dyspigmentation, or easy pluckability. Assess the skin for areas of drying, flaking, cracking, or pigment change. Swollen parotid glands, changes in saliva production, or an enlarged liver may indicate concern for nutritional status. Weight loss, temporal wasting or general muscle wasting, edema, mental apathy, and confusion all can lead the clinician to suspect malnutrition. Although signs of malnutrition, they are rather nonspecific and therefore only suggestive of malnutrition. When these signs are present in a patient, more sensitive and objective methods of assessment should be used to confirm or rule out compromised nutritional status. Following is a summary of some basic anthropometric measurements and their nutritional assessment value.

The assessment most commonly used and easiest to perform during the physical examination involves weighing and measuring stature and body circumference. Measurements of weight, height, and arm and waist circumference require little effort or time yet give important information. Because height and weight can vary with the time of day and the amount of clothing, the measurements should be performed in the same way each time and the pertinent information recorded so that serial measurements are meaningful. Bed scales can be used for weighing ventilator-dependent patients. The weight of any ventilator tubing or other devices and dressings should be subtracted from the total weight. A weight loss of 5% of the usual body weight or an unintentional weight loss of 10 lb or more indicates increased nutritional risk. Although body weight has limited value in detecting malnutrition, low body weights correlate with poor medical outcomes. The patient care team should evaluate for edema and ascites when assessing weight status, which can result in misinterpretation of actual weight status. If a fluctuation or change in weight of several pounds is observed during a 24-hour period, it is most likely caused by water retention or loss.

The BMI is the primary method for assessment of the appropriateness of weight for a given height. The BMI is determined by weight (kg)/height (m²). Figure 18-5 is a table for finding the BMI without having to calculate it. A BMI in the range of 20 to 25 is considered optimal. A BMI from 25 to 30 is considered overweight, 30 to 35 is stage 1 obesity, 35 to 40 is stage 2 obesity, and 40 to 45 is stage 3 obesity, also known as morbid obesity. As the BMI exceeds 27, the risk for weight-related problems begins to increase. BMIs that are below 19 are associated with malnutrition problems and increased pneumonia infections. BMI is shown to be significantly associated with FEV_1 and FEV_1 divided by vital capacity.[71] In patients with COPD, the best survival outcomes are associated with those who have higher BMIs and in whom low BMI is an independent risk factor for dying.[71-73] Prevalence of malnutrition may be as high as 30% in people with COPD (BMI < 20 kg/m²), and the risk for COPD-related death doubles with weight loss. Body composition differs from healthy controls even in those with BMI greater than 20 kg/m². Fat-free mass

and bone density are lower in people with COPD.[12] A quick estimate of ideal body weight can be determined from the following (Hamwi equation): allow 106 lb for the first 5 feet of height and 6 lb for each additional inch (men). For women, start with 100 lb for the first 5 feet and add 5 lb for each additional inch. This does not account for variations in frame size but is useful for rapid estimation as to appropriateness of a patient's weight. The ideal body weight can also be used for estimating a patient's anatomic dead space (1 mL/lb ideal body weight) or for determining a starting tidal volume for a ventilator-dependent patient (5 to 7 mL/lb ideal body weight). The term **ideal body weight** simply refers to the weight the patient probably should weigh.

Body weight is often divided into two types: fat weight and lean body weight (lean body weight = total weight − fat weight). The problem is never simply a weight problem. A patient weighs too much only when the percentage of total body weight made up of fat exceeds about 23% for males and 28% for females. A method for estimating the percent of body fat is the skinfold measurement.

Triceps Skinfold Thickness. Measurement of skinfold thickness with the use of calipers is a fairly simple procedure (proper technique is important) that yields data on the fat and protein reserves in the body. The triceps skinfold is the most common place of measurement; however, several other sites can be used, usually in addition to the triceps area. Skinfold thickness, coupled with measurements of the upper arm circumference, arm muscle circumference, and arm muscle area, provides accepted estimates of PEM. The arm fat area may also be calculated and improves the body fat weight estimate when used along with triceps skinfold measurements.[74] These measurements are all compared with standard normal values to assess the degree of malnutrition. As with other tests, the exact value obtained with any one measurement may not be as important as the trend seen with serial measurements. It is important to establish baseline data for a patient when first admitted. Then the first signs of malnutrition can be detected and appropriate treatment implemented before serious deficiency symptoms occur.

Other, more accurate methods for assessment of body fat include underwater weighing, body volume displacement, and electrical bioimpedance measurements.[75] Only the last has a role in the hospital setting because underwater weighing requires the patient to be healthy and to be able to hold the breath under water for a period of time, and body volume displacement requires the patient to be confined in a small chamber. Electrical bioimpedance readings can be obtained at the bedside.

Laboratory Biochemical Tests

Laboratory biochemical tests tend to reflect body changes more quickly and to be more accurate than anthropometric tests. Table 18-1 summarizes their relative sensitivities to body nutritional change and suggests guidelines for interpretation.

Height in Inches

↓	56	57	58	59	60	61	62	63	64	65	66	67	68	69	70	71	72	73	74	75	76
100	22	22	21	20	20	19	18	18	17	17	16	16	15	15	14	14	14	13	13	13	12
105	24	23	22	21	21	20	19	19	18	18	17	16	16	16	15	15	14	14	14	13	13
110	25	24	23	22	22	21	20	20	19	18	18	17	17	16	16	15	15	15	14	14	13
115	26	25	24	23	23	22	21	20	20	19	19	18	18	17	17	16	16	15	15	14	14
120	27	26	25	24	23	23	22	21	21	20	19	19	18	18	17	17	16	16	15	15	15
125	28	27	26	25	24	24	23	22	22	21	20	20	19	18	18	17	17	17	16	16	15
130	29	28	27	26	25	25	24	23	22	22	21	20	20	19	19	18	18	17	17	16	16
135	30	29	28	27	26	26	25	24	23	23	22	21	21	20	19	19	18	18	17	17	16
140	31	30	29	28	27	27	26	25	24	23	23	22	21	21	20	20	19	19	18	18	17
145	33	31	30	29	28	27	27	26	25	24	23	23	22	21	21	20	20	19	19	18	18
150	34	33	31	30	29	28	27	27	26	25	24	24	23	22	22	21	20	20	19	19	18
155	35	34	32	31	30	29	28	28	27	26	25	24	24	23	22	22	21	20	20	19	19
160	36	35	34	32	31	30	29	28	28	27	26	25	24	24	23	22	22	21	21	20	20
165	37	36	35	33	32	31	30	29	28	28	27	26	25	24	24	23	22	22	21	21	20
170	38	37	36	34	33	32	31	30	29	28	27	27	26	25	24	24	23	22	22	21	21
175	39	38	37	35	34	33	32	31	30	29	28	27	27	26	25	24	24	23	23	22	21
180	40	39	38	36	35	34	33	32	31	30	29	28	27	27	26	25	24	24	23	23	22
185	42	40	39	37	36	35	34	33	32	31	30	29	28	27	27	26	25	24	24	23	23
190	43	41	40	38	37	36	35	34	33	32	31	30	29	28	27	27	26	25	24	24	23
195	44	42	41	39	38	37	36	35	34	33	32	31	30	29	28	27	27	26	25	24	24
200	45	43	42	40	39	38	37	36	34	33	32	31	30	30	29	28	27	26	26	25	24
205	46	44	43	41	40	39	38	36	35	34	33	32	31	30	29	29	28	27	26	26	25
210	47	46	44	43	41	40	38	37	36	35	34	33	32	31	30	29	29	28	27	26	26
215	48	47	45	44	42	41	39	38	37	36	35	34	33	32	31	30	29	28	28	27	26
220	49	48	46	45	43	42	40	39	38	37	36	35	34	33	32	31	30	29	28	28	27
225	51	49	47	46	44	43	41	40	39	38	36	35	34	33	32	31	31	30	29	28	27
230	52	50	48	47	45	44	42	41	40	38	37	36	35	34	33	32	31	30	30	29	28
235	53	51	49	48	46	44	43	42	40	39	38	37	36	35	34	33	32	31	30	29	29
240	54	52	50	49	47	45	44	43	41	40	39	38	37	36	35	34	33	32	31	30	29
245	55	53	51	50	48	46	45	43	42	41	40	38	37	36	35	34	33	32	32	31	30
250	56	54	52	51	49	47	46	44	43	42	40	39	38	37	36	35	34	33	32	31	30
255	57	55	53	52	50	48	47	45	44	43	41	40	39	38	37	36	35	34	33	32	31
260	58	56	54	53	51	49	48	46	45	43	42	41	40	38	37	36	35	34	33	33	32
265	60	57	56	54	52	50	49	47	46	44	43	42	40	39	38	37	36	35	34	33	32
270	61	59	57	55	53	51	49	48	46	45	44	42	41	40	39	38	37	36	35	34	33
275	62	60	58	56	54	52	50	49	47	46	44	43	42	41	40	38	37	36	35	34	34
280	63	61	59	57	55	53	51	50	48	47	45	44	43	41	40	39	38	37	36	35	34

Weight in Pounds

FIGURE 18-5 The body mass index (BMI) is determined by aligning a patient's weight with his or her height. The BMI is found where the row of weight intersects the column of height. See text for more explanation. (From http://www.niddk.nih.gov.)

Creatine phosphate is used in muscle as an energy reserve molecule. When there is an increased demand for ATP, creatine donates a phosphate to adenosine diphosphate (ADP), making ATP. The more muscle mass there is in the body, the more creatine there will be. Creatine is metabolized to **creatinine**, the form in which it is largely excreted. The clearance of creatinine from the blood by the kidneys is a good indicator of renal function. Measurement of 24-hour urinary excretion of creatinine correlates with the patient's lean body weight (muscle mass): the greater the muscle mass, the higher the urinary excretion of creatinine. When expressed in terms of height, a measure generally unaffected by malnutrition, urinary excretion of creatinine can be used as a general measure of malnutrition. The CHI is a predictor of muscle mass but may not correlate well with arm muscle circumference, probably because of the many factors that govern the excretion of creatinine. In young females and older men, if the creatinine excretion is related to the total arm length, the ability to predict malnutrition is improved.

TABLE 18-1

Current Laboratory Biochemical Tests and Guidelines for Interpretation

Measurement of Index	Deficient	Normal	Sensitivity
Creatinine-height index (CHI) (%)	40	60	Poor
Serum albumin level (g/dL)	2.5	3.5-5.0	Limited because of long half-life (20 days) and because a negative acute phase protein will respond negatively to any physiologic stress
Serum transferrin level (mg/dL)	100	200-400	Poor; unpredictable response to refeeding
Total iron-binding capacity (TIBC) (mg/dL)	<250	250-350	Poor; increased in pregnancy, iron deficiency, oral contraceptive use; iron may bind to proteins other than serum transferrin
Nitrogen balance	Negative balance	Equilibrium	Good; although nitrogen excretion often underestimated. Must be carefully measured to be helpful.
Thyroxin-binding prealbumin (TBPA) (mg/dL)	<10	10-20	Limited; half-life short (2 days) but is a negative acute phase protein
Retinol-binding protein (RBP) (µg/dL)	<3	3-6	Limited; half-life short (12 hr) but is a negative acute phase protein
Total lymphocyte count (cells/mm³)	<1200	2000-3500	Limited; decreased in injury, chemotherapy, radiotherapy, surgery; increased in infection
Differential count for lymphocytes (%)		20-45	Limited
Skin antigen testing	Negative	Positive	Good

Levels of **serum albumin**, the major protein fraction of blood, correlate well with body protein reserves of muscle mass. The measurement of serum albumin levels provides a useful screening tool for detecting PEM. However, because the turnover of serum albumin is slow (half-life is 20 days), a change in nutritional status is not soon reflected by this measurement. The time lag of 1 to 2 weeks for the serum albumin level to show a change after a nutritional alteration has occurred is too long to effectively manage the nutrition of most critically ill patients. In addition, serum albumin is a negative acute phase protein that results in rapid depletion during physiologic stress and may not be indicative of nutritional status.

Prealbumin, also called thyroxin-binding prealbumin (TBPA) because it carries about one third of the body's thyroxin (thyroid hormone), also carries retinol-binding protein (RBP). These two proteins quickly reflect nutritional deprivation or refeeding treatment because of their short half-lives (TBPA, 2 days; RBP, 12 hours).[76] As with serum albumin, both are negative acute phase proteins and may not accurately reflect nutritional status. Either can be used for assessing nutritional repletion in critically ill patients because the response time for these values is 3 days or less.[77]

Serum transferrin, the protein that transports iron in the body, has a half-life of 4 to 8 days. However, because of its wide range of normal values and its unpredictable response to refeeding in depleted patients, it has limited clinical use in nutritional assessment. The total iron-binding capacity (TIBC) of transferrin may also be used. However, it may overestimate transferrin levels because iron can also bind to other proteins in the blood. Transferrin levels may be elevated during iron deficiency anemia, the second and third trimesters of pregnancy, estrogen therapy, or oral

contraceptive use. Other hormones and disease states have a variable effect on **serum transferrin** levels and TIBC.

Nitrogen balance measurements, using 24-hour urine specimens, are essential for protein assessment and are commonly performed in acute care settings. However, an underestimation of nitrogen excretion can occur in patients with burns, diarrhea, vomiting, or other nitrogen-losing conditions.[78] A commonly used clinical estimation is as follows:

$$\text{Nitrogen balance} = \text{grams of nitrogen intake} - (\text{24-hr grams of UUN} + 4\text{ g})$$

For repletion of protein stores, a positive +2/4 grams is suggested.

Immunocompetence, or being dependent on globulin proteins (as mentioned previously), can also be used to help assess PEM. Total lymphocyte count (lymphocytes make the immunoglobulins) or their function can be measured. An easy test of their function (which requires them to have adequate protein to make their antibodies) is to challenge them with skin antigen testing. Antigens used are those to which a patient is most likely to have been previously exposed. With these, a quick antigen-antibody reaction should be seen at the skin-testing site, much like a positive tuberculin skin test reaction. However, if the patient is protein deficient, the skin test reaction will be greatly diminished or absent.[79] It should be noted that an iron deficiency can also diminish the response.[80]

As can be seen, no one test constitutes a perfect assessment of a patient's nutritional status. But with the appropriate use of selected anthropometric and biochemical measurements, along with astute observations by respiratory care practitioners, an adequate nutritional profile can be developed. Other sources should be consulted for further discussion of nutritional assessment.[81]

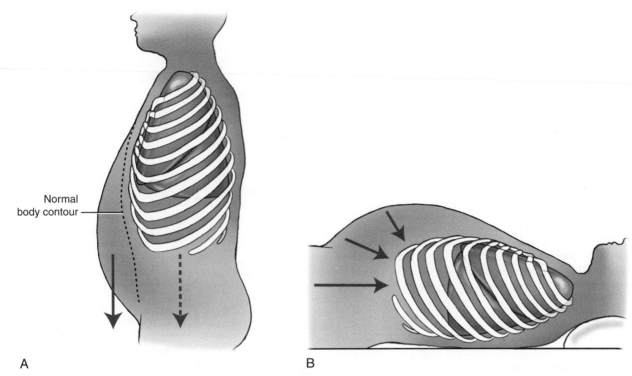

Normal
body contour

A

B

FIGURE 18-6 Effects of obesity on mechanics of breathing. **A,** In normal-weight persons, the weight of viscera is borne by the pelvic area, and the net weight force is in the direction of the *dotted arrow*. However, in obese people, the net force of the weight (*solid arrow*) is not supported by the pelvic area, and weight pulls directly down on the ribs. This favors the expiratory phase, making inspiration more difficult. **B,** In the supine position, the weight of viscera pushes up on the diaphragm, again making inspiration difficult.

SIMPLY STATED

No single measurement can determine the patient's nutritional status. A combination of the history, physical examination, and laboratory tests is often needed to determine the patient's nutritional needs.

Role of the Respiratory Therapist in Nutritional Assessment

Alert members of the patient care team not involved in direct nutritional assessment, including RTs, can contribute significantly to achieving good nutrition for patients with respiratory disorders. Signs or symptoms of potential nutritional problems should be sought during routine patient care.

In examining a patient with respiratory problems, the first step is to observe. Although malnutrition can never be diagnosed by simple inspection (except in extreme cases), much information can be learned by simply looking. During this time, various differential diagnoses can be formulated, which subsequent findings will confirm or disprove.

Inspection Findings

One should note the effects of body mass on breathing efficiency. Cachectic (nutritionally depleted) patients have readily outlined bony structures with depression of the intercostal spaces. Accessory muscles of respiration are often visible in these patients. Because severe muscle wasting can decrease lung function in those without lung disease, malnourished patients with COPD have compounded breathing difficulties. Patients who are obese have difficulty breathing in direct proportion to their excess fat weight. Obesity imposes a restrictive condition on top of whatever lung condition already exists. Figure 18-6 illustrates the effects of excess fat weight on the mechanics of breathing. Note the increased energy that must be expended during inspiration. Pregnancy can produce similar interference with the mechanics of breathing.

During inspection of the patient, the amount of effort that can be generated during coughing should be observed. Muscle weakness accompanies poor nutrition. Also, the viscosity of the sputum should be noted. This, along with jugular venous pressure (JVP) estimation, can give clues to fluid balance. Of course, in patients with right ventricular heart failure, the JVP will be elevated by factors other than simple fluid overload. In addition, a distended abdomen, as with ascites (fluid retention), may cause fluid balance as well as breathing problems. Edema of the extremities should also be noted; when present, it may require alterations in the patient's fluid and sodium intake.

Auscultation Findings

Coarse or fine crackles in the lung bases on auscultation can indicate either fluid overload or a loss of blood protein (oncotic pressure). Wheezing may be associated with some food intolerances or foods that contain yellow food coloring. As previously mentioned, alcohol can produce wheezing in some people. Aspirated food can also produce wheezing. The fine, late inspiratory crackles of atelectasis may result from decreased surfactant production resulting from malnutrition. Hearing the S_3 heart sound of congestive heart failure could suggest that fluid may be accumulating in the lungs. An S_4 heart sound can be associated with severe anemia.

Laboratory Findings

Decreases in pulmonary function measures, such as FVC or FEV_1, may indicate protein-energy deficiency or severe malnutrition. In morbidly obese patients, decreased FVC can also occur with excess adipose tissue weight because of adipose tissue's restrictive effects. Decreases in peak expiratory pressure (PEP) and peak inspiratory pressure (PIP) are also associated with poor nutrition. Altered lung compliance, as measured in the laboratory, or effective compliance, as measured when taking ventilator parameters, can result from fluid and serum albumin changes acutely or from chronic malnutrition.

Arterial blood gas (ABG) values can be altered with nutrition, as mentioned previously. Increased Pa_{CO_2} levels can result from excess parenteral infusion of glucose or simply from insufficient muscle energy to achieve adequate ventilation. The chemoreceptor set point can also be altered by changes in protein (amino acid) intake, thereby altering sensitivity to Pa_{CO_2} levels. Oxygenation parameters (oxygen saturation, oxygen content, hemoglobin) are all affected by nutritional status. Anemias can result from deficiencies in iron, folic acid, or vitamin B_{12}. Some patients may not be able to tolerate high intakes of fat or lipid infusions because of the resulting lowered Pa_{O_2}.

Changes in pH can indicate changes in dietary intake of potassium, sodium, or foods that leave an alkaline or acidic residue. Low Pa_{O_2} levels, with subsequent lactate production, can lower pH as well. As alluded to earlier, any change in the Pa_{CO_2} set point can alter acid-base balance.

The RT can become directly involved in the nutritional assessment of patients by measuring $\dot{V}_{O_2}$ in determining energy needs. In addition, the eating environment and conditions that may affect the eating process should be assessed. An effort should be made to have clean equipment in the patient's room, to empty suction bottles, and to remove or hide sputum cups during mealtimes. A prerequisite to good nutrition is a good appetite, and a good appetite is hard to invoke unless the surroundings are pleasant. The RT can further assist by helping patients receive adequate oxygen therapy during and after meals and by scheduling breathing treatments to not interfere with mealtimes. Patients who are using oxygen masks should have an order for oxygen via cannula while eating. Attending to the oxygenation of the patient is of great nutritional importance. A decrease in oxygen saturation while eating can occur in patients with severe COPD.[82] A patient who is short of breath may not eat, and if the patient does eat, food metabolism may be compromised.

A respiratory problem is rarely caused by poor nutrition alone; however, the RT will often see nutritional deficiencies complicating an existing lung problem. Being alert to the effect of nutrition on respiratory function may help stabilize the condition of a patient with lung disease that was previously deteriorating because of nutritional neglect.

KEY POINTS

▶ The use of food for energy at the cellular level requires oxygen to support a controlled combustion process that produces energy molecules of ATP, which are used in all of the body processes for energy.

▶ The metabolic rates of the tissues dictate the amount of oxygen needing to be picked up in the lungs. Oxygen uptake ($\dot{V}_{O_2}$) is a respiratory factor that can be measured in the laboratory or at the bedside.

▶ If $\dot{V}_{O_2}$ is measured while a person is in a resting state, upon awakening, the REE or RMR can be calculated.

▶ If the calorie intake is less than needed, there will be a decrease in weight, as is commonly seen in patients with COPD.

▶ Nutritional repletion in respiratory patients is often hindered by some of the necessary therapeutic actions. Bronchodilators may produce nausea; oxygen by nasal cannula disturbs the sense of smell and therefore taste because 70% of the taste of food is contributed by the sense of smell.

▶ The diaphragm, as the main muscle of respiration, needs adequate glycogen stores to be able to meet the metabolic demand of breathing, especially when the work of breathing is elevated.

▶ Protein is needed for maintaining the heart muscle, buffering acids, helping to make clotting factors in the blood, and transporting lipids and iron in the blood.

▶ Oncotic pressure (a form of osmotic pressure that tends to pull water into the blood vessels from the tissue) in the blood is maintained primarily by albumin, the major blood protein produced by the liver.

▶ Water is the major constituent of the blood and body cells. Sufficient water intake is necessary for proper circulation, clearing of waste from the body, and maintenance of blood pressure.

▶ The metabolic process can be divided into two pathways: those that break down molecules as energy is released (catabolism) and those that build up new molecules (anabolism) to be used in a structural or a functional role.

▶ The basic nutritional requirements include carbohydrate, protein, fat, vitamins, minerals, and water. Carbohydrate, protein, and fat provide the energy the body needs as well as the basic chemical skeletons on which structural and functional body systems are built.

▶ Patients with more severe COPD often do better with a higher fat content in the diet and less carbohydrate because there is less carbon dioxide production.

▶ Patients with cystic fibrosis tend to lack certain enzymes produced in the pancreas and needed for the digestion and absorption of fats. As a result, such patients generally need to take dietary supplements to compensate.

KEY POINTS—cont'd

▶ Adequate fluid intake is extremely important for patients with respiratory disorders. Proper function of the lungs' mucociliary clearance mechanism requires good hydration.

▶ The routes of nutritional administration can be either enteral or parenteral. The preferred route is enteral. If a patient is intubated and cannot take food by mouth, tube feeding is instituted through a nasogastric tube.

▶ When all other attempts at feeding are unsuccessful, the last resort is TPN. TPN is the feeding of patients by direct infusion of nutrients into either a peripheral or a central vein.

▶ The BMI is the primary method for assessment of the appropriateness of weight for a given height. The BMI is determined by weight (kg) divided by height (m^2).

▶ Cachectic (nutritionally depleted) patients have readily outlined bony structures with depression of the intercostal spaces. Accessory muscles of respiration are often visible in these patients.

▶ Patients who are obese have difficulty breathing in direct proportion to their excess fat weight. Obesity imposes a restrictive condition on top of whatever lung condition already exists.

CASE STUDY

The patient is a 58-year-old, white female presents to the emergency department (ED). She is retired from a cashier's position at a large chain store. She lives with her husband who is 59 years old and has a history of myocardial infarction (MI). Her chief complaints are extreme fatigue and difficulty completing activities of daily living (ADLs). Her past medical history reveals the following:

• Diagnosed with emphysema 4 years ago, before she had frequent episodes of bronchitis and upper respiratory infections
• Medications include ipratropium bromide and albuterol sulfate
• Smoker: 1 pack/day for more than 44 years; quit 1½ years ago
• Family history: significant for lung cancer in father and uncle
  A physical examination shows:
• General appearance: female in no acute distress
• Vitals: temperature, 98.6° C; heart rate 90 beats/min; respiratory rate, 23 breaths/min; blood pressure, 134/85 mm Hg
• Heart: regular rate and rhythm; mild jugular distension
• Neurologic: alert and oriented; cranial nerves intact
• Skin: warm and dry
• Extremities: mild pitting edema, 1+; no clubbing or cyanosis
• Chest/lungs: breath sounds decreased; on percussion, hyperresonant; wheezing with prolonged expiration; rhonchi; use of accessory muscles at rest
• Abdomen: normal exam
• Weight: 120 lb = 54.5 kg

• Height: 5 ft, 3 in
• Usual body weight: 140-150 lb (3 years ago)
• Ideal body weight: 115 lb
• BMI: healthy range
• Significant weight loss since diagnosis of COPD
• Edentulous with poorly fitting dentures

Patient was admitted to the hospital with an admitting diagnosis of acute exacerbation of COPD, increasing dyspnea, hypercapnia, rule out pneumonia

The plan includes the following:
• O_2 at 1 L/min via nasal cannula; O_2 saturation 90% to 92%
• IV fluids started at D_5 half-normal saline with 20 mEq KCl @ 75 mL/hr
• Medications: methylprednisone (Solu Medrol)
• Antibiotic: cephalosporin (Ancef)
• Bronchodilator: ipratropium bromide and albuterol sulfate
• ABGs q 6 hr, chest radiograph, sputum cultures, and Gram stain

The diagnosis is acute exacerbation of COPD with bacterial pneumonia, progressive COPD.

Laboratory Values

Chemistry Labs	FM Values	Normal Range
Albumin (g/dL)	3.3 ↓	3.5-5.0
Prealbumin (mg/dL)	15 ↓	16-40
Transferrin (mg/dL)	215	200-400
Sodium (mEq/L)	138	135-145
Potassium (mEq/L)	3.8	3.5-5.0
Chloride (mEq/L)	102	96-106
PO_4 (mg/dL)	3.3	3.0-4.5
Magnesium (mEq/L)	1.9	1.3-2.1
Total CO_2 (mEq/L)	31 ↑	23-29
Glucose (mg/dL)	90	
Total bilirubin (mg/dL)	0.5	0.3-1.9
BUN (mg/dL)	10	10-20
Uric acid (mg/dL)	4.0	3.5 and 7.2
Calcium (mg/dL)	9.3	8.5-10.2

Hematology Labs	FM Values	Normal Range
WBC × 10^3 (mm^3)	14	4.5-10
RBC × 10^6 (mm^3)	4.5	4.2-5.4
Hgb (g/dL)	11.6	12.3-15.3
Hct (%)	34.9	36.1-44.3

ABGs	Admission Values	Day 3	Normal Range
pH	7.28	7.5	7.38-7.42
$Paco_2$ (mm Hg)	51	41	38-42
Pao_2 (mmHg)	74	91	75-100
SO_2 (%)	92	95	94-100
HCO_3^- (mEq/L)	23	28	22-28

Her usual nutritional intake includes:
Breakfast: tea with sugar, ½ cup oatmeal
Lunch: ½ cup cottage cheese, small amount of canned fruit
Dinner: soup and crackers, eggs and toast
Drinking juices or caffeinated colas throughout the day
Complains of poor appetite, taste changes, and weight loss, fatigue when cooking meals.

Her nutritional diagnosis is inadequate oral/food intake and involuntary weight loss.

Interventions

Educate the patient regarding use of bronchodilators and caffeine intake.

Provide suggestions to ease preparation of foods/meals.

Increase intake of food throughout day, including small, frequent meals.

Increase nutrient density of meals and snacks without increasing volume.

Rest before and after meals.

Improve O_2 status before and after meals.

Schedule treatments at least 1 hour before meals; improve physical conditioning.

ASSESSMENT QUESTIONS

See Appendix for answers.

1. What gas is required for the optimal production of ATP?
   a. Carbon dioxide
   b. Oxygen
   c. Nitrous oxide
   d. Argon

2. Which of the following is an indicator of the energy requirements of the patient?
   a. $Pa_{O_2}/P_{A_{O_2}}$ ratio
   b. Minute ventilation
   c. $\dot{V}_{O_2}$ per minute
   d. Vital capacity

3. Which of the following is true about the REE?
   a. It requires a $\dot{V}_{O_2}$ measurement to calculate
   b. It gives an exact estimate of the patient's nutritional needs
   c. It cannot be measured in mechanically ventilated patients
   d. It should be measured daily

4. Measuring the patient's energy expenditure using oxygen consumption is referred to as which of the following?
   a. Direct calorimetry
   b. Indirect calorimetry
   c. Simple calorimetry
   d. Complex calorimetry

5. Which of the following is a pulmonary effect of starvation?
   a. Increased D_{LCO}
   b. Increased FEV_1
   c. Increased risk for pneumonia
   d. Catabolism of fats to meet glucose needs

6. Which of the following in excess quantities contributes to the most CO_2 production?
   a. Protein
   b. Carbohydrates
   c. Fat
   d. Calories

7. What element must be stored in sufficient quantities to meet the metabolic demands of the diaphragm?
   a. Arginine
   b. Glycogen
   c. 2,3-DPG
   d. Fat

8. Which of the following is true about anaerobic metabolism?
   a. It can cause a metabolic acidosis
   b. It results in reduced lactate production
   c. It results in reduced production of carbon dioxide

9. What is the RQ value of a patient on a pure carbohydrate diet?
   a. 0.60
   b. 0.70
   c. 0.85
   d. 1.00

10. In feeding the patient with pulmonary disease, how many grams of protein per kilogram of body weight are initially required?
    a. 1.5-2.0
    b. 1.2-1.5
    c. 0.8-1.0
    d. 0.6-0.8

11. Which of the following may be more difficult to achieve with a high-carbohydrate diet?
    a. Oxygenation
    b. Cellular gas exchange
    c. Oxygen transport
    d. Weaning from mechanical ventilation

12. Nitrogen balance is useful in determining:
    a. The adequacy of protein intake
    b. The adequacy of fat intake
    c. The need for vitamin supplementation
    d. Fluid and electrolyte balance

13. Which of the following is associated with a low-protein diet?
    a. Increased work of breathing
    b. Increased fixed acid load
    c. Immune compromise
    d. Increased stress on the kidneys

14. Which of the following is not associated with a high-fat diet?
    a. Increased risk for heart disease
    b. Decreased tissue oxygenation
    c. Decreased D_{LCO}
    d. Increased carbon dioxide production

15. What mineral plays a very important role in oxygen transport?
    a. Calcium
    b. Iron
    c. Zinc
    d. Magnesium

16. What route of nutritional feeding is considered as the first choice in feeding patients?
    a. Enteral
    b. Parenteral
17. Which of the following is not associated with an increased metabolism?
    a. Severe burns
    b. Severe infection
    c. Trauma
    d. Hypothyroidism
18. Which of the following might indicate poor nutritional status?
    a. BMI at normal weight
    b. Nitrogen balance
    c. Positive response to skin antigen testing
    d. Negative nitrogen balance
19. What factor may contribute to decreased colloid osmotic pressure and pulmonary edema?
    a. Hypoalbuminemia
    b. High-fat diet
    c. High magnesium levels
    d. Essential fatty acid deficiency
20. How does the cachectic patient appear physically?
    a. Central obesity only
    b. Very thin and malnourished
    c. Edematous around the face
    d. Very short of breath

References

1. Andreoli TE, Carpenter CCJ, Griggs RC, et al. *Andreoli and Carpenter's Cecil essentials of medicine.* 7th ed. Philadelphia: Saunders; 2007.
2. Gaultier C. *Lung development.* New York: Oxford University Press; 1999.
3. Girardet JPH, Viola S. Nutrition and severe chronic respiratory diseases: pathophysiologic mechanisms. *Pediatr Pulmonol Suppl* 2001;**23**:20.
4. Doley J, Mallampalli A, Sandberg M. Nutritional management for the patient requiring prolonged mechanical ventilation. *Nutr Clin Pract* 2011;**26**:232.
5. Swartz DB. Malnutrition in congestive obstructive pulmonary disease. *Respir Care Clin N Am* 2006;**12**:S21.
6. Orozco-Levi M. Structure and function of the respiratory muscles in patients with COPD: impairment or adaptation?. *Eur Respir J* 2003;**22**(Suppl. 46):415.
7. Benott RN, Bistrian B. Metabolic and nutritional aspects of weaning from mechanical ventilation. *Crit Care Med* 1989;**17**:181.
8. Budweiser S, Meyer K, Jorres RA, et al. Nutritional depletion and its relationship to respiratory impairment in patients with chronic respiratory failure due to COPD or restrictive thoracic disease. *Eur J Clin Nutr* 2008;**62**:436.
9. Murciano D, Rigud D, Pingleton S, et al. Diaphragmatic function in severely malnourished patients with anorexia nervosa: effects of renutrition. *Am J Respir Crit Care Med* 1994;**150**:1569.
10. Mason PJ, Lewis JF. Pulmonary surfactant. In: Mason RJ, Broaddus VC, Munroy JF, editors. *Textbook of respiratory medicine.* Philadelphia, PA: Elsevier Saunders; 2005.
11. Stacy KM. Pulmonary disorders. In: Urden LD, Stacy KM, editors. *Priority in critical care nursing.* 3rd ed. St. Louis: Mosby; 2000.
12. Academy of Nutrition and Dietetics. *Evidence Analysis Library, Chronic Obstructive Pulmonary Disease.* Retrieved February 24, 2012, from http://www.adaevidencelibrary.com/topic.cfm?cat=1401.
13. Wooley JA, Sax HC. Indirect calorimetry: applications to practice. *Nutr Clin Pract* 2003;**18**:434.
14. Academy of Nutrition and Dietetics. *Evidence Analysis Library, Critical Illness.* Retrieved February 25, 2012, from http://www.adaevidencelibrary.com/topic.cfm?cat=4063.
15. Lev S, Cohen J, Singer P. Indirect calorimetry measurements in the critically ill patient: facts and controversies—the heat is on. *Crit Care Clin* 2010;**26**:e1.
16. Weir JBV. New methods for calculating metabolic rate with special reference to protein metabolism. *J Physiol* 1949;**109**:1.
17. Haugen HA, Chan LN, Li F. Indirect calorimtery: a practical guide for clinicians. *Nutr Clin Pract* 2007;**22**:377.
18. Schwartz DD. Pulmonary and failure. *Contemporary nutrition support practice.* 2nd ed. Philadelphia: Saunders; 2003.
19. McClave SA, Snider HL. Use of indirect calorimetry in clinical nutrition. *Nutr Clin Pract* 1992;**7**:207.
20. Cohen RI, Marzouk K, Berkoski P, et al. Body composition and resting energy expenditure in clinically stable, non-weight losing patients with emphysema or chronic bronchitis in acute respiratory failure. *Chest* 2003;**124**:1365.
21. Mueller DH. Medical nutrition therapy for pulmonary diseases. *Krause's food and nutrition therapy.* 12th ed. St. Louis: Saunders; 2008.
22. Raguso CA, Luthy C. Nutritional status in chronic obstructive pulmonary disease: role of hypoxia. *Nutrition* 2011;**27**:138.
23. Koehler F, Doehner W, Hoernig S, et al. Anorexia in congestive obstructive pulmonary disease: association to cachexia and hormonal derangement. *Int J Cardiol* 2007;**119**:83.
24. Thorsdottir I, Gunnarsdottir I. Energy intake must be increased among recently hospitalized patients with chronic obstructive pulmonary disease to improve nutritional status. *J Am Dietetic Assoc* 2002;**102**:247.
25. Doekel RC, Zwillich CW, Scoggin CH, et al. Clinical semi-starvation: depression of hypoxic ventilatory response. *N Engl J Med* 1976;**295**:358.
26. Weissman C, Askanazi J. Nutrition and respiration. *Clin Consult Nutr* 1982;**2**(Suppl):5.
27. Fiaccadori E, Coffrini E, Fraccia C, et al. Hypophosphatemia and phosphorus depletion in respiratory and peripheral muscles of patients with respiratory failure due to COPD. *Chest* 1994;**105**:1392.
28. Sahebjami H, Vassallo CL, Wirman JA. Lung mechanics and ultrastructure in prolonged starvation. *Am Rev Respir Dis* 1978;**117**:77.
29. Lewandowski K, Lewandowski M. Intensive care in the obese. *Best Pract Res Clin Anaesthesiol* 2011;**25**:95.
30. Gieseke T, Gurushanthaiah G, Glauser FL. Effects of carbohydrates on carbon dioxide excretion in patients with airway disease. *Chest* 1977;**71**:55.
31. Sue CY, Chung MM, Grosvenor M, et al. Effect of altering the proportion of dietary fat and carbohydrate on exercise gas exchange in normal subjects. *Am Rev Respir Dis* 1989;**139**:1430.
32. Talpers SS, Romberger DJ, Bunce SB, et al. Nutritionally associated increased carbon dioxide production: excess total calories vs high proportion of carbohydrate calories. *Chest* 1992;**102**:551.
33. Saltzman HA, Salzano JV. Effects of carbohydrate metabolism upon respiratory gas exchange in normal men. *J Appl Physiol* 1971;**30**:228.

34. Hansen JE, Hartley H, Hogan RP. Arterial oxygen increase by high-carbohydrate diet at altitude. *J Appl Physiol* 1972;**33**:441.

35. Askanazi J, Rosenbaum SH, Hyman AI, et al. Respiratory changes induced by the large glucose loads of total parenteral nutrition. *JAMA* 1980;**243**:1444.

36. Swank RL, Nakamura H. Oxygen availability in brain tissues after lipid meals. *Am J Physiol* 1960;**198**:217.

37. Talbott GD. Frayser: Hyperlipidemia, a cause of decreased oxygen saturation. *Nature* 1963;**200**:684.

38. Williams AV, Higginbotham AC, Knisely MH. Increased blood cell agglutination following ingestion of fat, a factor contributing to cardiac ischemia, coronary insufficiency, and anginal pain. *Angiology* 1957;**8**:29.

39. Angelillo VA, Bedi S, Durfee D, et al. Effects of low and high carbohydrate feedings in ambulatory patients with chronic obstructive pulmonary disease and chronic hypercapnia. *Ann Intern Med* 1985;**103**:883.

40. Kuo CD, Shiao GM, Lee JD. The effects of high-fat and high-carbohydrate diet loads on gas exchange and ventilation in COPD patients and normal subjects. *Chest* 1993;**104**:189.

41. Chandra RK. Effect of vitamin and race-element supplementation on immune responses and infection in elderly subjects. *Lancet* 1992;**340**:1124.

42. Jain AM. Influence of vitamins and trace-elements on the incidence of respiratory infection. *Nutr Res* 2002;**22**:88.

43. Langkamp-Henken B, Bender BS, Gardner EM, et al. Nutritional formula enhanced immune function and reduced days of symptoms of upper respiratory tract infection in seniors. *J Am Geriatr Soc* 2004;**52**:3.

44. Chen R, Tunstall-Pedoe H, Bolton-Smith C, et al. Association of dietary antioxidants and waist circumference with pulmonary function and airway obstruction. *Am J Epidemiol* 2001;**153**:157.

45. Grievink L, Smit HA, Veer P, et al. Plasma concentrations of the antioxidants beta-carotene and alpha-tocopherol in relation to lung function. *Eur J Clin Nutr* 1999;**53**:813.

46. Wright RJ. Make no bones about it: increasing epidemiologic evidence links vitamin D to pulmonary function and COPD. *Chest* 2005;**128**:3781.

47. Grievink L, Smit HA, Ockä MC, et al. Dietary intake of antioxidant (pro)-vitamins, respiratory symptoms and pulmonary function: the MORGEN study. *Thorax* 1998;**53**:166.

48. Dietrich M, Block G, Norkus EP, et al. Smoking and exposure to environmental tobacco smoke decrease some plasma antioxidants and increase gamma-tocopherol in vivo after adjustment for dietary antioxidant intakes. *Am J Clin Nutr* 2003;**77**:160.

49. Fletcher AE, Breeze E, Shetly PS. Antioxidant vitamins and mortality in older persons: findings from the nutrition add-on study to the Medical Research Council Trial of Assessment and Management of Older People in the Community. *Am J Clin Nutr* 2003;**78**:999.

50. Bodner C, Godden D, Brown K, et al. Antioxidant intake and adult-onset wheeze: a case-control study. Aberdeen WHEASE Study Group. *Eur Respir J* 1999;**13**:22.

51. Cesari M, Pahor M, Bartali B, et al. Antioxidants and physical performance in elderly persons: the Invecchiare in Chianti (InCHIANTI) study. *Am J Clin Nutr* 2004;**79**:289.

52. Cesari M, Penninx BWJH, Lauretani F, et al. Hemoglobin levels and skeletal muscle: results from the InCHIANTI study. *J Gerontol A Bio Sci Med Sci* 2004;**59**:M249.

53. Goodman DS. Vitamin A and retinoids in health and disease. *N Engl J Med* 1984;**310**:1023.

54. Li T, Molteni A, Latkovich P, et al. Vitamin A depletion induced by cigarette smoke is associated with the development of emphysema in rats. *J Nutr* 2003;**133**:2629.

55. Michaud DA, Feskanich D, Rimm EB, et al. Intake of specific carotenoids and risk of lung cancer in 2 prospective US cohorts. *Am J Clin Nutr* 2000;**72**:900.

56. Riboli E, Norat T. Epidemiologic evidence of the protective effect of fruit and vegetables on cancer risk. *Am J Clin Nutr* 2003;**78**(Suppl):5598.

57. Kann Jr HE, Mengel CE, Smith W, et al. Oxygen toxicity and vitamin E. *Aerospace Med* 1964;**35**:840.

58. Cross CE, Hasegawa G, Reddy KA, et al. Enhanced lung toxicity of O_2: in selenium-deficient rats. *Res Commun Chem Pathol Pharmacol* 1977;**16**:695.

59. Richard C, Lemonnier F, Thibault M, et al. Vitamin E deficiency and lipoperoxidation during adult respiratory distress syndrome. *Crit Care Med* 1990;**18**:4.

60. Frank L. Antioxidants, nutrition, and bronchopulmonary dysplasia. *Clin Perinatol* 1992;**19**:541.

61. Fiaccadori E, Del Canale S, Coffrini E, et al. Hypercapnic-hypoxemic chronic obstructive pulmonary disease (COPD): influence of severity of COPD on nutritional status. *Am J Clin Nutr* 1988;**48**:680.

62. Mallampalli A. Nutritional management of the patient with chronic obstructive pulmonary disease. *Nutr Clin Pract* 2004;**19**(6):550.

63. Knekt P, Kumpulainen J, Jarvinen R, et al. Flavonoid intake and risk of chronic diseases. *Am J Clin Nutr* 2002;**76**:560.

64. Eid AA, Ionescu AA, Nixon LS, et al. Inflammatory response and body composition in chronic obstructive pulmonary disease. *Am J Respir Crit Care Med* 2001;**164**:1414.

65. Schwartz J. Role of polyunsaturated fatty acids in lung disease. *Am J Clin Nutr* 2000;**71**(Suppl):393.

66. Becker AB, Simons KJ, Gillespie CA, et al. The bronchodilator effects and pharmacokinetics of caffeine in asthma. *N Engl J Med* 1984;**310**:743.

67. Lebowitz MD. Respiratory symptoms and disease related to alcohol consumption. *Am Rev Respir Dis* 1981;**123**:16.

68. Geppert EF, Boushey HA. Case report: an investigation of the mechanism of ethanol-induced bronchoconstriction. *Am Rev Respir Dis* 1978;**118**:135.

69. Heinemann HO. Alcohol and the lung: a brief review. *Am J Med* 1977;**63**:81.

70. Dolly FR, Block JA. Increased ventricular ectopy and sleep apnea following ethanol ingestion in COPD patients. *Chest* 1983;**83**:469.

71. Chailleux E, Laaban JP, Veale D. Prognostic value of nutritional depletion in patients with COPD treated by long-term oxygen therapy: data from the ANTADIR observatory. *Chest* 2003;**123**:1460.

72. Bartolome RC, Cote CG, Marin JM, et al. The body-mass index, airflow obstruction, dyspnea, and exercise capacity index in chronic obstructive pulmonary disease. *N Engl J Med* 2004;**350**:1005.

73. Landbo C, Prescott E, Lange P, et al. Prognostic value of nutritional status in chronic obstructive pulmonary disease. *Am J Respir Crit Care Med* 1856;**160**:1999.

74. Frisancho AR. New norms of upper limb fat and muscle areas for assessment of nutritional status. *Am J Clin Nutr* 1981;**34**:2540.

75. Schols AM, Wouters EF, Soeters PB, et al. Body composition by bioelectrical impedance analysis compared with deuterium dilution and skin-fold anthropometry in patients with chronic obstructive pulmonary disease. *Am J Clin Nutr* 1991;**53**:421.

76. Gofferje H. Prealbumin and retinol-binding protein highly sensitive parameters for the nutritional state in respect to protein. *Med Lab* 1979;**5**:38.

77. Shetty PS, Jung RT, Watrasiewicz KE, et al. Rapid turnover transport proteins: an index of subclinical protein-energy malnutrition. *Lancet* 1979;**2**:230.

78. Blackburn GL, Bistrian BR, Maini BS, et al. Nutritional and metabolic assessment of the hospitalized patient. *J Parenter Enteral Nutr* 1977;**1**:11.

79. Vitale J. *Impact of nutrition on immune function: nutrition in disease series*. Columbus, OH: Ross Laboratories; 1979.

80. Strauss RG. Iron deficiency infections and immune function: a reassessment. *Am J Clin Nutr* 1978;**31**:660.

81. Peters JA, Burke K, White D. Nutrition in the pulmonary patient. In: Hodgkin JE, Zorn E, Connors G, editors. *Pulmonary rehabilitation: guidelines to success*. Woburn, MA: Butterworth; 1984.

82. Brown SE, Casciari RJ, Light RW. Arterial oxygen desaturation during eating in patients with severe chronic obstructive pulmonary disease (COPD) [abstract]. *Chest* 1979;**3**:346.

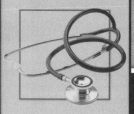

Chapter 19

Sleep and Breathing Assessment

ROBERT ALLEN AND ALBERT J. HEUER*

LEARNING OBJECTIVES

After reading this chapter, you will be able to:

1. Describe the role of the respiratory therapist in the assessment of patients for potential sleep-disordered breathing.
2. Identify the number of Americans affected by sleep disorders.
3. Describe the expected findings in the assessment of patients with sleep-disordered breathing.
4. Explain the correlation among sleep apnea, snoring, and excessive daytime sleepiness.
5. List the criteria used with the Epworth Sleepiness Scale and the Berlin Questionnaire surveys in assessing the presence of a sleep disorder.
6. Describe the normal stages of sleep with associated physiologic changes in the cardiopulmonary system.
7. List the clinical and assessment criteria for obstructive, central, and mixed sleep apnea.
8. Describe the role of a polysomnogram in providing a differential diagnosis for sleep-disordered breathing.
9. Describe the typical physiologic parameters monitored on a polysomnogram montage.
10. List the criteria used to classify sleep apnea as mild, moderate, or severe.
11. Identify the symptoms and assessment characteristics for children with sleep apnea.
12. Understanding basic treatment options and insurance coverage criteria.

KEY TERMS

apnea-hypopnea index (AHI)
arousal
Berlin Questionnaire
central sleep apnea (CSA)
EEG arousal
electroencephalogram
Epworth Sleepiness Scale
  (ESS)
excessive daytime sleepiness/
  somnolence (EDS)

hypopnea
micrognathia
mixed sleep apnea (MSA)
montage
non–rapid eye movement
obstructive sleep apnea (OSA)
polysomnogram
rapid eye movement
respiratory effort–related
  arousal (RERA)

retrognathia
sleep apnea
sleep architecture
sleep-disordered breathing
slow-wave sleep
snoring
STOP-BANG analysis
sudden infant death syndrome
  (SIDS)

---

*S. Gregory Marshal contributed some of the content of this chapter as contributor of the prior edition of this text.

According to the National Sleep Foundation, approximately 40 million Americans suffer from some type of sleep disorder. The National Heart, Lung, and Blood Institute estimates that of those with sleep disorders, nearly 18 million have some form of sleep apnea. There are more than 70 diagnosed sleep disorders. With 1 in 6 Americans afflicted with **sleep-disordered breathing** (SDB), respiratory therapists (RTs) must be prepared to identify sleep disorder symptoms in their patients. Critical thinking skills that relate a patient's known cardiopulmonary history to the presenting complaints and symptoms are key to identifying sleep-related complications or comorbidities.

RTs, sleep technologists, and sleep technicians are important members of the patient care team responsible for conducting a sleep assessments study, or **polysomnogram** (PSG), and related functions in sleep disorder centers throughout the country. RTs and sleep technicians and technologists working in these centers provide the diagnostic and therapeutic expertise needed to provide primary care physicians, board-certified sleep specialists, and other physician specialists with the information necessary to correctly diagnose and treat sleep disorders.

There are several pathways to entering the sleep profession. Although on-the-job trainees can function without licenses nor credentials in some states, an increasing number of states are requiring credentialing, licensure, or both. At least part of the reason for this is that the Centers for Medicare and Medicaid Services require that only specifically credentialed professionals, including but not limited to RTs, perform sleep studies for Medicare beneficiaries. An individual can be credentialed to perform sleep studies by several boards. The Board of Registered Polysomnographic Technologists grants the credential of Registered Polysomnographic Technologist. The American Board of Sleep Medicine (ABSM) offers credentialing as a Registered Sleep Technologist.

In addition, licensed and credentialed RTs can perform sleep studies, noninvasive positive-pressure titration, and related functions in all 50 states. Many RTs are employed in sleep disorder centers, and their specific background in ventilation, pulmonary anatomy and physiology, pharmacology, and cardiopulmonary diseases makes them valuable assets to the sleep community.

Although ideally providing physical and mental restoration, sleep may be a frustrating experience for many individuals with SDB. Worse yet, sleep disorders can actually exacerbate or compromise preexisting disease conditions during night hours and present life-threatening scenarios. This chapter provides the RT with information on normal sleep staging, the physiologic changes seen during normal sleep, the assessment of SDB, and a brief discussion of selected sleep disorders.

Normal Stages of Sleep

Although dictionary definitions of sleep may suggest a suspension of consciousness and muscular activity or a reduction of one's awareness of the environment, sleep is actually an active process with continuous stimulation of specific regions of the brain throughout the night.

Historically, sleep has been classified in various ways; however, current nomenclature recognizes only two primary states of sleep. For adults and children, the two major states of sleep are **non–rapid eye movement** (NREM) and **rapid eye movement** (REM), named for the absence and presence, respectively, of the rapid fluttering or rolling of the eyes and the loss or retention of muscle tone during each phase (Fig. 19-1). There are special states for newborns and infants up to 6 months of age because their brain wave patterns do not yet conform to standard adult classification. They include definitions such as active, quiet, and indeterminate sleep to illustrate the ambiguity of neural activity in the very young. NREM and REM stages cycle back and forth every 60 to 90 minutes for a total of four or five cycles for adults during a normal 8-hour sleeping period. With sleep occupying one third of our life, the quality and quantity of sleep have long-range health and quality-of-life implications.

Non–Rapid Eye Movement Sleep

Sleep normally begins with NREM and progresses to REM sleep. While in NREM, **electroencephalogram** (EEG) tracings demonstrate diminishing brain activity, suggesting a resting or restorative state. Until recently, NREM was described as four stages of sleep, but a recent reclassification has reduced NREM to three stages. They are differentiated by the amplitude, or wave height, and the frequency, or speed, of the EEG tracings. NREM stages are broken into N1, N2, and N3, the "N" standing for non-REM. With each progressive stage of NREM, the state of sleep is deeper.

As sleep progresses, children and adults normally begin with stage N1. During stage N1, slow rolling eye movements and low-amplitude and mixed-frequency EEG waves are noted. Only 5% to 10% of the sleep period is normally spent in N1. Within 2 to 10 minutes, sleep usually progresses to stage N2. EEG tracings show spikes called *K complexes* and *sleep spindles*. In adults, about 40% to 50% of the total sleep period is spent in stage N2.

Stage N3 (formerly stages 3 and 4) is considered the deepest stage of sleep and is about 25% of the sleep period. The EEG demonstrates **slow-wave sleep**, which is characterized by high-amplitude waves. *Delta sleep* is hypothesized to be physically restorative sleep. While in N3, sensitivity to external stimuli is diminished, and it is difficult to awaken a person out of this stage of sleep. In addition, the amount of time a person spends in N3 sleep tends to decrease with age, dropping by as much as 50% after puberty. Essential growth hormones are also released during this stage during childhood and adolescence, especially during the first half of the night.

During NREM sleep, the control of core body temperature and regulation of respiration are maintained, the respiratory rate slows, and tidal volume decreases, resulting in an

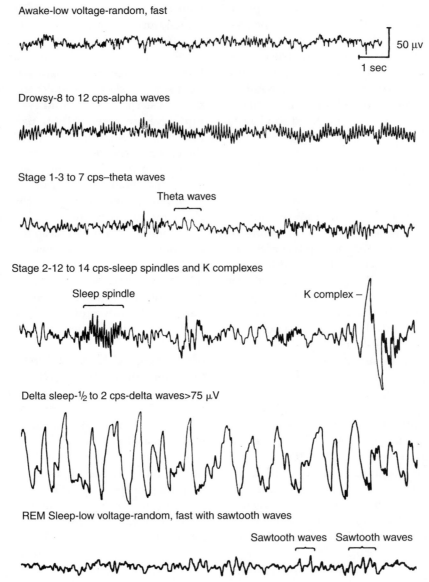

Awake-low voltage-random, fast

50 µv

1 sec

Drowsy-8 to 12 cps-alpha waves

Stage 1-3 to 7 cps–theta waves

Theta waves

Stage 2-12 to 14 cps-sleep spindles and K complexes

Sleep spindle   K complex —

Delta sleep-½ to 2 cps-delta waves>75 µV

REM Sleep-low voltage-random, fast with sawtooth waves

Sawtooth waves   Sawtooth waves

FIGURE 19-1 Human sleep stages. REM, rapid eye movement. (From Hauri P: *The sleep disorders: current concepts,* ed 2, Kalamazoo, MI, 1982, Upjohn.)

increase in arterial carbon dioxide partial pressure ($Paco_2$). As a result, the inspired minute ventilation is approximately 13% to 15% lower in NREM sleep than during wakefulness. This reduction in minute ventilation for normal human subjects causes an increase in the $Paco_2$ of 2 to 4 mm Hg. Systemic blood pressure may decrease during NREM sleep by 5% to 10% during stages N1 and N2, with a decrease of 8% to 14% during N3 sleep. With age, the percentage of time spent in stages N1 and N2 progressively increases, whereas stage N3 sleep decreases dramatically. Because stages N1 and N2 are lighter stages of sleep, a higher incidence of insomnia is understandably reported with age.

SIMPLY STATED

NREM occupies about 75% of the sleep period normally and includes restorative sleep known as slow-wave sleep.

Rapid Eye Movement Sleep

During REM, the brain is active, and dreaming almost always occurs. Throughout the night, REM episodes increase in duration and normally account for about 25% of the total sleep period. EEG tracings demonstrate low-amplitude mixed-frequency waves, similar to those seen in N1 sleep, except that patients in REM have rapid eye movements and a substantial decrease in muscle tone. At their lowest levels during REM, electromyography (EMG) monitoring of muscles of the chin (representative of skeletal muscle tone), demonstrates measurements that are similar to a paralyzed state. This partial paralysis results in a further decrease of the minute ventilation in healthy adults and children, producing associated episodes of hypoxemia and hypercapnia.

The loss of skeletal muscle tone during REM also affects pharyngeal muscles, resulting in increased upper airway resistance as pharyngeal tissues relax and the upper airway lumen is narrowed. Typically, relaxation of the tongue and soft tissues of the oropharynx are the cause of upper airway resistance that may lead to upper airway obstruction. Additionally, heart rate variability is increased, and cardiac arrhythmias are commonly seen during REM.

Characteristically during REM sleep, there is a loss of core body temperature regulation, whereas cerebral blood flow and cerebral temperature increase because of increased brain activity. Systemic blood pressure may become variable and somewhat elevated compared with levels during NREM. Understandably, the physiologic effects of REM may be more profound in patients with preexisting pulmonary or cardiac disease. Normal physiologic changes associated with REM may precipitate increased complications associated with altered ventilation, blood pressure, and heart rate for these particular patients.

SIMPLY STATED

REM occupies 25% of the sleep period and is characterized by active brain activity, dreaming, and partial paralysis of skeletal muscles.

Sleep architecture describes the pattern of various sleep stages that a patient enters throughout the night. Although the approximate percentage of sleep time spent in the three phases of NREM and REM previously described are representative of normal sleep architecture, each person has a distinct pattern particular to his or her own sleep cycle. This pattern can also vary based on the person's overall tiredness, physical excursion during waking hours, and overall lifestyle.

A histogram of the sleep architecture is part of each sleep study and visually depicts the time spent in each phase of sleep (Fig. 19-2).

SIMPLY STATED

Sleep architecture represents the sleep cycles entered during the sleep period. A histogram of the sleep architecture visually depicts the cycling of sleep stages.

In summary, during normal sleep, we begin at stage N1, progress to stage N2, and then reach stage N3 as sleep deepens. During NREM, the brain is in a state of rest, while the body can still move and respond to stimuli. Once REM sleep is initiated, the brain becomes more active, and the body experiences partial skeletal muscle paralysis, with ventilation, blood pressure, and heart rate becoming variable. Although obstructive-type breathing disorders can occur at any stage of sleep, for patients with such a disorder in REM, the soft tissues of the oropharynx relax because of partial paralysis, resulting in upper airway obstruction to airflow. With a loss of airflow and ventilation, the oxygen saturation as measured by pulse oximetry (SpO_2) declines, whereas the $PaCO_2$ rises. Because the brain is the most sensitive organ to changes in arterial oxygen partial pressure (PaO_2) and $PaCO_2$, it disrupts sleep at REM onset by "pulling the patient up" out of REM and back into stage N1 or N2 sleep. As the patient then regains muscular control in the NREM state, ventilation is restored, and PaO_2, $PaCO_2$, and pH values are more normalized; however, sleep has been disrupted to correct this acid-base balance and oxygenation issue. This disruption of sleep to restore oxygenation and acid-base balance is documented as an **EEG arousal** and usually occurs many times throughout the night.

It is understandable how physically exhausted a patient can become if every time he or she begins the transition into REM, sleep must be interrupted to resume breathing. As a result, such patients report they have not had dreams for years and experience early morning physical exhaustion and headaches as well as **excessive daytime sleepiness/somnolence (EDS)**. Sleep studies in such patients may document 400 to 600 EEG arousals per night and the absence of REM sleep. It should be apparent that when the sleep architecture is disrupted, EDS will result.

A full diagnostic PSG study is required to accurately identify a patient's sleep architecture. Once documented, RTs, sleep technologists, and sleep technicians can titrate positive airway pressure (PAP) devices to relieve SDB and return the patient to more normalized sleep architecture. The goal in the treatment of all SDB is to minimize

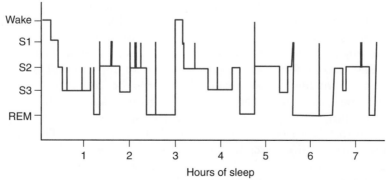

FIGURE 19-2 Histogram showing normal sleep architecture for each stage of the sleep period for a young, healthy adult. Beginning with the patient's awake state (WAKE), stage 1 NREM (S1) is followed by stage 2 NREM (S2), stage 3 NREM (S3), and REM. Note the cycling of stages throughout the sleep period between the various stages.

arousals and sleep disruptions, helping achieve normalized sleep architecture.

Assessment of Sleep-Disordered Breathing

Results of the physical examination are frequently nonspecific and unremarkable for the patient with SDB. Often, the symptoms of SDB may mimic those of other sleep disorders, leaving it hard to diagnose without proper testing. On inspection, patients most commonly present with obesity and hypertension, although many present with normal body habitus, skin coloring, and respiratory rate and no discernible features of SDB. If a severe and chronic SDB condition does exist, physical examination findings similar to cor pulmonale or congestive heart failure (CHF) may be evident. When conversing with the patient, symptoms of EDS may be present, and if left undisturbed, the patient may begin to quickly doze during an assessment. In some cases, the loss of sleep can produce lethargy or an inability to concentrate on tasks and questions.

SIMPLY STATED

Although the physical examination may appear normal for the SDB patient, the role of the RT is pivotal during routine patient assessment through questioning the patient's sleeping habits.

By far, the most common problem found in SDB is **obstructive sleep apnea (OSA)**. Sleep apnea is defined as the cessation of airflow for at least 10 seconds during sleep caused by an obstruction in the airway with increased diaphragmatic effort, a change in the EEG, or an EEG arousal, that is at least 3 seconds in length. Sleep apnea can be caused by multiple anatomic and physiologic conditions, and these aspects are discussed later. An EEG is the documented record of brain wave activity collected from electrodes placed on the head and face, using a measuring system referred to as the *international 10-20 system,* or simply "10-20," so-named because it uses percentages of 10 and 20 in relation to physical "landmarks" on the human head. The EEG waveforms are used to document brain wave activity and to identify the levels or stages of sleep during a sleep study. An EEG arousal occurs when a patient's sleep is momentarily disrupted and is documented by a change in the EEG tracings for at least 3 seconds during a sleep study. Many situations may cause an EEG arousal such as a loud noise, room temperature, a dream, body positioning in the bed, or an apnea episode. Patients will not be aware that they have sleep apnea but may comment that they often awaken from sleep with a gasp, snort, or loud snore.

One of the most common findings associated with sleep apnea is snoring. **Snoring** is the noise produced during inspiration during sleep as a result of soft tissue vibrations in the palate and pillar regions of the oropharynx. Snoring is never a healthy sign, and many snorers may eventually develop significant sleep apnea. Because patients are not aware of their snoring problem, a roommate or family member may be more likely to provide this portion of the medical history. Snoring may be the first sign of a sleep disorder in children and adults. Although families may jest about the snoring of a family member, perpetual snoring is an indicator for a medical examination and possibly a diagnostic sleep study.

Another common symptom associated with sleep apnea, and other SDBs, is EDS, which is difficulty maintaining wakefulness. Unlike sleep apnea, patients with EDS are very conscious of the fact that they have difficulty remaining awake during the day. EDS is a hallmark of sleep disorders. Everyone has experienced the difficulty of staying awake after a night of interrupted or shortened sleep. For individuals with sleep disorders, EDS is likely to be a daily experience that often interferes with the patient's ability to function. EDS ultimately increases the possibility of workplace or school accidents and has a negative impact on overall productivity.

Assessment of snoring and excessive somnolence issues can easily be obtained during the medical history and interview portion of the physical assessment. The inclusion of a few questions regarding snoring and daytime sleepiness will strengthen the assessment process and assist the RT in confirming other health-related issues associated with sleep disorders. Two instruments have been developed that can provide additional valuable information and insight. The **Epworth Sleepiness Scale (ESS)** is a tool used to assess daytime sleepiness, and the **Berlin Questionnaire** is a survey instrument used to identify risk factors associated with sleep apnea.

Epworth Sleepiness Scale

The ESS is a simple, eight-item questionnaire that measures daytime sleepiness and is essential for initial screening of sleep disorders. The ESS was developed by Dr. Murray Johns of the Epworth Hospital in Melbourne, Australia in 1991. The survey presents eight situations, and the patient is asked to rate the chances of dozing in each situation, with the value of 0 representing no chance of dozing; 1, a slight chance of dozing; 2, a moderate chance of dozing; and 3, a high chance of dozing. The sleepiness score is totaled, and if the ESS total is 1 to 6, sleep is appropriate and no EDS is noted. If the ESS total is 7 or 8, the score is considered average. An ESS score of 9 or greater indicates that the individual should consult a sleep specialist without delay because there is evidence of EDS (Fig. 19-3). The ESS questionnaire has been shown to have a high degree of reliability and internal consistency as an evaluation instrument.

Berlin Questionnaire

The Berlin Questionnaire is an outcome of the 1996 Conference on Sleep in Primary Care held in Berlin, Germany.

Epworth Sleepiness Scale

Name: _____ Today's date: _____

Your age (Yrs): _____ Your sex (Male=M, Female=F): _____

How likely are you to doze off or fall asleep in the following situations, in contrast to feeling just tired?

This refers to your usual way of life in recent times.

Even if you haven't done some of these things recently try to work out how they would have affected you.

Use the following scale to choose the most appropriate number for each situation:

> 0 = would never doze
> 1 = slight chance of dozing
> 2 = moderate chance of dozing
> 3 = high chance of dozing

It is important that you answer each question as best you can.

Situation	**Chance of Dozing (0-3)**
Sitting and reading _____	___
Watching TV _____	___
Sitting, inactive in a public place (e.g., a theatre or a meeting) _____	___
As a passenger in a car for an hour without a break _____	___
Lying down to rest in the afternoon when circumstances permit ____	___
Sitting and talking to someone _____	___
Sitting quietly after a lunch without alcohol _____	___
In a car, while stopped for a few minutes in the traffic _____	___

THANK YOU FOR YOUR COOPERATION

© M.W. Johns 1990-97

FIGURE 19-3 Epworth Sleepiness Scale (ESS) developed by Dr. M. W. Johns. An ESS score of 9 or greater suggests the need to see a sleep specialist because excessive daytime sleepiness is present. (Courtesy M. W. Johns, 1990-1997.)

More than 120 American and German pulmonary and primary care physicians developed the questionnaire from the literature to identify behaviors consistent with the presence of SDB. The focus of the instrument is deliberately limited to risk factors associated with sleep apnea. The 10-item survey is divided into three categories, with category 1 addressing snoring, category 2 identifying EDS, and category 3 assessing current blood pressure and body mass index (BMI) (Fig. 19-4). To be classified as at high risk for sleep apnea, an individual must qualify for at least two categories. The Berlin Questionnaire has a high degree of sensitivity and specificity for predicting sleep apnea in individuals.

The usefulness of the ESS and the Berlin Questionnaire is critical to the assessment of possible sleep disorder complications in the cardiopulmonary patient. Inclusion of one or both surveys during the patient assessment will provide the RT with information crucial to identifying patient symptoms. A description of signs and symptoms associated with selected SDBs is provided later in the chapter. Before focusing on specifics of SDB, the normal stages of sleep should be examined to better understand the health impact of disrupted sleep.

STOP-BANG Assessment

Created in 2008 by a group of anesthesiologists, the STOP-BANG assessment is rapidly becoming the standard for quickly and effectively identifying a person's likelihood of having obstructive sleep apnea. The questions revolve around different factors—some symptomatic, some physical

Berlin *Questionnaire*

© 1997 IONSLEEP

SLEEP EVALUATION IN PRIMARY CARE

Category 1

1. Complete the following:
Height _____ Age _____
Weight _____ Male/female ____

2. Do you snore?
☐ Yes
☐ No
☐ Don't know

If you snore:

3. Your snoring is?
☐ Slightly louder than breathing
☐ As loud as talking
☐ Louder than talking
☐ Very loud. Can be heard in adjacent rooms.

4. How often do you snore?
☐ Nearly every day
☐ 3-4 times a week
☐ 1-2 times a week
☐ 1-2 times a month
☐ Never or nearly never

5. Has your snoring ever bothered other people?
☐ Yes
☐ No

6. Has anyone noticed that you quit breathing during your sleep?
☐ Nearly every day
☐ 3-4 times a week
☐ 1-2 times a week
☐ 1-2 times a month
☐ Never or nearly never

Category 2

7. How often do you feel tired or fatigued after your sleep?
☐ Nearly every day
☐ 3-4 times a week
☐ 1-2 times a week
☐ 1-2 times a month
☐ Never or nearly never

8. During your waketime, do you feel tired, fatigued, or not up to par?
☐ Nearly every day
☐ 3-4 times a week
☐ 1-2 times a week
☐ 1-2 times a month
☐ Never or nearly never

9. Have you ever nodded off or fallen asleep while driving a vehicle?
☐ Yes
☐ No

If yes, how often does it occur?
☐ Nearly every day
☐ 3-4 times a week
☐ 1-2 times a week
☐ 1-2 times a month
☐ Never or nearly never

Category 3

10. Do you have high blood pressure?
☐ Yes
☐ No
☐ Don't know

BMI =

Scoring questions: Any answer within box outline is a positive response.

Scoring categories:
Category 1 is positive with 2 or more positive responses to questions 2-6 ☐
Category 2 is positive with 2 or more positive responses to questions 7-9 ☐
Category 3 is positive with 1 positive response and/or a BMI >30 ☐

Final result: 2 or more positive categories indicates a high likelihood of sleep disordered breathing.

FIGURE 19-4 The Berlin Questionnaire predicts risk factors associated with sleep apnea. (The Berlin Questionnaire is the outcome of the Conference on Sleep in Primary Care held in Berlin, Germany, April, 1996)

features. These symptoms and features include snoring, high blood pressure, observed pauses in breathing, daytime sleepiness, BMI, age, neck size, and gender. These factors are measured by asking eight questions. The likelihood of SDB is based on the respondent's answering greater than or less than three questions positively. The major factors considered in a **STOP-BANG analysis** are summarized in Box 19-1.

SIMPLY STATED

The ESS assesses daytime sleepiness, the Berlin Questionnaire and STOP-BANG assessment tool identify sleep apnea risk factors.

The Polysomnogram

Guidelines for conducting and evaluating sleep studies are established by the American Academy of Sleep Medicine (AASM) and specifically pertain to Medicare patients but may also provide some insight regarding best practices for all patients. The term *polysomnogram* is best understood by dissecting the word for its root meaning: *poly* means "many," *somno* means "sleep," and *gram* means "writing." Combined together, these terms mean "many sleep writings," which is an accurate description of how the test looks on the computer screen. The arrangement or configuration of the various physiologic tracings on the PSG

Box 19-1	STOP-BANG Questionnaire

1. Snoring

Do you snore loudly (louder than talking or loud enough to be heard through closed doors)?

Yes   No

2. Tired

Do you often feel tired, fatigued or sleepy during daytime?

Yes   No

3. Observed apnea

Has anyone observed you stop breathing during your sleep?

Yes   No

4. Blood Pressure

Do you have or are you being treated for high blood pressure?

Yes   No

5. BMI

Is your body mass index more than 35 kg/m^2?

Yes   No

6. Age

Are you older than 50 years?

Yes   No

7. Neck circumference

Is the circumference of your neck greater than 40 inches?

Yes   No

8. Gender

Are you a male?

Yes   No

Answering yes to three or more of these questions indicates a high likelihood for having sleep-disordered breathing.

(From Chung F, Yegneswaran B, Liao P, et al: STOP questionnaire: a tool to screen patients for obstructive sleep apnea. *Anesthesiology* 108:812-821, 2008)

the EEG tracings and scores the sleep study by staging the NREM and REM periods. All abnormal breathing, including apneas, hypopneas, arousals, and oxygen desaturations, are noted, and calculations are made relative to each event. The scored sleep study is forwarded to a physician trained in interpreting sleep studies, such as a board-certified sleep physician (D-ABSM). Sleep physicians may have a background in neurology, pulmonary medicine, internal medicine, otolaryngology, cardiology, or other related areas. Once the PSG study is interpreted, the results are returned to the prescribing physician, and the patient is informed of the results. If the PSG study demonstrates the need for treatment, such as PAP, the sleep laboratory or physician will contact a durable medical equipment (DME) company. The DME employs RTs, who will fit the patient with the proper continuous PAP (CPAP) or bilevel PAP interface (nasal mask or pillows), instruct the patient how to use the PAP equipment, and provide education on the patient's specific SDB. Patient follow-up is provided by the DME and sleep physician for PAP or treatment compliance issues. Patient compliance is important to improve quality of life as well as to help ensure equipment supplier reimbursement.

SIMPLY STATED

A sleep study continuously records physiologic data from at least 17 sources on the patient's head and body. The arrangement of these data on a single page is called a montage.

RTs and sleep technologists conducting PSG studies must strictly adhere to specific criteria to properly complete the study and titrate PAP to the appropriate treatment pressure to correct patient apneas and hypopneas. The apneas and hypopneas must be counted during each hour of the sleep study and specific calculations made. The primary index defining the presence of apneas and hypopneas is the **apnea-hypopnea index (AHI)**, or the number of hypopneas and apneas per hour of sleep time. Classifying sleep disorder severity involves many factors, but sleep specialists generally agree that the degree of AHI corresponds to the severity of sleep apnea. An AHI of less than 5 means the sleep study documented fewer than five hypopneas and apneas per hour, which is within normal range. According to the AASM, an AHI of 5 to 15 is termed *mild sleep apnea* and does not necessarily warrant treatment. An AHI of 15 to 30 describes moderate sleep apnea, and an AHI greater than 30 denotes severe sleep apnea in the adult population, both of which typically need to be treated. Other criteria and symptoms must also be considered by the sleep specialist to completely evaluate or score a patient's sleep study. Certainly, patients with a pulmonary or cardiac disease history in addition to sleep apnea will present a more complicated patient scenario and require additional assessment for treatment options.

page or screen is called a **montage**. A typical montage has a minimum of 17 channels of information or tracings, similar to an electrocardiogram (ECG) tracing (Fig. 19-5). In fact, the ECG channel is always monitored during a PSG study, along with three channels recording the EEG tracings to identify NREM or REM sleep stages, two channels documenting right and left eye movement, one channel monitoring chin movement, two channels recording right and left leg movement, and seven more channels recording snoring, airflow, thoracic-abdominal movement, SpO_2, heart rate, and body position (Fig. 19-6).

When SDB is suspected, a PSG study should be ordered directly by the physician or through a referral to a board-certified sleep specialist, and the patient is then scheduled for a sleep study. When the patient arrives at the sleep center, the RT or sleep technologist attaches electrodes with electrolyte gel in specific locations on the patient's body to gather the physiologic data during the sleep study. As the patient sleeps, the PSG records physiologic changes during the sleep period. At the conclusion of the sleep study the next morning, the patient is awakened and instructed to check with his or her prescribing physician for the final PSG report. The RT or sleep technologist then analyzes

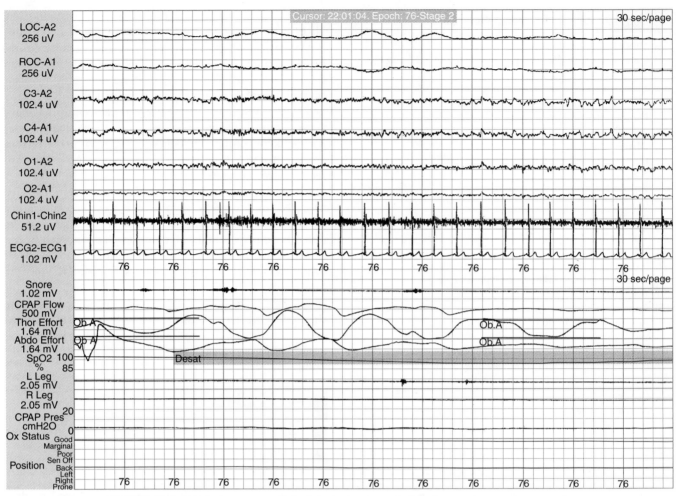

FIGURE 19-5 A typical montage of physiologic data recorded during a polysomnogram study.

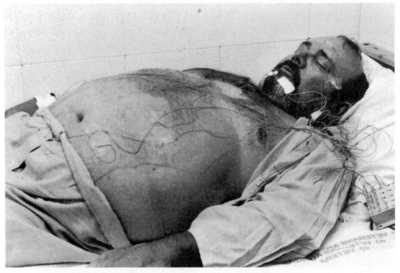

FIGURE 19-6 Patient with sleep-disordered breathing ready for a sleep study with electrodes attached to detect chest and abdominal movement, electrocardiogram (ECG) leads on the chest, electroencephalogram (EEG) leads on the head and face, electrodes above and below the eyes and on the chin and cheek, and leads going down to the right and left legs.

For infants and children, an AHI greater than 1 is considered abnormal, with an end-tidal carbon dioxide greater than 53 mm Hg or SpO_2 less than 92%. In the same way that pulmonary function tests are used to definitively diagnose the presence of chronic obstructive pulmonary disease (COPD), PSGs are used to identify SDB conditions. Whether the SDB is anatomic or neurologic, AHI determination is considered the primary factor in diagnosing SDB related to apneas and hypopneas.

SIMPLY STATED

The AHI is the primary diagnostic calculation used to confirm the presence of sleep apnea and to classify it as mild, moderate, or severe. All such patients should be assessed for the need for appropriate treatment, and those with an AHI score above 15 generally require some form of treatment.

Sleep-Disordered Breathing

With more than 70 different sleep disorders, the range of disorders can vary from insomnia and jet lag syndrome to sleep apnea and sleepwalking. Although anatomic or chemical predisposing factors may be responsible for SDB development, sleep disorders can occur at any age, may be present at birth, and warrant a PSG for proper diagnosis and treatment. The RT will frequently encounter cardiopulmonary patients with sleep disorder issues, whether diagnosed or undiagnosed. Like patients with COPD, sleep disorder patients have symptoms that may present blatantly or occultly. The role of the RT assessor is critical in identifying SDB issues for the patient and physician. This section focuses on SDB related to obstructive, central, and mixed sleep apneas as well as on the effects of snoring and upper airway resistance.

Definitions

As previously stated, one of the most distinguishing symptoms of SDB is **sleep apnea**. All forms of sleep apnea must meet stated definition criteria but can be further differentiated into three types of apnea according to the etiology: obstructive, central, and mixed. OSA is 10 seconds of apnea with continued thoracic-abdominal efforts caused by an obstruction in the airway. **Central sleep apnea (CSA)** is 10 seconds of apnea in the absence of thoracic-abdominal effort. The lack of the physiologic drive to breathe is the etiology of CSA, which is most likely to occur at sleep onset or during REM sleep. **Mixed sleep apnea (MSA)** has components of both OSA and CSA present during the sleep period.

A term associated closely with all types of apnea is **hypopnea**, defined as a reduction of airflow greater than 30% of the baseline airflow for at least 10 seconds with at least a 4% reduction in the SpO_2 or a 3% decrease or an EEG arousal of at least 3 seconds with a decrease in airflow of at least 50%. It should be noted that based on AASM recommendations, Medicare guidelines require a 4% reduction in SaO_2, regardless of arousal. If the reduction in airflow is greater than 90%, the event is scored as an apnea. Hypopneas and apneas can cause a sleep **arousal,** defined as an interruption of sleep continuity. A **respiratory effort–related arousal (RERA)** is similar to a hypopnea, but with any reduction in airflow and an oxygen desaturation of less than 3%. RERAs are classified by the EEG arousal that they cause. They tend to be caused by minor airway resistance, but not to the degree of an obstructive event, like apnea or hypopnea.

Obstructive Sleep Apnea

By far, the most common form of SDB in adults is OSA. The etiology of OSA is anatomic and may include abnormalities such as enlarged tonsils; a large tongue; a small mandible, known as **micrognathia**; a deviated septum; or a recessed lower jaw, known as **retrognathia**. As REM sleep is approached and partial paralysis of skeletal muscles occurs throughout the body, the decrease in muscle tone and relaxation of muscles throughout the oropharyngeal region result in a change in the airway lumen. Anatomic airway narrowing may also produce a complete airway obstruction, resulting in an apnea event, or a partial obstruction, producing hypopnea.

During apnea, the patient with OSA will continue to make ventilation efforts despite airway obstruction. As the diaphragm drops and negative intrapleural pressures attempt to ventilate the patient, the chest and abdomen move paradoxically, producing a seesaw movement. PSG tracings document the obstructive event by showing no airflow and active thorax contractions working in opposition of abdominal movements with a declining SpO_2 (Fig. 19-7). The drop in SpO_2 results in an EEG arousal, and the patient often gasps and sits up in bed to open the airway. If the patient was entering or in REM sleep when this event occurred, the patient would likely revert back to stage N1 or N2 sleep. Most patients are not aware that they sit up in bed, gasp, or cough but merely lie back down only to repeat the process throughout the night.

SIMPLY STATED

OSA occurs when an obstruction of airflow in the upper airway causes air movement into the lungs to cease while thoracic-abdominal efforts to breathe continue.

If the airway obstruction is partial, a hypopnea may result, and this process is repeated with only shallow, ineffective ventilation instead of an apnea event. Hypopneas frequently result in an EEG arousal and repositioning in the bed before resuming sleep (Fig. 19-8). Incomplete airway obstruction may be due to airway narrowing, such as is thought to result in RERAs (Fig. 19-9). During RERAs, the thorax and abdomen move in a diminished, asynchronous manner, although the SpO_2 remains stable. RERAs usually result in an EEG arousal, and the patient's sleep stage is disrupted.

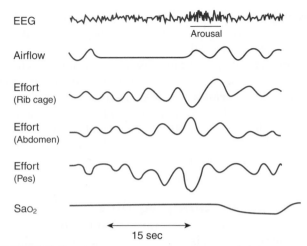

FIGURE 19-7 Polysomnogram representation of obstructive sleep apnea with absence of airflow for 10 seconds and paradoxic movement of the rib cage and abdomen in response to an obstructed airway. The electroencephalogram arousal signals the patient gasping for breath to reestablish the airway and resume ventilation. (From Kacmarek RM, Stoller JK, Heuer AJ: *Egan's fundamentals of respiratory care,* ed 10, St. Louis, 2013, Mosby.)

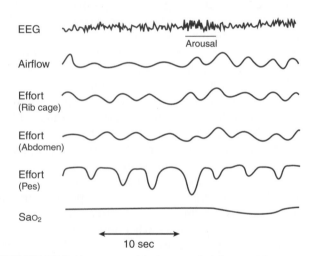

FIGURE 19-8 Hypopnea with decreased airflow and increasing respiratory efforts until an electroencephalogram arousal occurs to awaken the patient as the airway is reestablished. (From Kacmarek RM, Stoller JK, Heuer AJ: *Egan's fundamentals of respiratory care*, ed 10, St. Louis, 2013, Mosby.)

Mallampati Score

The Mallampati score was first described by Dr. S. R. Mallampati to categorize the amount of open space in the oropharynx when certain anatomic structures are visualized by looking in the mouth. Scoring of the Mallampati from direct visualization is as follows: class 1—full visibility of tonsils, uvula, and soft palate; class 2—visibility of hard and soft palate, upper portion of tonsils, and uvula; class 3—soft and hard palate and base of the uvula are visible; and class 4—only hard palate is visible (Fig. 19-10). A Mallampati score of class 1 would be considered normal. Because of the high association of OSA and oropharyngeal lumen space, a

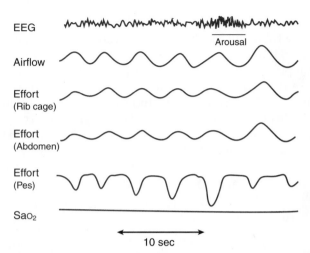

FIGURE 19-9 Respiratory effort–related arousal in which airflow, chest, and abdominal movements appear normal, but respiratory efforts increase until an electroencephalogram arousal reestablishes the airway. (From Kacmarek RM, Stoller JK, Heuer AJ: *Egan's fundamentals of respiratory care*, ed 10, St. Louis, 2013, Mosby.)

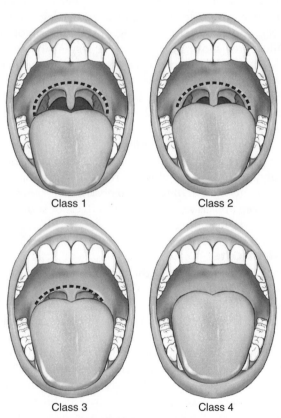

FIGURE 19-10 Mallampati scores.

high Mallampati score has been correlated with a high risk for OSA, especially in the presence of nasal obstruction.

SIMPLY STATED

The Mallampati score can be easily determined through assessment and a class 3 or 4 score is highly associated with OSA issues.

Signs, Symptoms, and Additional Health Consequences

Symptoms and signs of OSA in adults may include loud snoring, apnea periods (as reported by sleep partners), chronic morning tiredness regardless of the length of sleep, EDS, morning headaches, recent weight gain, limited attention, memory loss, changes in judgment or personality, lethargy or sluggishness, hyperactive behavior, the need to take naps, depression, slowed responses, decreased libido, frequent falling asleep while driving, high blood pressure, automatic behavior (performing actions by rote), and swelling of the feet or legs. Symptoms associated with apnea and hypopnea are generally most profound when the sleeping patient is supine and can be worsened if the patient is suffering from sleep deprivation, has consumed alcohol before going to bed, or has used sedatives.

In addition to the signs and symptoms of OSA, the additional health consequences of untreated OSA are significant. Beyond daytime somnolence, disruption of normal sleep cycles can result in impaired mental function as well as psychosocial problems. In addition, arterial desaturation during apneic episodes can place stress on the organ systems, including the pancreas, which may contribute to development or worsening of diabetes. It is also suspected that disruption of sleep-wake cycles may increase the release of stress hormones, including sympathetic mediators, which can increase both blood pressure and heart rate. Furthermore, decreases in alveolar ventilation during repeated apneic periods can contribute to pulmonary vasoconstriction and polycythemia, which can lead to cor pulmonale. Other consequences include erectile dysfunction and a decreased libido, coronary artery disease, myocardial infarction, heart failure, and stroke.

Box 19-2 summarizes the signs, symptoms, and other health consequences of untreated OSA.

OSA has historically been found most frequently in elderly obese men with a neck size greater than 17 inches and with a shortened neck. Heavy snoring that begins soon after falling asleep is the classic picture of a patient with OSA. Typically, the snoring becomes louder and is then interrupted by a period of apnea followed by a loud snort or gasp. After reestablishing the airway, snoring returns, and the cycle repeats. The snoring and gasping events may drive the spouse or sleep partner from the bed to another room. Some assessments note whether the sleep partner sleeps one room, two rooms, or three rooms away from the snoring patient. Risk factors associated with worsening of OSA include a BMI of 25 or higher, alcohol consumption before bedtime, smoking, nasal congestion at night, and large tonsils (Box 19-3).

Physical Assessment

When assessing the patient with OSA, the RT or other member of the patient care team may note physical signs such as EDS, lethargy, poor concentration, obesity, large or short neck, or retrognathia or micrognathia. If SDB is

---

Box 19-2 Obstructive Sleep Apnea Quick Facts

SIGNS AND SYMPTOMS OF UNTREATED OSA
- Habitual, loud snoring
- Breathing pauses while asleep
- Falls asleep while driving
- Struggles to stay awake when inactive, such as when watching television or reading
- Difficulty paying attention or concentrating at work, school, or home
- Performance problems at work or school
- Often told, "you look sleepy"
- Difficulty remembering information
- Slowed responses
- Difficulty controlling emotions
- Need to take naps almost every day
- Morning tiredness and feeling a lack of rest even after sleeping
- Morning headaches
- Depression

CONSEQUENCES OF UNTREATED OSA
- Daytime sleepiness impairing ability to operate machinery or a vehicle
- Decreased physical performance
- Decreased academic performance due to attention issues
- Diabetes
- Psychosocial problems
- Erectile dysfunction and decreased libido
- Decreased ability to concentrate
- Reduced quality of life
- High blood pressure
- Coronary artery disease
- Myocardial infarction
- Cor pulmonale
- Heart failure
- Stroke

Box 19-3 Risk Factors for OSA

- Excessive body weight (BMI ≥25)
- Alcohol consumption before bedtime
- Smoking
- Nasal congestion at night
- Increased neck size (≥17 inches in males and ≥16 inches in females)
- Large tonsils
- Males >40 years of age

BMI, body mass index.

---

suspected, the patient should be questioned about his or her sleep habits and either the STOP-BANG assessment, ESS, or Berlin Questionnaire should be completed by the patient. During the physical examination, the patient's throat should be visualized and the Mallampati score documented. Systemic arterial blood pressure is elevated in more than 50% of patients with OSA, and the resting blood pressure should be assessed. Finally, signs of CHF and pulmonary hypertension should be assessed by inspection and palpation.

As indicated earlier, untreated OSA can lead to multiple organ and system dysfunction. As a result, the RT or other clinician should be on the alert for long-term health consequences of untreated OSA, including pulmonary hypertension, right heart failure, CHF, polycythemia, insulin resistance, and hyperinsulinemia. In addition, a wide variety of cardiac dysrhythmias are commonly seen in OSA patients, with swings from bradycardia to tachycardia during apnea and hypopnea events. Finally, cerebrovascular accident and hypertension are twice as likely to develop in OSA patients compared with healthy subjects of the same age. RTs and other clinicians should be aware of these conditions associated with OSA because with proper diagnosis and treatment, they can be effectively treated in most cases.

Children and Infants with OSA

As with adults, the primary symptom of OSA in children is snoring. The presentation of OSA in children and infants is quite different from that in adults. Certainly, anatomic features of the airway lumen are the primary issue, but OSA can be found in children of any body size. Symptoms are also quite different from those in adults, and the clinical features addressed in the ESS and Berlin Questionnaire are not applicable to children. Children with OSA may present as sleepy or hyperactive, which may confuse parents and teachers. Additionally, OSA may cause children to exhibit social withdrawal, poor academic performance, and aggressive behavior.

> **SIMPLY STATED**
>
> Children with OSA present with different symptoms than expected with adults and may include hyperactivity, aggressive behavior, social awkwardness, poor attention span, poor academic performance, or characteristics of attention deficit/hyperactivity disorder (ADHD).

Central Sleep Apnea

As previously mentioned, CSA is sleep apnea in which there is a lack of thoracic-abdominal effort for at least 10 seconds (Fig. 19-11). The basis for apnea is not due to obstruction of the airway; rather, it is the physiologic lack of the drive to breathe. CSA is responsible for only about 10% of all adult SDB but is more common in children and infants. CSA is observed most often in stage 1 NREM or during REM sleep. The cause of CSA can be quite varied and complex. The neurologic control of breathing, located in the brainstem, may be injured because of stroke, brainstem lesion, encephalitis, neurodegeneration, radiation treatments to the cervical spine region, or CHF.

The drive for ventilation, called the *hypercapnic drive*, is normally controlled by the amount of CO_2 dissolved in the blood. The secondary, or backup, ventilation drive mechanism, termed the *hypoxic drive*, is based on the amount of

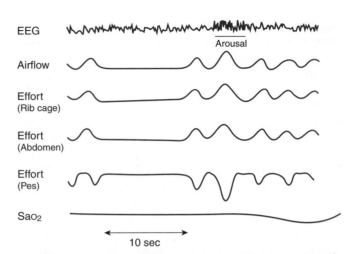

FIGURE 19-11 Central sleep apnea in which there is cessation of airflow for at least 10 seconds in the absence of thoracic and abdominal movement until an electroencephalogram arousal resynchronizes respiratory effort. (From Kacmarek RM, Stoller JK, Heuer AJ: *Egan's fundamentals of respiratory care*, ed 10, St. Louis, 2013, Mosby.)

oxygen in the blood. During sleep, both the hypoxic and hypercapnic ventilatory drive mechanisms are suppressed. It is thought that, during sleep, the control of ventilation is closely associated with metabolic pathways, making body chemistry primarily responsible for ventilation.

> **SIMPLY STATED**
>
> CSA results from a lack of physiologic stimulation to breathe causing cessation of airflow and is characterized by the absence of thoracic-abdominal efforts.

Signs and Symptoms

The signs of CSA are not as apparent as those of OSA. Individuals with CSA are most often not obese and do not have a large neck circumference size. Snoring is not usually present; however, EDS may be reported as a result of the lack of restorative sleep from frequent awakenings during apnea periods. Because CSA is closely associated with neurologic issues, patients may report symptoms such as difficulty swallowing, a change in the ability to use their voice, or other body weakness or numbness. Any of these neurologic symptoms should be immediately reported to a physician for complete assessment and diagnostic investigation.

One of the more common signs of CSA is the presence of Cheyne-Stokes respirations. Cheyne-Stokes respirations are periodic breathing in which respiratory efforts gradually increase in depth and frequency, followed by a decrease in depth and frequency punctuated by an apneic period. The pattern of increasing and decreasing depth and rate is also known as the *waxing and waning pattern*. The proper way to describe the Cheyne-Stokes event during an assessment is to record the time of the waxing and waning phase and the apneic episode. It is not uncommon for the apnea periods or waxing and waning phases to vary, with each cycle lasting 30 seconds to 2 minutes in length.

Children with Central Sleep Apnea

Although CSA is much less common in children, it is often found in premature infants born before 37 weeks' gestation. CSA is also found with congenital cardiac disorders that cause an elevation of the $Paco_2$. As with adults, hypercapnic drive centers in the brainstem may be insensitive or too immature to trigger corrective breathing commands to respiratory muscles, resulting in periods of apnea. Multiple disorders may precipitate CSA in children and infants, including neuromuscular, neurologic, metabolic, gastrointestinal, or hematologic abnormalities or an infection with an accompanying fever.

Sudden infant death syndrome (SIDS) is thought by some experts to be associated with CSA, but no clinical evidence that the two are linked has been presented to date. SIDS is defined as "the sudden death of an infant under 1 year of age, which remains unexplained after a thorough case investigation, including performance of a complete autopsy, examination of the death scene, and review of the clinical history." Although the etiology is unknown, the majority of reported SIDS cases occur in the first 6 months of age, with a peak incidence between 2 and 4 months of age. SIDS has been shown to have a familial relationship to OSA, positional sleeping, and families with a history of apparent life-threatening events rather than CSA. Recent SIDS research during the past decade has linked it to significant risk factors such as prone sleeping position, bed sharing, maternal substance abuse, and cigarette smoking. Despite a decrease in SIDS incidence of 38% in the United States, it remains the leading cause of death in children younger than 1 year.

Mixed Sleep Apnea

As the name implies, MSA is the combination of OSA and CSA in the same patient. Typically, the diagnostic sleep study presents with a CSA component initially, followed by an OSA phase (Fig. 19-12). In some cases, as PAPs are being titrated for a patient to relieve the obstructive apneas, an underlying CSA episode is seen. Without the PSG diagnostic and titration study, MSA is virtually impossible to confirm. Once the MSA patient's OSA component is treated with PAP, the CSA component can be addressed by providing a backup rate controller on the PAP device. Use of pharmaceuticals to relieve CSA symptoms may be attempted empirically, but complete resolution is difficult and challenging at best.

Comparison of the PSG tracing of airflow through the nose or mouth with respiratory effort tracings is the primary way to differentiate among OSA, CSA, and MSA. During OSA, the obstructed airway results in the cessation of airflow while respiratory efforts continue. During CSA, neither airflow nor respiratory efforts are present. With MSA, the tracings reflect the typical CSA lack of airflow or respiratory effort followed by respiratory effort and no airflow, as seen with OSA.

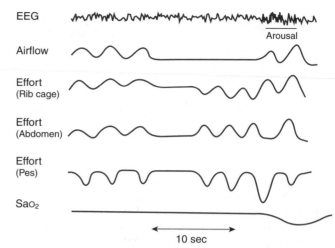

FIGURE 19-12 Mixed sleep apnea in which an initial central sleep apnea episode gives way to an obstructive sleep apnea episode until an electroencephalogram arousal reestablishes the airway and resynchronizes respiratory efforts. (From Kacmarek RM, Stoller JK, Heuer AJ: *Egan's fundamentals of respiratory care,* ed 10, St Louis, 2013, Mosby.)

SIMPLY STATED

MSA is a combination of OSA and CSA. When OSA is treated, CSA remains the cause of sleep apnea.

KEY POINTS

▸ Assessment skill development and awareness of the impact of unidentified and untreated sleep disorders are more critical than ever. During the patient interview and assessment process, a few simple questions regarding the quality and quantity of the patient's sleep may redirect the physical assessment.

▸ Approximately 1 in 6, or more than 40 million, Americans suffers from some type of sleep disorder, with an estimated 18 million having some form of sleep apnea.

▸ RTs are valuable assets to the sleep community because they are a major segment of the workforce conducting sleep studies in sleep disorder centers throughout the country, and they have a unique background in ventilation, pulmonary anatomy and physiology, pharmacology, and cardiopulmonary diseases.

▸ Although the results of inspection, palpation, percussion, and auscultation during a physical assessment are frequently nonspecific and unremarkable for the patient with SDB, the associated signs and symptoms are quite specific and may include EDS, lethargy, poor concentration, obesity, large or short neck, retrognathia or micrognathia, morning headache, loss of memory or concentration, recent weight gain, erectile dysfunction, nocturnal enuresis, pedal edema, or general tiredness regardless of how many hours of reported sleep.

▸ Diagnostically, sleep apnea is defined as the cessation of airflow for at least 10 seconds during sleep caused by an obstruction in the airway. Although patients may be unaware they have sleep apnea, it is likely they have been told they snore.

▸ Snoring is the noise produced during inspiration during sleep as a result of soft tissue vibrations in the palate and pillar regions of the oropharynx and may eventually lead to the development of significant sleep apnea.

KEY POINTS—cont'd

▶ EDS is difficulty staying awake during the day. Patients with sleep apnea will be very conscious of the effects of daytime somnolence on their lifestyle.

▶ The ESS is an eight-item questionnaire that measures daytime sleepiness for the initial screening of sleep disorders. The Berlin Questionnaire focuses on the risk factors associated with sleep apnea and has a high degree of sensitivity and specificity for predicting sleep apnea.

▶ The STOP-BANG assessment is rapidly becoming the standard for a quick way to effectively identify a person's likelihood of having obstructive sleep apnea.

▶ The two major states of sleep, NREM and REM, cycle back and forth every 60 to 90 minutes for a total of four or five cycles during a normal 8-hour sleeping period. Usually, sleep begins at stage 1 NREM, progresses to stage 2, and is followed by stage 3 NREM as sleep deepens. During NREM, the brain is in a state of rest while the body can still move and respond to stimuli.

▶ As REM sleep is initiated, the brain becomes more active, and the body experiences partial skeletal muscle paralysis with changes in ventilation, blood pressure, and heart rate.

▶ During an OSA event, the obstructed airway results in the cessation of airflow while respiratory efforts continue. With CSA, neither airflow nor respiratory efforts are present; and in MSA, the tracings reflect the typical CSA lack of airflow or respiratory effort, followed by respiratory effort and no airflow as seen with OSA.

▶ A typical montage has a minimum of 17 channels of physiologic data, including ECG, EEG, right and left eye movement, chin movement, right and left leg movement, snoring, airflow, thoracic movement, abdominal movement, SpO_2, heart rate, and body position.

▶ Based on the PSG study, a calculated AHI of less than 5 is considered within normal range. Mild sleep apnea is defined by an AHI of 5 to 20, moderate sleep apnea describes an AHI between 20 and 40, and an AHI greater than 40 denotes severe sleep apnea in adults.

▶ The primary symptom of OSA in children is snoring, but children with OSA may present as hyperactive or sleepy; exhibit social withdrawal, poor academic performance, or aggressive behavior; or may be misdiagnosed as having ADHD.

▶ Beyond daytime somnolence, disruption of normal sleep cycles that comes with OSA can result in impaired mental function, psychosocial problems, diabetes, hypertension, heart failure, stroke, and other conditions.

CASE STUDY

A 23-year-old male who plays football for a local university as a defensive lineman has difficulty staying awake in class and in football meetings, where he quickly falls asleep. Complaining of severe fatigue, he visited his attending physician. A teammate accompanying him states that when the team is on road trips, none of the other team members can sleep in the same room with him because of his very loud snoring with pauses in breathing and gasping. He has a present medical history of hypertension and a past history of a nasal fracture, which was corrected with nasal

surgery. His physician ordered a diagnostic sleep study to determine the potential presence of SDB.

Physical Assessment

The patient is 76 inches tall and weighs 350 lb for a BMI of 42.6 kg/m². He is a nonsmoker who consumes one caffeinated beverage daily and three to four alcoholic beverages weekly. He gets regular exercise 4 days per week. His vital signs at rest are blood pressure: 145/88 mm Hg; respiratory rate: 26 breaths/minute; and heart rate: 112 beats/minute.

On inspection, the patient has a short, 19-inch neck. His enlarged tonsils and the narrowed hypopharynx result in a Mallampati score of class 3, and he appears to be primarily a mouth breather. Chest assessment reveals a large, muscular thorax with normal, bilateral chest wall movement noted. There is no digital clubbing or cyanosis present. Palpation reveals bilateral chest wall movement with normal intercostal spacing for thorax size. Tactile fremitus is somewhat diminished because of the large BMI. Percussion is all within normal limits for thorax size. Auscultation reveals somewhat diminished but normal breath sounds. No abnormal heart sounds were noted.

The ESS and Berlin Questionnaire were administered, with an ESS score of 22 and three positive categories for the Berlin survey. When asked to comment on his sleeping habits, he stated that he is always tired regardless of how much time he spends in bed trying to get rest. The patient also stated that he usually awakes about 2:00 or 3:00 AM and has a difficult time going back to sleep. He stated he has difficulty driving during the day or night without "dozing at the wheel."

Polysomnogram

A complete PSG with a digital sleep system was used, along with the international 10-20 system of electrode placement for recording EEG, EMG, electro-oculogram (EOG), ECG, respiratory effort, oximetry, body position, airflow, snoring sound, pulse rate, and limb movement channels. Sleep study results revealed the following:

Total REM sleep	16% (normal 15%-20%)
Stage 1 NREM	6.1% (normal 5%-10%)
Stage 2 NREM	63% (normal 40%-50%)
Stage 3 NREM	14.9% (normal 25%)

Interpretation and Impression

The patient meets diagnostic criteria for OSA, upper airway resistance, periodic limb movement syndrome, and primary snoring. Severe OSA is present with an AHI of more than 40. The arousal index of 76.1 per hour substantiates the patient's complaint of EDS. Sleep distribution and sleep architecture are abnormal and consistent with frequent arousals. Delta sleep during stage 3 NREM is limited, with prolonged stage 2 NREM sleep.

Recommendations

• PAP titration PSG study ordered
• Clinical follow-up
• Dietary consultation not appropriate at this time because of sports involvement

CASE STUDY

A 44-year-old female who complains of chronic fatigue and morning headaches made an appointment with her physician. Her husband states that she snores very loudly during the night with frequent pauses in her breathing that frighten him. He has tried to awaken her to take a deep breath, but sometimes it takes several attempts to wake her up. He is not resting well himself because of her sleeping habits. Her present medical history includes hypertension, hypothyroidism, and CHF. After the patient interview and assessment, her physician ordered a split-night PSG study that will include a diagnostic sleep study and a PAP titration trial, if indicated.

Physical Assessment

The patient is 61 inches tall and weighs 235 pounds for a BMI of 63.5 kg/m^2. She is a nonsmoking mother of two teenagers who consumes six to seven caffeinated beverages daily and one to two alcoholic beverages weekly. She does not regularly exercise. Her resting vital signs are blood pressure: 162/90 mm Hg; respiratory rate: 24 breaths/minute and heart rate: 122 beats/minute.

On inspection, she has a short, thick neck that is 17.5 inches in circumference. She has large tonsils, a large tongue, and a long uvula with a Mallampati score of class 4. Her neck and throat area seem enlarged for her body size. Chest assessment reveals normal, bilateral movement with no digital clubbing or cyanosis. All other findings are within normal limits. Her feet and legs appear to be edematous. Palpation reveals bilateral chest wall movement and diminished tactile fremitus. Her feet and legs show 2+ pitting edema. Percussion is all within normal limits, and auscultation reveals diminished, normal breath sounds. A pronounced P$_2$ heart sound is noted over the precordium.

The ESS score for the patient was 18, and she had three positive categories for the Berlin survey, indicating EDS and significant sleep apnea factors, respectively. She also states she was diagnosed with hypothyroidism several years ago but has not been taking her medication. She reports a weight gain of 60 lb in the past 3 years.

Polysomnogram

A standard PSG study with a digital sleep system was performed with the international 10-20 system of electrode placement for recording EEG, EMG, EOG, ECG, respiratory effort, oximetry, body position, airflow, snoring sound, pulse rate, and limb movement channels. After 4 hours, the sleep study results revealed the following:

Total REM sleep	2% (normal 15%-20%)
Stage 1 NREM	4% (normal 5%-10%)
Stage 2 NREM	76% (normal 40%-50%)
Stage 3 NREM	18% (normal 25%)

Pretreatment Interpretation and Impression

The patient meets diagnostic criteria for OSA, hypoxemia, upper airway resistance, absence of REM sleep, periodic limb movement syndrome, and primary snoring. Severe OSA is present with an AHI of more than 40. The arousal index of 83.4 per hour substantiates the patient's complaint of EDS. Sleep distribution and sleep architecture are abnormal, consistent with frequent arousals. Delta sleep during stage 3 NREM is limited with prolonged stage 2 NREM sleep, and REM sleep is absent.

Pap Titration Study

After the 4-hour PSG study, the technician fitted the patient with an appropriate nasal CPAP mask, and after lights out, the patient was returned to sleep. At 12:35 AM, CPAP was initiated at 5 cm H$_2$O and increased incrementally to BiPAP of 19/16 cm H$_2$O. At this level of PAP support, only one hypopnea was recorded, and the AHI was reduced to 2.4; normal is less than 5. The lowest SpO$_2$ recorded at this setting was 92%, and the mean SpO$_2$ was 94%. The therapeutic pressure to reverse sleep apnea was a BiPAP setting of 19/17 cm H$_2$O.

Recommendations

- BiPAP for home use with a preset pressure of 19/17 cm H$_2$O
- Clinical follow-up
- Dietary consultation with nutritionist
- Consult with endocrinologist for thyroid condition
- Consult with cardiologist for CHF
- Recommend exercise program

ASSESSMENT QUESTIONS

See Appendix for answers.

1. Which of the following will assist the RT in predicting sleep apnea?
   a. ESS
   b. Berlin Questionnaire
   c. Inspection of the chest
   d. ECG
2. All of the following are symptoms of OSA in adults, except:
   a. Morning headaches
   b. Memory loss
   c. Hyperactive behavior
   d. Depression
3. In which stage of sleep is "restorative sleep" thought to occur?
   a. Stage 1 NREM
   b. Stage 2 NREM
   c. Stage 3 NREM
   d. REM
4. To meet the definition criteria for sleep apnea, how many seconds of airflow cessation during sleep must be documented?
   a. 4 seconds
   b. 6 seconds
   c. 8 seconds
   d. 10 seconds

5. Which of the following is not a physiologic parameter routinely monitored during the PSG study?
   a. SpO$_2$
   b. ECG
   c. EEG
   d. Right and left arm

6. If on assessment the Mallampati score is class 4, the patient would be at high risk for which type of SDB?
   a. CSA
   b. OSA
   c. MSA
   d. SIDS

7. A reduction in airflow greater than 30% 10 seconds during sleep defines which of the following?
   a. Apnea
   b. RERA
   c. Arousal
   d. Hypopnea

8. Which of the following diagnostically defines the presence of moderate sleep apnea?
   a. AHI of 3
   b. AHI of 12
   c. AHI of 28
   d. AHI of 44

9. Which of the following is not true regarding SIDS?
   a. Involves infants younger than 1 year
   b. Peaks at 8 months of age
   c. Familial relationship to OSA
   d. Incidence has decreased by 35% in the United States

10. Which of the following is the first sign of SDB?
    a. Snoring
    b. EDS
    c. Obesity
    d. Hypertension

Bibliography

Chung F, Yegneswaran B, Liao P, et al. STOP questionnaire: a tool to screen patients for obstructive sleep apnea. *Anesthesiology* 2008;**108**:812–21.

Farney RJ, Walker BS, Farney RM, et al. The STOP-BANG equivalent model and prediction of severity of obstructive sleep apnea: relation to polysomnographic measurements of the apnea/hypopnea index. *J Clin Sleep Med* 2011;**7**:459.

Kacmarek RM, Stoller JK, Heuer AJ. *Egan's fundamentals of respiratory care*. 10th ed. St. Louis: Mosby-Elsevier; 2012.

Liistro G, Rombaux P, Belge C, et al. High Mallampati score and nasal obstruction are associated risk factors for obstructive sleep apnea. *Eur Respir J* 2003;**21**:248.

Sharma BR. Sudden infant death syndrome: a subject of medicolegal research. *Am J Forensic Med Pathol* 2007;**28**:69.

Spriggs WH. *Principles of polysomnography*. 1st ed. Salt Lake City: Sleep Ed; 2003.

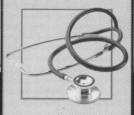

Chapter 20

Home Care Patient Assessment

ALBERT J. HEUER

CHAPTER OUTLINE

The Evolution and Importance of Respiratory
    Home Care
The Home Care Patient
Home Care Assessment Tools
    and Resources
Role and Qualifications of the Home Care
    Respiratory Therapist

Assessment and the Home Visit
    Initial Visit and Assessment
    Home Care Equipment
    Patient Education and Training
    Plan of Care
    Follow-Up Care
    Discharging the Patient

LEARNING OBJECTIVES

After reading this chapter, you will be able to:
1. Describe the evolution and advantages of respiratory home care.
2. Explain the several major legislative and policy guidelines affecting home respiratory care.
3. Identify the type of patients who receive home respiratory care.
4. Describe the role of the respiratory therapist in home care.
5. List major tools and resources used in respiratory home care assessment.
6. Identify the key elements involved in assessing the respiratory home care patient.
7. Identify the components of the initial evaluation of the patient and home environment.
8. Describe respiratory equipment commonly used to assess and treat patients at home.
9. Review the guidelines for qualifying a patient for home oxygen therapy reimbursement.
10. Explain the purpose and the procedure for developing a plan of care.
11. Describe strategies for educating patients in the home setting.
12. Explain the importance of follow-up care.

KEY TERMS

Centers for Medicare and
    Medicaid Services (CMS)
home medical equipment
    (HME)

Hospital Consumer
    Assessment of Healthcare
    Providers and Systems
    (HCAHPS)

plan of care
respiratory home care
The Joint Commission

L egislation that established Medicare in the 1960s also introduced a reimbursement structure for health care services provided in the home and at other alternative settings. More recently, the implementation of governmental policies and formal legislation has provided incentives to help successfully provide care for patients with chronic disease outside of the acute care setting. More specifically, the **Hospital Consumer Assessment of Healthcare Providers and Systems (HCAHPS)** survey process has been adopted and implemented by the **Centers for Medicare and Medicaid Services (CMS).**

Under HCAHPS, health care providers receive financial rewards for positive outcomes, including appropriately providing care for patients at home and preventing hospital readmissions. Provisions of the Patient Protection and Affordable Care Act of 2010 further strengthen the implications for adherence to HCAHPS and optimizing outcomes. It is because of these provisions and other trends, including the aging population, that the number of patients receiving care at home increased to more than 10 million in 2010, this trend is likely to continue in the future.[1]

Many patients needing home care suffer from respiratory conditions such as chronic obstructive pulmonary disease (COPD), which is ranked as the third most common cause of death in the United States.[2,3] Patients with acute exacerbations of diseases, such as COPD, asthma, and cystic fibrosis, are initially treated in a hospital or a similar facility. However, a common goal of the care plan for such patients and the purpose of incentives under HCAHPS is to successfully treat their acute illness and discharge them to the home setting or other alternate site, and to help prevent readmission to the hospital. Not surprisingly, home care is not only cost-effective but also enhances patients' quality of life, can have a positive influence on their psychosocial well-being, and minimizes their exposure to nosocomial infections and in-hospital hazards.

The American Association for Respiratory Care (AARC) defines **respiratory home care** as "prescribed respiratory services provided in a patient's personal residence." It should be noted that the term *home care* is not limited to care provided in a patient's house, condo, or apartment and may also include other forms of personal residences, such as group homes and assisted living facilities. In addition, many of the concepts in this chapter can be applied to other alternative settings such as skilled nursing facilities. The AARC also states in regard to home care that "prescribed respiratory care services include, but are not limited to, patient assessment and monitoring, diagnostic and therapeutic modalities and services, disease management and patient and caregiver education."[4] On the surface, these services may appear to be similar to those provided in traditional acute care facilities. However, the way in which such services are performed and the resources immediately available require adjustments when applied by the respiratory therapist (RT) in a home care environment. In fact, there are many career opportunities for RTs in home care, primarily with **home medical equipment** (HME) companies. However, success as a home care RT not only depends on clinical competency in patient assessment and treatment but also requires strong skills related to patient education, communication, time management, ability to work independently, and resourcefulness. These and other qualifications of the RT working in home care are discussed in more detail later in this chapter.

The Evolution and Importance of Respiratory Home Care

As a result of skyrocketing medical costs, pressure from third-party payers such as Medicare and health insurance companies, and the desire to enhance the patient's quality of life, a strong emphasis is now placed on reducing the length of a patient's stay in an acute care facility. Some suggest that the plan to discharge a patient from a hospital or similar setting to their home should begin when they are first admitted. This significant increase in the number and complexity of home care patients has affected respiratory home care. In essence, there are now more respiratory patients being cared for at home, and they tend to be sicker and need a greater variety of medical interventions. A greater number of patients are receiving relatively common modalities, such as home oxygen therapy, and others require procedures that were once only performed in an acute care facility. In addition, tracheostomy tube changes, aerosolized antibiotic treatments, and ventilator weaning are now being done in the patient's home. The availability of such services and the personnel to perform them not only enables physicians to discharge their patients earlier but also not admit them at all. This presents RTs in home care with some interesting challenges.

In addition to offering the advantage of decreased medical costs, home care tends to enhance a patient's quality of life by enabling a patient to participate in his or her own care, spend more time with loved ones and friends, and potentially avoid the need to be placed in a long-term care or similar facility. All of these advantages are particularly noteworthy in light of the projection that the number of people receiving home care services will rise to more than 12 million by 2016.[5] When coupled with the fact that respiratory diseases account for the fifth largest reimbursement category under Medicare, it is expected that home care will also provide RTs with many new opportunities for the future.[6] However, to successfully pursue such opportunities, RTs need to excel in many areas, including those related to assessing the patient and the environment of care, as discussed in the next sections.

The Home Care Patient

The notion of a typical home care patient does not exist because all are unique in some way. However, there are certain diseases and therapeutic modalities that are much more likely to be found in alternate settings, including the home. Thus, assessments and care plans done for home care patients should address clinical findings most commonly associated with such conditions.

From the standpoint of such diseases, the home care RT most often sees patients with some form of a chronic lung condition. Emphysema, asthma, and chronic bronchitis are health problems the RT is likely to encounter daily. Sleep-disordered breathing, infant apnea, neuromuscular diseases, and other debilitating illnesses also are seen. Box 20-1 lists some of the most common respiratory disorders seen in home care.

Oxygen is the most common respiratory therapy modality seen in home care. A patient with an acute exacerbation of COPD may need short-term home care services designed to instruct and evaluate the patient on the use of home oxygen equipment, compressor nebulizer therapy, or a new medication schedule. Assessments should be performed to determine need, response to therapy, and compliance and to identify emergent problems that could lead to a rebound hospitalization. Goals might relate to assisting the patient

Box 20-1	Disorders Commonly Encountered in Respiratory Home Care

- COPD
- Acute and chronic bronchitis, bronchiolitis
- Stable and unstable asthma
- Acute and resolving pneumonia
- Restrictive lung diseases
- Sleep-disordered breathing
- Acute upper respiratory infections
- Airway clearance problems
- Neuromuscular and other ventilatory insufficiency disorders
- Infant apnea, apnea of prematurity

in becoming independent with his or her care: to self-administer nebulizer treatments as prescribed, to use and maintain the oxygen equipment as instructed, and to know when to call the oxygen provider and how to respond to emergency situations. Once these goals are accomplished, the patient will generally be discharged from services.[7]

Conversely, a patient needing mechanical ventilation for life support requires home care services for as long as he or she remains at home. The technical nature of home ventilators and ancillary equipment necessitates that evaluation and maintenance be done often to ensure that they function properly. Home ventilator users also require frequent physical assessment to determine compliance with treatment and response to therapy and to identify emergent problems.[8]

In the middle of the spectrum are patients who require limited home care services for days, weeks, or months for the treatment of infections, management of a tracheostomy, newly prescribed oxygen therapy, or stabilization on a program of noninvasive ventilation. Home care services are terminated once the need no longer exists; however, the patient whose condition has changed or who has had a change in caregivers, environment, or equipment may need to have those services restarted.

SIMPLY STATED

The home care RT sees a great variety of patients at home; they tend to be medically complex and often require several treatment modalities.

Home Care Assessment Tools and Resources

The home care RT uses many of the methods of assessment used in the acute care setting. Several of the techniques of physical examination described earlier in this book are used in home care (see Chapters 4 and 5). Likewise, the equipment used in assessing the home care patient is also similar to that employed in the bedside evaluation of many hospitalized patients. However, the home care RT needs to become especially proficient in the use of basic

equipment (e.g., stethoscope) and techniques because of the limited availability of high-tech assessment resources such as radiographic images (x-rays or computed tomography scans), bronchoscopy, serial arterial blood gases (ABGs), and complete pulmonary function testing (PFTs). In essence, the absence of such advanced resources in home care means that each assessment tool and technique available needs to be used correctly and all the results properly considered by the RT.

Perhaps the most important assessment resources available to the home care RTs are their own senses, including what they see, hear, feel, and smell. Changes in the patient's overall appearance, skin color, breath sounds, and chest expansion are strong clues that the care plan needs adjustment.

The devices most commonly used to assess home care patients are a stethoscope, sphygmomanometer, and pulse oximeter. Peak flowmeters and respirometers may also be useful in assessing basic pulmonary function on select patients such as patients with asthma and ventilator-assisted patients. End-tidal carbon dioxide ($etCO_2$) monitors and portable diagnostic sleep-recording devices are used for select patients. Beyond patient assessment, other devices, such as oxygen analyzers, flowmeters, and calibrated pressure gauges, are used to monitor the function of home respiratory equipment, including oxygen concentrators and home ventilators.

It is important to understand the limitations of these portable assessment instruments used in the home and other alternate sites. Most important, each parameter assessed must be taken as part of the whole, and the RT must understand that an abnormal reading may not be abnormal for a particular patient, given that patient's baseline values. For example, a chronically ill patient's baseline vital sign measurements may be slightly above the normal ranges, such as in a COPD patient whose heart rate and respiratory rate are typically 110 beats/minute and 22 breaths/minute, respectively. This is why it is so important to perform an initial assessment on each patient and establish baseline parameters.

The tools themselves have limitations. Blood pressure measurements usually are done using a sphygmomanometer and cuff. Blood pressure measurements can be inaccurate if performed improperly. Using a cuff that is too narrow or applying the cuff too tightly results in erroneously high readings. Some automated blood pressure monitoring devices are prone to error. The RT should also take care not to press on the brachial artery too forcefully with the head of the stethoscope because this could result in erroneously high diastolic pressure readings. Some patients use self-administered blood pressure units to monitor their blood pressure. Used correctly, these units are generally accurate. However, it is fairly easy to use them incorrectly, which can give the patient inaccurate results.[9] The RT should review the patient's technique and review the manufacturer's instructions to ensure that the equipment is being used properly. It is also useful to periodically compare an automated unit's readings with those obtained using the RT's blood pressure cuff. It is important for the patient to take his or her blood pressure readings at the same time each day, using the same arm, after a short rest period, and sitting in the same position each time.

Peak flowmeters are commonly used for generally stable patients at home. In fact, daily peak flow measurements are often included in asthma management programs, particularly for children.[10] Reductions in peak flow readings may be a good indicator of changes in airway reactivity and patency associated with asthma. Proper technique is essential to obtain accurate readings, and the patient should be instructed to use the peak flowmeter on waking in the morning before using a bronchodilator. Each patient should have his or her own peak flowmeter; however, there is variability between models and brands, which may lead to inconsistent results.[11]

Pulse oximetry is also used in home care as an indicator of the adequacy of hemoglobin oxygen saturation (SpO_2). It is generally considered medically unnecessary for most home care patients to have ongoing or continuous pulse oximetry monitoring, and most insurance companies will not pay for oximeters for home use. Consequently, the home care RT or nurse may simply bring a pulse oximeter unit to monitor SpO_2 during periodic visits. However, a few home care patients on more sophisticated modalities, including mechanical ventilation, may have a pulse oximeter at home. In such instances, the patient or caregiver will need to be instructed on how to obtain an accurate reading and how to avoid inaccurate readings. For example, if the patient's hands are cold, the oximetry readings could be erroneously low, or a reading may be altogether unobtainable. If the patient smokes, the readings could be erroneously high. Excessive movement, high levels of ambient light, or a low battery in the oximeter can also result in inaccurate readings. The user must understand these issues and be instructed to interpret the oximetry readings as part of a whole assessment; recommended changes should not be based on oximetry readings alone.[12]

Oxygen analyzers are commonly used in home respiratory care, but like oximeters, they are not necessary for continuous monitoring in most cases. Oxygen analyzers are used most often to evaluate the function of oxygen equipment during servicing or troubleshooting. They must be calibrated according to the manufacturer's recommendations, and the RT must use care when carrying an oxygen analyzer in his or her car to avoid damaging it.

Other equipment used in respiratory home care includes $etCO_2$ monitors, which can be particularly useful in patients with COPD and neuromuscular disorders. In rare instances, arterial blood sampling and analysis is performed in the home by mobile blood gas laboratories or by using point-of-service analyzers. Sputum and venous blood samples can be collected, and even electrocardiograms are occasionally obtained in the home. Once again, all of the devices used in assessing the home care respiratory patient have limitations and should be used with these issues in mind. On the other hand, the ability to properly use these tools may eliminate the need to transport the patient to a health care facility for a diagnostic procedure. More important, the ability to collect an array of clinical information often helps form a clinical picture and may warrant that the RT recommend a change to the patient's care plan that may avoid hospitalization of the patient.[13]

> **SIMPLY STATED**
>
> The limited availability of high-tech assessment tools, such as radiographic images (x-rays), in home care means that each assessment tool and technique available needs to be used correctly and all results properly considered by the RT.

Role and Qualifications of the Home Care Respiratory Therapist

The role of the home care RT depends in part on whether the HME company provides only HME services or also handles clinical respiratory services under The Joint Commission accreditation guidelines. **The Joint Commission**, formerly known as the Joint Commission on Accreditation of Healthcare Organizations, or JCAHO, is a private organization recognized by the federal government that surveys and evaluates more than 90% of all HME companies in the United States for accreditation. If a home care company is accredited to provide only HME services, then the RT's role is mainly educating and ensuring safe use of home respiratory equipment such as oxygen concentrators (discussed later in this chapter). However, if the HME company also furnishes clinical respiratory services, then the RT's function typically includes performing clinical patient assessment, testing, and administering treatment to patients at home.[14] Most HME firms provide both types of services; thus, home care RTs must be qualified in both areas.

The primary role of the home care RT is to help set up respiratory equipment and train the patient and caregiver on the equipment's safe and effective use and maintenance. The RT also monitors the patient's overall clinical status and changes in condition as well as the patient's response to home therapy. Several skills and qualifications are needed to fulfill this role. Foremost, a home care RT must have outstanding clinical abilities to properly assess and treat the home care patient, as well as being well versed in all respiratory therapy modalities. In applying their clinical skills, RTs must be extremely resourceful and versatile and possess good critical thinking skills because home care RTs generally perform most of their daily work functions without the presence of other clinicians. Being "on the road," the home care RT mainly has access to the medical equipment and devices that he or she brought or that were previously delivered to the patient's home. It is not uncommon for the job to require creative adjustments or adaptations within the realm of appropriate clinical care. Despite often operating by oneself, the home care RT must also be a team player, acting as just one important member of the patient care team and representing just one of several health disciplines responsible for devising and executing the patient care plan. Other members of the patient care team often include home health nurses; speech, physical, and occupational therapists; social workers; dietitians; home health aides; lay caregivers; and most important, the patient. Cooperation and collaboration among team members is vital to optimizing outcomes; the home care RT must also excel in communication and interpersonal skills. Communication skills, coupled with an organized approach, attention to detail, and sensitivity to cultural and age-specific considerations, are quite helpful in teaching a patient to use, maintain, and troubleshoot a complex piece of medical equipment. These same skills will also help the RT uncover changes in clinical status and promptly recommend appropriate modifications in the plan of care.[15] It may be the quick recognition of, and response to, changes in a patient clinical status that can help prevent a hospital readmission, thus improving both the patient's quality of life and the outcomes included as part of HCAHPS. In extreme situations, such as a patient whose condition has severely worsened, the RT may need to use several skills simultaneously, within the context of his or her limitations. The RT should quickly recognize the seriousness of the situation and promptly activate emergency medical services (calling 9-1-1), administer cardiopulmonary resuscitation if appropriate, and later notify other team members, including the physician.

In addition, the RT should have a basic working knowledge of major guidelines, rules, and regulations pertaining to patient assessment and therapy in the home setting. Among these, the RT should have a solid understanding the AARC Clinical Practice Guidelines, especially those that pertain to patient assessment, as well as home care therapy and equipment. In addition, the RT should be familiar with certain rules and regulations set forth by the CMS. One such rule pertains to qualifying patients for home oxygen reimbursement by CMS. Under these rules, the home care patient must meet certain thresholds regarding arterial oxygen desaturation, either by pulse oximetry or ABG results, in order to be eligible for such reimbursement. Figure 20-1 is an example of a Certificate of Medical Necessity for home oxygen, whereby the physician verifies that the patient has met such threshold by completing and signing the form. It is important to note that the RT representing the home care company providing the home oxygen should not be directly involved in assessing or qualifying the patient for home oxygen reimbursement to avoid any appearance of a conflict of interest. Instead, such assessment should be performed by the prescribing physician or an RT with no affiliation with the company providing the oxygen equipment.

Finally, it is helpful for the home care RT to have basic skills relating to insurance reimbursement. The acute care RT has little need to know the cost of therapy or a medical device or reimbursement limits and procedures. However, it can be helpful for the home care RT to have a general understanding of the rules and guidelines for reimbursement. The RT who knows the major relevant provisions of Medicare and private health insurance can help provide efficient quality care to home care patients that maximizes the use of limited resources.

SIMPLY STATED

The home care RT must be quite familiar with respiratory care procedures, as well as possess some familiarity with many nursing care procedures, nonrespiratory equipment, and reimbursement policies.

Assessment and the Home Visit

Assessment is one of the most important aspects of respiratory home care because it can affect all aspects of the patient's care. The home care RT needs to be proficient in assessing both the patient and the environment of care. A thorough evaluation includes assessing the type of equipment required, instruction needs of the patient and caregivers, whether other medical services are necessary, the type of monitoring and follow-up needed, and the safety and adequacy of the home environment. This section covers proper clinical assessment of the home care patient and describes the major considerations in evaluating the home care environment.

In general, the RT makes an initial home visit because the patient has a respiratory problem that can be treated at home with the appropriate respiratory equipment. After the physician writes the order for home therapy, a referral is typically made to the HME provider who contacts the insurance company or Medicare to receive approval. In the case of home oxygen, the patient's blood oxygen levels will need to be assessed to ensure that they meet criteria to qualify for insurance or Medicare reimbursement. Again, it is important to note that, in such instances, the assessment of blood oxygen levels should not be performed by the RT working for the HME provider to avoid any possible conflict of interest. Once approval is received by the HME company, arrangements are made to deliver the equipment, and the RT is notified to schedule an initial visit. It should be noted that health insurance reimbursement in most cases is only permitted for respiratory equipment and that generally no payments are made to the HME company for the RT's hourly wage.

SIMPLY STATED

An assessment of the physical environment should always be performed during the initial visit, even if a physical assessment of the patient is not going to be performed.

CERTIFICATE OF MEDICAL NECESSITY
CMS-484 — OXYGEN

DME 484.03

SECTION A   Certification Type/Date: INITIAL ___/___/___   REVISED ___/___/___   RECERTIFICATION___/___/___

PATIENT NAME, ADDRESS, TELEPHONE and HIC NUMBER	SUPPLIER NAME, ADDRESS, TELEPHONE and NSC or applicable NPI NUMBER/LEGACY NUMBER
(___) ___ ___ - ___ ___ HICN _____	(___) ___ ___ - ___ ___ NSC or NPI #_____

PLACE OF SERVICE_____	HCPCS CODE	PT DOB ___/___/___ Sex ___ (M/F)
NAME and ADDRESS of FACILITY *if applicable (see reverse)*	_____ _____ _____ _____	PHYSICIAN NAME, ADDRESS, TELEPHONE and applicable NPI NUMBER or UPIN (___) ___ ___ - ___ ___ UPIN or NPI #_____

SECTION B   Information in This Section May Not Be Completed by the Supplier of the Items/Supplies.

EST. LENGTH OF NEED (# OF MONTHS): _____ 1–99 *(99=LIFETIME)*   DIAGNOSIS CODES (ICD-9): _____ _____ _____ _____

ANSWERS	ANSWER QUESTIONS 1–9. (Circle Y for Yes, N for No, or D for Does Not Apply, unless otherwise noted.)
a)_____mm Hg b)_____% c)___/___/___	1. Enter the result of most recent test taken on or before the certification date listed in Section A. Enter (a) arterial blood gas PO2 and/or (b) oxygen saturation test; (c) date of test.
1 2 3	2. Was the test in Question 1 performed (1) with the patient in a chronic stable state as an outpatient, (2) within two days prior to discharge from an inpatient facility to home, or (3) under other circumstances?
1 2 3	3. Circle the one number for the condition of the test in Question 1: (1) At Rest; (2) During Exercise; (3) During Sleep
Y N D	4. If you are ordering portable oxygen, is the patient mobile within the home? If you are not ordering portable oxygen, circle D.
_____LPM	5. Enter the highest oxygen flow rate ordered for this patient in liters per minute. If less than 1 LPM, enter a "X".
a)_____mm Hg b)_____% c)___/___/___	6. If greater than 4 LPM is prescribed, enter results of most recent test taken on 4 LPM. This may be an (a) arterial blood gas PO2 and/or (b) oxygen saturation test with patient in a chronic stable state. Enter date of test (c).
	ANSWER QUESTIONS 7-9 **ONLY** IF PO2 = 56–59 OR OXYGEN SATURATION = 89 IN QUESTION 1
Y N	7. Does the patient have dependent edema due to congestive heart failure?
Y N	8. Does the patient have cor pulmonale or pulmonary hypertension documented by P pulmonale on an ECG or by an echocardiogram, gated blood pool scan or direct pulmonary artery pressure measurement?
Y N	9. Does the patient have a hematocrit greater than 56%?

NAME OF PERSON ANSWERING SECTION B QUESTIONS, IF OTHER THAN PHYSICIAN (Please Print):
NAME: _____   TITLE: _____   EMPLOYER: _____

SECTION C   Narrative Description of Equipment and Cost

(1) Narrative description of all items, accessories and options ordered; (2) Supplier's charge and (3) Medicare Fee Schedule Allowance for each item, accessory and option. (See instructions on back.)

SECTION D   Physician Attestation and Signature/Date

I certify that I am the treating physician identified in Section A of this form. I have received Sections A, B and C of the Certificate of Medical Necessity (including charges for items ordered). Any statement on my letterhead attached hereto, has been reviewed and signed by me. I certify that the medical necessity information in Section B is true, accurate and complete, to the best of my knowledge, and I understand that any falsification, omission, or concealment of material fact in that section may subject me to civil or criminal liability.

PHYSICIAN'S SIGNATURE _____   DATE ____/____/____

Signature and Date Stamps Are Not Acceptable.

Form CMS-484 (09/05)

FIGURE 20-1 A Certificate of Medical Necessity for home oxygen therapy reimbursement under the Centers of Medicare and Medicaid (CMS) guidelines. (Instructions for completing the Certificate can be found online http:// www.medicare.gov/ - form CMS-484 (09/05). Dept. of Health and Human Servies, Centers for Medicare and Medicaid Services,CMS Baltimore MD)

Box 20-2	Key Elements of the Initial Evaluation
Patient	**Environment**
Past and current medical history	Cleanliness, safety, hazards
Symptom profile	Smoke alarm, fire extinguisher
Medication review	Adequate electricity
Physical examination	Heating, cooling
Evaluation of functional limitations	Space for equipment, supplies
	Adequate cleaning facilities
Psychosocial evaluation	Telephone
Nutritional status	Emergency access
Caregiver evaluation	Equipment needs
Advance directives	

Initial Visit and Assessment

The purpose of the initial visit is to assess the patient and home environment as well as to set up the prescribed respiratory equipment if not already done and instruct the patient and caregivers on how to use it. In some instances, the equipment has been set up before the RT's arrival. Most HME providers use specially trained service technicians to deliver, set up, and train the patient in the use of certain types of respiratory equipment such as home oxygen equipment. The RT then sees the patient, usually within 24 to 48 hours.

After the equipment has been set up and the patient and caregiver have been properly instructed, the RT will perform a comprehensive evaluation of the patient. The results of this assessment affect all other aspects of the patient's home care program. The assessment also establishes a baseline from which the patient is compared during subsequent visits. Box 20-2 highlights the elements of the comprehensive initial evaluation.

Medical History

If possible, the RT begins reviewing the portions of the medical record received by the HME provider before the initial visit to become familiar with the patient's medical history and current medical condition. This previsit review can also help the RT anticipate if there will be additional equipment or services needed. To build on this foundation, the RT interviews the patient and caregivers and then examines the patient during the initial visit. The patient interview is conducted to help disclose relevant existing conditions and establish the patient's current medical status and symptom profile. Smoking status, pulmonary risk factors, and previous medical history (including preexisting conditions, surgeries, and hospitalizations) should be determined. Any treatments or therapies the patient is undergoing should also be identified. The RT should also ask the patient whether his or her immunization record for influenza and pneumococcal vaccines is current and to identify any drug allergies. A medical history of the patient's family should also be obtained and recorded because certain respiratory conditions (such as cystic fibrosis) are believed to have a genetic link.

Physical Examination

After the medical history has been obtained, the RT should assess the patient's cardiopulmonary status and examine other clinical findings. Initially, the patient's age, height, weight, and general appearance are recorded, followed by an assessment of vital signs, including blood pressure, pulse rate, respiratory rate and quality, and pulse oximetry, as previously noted in this text. It is important to note that pulse oximetry should generally be done only with a physician's order. Often, this is handled by ensuring that the physician's standing orders that allow the RTs to perform oximetry on their patients are in place. Auscultation, palpation of the chest, and observation for cyanosis, clubbing, and peripheral edema are also done. Abnormal findings or those that suggest a change in clinical status should be documented and reported to the physician, if appropriate. Many of these examination techniques are similar to those used in an acute care setting and described throughout this text.

Some aspects of the physical examination may need to be altered to protect the patient's privacy. The home care therapist may be the only person in the room with the patient when the examination is being performed. Therefore, it may be considered improper for the RT to ask the patient to disrobe for auscultation of the lungs, especially when an RT examines a patient of the opposite gender. In such cases, auscultation must be performed over the patient's shirt or nightclothes, keeping in mind that extraneous sounds may occur when the patient's clothing rubs against the chest piece of the stethoscope. Obtaining the patient's permission to perform the physical examination is essential to making the encounter comfortable for both the patient and the RT.

Part of the physical examination often includes some form of diagnostic testing. Basic PFTs, such as peak flow, tidal volume, negative inspiratory force, and forced vital capacity, may be appropriate for patients with asthma or certain neuromuscular disorders.[10] It is also becoming more common for an $etCO_2$ breath sample to be ordered for a patient with suspected ventilatory insufficiency. A change in sputum production may prompt a physician's order for sputum sample collection and analysis.

HME providers that are accredited by The Joint Commission for clinical respiratory services can allow the RT to perform a patient's initial physical assessment without a physician's order; however, the RT can only perform ongoing physical assessments of the patient under written orders by the patient's physician.

Physical and Functional Limitations

Evaluation of physical and functional limitations is performed to identify any physical or functional problems that could reduce the patient's ability to perform self-care. In addition, such problems predispose the patient to falling and sustaining related injuries. Consequently, specific precautions should be followed to minimize the risk for falls and other household accidents.[16]

To help reveal such limitations, the RT should become aware of preexisting conditions noted in the medical record, as well as examine the patient to uncover physical deficits in eyesight, hearing, speech, strength, endurance, and mobility. The RT must also evaluate a patient's cognitive abilities. Any physical or cognitive problems could affect the patient's ability to perform self-care and limit his or her ability to safely manage any medical equipment that has been prescribed. If the patient has other caregivers assisting with his or her care, consideration must be given to any functional or physical limitations those caregivers may have.

Several functional areas must be considered. The patient's ability to independently perform basic activities of daily living should be assessed. Such activities include personal care, cooking, and independent or assisted mobility within the home. For example, the patient with COPD may appear unkempt because he or she cannot bathe and dress without severe shortness of breath. The patient may not use the portable oxygen tank because of lack of hand strength to turn on the oxygen regulator. Perhaps the patient cannot walk from the living room to the bathroom without stopping or assistance or does not have enough strength to get up out of a chair. The same patient may have difficulty seeing the calibration markings on an oxygen tank or a medication eyedropper. The RT may even have had difficulty scheduling the initial visit because the patient could not hear the telephone ringing. The presence of any of these limitations should be noted in the initial assessment, and the RT should follow-up to ensure they have been properly addressed.

It is also important to assess cognitive function. A patient with short-term memory problems may have difficulty remembering the RT's instructions on how to fill the portable oxygen tank. A patient who is depressed may not listen to instructions or may refuse the oxygen altogether. Cognitive impairment caused by stroke or even some types of medications can interfere with the patient's ability to use HME safely or without caregiver assistance. It is also important to note that moderate to severe hypoxemia or hypercarbia may cause acute cognitive impairment and may signify that the patient's condition has worsened or that the equipment has either malfunctioned or is not being used properly. Any of these circumstances would require immediate action by the RT and a prompt modification to the care plan. Finally, caregivers in the home will need a basic evaluation to ensure that they have the cognitive abilities to help manage the patient's care and equipment.

Medication Review

The RT and other clinicians, such as home health nurses, should review the patient's current medication regimen. This review identifies all prescription, over-the-counter, and herbal remedies the patient is taking. Special attention should be given to medications that have similar names such as salmeterol and Solu-Medrol. The RT evaluates the patient's level of understanding about how he or she should be taking each medication and assesses the patient's compliance with the treatment plan. It may be helpful to ask the patient how he or she keeps track of medications and suggest the use of a medication scheduling pill holder for simplification, if needed. The RT should also ask to see the patient's technique for using metered-dose inhalers, dry powder inhalers, and medication nebulizers. If the RT determines that the patient is not using the medications as prescribed, the RT should inform the patient's physician and document this point. The RT can also recommend that the patient consult with a pharmacist for advice and clarification. Issues regarding medications should be communicated to other members of the patient care team, such as the home health nurse, and addressed in the patient's care plan.

Psychosocial Evaluation

It is relatively common for patients with chronic lung disease to also have psychosocial issues such as anxiety and depression. As a result of this and because such issues can affect other aspects of the patient's health, a review of the home care patient's psychosocial status should be included in the initial home patient assessment. This assessment includes the patient's self-image, outlook on the present and future situation, home status and support systems, and work history.[17] Home care patients can be anxious, embarrassed, angry, or depressed over their state of health and may feel that they are a burden to their families. They may have difficulty coping with being dependent on others for help with basic activities of daily living, particularly when this dependence involves role reversal. For example, a male patient who has always had control and authority may have difficulty coping with losing that control and having to be assisted by his wife or being told what to do by health care workers. This patient may deny his condition or try to exert control by not complying with treatment regimens or refusing treatment altogether, to the detriment of his health.

Patients forced to retire because of declining health may become depressed at the loss of their role as breadwinner. They may become so concerned about finances that they refuse medications or equipment because they feel they cannot afford them. They feel that they have become a physical and financial burden on their families. Depression can lead to hostility toward caregivers, refusal of care or treatment, and verbal expression of suicidal thoughts. Anxiety can lead to medication abuse, increased shortness of breath, insomnia, and other health problems.

Caregivers in the home can also suffer from depression, anxiety, and burnout. The spouse of a patient with COPD may have to quit work to care for the patient and may be concerned with financial problems while also having to worry about the patient's health. The asthmatic child's mother may overuse emergency services because of her fear of a life-threatening asthma attack.

It is important that the RT look for signs of caregiver depression, anxiety, and burnout such as abuse and neglect.

Box 20-3 lists some behavioral clues the RT should look for during this evaluation.

The RT should notify the patient's physician of any psychosocial problems and ultimately the involvement of a mental health clinician, such as a social worker, may be indicated. The social worker can assist the patient and family with financial issues, caregiver burnout, and adjustment problems. The social worker can also assist the patient and family with decisions about advance directives if these have not been made.

Box 20-3	Signs and Symptoms of Psychosocial Problems in the Home

- Excessive expression of fear, shame, or embarrassment
- Poor hygiene and/or sloppy appearance
- Patient indicates he/she feels depressed
- Evasive or withdrawn behavior
- Signs of physical or emotional abuse

QUESTIONS TO ASK

Physical and Functional Limitations in Patients and Caregivers

Ask yourself the following questions when assessing the limitations of patients and caregivers:

- Is the patient able to walk unaided or does he/she need a walker, cane, or other walking aid? Is the patient able to walk without significant shortness of breath? Is the patient able to climb a flight of stairs if the home has stairs? Does the patient have any weakness, arthritis, pain, swelling, or reduced range of motion in his/her feet, ankles, or legs?
- Does the patient have arthritis in his/her hands? Is the patient able to make a fist? Does the patient need assistance when performing an activity with his/her hands? Do the patient's hands shake? Does the patient have the strength to lift a portable oxygen tank or nebulizer?
- Does the patient have any hearing or vision problems? Can the patient read medication containers accurately? Is the patient able to read the gauges, flowmeters, or other indicators on the HME? Can the patient read the written instructions provided with his/her medications and equipment? Can the patient hear the alarms made by the equipment? Can the patient hear the telephone, doorbell, or normal speaking voices?
- Can the patient shower or bathe without assistance? Can the patient dress without assistance? Is the patient exhausted or short of breath after bathing or going to the toilet? Does the patient using oxygen need a higher flow rate during these activities?
- Is the patient able to make his/her own bed? Does the patient do his/her own cleaning and laundry?
- Is the patient able to prepare meals? Does the patient need assistance with food shopping? How many meals does the patient eat per day?
- Does the patient have difficulty remembering how to use any of the medical equipment? Does the patient remember which HME company has provided his/her equipment? Can the patient remember when was his/her last bronchodilator treatment? Can the patient remember how many times a day to take each of his/her medications?
- Do the patient's breathing problems limit his/her lifestyle in any way? Is the patient homebound? (Adapted from Dunne PJ, McInturff SL: The home visit. In Dunne PJ, McInturff SL: Respiratory home care: the essentials, Philadlphia, 1997, FA Davis)

Nutritional Review

The patient's nutritional status is also evaluated in the initial visit, and the RT should inquire about any dietary restrictions (e.g., sodium, sugar, fat, or calories). The RT should determine how many meals the patient eats per day mainly because it is common for patients with pulmonary disease to eat poorly or decline food rather than suffer the dyspnea associated with its preparation and consumption. Such a patient would benefit from instruction in energy conservation techniques to help him or her prepare food and eat it. An important question to ask during the nutritional assessment is whether the patient leaves the oxygen cannula on during cooking and eating. It is common to discover that patients remove their oxygen cannula while cooking because they are afraid of the danger of using oxygen around sources of heat. Many patients also remove their oxygen cannula during meals, often for cosmetic reasons. Identifying these issues would prompt problem solving by the RT and patient. For example, a visit by a home health dietitian could be suggested, or the patient could be encouraged to use a local meal preparation and delivery service such as Meals on Wheels. A review of oxygen safety, including keeping oxygen tubing a safe distance from open cooking flames, would also be appropriate. Chore workers or personal attendants can be hired to assist the patient with meal preparation. The dietitian may ultimately recommend that the patient be started on parenteral or enteral nutrition.[18] The RT can also reinforce any dietary recommendations that have already been made for the patient (see also Chapter 18).

Cultural, Ethnic, and Religious Considerations

Cultural, ethnic, and religious beliefs can also affect the patient's home care program. Language differences can make it difficult for the patient and the RT to communicate. The RT may need to locate an interpreter or use an outside service to translate; however, there may be a family member available who can also perform this role. Additionally, many equipment user manuals and other written instructional materials are now written in several languages to help overcome this problem.

Some cultures encourage extended families to live together in a single dwelling. This can be advantageous because it increases the number of potential caregivers and reduces the feeling of isolation suffered by some patients.

It can be less of an advantage when care must be divided among a limited number of family members, particularly if this involves small children. Some customs dictate that shoes be removed before entering the home. Other patients may have religious beliefs that require an alteration in the home care program (e.g., a patient may decline visits on days of worship or may decline treatment on religious grounds). A patient may request religious counsel as part of his or her health care team or request that prayers be said for him or her. In all cases, the RT should try to identify and respect the patient's spiritual, cultural, and ethnic customs and preferences.

Environmental Assessment

An environmental assessment is done to determine whether problems exist in the physical environment that would affect patient care. The home is inspected to identify health, fire, and safety hazards.[19] The home's walkways should be free of anything that could cause the patient to stumble and fall (e.g., throw rugs should be removed if the patient has gait problems or uses a walking aid). Halls and doorways should be wide enough for the patient to pass through, particularly when he or she uses a walker. Emergency exit routes must be identified, and a plan for the quick removal of the patient should be developed and posted for all caregivers and emergency personnel.

Many older homes have electrical outlets that are not grounded properly. Patients often use multiplug adapters that are overloaded or in ill repair. Depending on the amount of medical equipment the patient needs, the home may not supply enough amperage on a circuit to power the equipment and the other appliances the patient wants to use. In extreme cases, some patients do not have electricity at all or "borrow" it from neighbors through extension cords. Inspection by a professional electrician may be needed to determine whether modifications are necessary to support the patient's equipment needs. In some cases, it may not be possible to safely place equipment in the home.

The home should be inspected for functioning smoke alarms and fire extinguishers. There should be plenty of room for all equipment and supplies the patient will need; this is critical when oxygen is going to be used. Oxygen equipment must be placed at least 6 feet away from any heat sources and should not be placed on or near heater vents or in closets. Equipment powered by compressors, such as oxygen concentrators, nebulizers, and ventilators, must have enough free space around it to allow for adequate air intake and cooling. Other furniture may need to be removed to make space for hospital beds and other large equipment.

The home should have a working telephone. Touch-tone telephones with oversized numbers are available for patients with poor vision, and telephones with amplifiers or lights are helpful to patients with hearing deficits. Cordless and cellular telephones are ideal for patients who become short of breath trying to get to a ringing phone.

Cordless and cellular phones also are handy to keep at the patient's bedside; this enables the caregiver to stay at the patient's side instead of having to leave the room to make a call, particularly in an emergency. However, cordless phones and other electronic devices should not be placed on or too close to equipment, such as ventilators or apnea monitors, because of the potential for electromagnetic interference, which can affect the functioning of such equipment.

Patients with pulmonary impairment may not tolerate wide fluctuations in ambient temperature, so the home should be evaluated for its heating and cooling systems. Wood-burning stoves and fireplaces can aggravate lung problems, particularly asthma, as can stoves or heaters that are not vented. When inspecting the home of an asthmatic patient, the RT must be particularly careful to identify possible triggers such as old carpeting, pets, mold, and wood fires.[20]

SIMPLY STATED

A comprehensive initial evaluation will help the RT determine the most appropriate respiratory and HME for the patient.

Home Care Equipment

The nature of the patient's illness generally dictates the respiratory and other medical equipment needs of the home care patient. Respiratory equipment commonly used at home is listed in Box 20-4. However, the practitioner's assessment of the patient and the home environment may reveal that equipment-related modifications or additions should be pursued. For example, the RT's assessment may show that the functional ability of a patient with an standard oxygen concentrator may have improved, and as a result, an oxygen-conserving device used with either a

---

Box 20-4	Respiratory Equipment Necessitating a Home Care Respiratory Therapist Visit

- Oxygen therapy equipment
- Invasive and noninvasive ventilators
- Compressor nebulizers
- Bland aerosol therapy
- Continuous positive airway pressure (CPAP) and bilevel pressure devices
- Suction machines for oral, endotracheal, and intermittent gastric suction
- Mechanical airway clearance devices (percussors, flutter valves, or exsufflation devices)
- Apnea monitors
- Portable sleep-recording devices
- Oximeters
- Airway adjuncts (tracheostomy tubes, laryngectomy tubes, or transtracheal oxygen catheters)

portable concentrator or a stationary liquid oxygen system and refillable portable unit may be a better choice because it facilitates ambulation. Likewise, an evaluation of the home environment may show an inadequate number of electrical outlets or amperage, suggesting the use of a liquid oxygen system rather than an electrically powered oxygen concentrator. Careful observation of where and how the equipment will be used is essential.

The patient using a home ventilator will likely need battery-powered equipment as a backup, especially if he or she lives in an area with frequent power outages. A patient who lives in a small mobile home may not have enough room for a hospital bed, and if that patient suffers from orthopnea, arthritis, or another need for frequent changes in body position, it will be necessary to find other ways to elevate the head during sleep or to facilitate positioning.

If the functional assessment reveals that the patient has difficulty with personal care, such as bathing or using the toilet, adaptive equipment can make these activities less taxing and, more important, less hazardous. Bath seats, shower chairs, handheld shower attachments, and grab bars can make bathing and washing safer and much easier. In such instances, the RT can recommend that a physical therapist perform a home evaluation to ensure that the patient's environment permits him or her to function as independently and safely as possible.

Equipment Maintenance

An essential aspect of home care is ensuring proper maintenance of home respiratory equipment. As a result, the RT not only needs to assess the patient and set up the equipment but also should instruct the patient and caregiver and evaluate their ability to use and maintain the equipment (see next section). To accomplish this, equipment maintenance and basic troubleshooting should be thoroughly covered on the initial visit and reinforced during subsequent visits.

With regard to medical equipment maintenance, it is important to note that each manufacturer has specific guidelines for periodic preventive maintenance and servicing. Home ventilators also must be replaced periodically for more extensive maintenance, usually after specified hours of operation or a specific time period. Oxygen equipment also needs routine monitoring and maintenance. Output concentration and flow rates of oxygen concentrators must be checked and external and internal filters replaced. Flow rates of liquid oxygen equipment must be checked routinely for accuracy, and seals must be replaced periodically. An electrical safety check should be performed on all electrically powered equipment at least every 12 months.

Some types of home oxygen equipment include monitoring devices to assist with equipment maintenance. Oxygen concentrators can be equipped with *oxygen concentration indicators* (OCIs), which alert the user if the concentration output drops below a certain level. OCIs are helpful in ensuring that the patient is always receiving an adequate concentration of oxygen (e.g., an oxygen concentrator without an OCI may still put out the prescribed flow of 2 L/minute, but the concentration of that flow may be 80%, 75%, or even lower). In this instance, the patient has no way to know that the inspired oxygen level is too low except that he or she may not feel as good. As a result, patients and caregivers should be instructed on the significance of OCIs.

Patient Education and Training

Assessment is one of the most important skills that an RT can have, although the ability to teach runs a close second. Part of the initial and subsequent home visits should be spent training the patient and caregivers on basic assessment techniques and how to use and maintain the prescribed medical equipment, as well as performing the related respiratory care procedures. Indeed, RTs have been shown to be uniquely effective in teaching patients.[21] The RT must be able to convey technical information in a simple and meaningful way and to verify that what was taught was also understood. Each person learns differently, and the RT must determine how each particular patient learns best. Some patients learn best by visualization or by reading. Others learn best by listening, and some learn best by doing.[22] The RT probably will use a combination of these methods during training. In any event, it is generally useful to give the patient printed material that covers the key points in an easily understandable manner. Some patients and caregivers may benefit from audiovisual or Internet-based educational resources. It may also be helpful to select a "teachable moment," which is a moment relatively free from outside stimuli and other distractions. Box 20-5 outlines some useful teaching strategies.

In general, the caregivers and even the patient can be taught to obtain and record basic vital signs, such as heart and respiratory rate and regularity, blood pressure, and temperature. They should also be instructed on basic emergency procedures, including those to follow in a

Box 20-5	Helpful Strategies to Use During Patient Education and Training

- Select a "teachable moment" to ensure the learner's attention.
- Present only the necessary information.
- Use simple or lay terms.
- Demonstrate the procedure exactly as it should be performed.
- Have the learner practice several times.
- Ask for a return demonstration from the patient or caregiver.
- Try to limit each training session to 30 to 60 minutes.
- Encourage the learner to ask questions.
- Use video, audio, and web-based material.
- Leave printed instructions.
- Leave a 24-hour telephone number.

TABLE 20-1		
Sample Plan of Care		
Problem	**Goal**	**Action**
Hypoxia by O_2 saturation	Patient will maintain O_2 saturation above 90%	Monitor O_2 saturation by pulse oximetry monthly and as needed
Patient cannot see flowmeter on concentrator	Patient will use O_2 at 1 L/min at rest and 2 L/min with activity	Instruct patient's family in how to verify flow rate on concentrator as prescribed
Patient cannot carry portable O_2 tank	Patient will use portable O_2 as prescribed when away from house	Supply patient with smallest aluminum O_2 cylinder with O_2-conserving device
Patient refuses to wear O_2 cannula in public	Patient will wear O_2 as prescribed	Review health problems associated with hypoxia, provide patient with clear nasal cannula, encourage patient to carry portable cylinder in backpack or other carrying bag

natural catastrophe or an apparent medical emergency. In addition, patients and caregivers should be taught to use, maintain, and perform basic troubleshooting on respiratory equipment in place at the home. Patients who have a functional limitation that prevents them from doing the procedure or using the equipment may still be involved in the training.

Whether the training or education involves assessment, equipment use, or emergency procedures, it is important that the RT evaluate how much the patient and caregiver have understood and provide additional training as necessary.[22] Generally, competency to perform such procedures can be shown through a return demonstration given by the caregiver or patient and recorded by the RT. To get to that point, however, it may be necessary for the RT to visit the patient's home two or three times to continue the training sessions, particularly when there are several concepts to be covered relating to assessment and multiple pieces of equipment. It is common for patients and families to be overwhelmed during the RT's initial visit and for them not to remember all the instructions the RT may give them. It is important for the RT to factor this into the plan of care and to use follow-up visits to provide additional training and monitor the patient's condition and the caregiver's ongoing performance.

Plan of Care

One of the primary objectives of the initial assessment and evaluation is for the RT to gather information that will help develop an individualized plan of care for the patient. The **plan of care** is developed from issues and problems identified during the initial evaluation. From there, goals and desired outcomes are identified along with activities that will help achieve them. Goals should be specific, measurable, attainable, realistic, and within a specified time frame. As time passes and the patient has been home for some time, the plan of care is generally modified to reflect changes in the patient's condition, needs, or environment of care. Likewise, the physician's orders should reflect the initial goals, and the RT should recommend any appropriate changes over time.

For example, during the initial evaluation, the RT may notice that the patient is having difficulty reading the flowmeter on the oxygen concentrator or that the patient is too weak to carry a portable oxygen tank. In other cases, the patient may admit to the RT that he or she is embarrassed to wear an oxygen cannula in public and so refuses to use the portable oxygen system outside the house. In these instances, the plan of care should list these issues or problems and include goals and corrective actions. Table 20-1 shows a sample plan of care for a patient with home oxygen based on the physician's order for treatment.

SIMPLY STATED

Some of the best ways to help ensure that a patient or caregiver is competent to perform a procedure related to assessment of equipment is to instruct them thoroughly, let them practice and ask questions, and then have them give a good return demonstration.

Follow-Up Care

The plan of care or service should also include the RT's plan for follow-up care. Based on the issues identified during the initial evaluation and the desired outcomes, including the prevention of hospital readmissions, the patient may or may not need ongoing physical assessment and evaluation. This is usually a function of how ill or unstable the patient is or what type of equipment the patient is using. For example, the RT probably would not perform ongoing assessments on a patient using a compressor nebulizer or, if follow-up is indicated, it should be for a short duration. The RT may have found during the initial evaluation that the patient seemed to have difficulty remembering how to schedule the treatments, and a follow-up visit should be made. Once it is established that the patient is taking treatments as prescribed, the patient no longer needs regular follow-up.

It is ideal to reassess the patient completely during each follow-up visit, particularly when the home visits are done less frequently. The RT often will identify something that has changed from the initial evaluation, and emergent

TABLE 20-2		
Interpretation of Signs and Symptoms in the Home Care Patient		
Finding	**Possible Cause**	**Action**
Dyspnea, cyanosis	Malfunction of equipment, poor compliance with treatment, change in physical status	Check O_2 equipment, assess patient, review energy conservation techniques and pursed-lip breathing, contact physician
Wheezing	Bronchospasm, congestive heart failure, pulmonary infection	Examine patient, verify compliance with medication regimen, review medication nebulizer procedures, contact physician
Increased sputum or change in sputum color	Lung or airway infection	Assess patient, check temperature, check compliance with therapy and cleaning of equipment, contact physician
Pedal edema	Heart failure, fluid overload	Assess patient, verify function of O_2 equipment, check compliance with O_2 therapy, verify compliance with medication regimen, contact physician
Poor appetite	Depression, dyspnea, fever	Assess patient, examine medication schedule, review energy conservation techniques, contact physician

problems are found this way. It may be during a periodic visit to evaluate the oxygen equipment that the RT notices a change in the patient's shortness of breath or an increase in pedal edema. The RT may have found that the patient is using portable cylinders faster than expected or that the patient is not using as much oxygen as he or she should, as evidenced by the hour meter on the concentrator. The essence of the follow-up visit is that the RT will generally find something that has changed about the patient, equipment, or environment, and thus the plan of care is continually evolving based on the goals that are met and new issues that arise. Table 20-2 reviews physical changes that may be found during a follow-up visit and the recommended actions for the RT.

A growing trend in follow-up care is telemonitoring, which is usually done by telephone modem on equipment specially designed for remote monitoring. This equipment collects and stores data that can track use and compliance and identify and categorize events such as breathing problems or heart arrhythmias. Some telemonitoring equipment also has video capabilities that allow the health care professional not only to interview the patient but also to monitor blood pressure, listen to the patient's lungs, inspect wounds, and perform other physical assessment tasks. Telemonitoring reduces the amount of time required for a visit because it eliminates the driving time involved, allowing the health care professional to see more patients in a day.[23] Telemonitoring is not yet widely used, partly because of the expense involved in providing the equipment, which is generally not reimbursable.

Discharging the Patient

Most home care patients are not followed by the RT indefinitely. The ultimate goal of respiratory home care is to provide the patient with the tools to manage his or her own care. These tools include the knowledge base, equipment, procedures, and self-monitoring capability.

The plan of care is established to work through the problems and issues found during the RT's home visits.

As problems are identified, goals are set to achieve desired outcomes and correct the problems. For most patients, the goals are achieved, and the patient becomes capable of self-monitoring. At this point, the patient is discharged from respiratory care services.

If the patient continues to use medical equipment, such as oxygen, ventilators, and apnea monitors, he or she will at least continue to need service visits to monitor the function of that equipment. Those services may or may not be performed by the RT. Some HME providers use specially trained service technicians to make these service calls, and others use RTs to service life support equipment and service technicians to monitor oxygen and nebulizer equipment. These service technicians are trained to identify and report back any problems that might require patient contact by the RT.

KEY POINTS

▶ Several factors, including technologic advancements, our aging population, and increasing demands on health care resources and quality initiatives such as HCAHPS, have resulted in a greater number of patients receiving respiratory therapy at home.

▶ For RTs, home care is a viable career path and an alternative to working in an acute care facility.

▶ In addition to outstanding clinical abilities, the successful home care RT needs to possess an array of other competencies, including critical thinking skills and resourcefulness, as well as time management and communications skills.

▶ Respiratory conditions that are commonly encountered in home care include COPD, sleep disorders, and neuromuscular diseases.

▶ Treatment modalities that are often used in home care include long-term oxygen, continuous positive airway pressure (CPAP), bronchodilator therapy, and mechanical ventilation.

▶ The initial assessment of a home care patient should include an evaluation of the medical history, a physical

KEY POINTS—cont'd

examination, review of medications, and an assessment of psychosocial and nutritional status as well as cultural, ethnic, and religious needs.

▶ An environment of care evaluation done by the RT should focus on identifying and addressing potential hazards, ensuring the adequacy of space and electrical service, and devising a plan for responding to emergencies such as power outages and fires.

▶ Patient and caregiver training and education initiatives done by the RT should focus on basic patient assessment as well as proper use, cleaning, and maintenance of all respiratory equipment.

▶ The RT should be aware of the guidelines pertaining to qualifying a patient for home oxygen therapy reimbursement under CMS and should never be directly involved in the assessment process if affiliated with the home oxygen company.

▶ The RT should ensure that an appropriate plan of care be developed that includes obtainable goals and activities focused on achieving those goals and should recognize active participation by the patient and/or caregivers.

▶ To optimize care and help ensure the best possible quality of life for the patient, the plan of care should be periodically reviewed and revised based on changes uncovered through patient follow-up.

ASSESSMENT QUESTIONS

See Appendix for answers.

1. All of the following factors have contributed to the rise in respiratory home care, *except*:
   a. Legislation relating to reimbursement and quality outcomes
   b. Desire to enhance quality of life for chronically ill patients
   c. Home care is easier for the RT than acute care
   d. Cost-effectiveness

2. Which of the following conditions is/are commonly seen in the home care setting?
   a. COPD
   b. Sleep disorders
   c. Neuromuscular patients with ventilatory insufficiency
   d. All of the above

3. All of the following respiratory modalities are commonly found in home care, *except*:
   a. Long-term oxygen therapy
   b. Continuous positive airway pressure (CPAP)
   c. Bronchodilator therapy
   d. High-frequency jet ventilation

4. All of the following are important attributes of the home care RT, *except*:
   a. Outstanding clinical assessment skills
   b. Extensive knowledge of home respiratory equipment

   c. In-depth understanding of the evolution of home care
   d. Excellent communication and interpersonal abilities

5. Which of the following procedures would generally *not* be assessed during a respiratory home care visit?
   a. Vital signs
   b. Mixed venous blood gas analysis
   c. Physical inspection of the patient
   d. Breath sounds

6. When should an RT working for an HME provider assess pulse oximetry specifically to determine whether the patient qualifies for home oxygen reimbursement under Medicare?
   a. Never
   b. After first signing a disclaimer
   c. Only if the HME company gets to set up oxygen on that patient
   d. If the patient had a lung transplantation

7. Which of the following is/are potential signs and symptoms of psychosocial problems in the home?
   a. Evasive answers
   b. Physical signs of abuse
   c. Unwarranted fear
   d. All of the above

8. Which of the following is true about the RT's evaluation in an initial home care visit?
   a. It often includes clinical evaluation of the patient
   b. It is performed by a physician
   c. It involves educating the patient and caregiver on the equipment and ongoing care
   d. Both a and c

9. Which of the following is true about the patient's plan of care?
   a. It identifies issues and establishes goals for the patient
   b. It includes activities consistent with attaining such goals
   c. It should be reviewed and updated to reflect changing patient needs
   d. All of the above

10. Which of the following would *not* be a part of the environmental assessment?
    a. Assessment of vital signs
    b. Determining adequacy of electrical service to accommodate electrically powered equipment
    c. Identifying potential safety hazards and recommending potential remedies
    d. Evaluating space requirements for ambulation and equipment

11. Which of the following is part of follow-up care?
    a. Helping the patient become as actively involved in his/her care as possible
    b. Reviewing and modifying the treatment plan
    c. Assessing the patient's compliance with the therapy
    d. All of the above

12. Appropriate ways to help ensure that a patient or caregiver is competent to perform a procedure is to do which of the following?
    a. Instruct them thoroughly
    b. Let them practice and ask questions
    c. Have them perform a good return demonstration
    d. All of the above

13. When your assessment of a home oxygen patient reveals that they have increased mobility and the desire to ambulate, what type of oxygen equipment would you recommend?
    a. Stationary oxygen concentrator
    b. Portable/refillable liquid system with a conserving device
    c. Stationary liquid oxygen system
    d. Oxygen cylinders

References

1. National Association for Home Care and Hospice. *Basic statistics about home care* Washington, DC: National Association for Home Care; 2010.
2. National Center for Health Statistics. *FastStats: deaths/mortality*. Washington, DC: Centers for Disease Control and Prevention; 2010.
3. Mannino DM, Buist AS. Global burden of COPD: risk factors, prevalence, and future trends. *Lancet* 2007;**370**(9589):765.
4. American Association for Respiratory Care Position Statement. *Home respiratory care services*. Dallas: AARC; 2010.
5. National Center for Health Statistics. *National home and hospice care survey*. Washington, DC: Centers for Disease Control and Prevention; 2007.
6. American Medical Association. *Medical management of the home care patient: guidelines for physicians*. 3rd ed. AMA: Chicago: AMA; 2007.
7. American Association for Respiratory Care. Clinical practice guideline: oxygen therapy in the home or alternate site health facility. *Respir Care* 2007;**52**:1.
8. American Association for Respiratory Care. Clinical practice guideline: long-term invasive mechanical ventilation in the home. *Respir Care* 2007;**52**:1.
9. Palantini P, Frick GN. Techniques for self-measurement of blood pressure: limitations and needs for future research. *J Clin Hypertens* 2012;**14**:139.
10. Woods ER, Bhaumik U, Sommer SJ, et al. Community asthma initiative: evaluation of a quality improvement program for comprehensive asthma care. *Pediatrics* 2012;**129**:465.
11. Pesola GR, O'Donnell P, Pesola Jr GR, et al. Comparison of the TAS versus EU Mini Wright peak flow meter in normal volunteers. *J Asthma* 2010;**47**:1067.
12. McMorrow RC, Mythen MG. Pulse oximetry. *Curr Opin Crit Care* 2006;**12**(3):269.
13. Schultz MZ. Outpatient management of severe COPD. *N Engl J Med* 2010;**363**:494.
14. The Joint Commission. *Standards for home medical equipment and clinical respiratory*. Oakbrook Terrace, IL: The Joint Commission; 2012.
15. Mishoe SC. Critical thinking in respiratory care practice: a qualitative research study. *Respir Care* 2003;**48**(5).
16. Carpenter CR. Evidence-based emergency medicine/systematic review abstract: preventing falls in community-dwelling older adults. *Ann Emerg Med* 2009;**55**:296.
17. Coultas DB, Edwards DW, Barnett B, et al. Predictors of depressive symptoms in patients with COPD and health impact. *COPD* 2007;**4**(1):23.
18. DiBaise JK, Scolapio JS. Home parenteral and enteral nutrition. *Gastroenterol Clin North Am* 2007;**36**(1):123.
19. McCullagh MC. Home modification. *Am J Nurs* 2006;**106**(10):54.
20. Richardson G, Eick S, Jones R. How is the indoor environment related to asthma? Literature review. *J Adv Nurs* 2005;**52**(3):328.
21. Stoller JK. Are respiratory therapists effective? Assessing the evidence. *Respir Care* 2001;**46**:1.
22. De Blasio F, Polverino M. Current practice in pulmonary rehabilitation for chronic obstructive pulmonary disease. *Ther Adv Respir Dis* 2012;**41**:658.
23. Whitten P, Mickus M. Home telecare for COPD/CHF patients: outcomes and perceptions. *J Telemed Telecare* 2007;**13**(2):69.

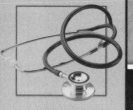

Chapter 21

Documentation

DAVID GOURLEY

CHAPTER OUTLINE

LEARNING OBJECTIVES

After reading this chapter, you will be able to:
1. Recognize the general reasons why documentation is important.
2. Identify the expectations for documentation in the patient's medical record required by The Joint Commission standards.
3. Explain the legal definition of negligence.
4. Identify the three major types of medical record documentation for respiratory therapists.
5. Describe the use of the subjective, objective, assessment, and plan method for documentation in the patient's medical record.
6. Explain the assessment, plan, implementation, and evaluation method and the problem, intervention, and plan method for documentation of patient assessment data.
7. Review the use of the situation, background, assessment, and recommendation format in patient assessment.
8. Explain the federal electronic medical record mandate.
9. Identify the advantages and disadvantages of the electronic medical record.

KEY TERMS

Center for Medicare and
    Medicaid Services (CMS)
confidentiality
critical thinking
electronic medical record
    (EMR)
electronic health record (EHR)

negligence
objective
privacy
situation, background,
    assessment, and
    recommendation charting
    (SBAR)

subjective, objective,
    assessment, and plan
    charting (SOAP)
subjective
The Joint Commission (TJC)

This chapter describes the reasons that so much time and energy are spent documenting patient care. The time spent documenting may appear counterproductive because it takes time away from providing direct patient care. However, documentation of the care provided and the patient's response is an essential element of the entire process of health care. This chapter reviews the medical-legal aspects of patient care documentation, with emphasis on The Joint Commission (TJC) requirements. The recent requirements for an electronic medical record (EMR) are also reviewed.

There is no one method of documentation that is preferred or required. Several different charting methods are presented here. The reader will appreciate how good documentation is essential from a legal perspective and, more important, how it provides better communication among members of the health care team and ultimately improves patient care.

General Purposes of Documentation

Once the respiratory therapist (RT) has completed the bedside patient assessment, consulted other members of the health care team, taken notes, reviewed the information in the medical record, and discussed the information with the patient's physician, it is time to record the assessment and plan into the medical record. The process of collecting the data involves the mental process called **critical thinking**. The critical thinking process requires many skills, including interpretation, analysis, evaluation, inference, explanation, and self-regulation.[1] The difficult part of assessment is over, and now all the RT has to do is describe the findings and thoughts in a concise and professional manner. Because the medical record is a legal document, the RT needs to understand some fundamental principles before making an entry into the patient's medical record.

The reasons for creating a record of the patient's interactions with any health care organization (HCO) include the following:

- To serve as a legal record of the care and service provided. The medical record is more than just a collection of data; it is a legal document.
- To collect evidence in support of the patient's problems and needs. When the clinical facts about the patient's condition are collected, the correct diagnosis can be confirmed, and the patient's clinical progress can be better monitored.
- To provide communication between members of the health care team. The clinical notes, reports, flow sheets, vital signs, and test results enable the physician and other members of the team to document that the patient has received high-quality care according to each profession's standards of care or hospital policies. Each discipline has unique perspectives to bring to the discussion of a patient's care plan.
- To support appropriate reimbursement. The hospital is a business that must collect revenues. As a result, the medical record is also a financial document. The medical record must clearly show the nature of the patient's needs in the form of the diagnosis. Hospital coders use the medical record to review information and assign appropriate codes in order to produce a bill. Medicare and other payers reimburse the hospital based on the patient's diagnosis.
- To support the operation of the HCO and its allocation of internal resources and to provide documentation of compliance with TJC and regulatory standards of care. This type of documentation provides data for legally mandated reports to state and federal governmental agencies. These reviews of the medical records and related financial records, as well as the subsequent reports from these reviews, are used to show the hospital's administration that the business is functioning effectively and in compliance with accreditation and regulatory bodies.
- To serve as an educational tool. Every health care professional must learn how to use the medical record correctly. At first, the medical record can be very intimidating, but with time, it becomes more familiar. The initial problem is often just finding the information you need. The medical record provides documentation of the clinical manifestations, course of the disease process, and the patient's responses to interventions. For this reason, even the experienced health care worker can learn from a good medical record. By reviewing a patient's record, you can learn what has and has not been effective for this particular patient. Furthermore, by reviewing large numbers of patient medical records, the RT or other member of the patient care team can learn how to more accurately describe each patient's condition and determine how to better treat patients with specific diseases. Most human research is based on or related to medical records. Extracting data from medical records is a complex process that requires skill, diligence, and attention to detail.

As noted, the patient's medical record is subject to review by different professionals for multiple reasons. By far the most common and compelling reason to scrutinize a patient's record, or the HCO's handling of medical records in general, is to monitor and improve the quality of medical care.

SIMPLY STATED

A retrospective review of patient charts can provide RTs and other health care professionals with the opportunity to see how patients with a certain problem were diagnosed, what treatment was given, and how the patients responded to that treatment.

The Joint Commission and Legal Aspects of the Medical Record

The Joint Commission (TJC), formerly known as the *Joint Commission on Accreditation of Healthcare Organizations (JCAHO)*, is the largest accreditation organization in the United States. It is an independent, nonprofit organization that accredits more than 19,000 health care providers and programs in all care settings. Their mission is "to continuously improve health care for the public, in collaboration with other stakeholders, by evaluating health care organizations and inspiring them to excel in providing safe and effective care of the highest quality and value." TJC's vision statements is "All people always experience the safest, highest quality, best-value health care across all settings" and their position statement is "Helping Health Care Organizations Help Patients."

TJC performs on-site surveys of HCOs to assess the quality of patient care and improve patient safety. If any HCO fails to comply with TJC standards, they will require action plans, follow-up, and evidence of compliance. If an HCO does not meet the requirements of TJC, the organization may be denied accreditation. TJC is authorized by the **Center for Medicare and Medicaid Services (CMS)** to monitor hospitals for compliance with the federal Conditions of Participation; thus, hospitals not accredited by TJC risk losing reimbursement through Medicare and Medicaid. In addition, many state health departments use TJC survey as their on-site inspection, so there could be regulatory ramifications as well.

TJC surveyors review patient records for documentation of safe and high-quality patient care. The Information Management and Record of Care, Treatment, and Services sections of The Joint Commission Comprehensive Accreditation Manual for Hospitals (CAMH) outlines how the organization "…manages internal and external information, including the medical record, and includes the components of a complete medical record."[2] The individual elements required in the medical record are provided and organized in common groups. The chapter also includes the medical record structure and details for management of the medical record. How each organization accomplishes these tasks is left up to that facility. TJC's on-site survey team evaluates an HCO's compliance with these requirements and reviews patients' medical records to assess the level of compliance. The survey team members may also provide consultation, including samples of how other organizations have complied with the standards. TJC survey team's objective is to assist the HCO to comply with the standards, not to be punitive toward individuals or the organization.

The following are TJC standards from the 2012 CAMH regarding the required medical record elements.[2] Periodically, there are revisions to these standards, but the basic principles of information management and documentation have remained unchanged.

- IM.02.01.01 The organization protects the privacy of health information.
- IM.02.01.03 The organization maintains the security and integrity of health information.

These standards are directed toward guarding the patient's rights to **privacy** (the individual's right to limit the disclosure of personal information) and **confidentiality** (the safekeeping of data and information so as to restrict access to individuals who have need, reason, and permission for such access).[2] These standards are consistent with both state and federal laws and regulations. Violations of these standards, or of related laws and regulations, can result in

legal action with fines for the institution or civil or criminal prosecution of the offenders (depending on the details of the incident). This legal action could result in personal fines, loss of job, loss of professional license, and possibly even jail time. The federal law, known as the Health Insurance Portability and Accountability Act of 1996 (HIPAA), details the legal expectations and professional standards regarding the transmission (verbal, written, or electronic) of protected health information (PHI).

In summary, these professional standards state that what you learn about a patient is on a "need to know" basis and you are not to share that information outside of that professional context. Generally, the RT needs to refer almost all questions coming from relatives and friends to the other professional team members such as the nurse, social worker, and naturally, the physician. These issues become complex at times, particularly when dealing with a culturally diverse environment.

- IM.02.02.01 The organization effectively manages the collection of health information.

This standard describes the use of standardized terminology, definitions, abbreviations, and symbols, including abbreviations that are prohibited.[2]

- RC.01.01.01 The organization maintains complete and accurate patient records for each individual patient. This standard describes the general components of the medical record.
- RC.01.02.01 Entries in the medical record are authenticated.

This standard describes who can make entries into the medical records and how the entries are authenticated.

- RC.01.03.01 Documentation in the patient record is entered in a timely manner.
- RC.02.01.01 The patient record contains information that reflects the patient's care, treatment, and services.

This standard defines in detail demographic and clinical information that must be contained in the patient record. It also includes a listing of additional documents that are required, when applicable.

- RC.02.03.07 Qualified staff receive and record verbal orders.

Communication problems during the receipt of verbal and telephone orders have resulted in serious medical errors. This alarming problem has resulted in TJC including the expectation that all verbal orders are to be read back to the person giving the order as part of the National Patient Safety Goals. This is meant to verify that the complete and correct order is being recorded and implemented. The person who gave the order, within a specified time frame, must authenticate all verbal orders. Because of these inherent problems regarding verbal orders, there is a general movement in the health care industry to discourage the use of verbal orders.

Guidelines regarding the authority to accept verbal orders are outlined in the respiratory care practice acts in most states. The general rule is that RTs can accept orders only for those treatments and services that they directly provide. This excludes drugs that RTs do not directly administer. RTs can, however, take orders for routine laboratory tests, chest radiographs, and standardized multidisciplinary protocols that are related to respiratory care practice.

All orders (written and verbal) must be dated and timed, identifying the names of the individuals who gave and received the order. Under certain circumstances, two persons should be present to take a verbal order or be on the phone line, and then one of these persons needs to repeat the order back to the physician before recording and carrying out the order. Both persons who heard the verbal directive should cosign the order in the medical record. The medical record must also indicate who implemented the order and what time the order was carried out.

- PC.01.02.01 The organization assesses and reassesses its patients.
- PC.01.02.03 The organization assesses and reassesses the patient and his or her condition according to defined time frames.
- PC.01.03.01 The organization plans the patient's care.
- PC.02.02.01 The organization coordinates the patient's care, treatment, or services based on the patient's needs.

RTs should integrate the information from various assessments of the patient, such as those of the physician, nurse, and other allied health professionals, to identify and assign priorities to the patient's care needs. Then the RT should base care decisions on the identified patient needs and care priorities. Attention should be paid to treating symptoms, such as dyspnea, and using accepted professional standards of practice, such as the American Association for Respiratory Care (AARC) Clinical Practice Guidelines.

TJC also requires that there be reassessments at regular intervals in the course of care to determine a patient's response. Furthermore, any significant change in a patient's condition should result in a reassessment, and the results or observations should be communicated to the other health care team members as appropriate.

These professional expectations are scrutinized carefully when the patient or family believes that the patient did not receive high-quality care or, more specifically, when it is believed that there has been some form of negligence.

SIMPLY STATED

TJC standards for documentation provide direction to all clinicians about what should be charted, how often, and to what level of detail. Without such standards, documentation would vary so much between health care facilities that patient records would be of little value.

Negligence is defined as an instance of failure to use the reasonable standard of care ("ordinary prudence") that results in injury or damages to another. Negligence has been committed when someone (who becomes the defendant) has failed to live up to a required duty of care owed to another person (the plaintiff). Generally, the legal definition of negligence requires the presence of the following four conditions:

- The defendant owed a duty of care to the plaintiff.
- The defendant breached that duty.
- The plaintiff suffered a legally recognizable injury.
- The defendant's breach of duty of care caused the plaintiff's injury.

SIMPLY STATED

Negligence is when a clinician or other caregiver has failed to live up to a duty of care owed to another person.

As an RT, you have a duty of care to your patients. The scope of your duty to a patient is outlined by your professional standards (e.g., the AARC Clinical Practice Guidelines, your state's respiratory care practice act and regulations, and TJC standards). Your scope of practice is further defined or limited by your job description in your place of employment. Functioning within your job description, the limits of your state's practice act, and the professional expectations keeps you professionally safe.

Concerns regarding ethical situations or clinical conflicts between disciplines should not be entered into the patient's medical record. Issues such as this need to be referred to the institutions' quality assessment or risk management department. Every HCO is required by TJC to have a performance improvement process that ensures that patient safety and quality of care issues can be brought up in a manner that is not punitive and that every employee is instructed on how to report or access this process.

- The absence of information or the lack of documented recognition of specific problems could constitute malpractice. Essentially, if a treatment, assessment finding, or clinical problem was not charted, it is generally considered not to have been done or detected.

If it was not charted, it was not done. For example, if it were not recognized that a patient on a ventilator had severe chronic obstructive pulmonary disease (COPD) and was at very high risk for auto–positive end-expiratory pressure (auto-PEEP) and the patient suffered injury or death, possibly as a result, the potential exists for legal liability. However, if the following occurred:

- Clinical notes show that auto-PEEP was being monitored with every ventilator parameter.
- There was documentation of communication among the patient care team members, including the RT, physician, and nurse, about the auto-PEEP problem.
- Bronchodilator therapy was started and ventilator changes were made (both in an attempt to decrease auto-PEEP).

Then the presumption would be that appropriate care was taken and the patient's injury or death was not caused by neglect or malpractice in this regard.

The medical record must accurately reflect the course and results of the patient care provided. Therefore, the accurate recording of the date, time, and place of events is essential. Late entries into the medical record are sometimes necessary but not a recommended practice. The standard calls for all information to be entered into the medical record in a timely manner. The definition and interpretation of *timely* is not always clear. In one case (*Joseph Brant Memorial Hospital v. Koziol* [1978]), a nurse did not chart her observations for 7 hours for a postoperative patient who then died during her shift. The delay in charting was interpreted by the court as the nurse not having made the observations. Vital signs and parameters should be charted immediately. Late entries of clinical notes or observations should be clearly marked as late entries and show the time entered and the time or period covered in the note.

SIMPLY STATED

Important information about patient assessment must be entered into the medical record in a timely fashion. If a therapeutic or diagnostic intervention is not charted, it is generally assumed not to have been done.

Types of Medical Records

The different kinds of entries into the medical record depend on the purpose of that entry. The major types that are most familiar to the RT are treatment records, flowcharts or parameter sheets, and test results.

Treatment records are concerned with a single event at a specific time. The treatment record shows when, how, and with what drugs or equipment a treatment was given. The patient's response to the therapeutic intervention must also be included in the treatment record. The record can contain patient-subjective information on the response to the treatment, but most of the treatment record is objective information. This type of documentation should include the following:

- Date and time of test or treatment
- Type of test or treatment
- Drugs and their dosages, if used
- Result, or response to treatment, including adverse reactions
- Goals, objectives, or end-point criteria for the treatment

This type of documentation is ideal for aerosolized medications, secretion clearance therapy, and tracheostomy care.

Flowcharts or parameter sheets have similar requirements for dates, times, changes in equipment settings, and, most important, the patient's responses to the therapeutic intervention. Flowcharting and parameter charting have become increasingly important in the sophisticated environment of the intensive care unit (ICU). This type of documentation is designed to show that the clinician assessed and responded to data or trends identified. In addition, it shows that the RT responded to opportunities to reduce invasive procedures and medications or adverse events. The importance of recording accurate ventilator and monitor alarm settings is often overlooked by busy clinicians. If a patient were to die from a massive tension pneumothorax after a period of high peak pressures with an inappropriately set high peak pressure alarm, a strong case could be made for malpractice. However, accurate and timely documentation will verify that the RT appropriately assessed the patient-ventilator interface. This type of documentation is best suited for ventilator parameter monitoring, serial vital signs, or oximetry readings.

Tests are mostly objective observations of clinical laboratory results (e.g., arterial blood gas [ABG] levels or electrolytes) or physiologic responses to clinical challenges (e.g., fluid challenges or optimal PEEP studies). Because tests are seen as integral to the clinical course of the patient's care, the date and time of the test and its subsequent reporting to the physician are very important.

Treatment records, parameter sheets, and test result forms are standard practice in most hospitals and typically do not pose a problem for most members of the patient care team. However, some RTs find documentation of patient assessments to be a challenge. Assessment notes, medical histories, and clinical notes are extremely important in conveying information and documenting that appropriate care has been given. These types of documentation demonstrate the efforts to collect all of the information about the patient and determine his or her medical needs.

Historically, the medical record was a binder or similar device stored in the nurses' station, containing all the required and appropriate paper documents. During the past several decades, there has been a transition to a "computerized medical record," more commonly known today as an **electronic medical record (EMR)** or **electronic health record (EHR)**. The EMR stands to increase efficiencies in the health care system and improve quality of care and patient safety. Most HCOs are actively moving toward a full EMR. Most, however, are still operating with a "hybrid," or combination of electronic and paper records. This will be rapidly changing to the full EMR over the next several years.

In addition to all the obvious advantages to the EMR, the federal government also introduced financial incentives to implementation of a full EMR. Under the Health Information Technology for Economic and Clinical Health (HITECH) Act, enacted as part of the American Recovery and Reinvestment Act of 2009 (ARRA), Medicare and Medicaid payments will require "meaningful use" of an EMR, accredited by a proper certification authority. The use of an EMR by 2015 is required in order to avoid losing a portion of Medicare reimbursement.

The advantages of the EMR include the following:

- Legibility
- Increased storage capacity for longer periods of time
- Accessibility from remote sites
- Information that is concurrently available

- Built-in "alert" systems for critical tests and values
- Customized views for various users
- Increased management monitoring capabilities
- Increased accuracy

Although the advantages of EMR are significant, implementation and use of EMR is not without challenges. TJC outlined some of these concerns in Sentinel Event # 42 entitled "Safely Implementing Health Information and Converging Technologies." The disadvantages of the EMR include the following:

- High start-up and maintenance costs
- Significant learning curve for staff
- Confidentiality and security
- Lack of standardization among systems

Organizing Patient Information

There is no single best way to document medical information, especially patient assessment. The challenge that RTs face clinically is to organize patient information and assessment in a logical, professional presentation.

One of the most frequently used methods of documenting patient assessments is the **subjective, objective, assessment, and plan charting (SOAP)** method. We will start with the SOAP format to demonstrate how to document a patient assessment because this format is an excellent teaching tool.

Step 1: Data Collection

As one astute physician has pointed out, "Data collection has been likened to picking flowers rather than mowing a lawn" (author unknown). For novices, a great deal of time and effort goes into collecting and organizing data without knowing its relevance. Novices do this because they do not know which information is valuable and which is not. As members of the patient care team become more experienced, they spend less time and effort in the collection of data because they know which data are clinically meaningful. The collection and organization of relevant data to make correct decisions is complex. The goal of data collection is to come to an accurate conclusion about the patient's condition, problems, and needs. To do so, it is necessary to start with proper bedside examination techniques. Poor examination methods lead to invalid data and inaccurate conclusions.

The first two steps of this system call for subjective and objective data collection (the S and O of SOAP). **Subjective** information is what the patient can tell you about how he or she feels. According to experts, obtaining a good medical history from the patient can give you a reasonable chance of correctly identifying a patient's problem before doing a single test. It is also evidence of the patient's level of consciousness. If the patient is comatose, that is all the subjective information you can gather; any additional information must be objective. Other people's observations can be included in this section because they may be able to fill in some of the following questions. Remember, when another person's report

about a subjective issue is used, it is always hearsay. Hearsay information can be entered into the SOAP only if the RT documents who was the source of the information.

The major questions to answer in the subjective section include the following:

- What is the patient's level of consciousness?
- What is the patient's chief complaint?
- How does the patient feel at the time of the assessment?
- Can the patient contribute any information that affects his or her diagnosis or treatment plan?

> ### SIMPLY STATED
>
> Subjective data are limited to what the patient tells you about his or her medical problems. Such documentation often is best put in terms of what the patient actually says during the interview.

The O in SOAP stands for **objective**. This is everything the RT or other member of the patient care team can measure and learns from tests and procedures. This part of the data collection can include the following:

- Vital signs (see Chapter 4)
- Physical examination of the head and neck, abdomen, and extremities for physical evidence of respiratory abnormality
- Physical examination of the thorax (heart and lungs) by inspection, palpation, percussion, and auscultation (see Chapter 5)
- Review of clinical laboratory studies (see Chapter 7)
- Review of ABG levels (see Chapter 8)
- Review of pulmonary function tests (see Chapter 9)
- Review of radiologic procedures, such as chest radiographs, computed tomography, and magnetic resonance imaging (see Chapter 10)
- Review of electrocardiograms (ECGs) (see Chapter 11)
- Review of ICU vascular pressure and cardiac outputs (see Chapters 15 and 16)
- Review of respiratory mechanics monitoring (see Chapter 14)

Step 2: Assessment

The RT's assessment of the patient's data involves critical thinking. This includes applying clinical and scientific reasoning processes and forming a hypothesis about the nature and cause of the patient's problems. This hypothesis is used to form a "problems/needs list," which helps focus on the patient's problems and needs. Case Study 21-1 is used to illustrate how to develop a problem/needs list (Box 21-1).

Problems can also fit into the following additional categories:

- Current versus potential problems. Potential problems include events or outcomes that RTs want to prevent, such as volutrauma, tracheal-esophageal fistulas, and reduced cardiac outputs from excessive mechanical ventilation.

Box 21-1	Assessment and the Development of a Problems/Needs List

How do you organize and report the information in Case Study 21-1 so that you can quickly identify the patient's problems and needs? All of this information can be used as the subjective and objective information of the SOAP. You can start with almost any sign or symptom you want; just make sure you use all the information you have. As you review each piece of information, ask yourself the following questions:

- Are the data normal or abnormal? (As a corollary, are the data normal in an abnormal setting?) As an example, a $Paco_2$ of 40 mm Hg is textbook normal, but if it is associated with a minute ventilation of 15 L, the patient probably has a severe dead space disease process. In this case, a $Paco_2$ of 32 mm Hg is not normal for a patient with dyspnea and a low Pao_2.
- If the findings are abnormal, are they mildly, moderately, or severely out of the norm? In this case, the acid-base and carbon dioxide levels are mildly out of line with normal ABG values, but the Pao_2 of 53 mm Hg is moderately reduced.
- Is this an acute or chronic problem for the patient? Does the patient have an acute episode superimposed on a chronic problem? For example, in this case, the hypoxemia may be a worsening of a chronic problem. More data are needed for further evaluation.
- Are any of these signs and symptoms related to each other? In this case, the patient is complaining of pain in his right elbow, but this sign probably is not related to his primary cardiopulmonary disease process. However, his fine inspiratory crackles and the leg pain have a high probability of being related to his cardiopulmonary disease process.
- Do the data indicate that there is something you can do about the patient's condition? Obviously, you can do something about the oxygenation problem, but you may not be able to administer the needed intravenous drugs because your scope of practice limits what you can and cannot give the patient.

- Respiratory versus nonrespiratory problems. The non-respiratory problems that RTs are interested in include cerebral blood flow, infections, ascites, and causes of metabolic acidosis. RTs need to know enough about these and similar topics to identify how nonrespiratory problems result in cardiopulmonary signs and symptoms.

Another important factor is to not confuse the cause or diagnosis with the patient's problem. For example, the cause is smoking, the diagnosis is heart and lung disease, and the patient's problem is chronic hypoxemia.

Ultimately, it is up to the physician to make an official diagnosis. However, the RT and other members of the patient care team may assist in making an accurate diagnosis by objectively identifying patient problems and describing their signs and symptoms. There may be a subtle difference at times, but it is a necessary distinction for medical-legal reasons. If RTs perform in a competent manner within their areas of expertise and scope of practice, they will generally be on safe medical-legal ground.

RTs can define the problems they identify using the following five major types:

- *Airway management:* from the nose and mouth down to the terminal respiratory bronchiole. This includes any problem that can be treated with artificial airways, pulmonary hygiene, cough assisting, suctioning, postural drainage, and in some circumstances, even PEEP.
- *Ventilation:* the act of ventilating the patient's lungs. Acute and chronic hypoventilation problems fall into this area and can be treated with invasive or noninvasive positive-pressure ventilation.
- *Oxygenation:* the process of delivering oxygen (O_2) down to the cellular level. This includes cardiac output as a component of delivered oxygenation. These conditions would typically be treated with O_2 therapy.
- *The work of breathing (WOB):* the mechanics of both spontaneous and artificial ventilation of the lungs. Most respiratory treatments have a direct or indirect positive effect on WOB; for instance, O_2 therapy reduces the amount of cardiopulmonary work the patient must perform to maintain a certain amount of ventilation or partial pressure of arterial O_2 (Pao_2). RTs can measure the WOB for a mechanically ventilated patient in joules per breath or joules per minute, but measuring the O_2 cost of breathing is generally too difficult to perform clinically.
- *Signs of acute cardiopulmonary problems that do not have a respiratory cause:* a good example is diabetic ketoacidosis with Kussmaul breathing in which the pulmonary manifestation is relieved with the administration of insulin.

From this perspective, it is clear that RTs provide a highly specialized focus on a fairly narrow scope of practice. Furthermore, this short problem list is clearly integrated into the full range of therapeutic interventions, from life support and emergency issues to daily supportive therapies such as simple O_2 therapy.

Documenting the problem in the medical record helps to prioritize patient needs and improve communication between the different disciplines. This method of linking the data with problem identification is a crucial learning step and cannot be stressed enough. If the RT documents the relationships between the data and the identified problem, other members of the health care team can follow your logic (Box 21-2).

SIMPLY STATED

The assessment part of the SOAP record is not used by RTs to diagnose the patient's problem but rather to formulate a list of the patient's cardiopulmonary problems and needs in order of severity.

Step 3: The Plan

Now that the patient's problems have been listed, each patient problem should indicate an intervention and

Box 21-2	Problem List for the Patient in Case Study 21-2

1. Hypoxemia: Pa_{O_2}, 56 mm Hg; Sa_{O_2}, 89%; cyanosis of the lips
2. SOB, pursed-lip breathing, and tachypnea
3. Fine crackles in both bases
4. Unresponsiveness to bronchodilators: peak flow 50% before and after treatment
5. Edema of the lower extremities
6. Tachycardia with irregular beats

Box 21-3	The Plan (Physician Orders) for the Patient in Case Study 21-1

1. O_2 via nasal cannula at 2 L/min continuously; titrate to keep Sp_{O_2} 92% or greater; ABG to follow
2. Morning ABG, also PRN if condition worsens; Sp_{O_2} q4h
3. CBC, CPK, electrolytes
4. Chest radiograph
5. ECG
6. Four puffs Atrovent qid
7. Four puffs Proventil, q4h PRN for SOB
8. Lasix 40 mg PO bid
9. Monitor I&O of fluids

therapeutic objective. For example, in Case Study 21-1, the hypoxemia should be treated with O_2. The amount of O_2 and the therapeutic objective must be discussed with the physician. The physician's order becomes the plan (e.g., "O_2 at 2 L/min via nasal cannula continuously; titrate to keep Sp_{O_2} at 92% or greater").

Consulting with the physician regarding orders is very important. The RT who repeatedly demonstrates effective data collection, problem identification, and appropriate therapeutic suggestions and communicates effectively with the physician will build a professional relationship based on trust. This trust between the physician and the therapist contributes to the reputation of the respiratory care department and our profession.

The following information is evident in Case Study 21-1 from the data gathered:
- The patient is acutely ill and requires interventions that may necessitate admission to the hospital for further evaluation.
- This may not be primarily a respiratory problem, and further information is needed to identify the underlying cause of the patient's symptoms.

A good medical plan must include a goal to measure against. Factors to consider when establishing or evaluating an objective include the following:
- *The purpose of the treatment.* By stating a goal for the treatment or therapy, the RT is meeting the expectations of the ordering physician and the needs of the patient. Every RT should know how to judge the effectiveness of the therapies he or she is administering and be able to guide both physicians and nurses in understanding the rationale for these goals.
- *Responsiveness of the patient.* If the therapy is administered correctly, the patient should respond in a predictable fashion. Assuming that the treatment was done correctly, if the patient does not meet the therapeutic goal, there are the following two basic possibilities:
  - The patient problem was not identified correctly, and the patient has a different problem.
  - The patient's condition is worse than originally thought. A good example would be status asthmaticus, which is asthma that does not respond to conventional treatment.

Objectives are critical for knowing when to make decisions or perform further interventions. When ordered to give a β_2-adrenergic bronchodilator to improve the shortness of breath (SOB), it might be wise to evaluate the patient's responsiveness by comparing the current PEF against the prior PEF. Objectives can be used as end-point criteria for the termination of the therapy. For example, if a patient reaches a Pa_{O_2} of 110 mm Hg on 1 L/minute nasal cannula, it is probably time to discontinue the O_2.

A number of barriers to correctly setting up patient plans are as follows:
- Inadequate data collection to make correct decisions (most common)
- Failure to recognize patient problems
- False assumptions about relationships between the data and the identified problem
- Confusing the disease with the problem, or confusing the cause with the problem; this barrier leads to ineffective intervention (Box 21-3)

The physician has continued the assessment by including additional tests (information collection) to assess cardiac signs and symptoms (e.g., ECG, chest radiograph, creatine phosphokinase [CPK], and heart sounds) and to confirm or eliminate additional diagnoses. The physician has recognized that there is a high probability that there is a cardiac problem. The RT cannot state that there is a cardiac problem because that is a diagnosis and out of the RT's scope of practice. An RT, however, can correctly relate the signs of a cardiac problem (e.g., tachycardia, irregular heartbeat, and edema of the lower extremities) and the signs of cellulitis.

Step 4: Implementation of the Plan

The next step is to actually give the treatment or perform the test. During the administration of bedside treatment, the RT still has to use critical thinking skills to perform the procedure or test correctly. Furthermore, the RT needs to keep in mind the technical aspects of equipment operation necessary for safe and effective care.

As the RT does the treatment or test, he or she continues to collect data through assessment to move on to the next step of evaluating the effectiveness of the plan.

Step 5: Evaluation of the Results of the Plan and Implementation

An important question to ask is whether the problem has been correctly identified. To answer this, it is necessary to go through another couple of questions, as follows:

- Was there any evidence of adverse effects?
- Was the response expected, given your knowledge of the patient and the technology used?

By actively seeking answers to these and similar questions and then acting on the observed results, the RT is returning to the data collection, assessment, plan, and implementation steps outlined earlier. This cycling through the steps of the scientific process is essential for good patient care.

> **SIMPLY STATED**
>
> RTs and other members of the patient care team who blindly follow physician orders are doing a disservice to their patients. The competent RT is constantly evaluating the effects of therapy and documenting the results in the patient's medical record. It may be necessary to contact the physician if serious adverse effects occur or if the patient requires a change in therapy.

Charting Methods

Most charting systems in use today are based on some variation of the problem-oriented medical record. All of the following charting systems require a clear outline of the patient's problems and corresponding physician orders or professional care plans to address those problems. Patient assessments can be written either on profession-specific forms or in the multidisciplinary progress notes, depending on the hospital standards. Four popular formats for writing progress notes are described in this section. The HCO will determine which of the following methods is acceptable.

> **SIMPLY STATED**
>
> The RT typically documents the results of tests and treatment on treatment records, flowcharts, and test records. Failure to do so may call into question whether the tests or treatments were actually done.

Subjective, Objective, Assessment, and Plan (SOAP) Charting

As noted earlier, SOAP charting is one of the most frequently used documentation methods, in part because it is believed to be the best presentation of the patient's conditions and clearly shows how the physician or other member of the patient care team arrives at his or her professional conclusions.

Assessment, Plan, Implementation, and Evaluation (APIE) Charting

A primary goal of the assessment, plan, implementation, and evaluation (APIE) method is to condense the data-collection statements and emphasize evaluation of the effectiveness of the interventions.

Problem, Intervention, and Plan (PIP) Charting

At the other extreme from the detailed presentation of SOAP charting is the minimalist approach: problem, implementation, and plan (PIP) charting. PIP charting is based on the assumption that the data collection has already been done in the medical record and that the subjective and objective information gathering of SOAP charting is redundant. Some people dislike this method because they like to see the evidence and logic leading to the assessment and resulting order. However, the PIP method works well for the experienced clinician who is pressed for time, wants to meet charting requirements, and needs to be brief. Under the "Problem" section, the patient's problem is stated simply, often with reference to the evidence that brought the author to this conclusion. Next is the "Intervention" section, which describes what is being done for the patient. This is often identical with the physician orders or standards of care for the services being provided. The "Plan" section shows how the intervention will be assessed or carried out, depending on the intervention.

Situation, Background, Assessment, and Recommendation (SBAR) Charting

The **situation, background, assessment, and recommendation charting (SBAR)** is one of the newer methodology for communication in health care. The SBAR format was originally modeled in aviation and military hand-off. Poor communication is identified as one of the root causes in the majority of sentinel events reported to TJC; thus, the SBAR method was well received in the health care community. The use of a standardized communication and documentation technique for all health care team members will ensure patient safety and quality outcomes. The SBAR format is meant to promote a structured situational briefing, regardless of different communication styles. The parts of the acronym SBAR stand for the following:

- *Situation:* What is happening now? (chief complaint or acute change)
- *Background:* What factors led to this event? (admitting diagnosis, history, vital signs, laboratory results, or other pertinent clinical findings)
- *Assessment:* What do you see? What do you think is going on?
- *Recommendation:* What action do you propose? What do you think should be done?

The SBAR method has proved highly successful in critical situations and has been promoted with the implementation of *medical emergency teams*, also known as *rapid response teams*. It is most successful for summary information with less than five key points. It is not as effective for broad communication or for in depth coverage of many related topics.

See the Case Studies for illustrations of each of these different charting styles.

KEY POINTS

▶ The role of the RT in the documentation of the patient assessment is well defined. The RT must be able to not only assess the patient's condition accurately but also document the findings in the patient's medical record using a prescribed format that meets the HCO, TJC, and legal requirements.

▶ The documentation of patient assessments serves a variety of purposes that are important to the business of the HCO.

▶ The absence of information or the lack of documented recognition of specific problems could constitute malpractice.

▶ If a treatment, assessment finding, or clinical problem was not charted, it is generally considered not to have been done or detected.

▶ A variety of documentation formats are available, each of which has its own advantages. Regardless of the method chosen, each recording in the patient chart must be accurate, concise, and available to other clinicians for review.

▶ Subjective information is what the patients can tell you about how they feel, whereas objective information is what you can measure, such as laboratory test results or vital signs.

▶ High-quality documentation after each patient encounter promotes improved communication within the HCO and promotes improved patient outcomes.

CASE STUDY 21-1

You are called to the emergency department to see a patient who is complaining of SOB. An order has been written for bronchodilator treatment. On arrival, you find a 65-year-old moderately obese man sitting upright on the examination table in a single-patient examination room. You observe that his respiratory rate is about 20 breaths/minute, with pursed-lip breathing and slight cyanosis around the lips, and he is unable to say more than a few words per breath. He is complaining of right elbow pain. His heart rate is 126 beat/minute and irregular. On auscultation, you hear fine crackles in both lung bases. He reports a nonproductive cough for the last 2 days, with increasing SOB, an inability to lie flat, and increasing leg pain. You notice that he is unable to tie his shoes because his feet are swollen and that his legs are very red, shiny, and painful to the touch. His current PEF is 50% of predicted. A room air ABG was done before your arrival: pH, 7.47; $Paco_2$, 32 mm Hg; Pao_2, 53 mm Hg; HCO_3^-, 23 mEq; BE, 0; Sao_2, 89%. No chest radiograph has been ordered yet.

You give the ordered bronchodilator treatment with O_2, but the patient reports no subjective relief. No changes in vital signs are noted. His color does improve a little during the treatment (O_2 at 6 L/minute via small-volume nebulizer), and his breath sounds are unchanged. His cough is nonproductive, and there is no measurable change in the peak flow after treatment.

SOAP Format Example

Date: 2/27/12
Time: 0950
S: Pt. c/o SOB and right elbow pain
O: Patient is a moderately obese male, orthopneic, pursed-lip breathing with cyanosis around lips. Can only speak a few words per breath. Fine crackles at bases, nonproductive cough × 2 days. Heart rate 126 beats/min and irregular. Bilateral pedal edema noted and painful to touch. Pao_2 53 on room air.
A:

1. Hypoxemic with Pao_2 53 on room air. Slight hyperventilation
2. Crackles auscultated with nonproductive cough
3. Pedal edema with pain to touch
4. Reduced peak flow, unchanged with bronchodilator

P:

1. Chest radiograph to be performed ASAP
2. Start on 2 L/min nasal cannula: done
3. Repeat ABG on O_2
4. ECG stat
5. Repeat bronchodilator

APIE Format Example

Date: 2/27/12
Time: 0950
A:

1. Signs and symptoms of respiratory distress and hypoxemia
2. Probable bronchospasm, unrelieved by bronchodilator
3. Tachycardia at 126, irregular
4. Pedal edema, painful to touch

P:

1. Chest radiograph ASAP
2. O_2 at 2 L/min nasal cannula
3. Repeat ABG
4. ECG

I:

1. Consultation with physician
2. O_2 at 2 L/min nasal cannula started
3. ECG performed

E: At 1030: Patient continues SOB, color improved. Pao_2 increased to 68 mm Hg on O_2

PIP Format Example

Date: 2/27/12
Time: 0950
P:

1. Signs and symptoms of respiratory distress and hypoxemia
2. Fine crackles, probably bronchospasm
3. Tachycardia at 126, irregular

CASE STUDY—cont'd

I:

1. O_2 at 2 L/min nasal cannula: PaO_2 increased to 68 mm Hg on O_2
2. Chest radiograph ASAP
3. ECG stat

P:

1. Continue O_2 therapy and monitor patient's ABG
2. Consult with physician for ongoing bronchodilator therapy

SBAR Format Example

Date: 2/27/12

Time: 0950

S: Patient is dyspneic and orthopneic, with nonproductive cough, severe pedal edema, painful to touch

B: Patient is an obese male. Nonproductive cough × 2 days

A: Patient is orthopneic at 20 breaths/min. Heart rate 126/min and irregular. PaO_2 53 on room air. Fine crackles bilaterally with nonproductive cough. Pedal edema severe and painful to touch. Peak flow 50% predicted, unchanged postbronchodilator

R: O_2 at 2 L/min via nasal cannula

Stat ECG

Repeat ABG

Continue bronchodilator therapy

CASE STUDY 21-2

The charge nurse calls you to the medical floor on the night shift because a patient has awakened with SOB. You find a 65-year-old man sitting upright in his bed, leaning forward on the nightstand. He is pursed-lipped and using accessory muscles to breathe, with a prolonged expiratory phase, at a rate of 16 to 18 breaths/minute. In the dim light of his semiprivate room, it is hard to see his color, but his skin is warm and moist over his upper torso, and his chest has an increased anteroposterior diameter. His SpO_2 is 86% on room air. On auscultation, you hear fine crackles in the right base and expiratory low-pitched wheezing in the upper lung fields bilaterally. Breath sounds in the left lung base are diminished. He has expectorated at least 10 mL of thick greenish-yellow sputum; no blood is seen. By palpation, his pulse is rapid and occasionally irregular. He was admitted 6 hours earlier for a knee fracture incurred during a fall that afternoon. When interviewed, he relates that he has COPD but has not been receiving any treatment for it for the last 6 months. When he was taking medication, it was only one MDI, 4 puffs in the early morning and afternoon, but he does not remember the name of the medication. The physician has been called, and you are awaiting a return phone call. You and the nurse agree to do the following:

1. Start O_2 therapy at 2 L/min via nasal cannula
2. Repeat SpO_2 after O_2 therapy
3. Get an ECG stat
4. Call the physician again and call the nursing and respiratory supervisors

Immediately after completing these interventions and telling your supervisor what you have done, you sit down to chart your assessment and what has transpired.

SOAP Format Example

Date: 2/27/12

Time: 0130

S: "I can't breathe," "I'm not on any inhalers at this time," "I have COPD"

O: Patient has SOB, skin is warm and moist. Using accessory muscles, pursed-lip breathing, and long expiratory phase. Expectorated 10 mL of thick yellow and greenish sputum. Fine crackles in right base, left base diminished, low-pitched wheezing throughout. SpO_2 on room air 86%.

A:

1. Signs and symptoms of respiratory distress and hypoxemia
2. Retained secretions, possible bronchospasm

P:

1. Call physician and appropriate supervisors: done
2. Start on 2 L/min nasal cannula: done
3. Repeat SpO_2: done at 0155: 89%
4. ECG: done at 0145
5. Request orders for above, stat ABG, bronchodilator therapy, and sputum culture and sensitivity

APIE Format Example

Date: 2/27/12

Time: 0130

A:

1. Signs and symptoms of respiratory distress and hypoxemia
2. Retained secretions, possible bronchospasm

P:

1. Call physician and hospital supervisors
2. Start on 2 L/min nasal cannula
3. Repeat SpO_2
4. ECG
5. Request orders for above, stat ABG, bronchodilator therapy, and sputum C&S

I:

1. Calls made
2. Started on 2 L/min nasal cannula
3. ECG done

E: At 0210: Patient's SOB decreased but not totally reversed; SpO_2 89% on O_2

PIP Format Example

Date: 2/27/12

Time: 0130

P:

1. Signs and symptoms of respiratory distress and hypoxemia.
2. Retained secretions, possible bronchospasm.

I:

1. Call physician and hospital supervisors: done
2. Start on 2 L/min nasal cannula: done and SpO_2 89% at 0155
3. ECG: done at 0145

CASE STUDY—cont'd

P:

1. Continue O_2 therapy and monitor patient's level of SOB and Sp_{O_2}
2. Request orders for above, stat ABG, and bronchodilator therapy

SBAR Format Example

Date: 2/27/12

Time: 0130

S: Patient has increased SOB

B: Patient has a history of COPD. He was admitted today after a fall that resulted in a fractured knee.

A: Patient is orthopneic: 18 breaths/min. Skin is warm and moist. Sp_{O_2} is 86% on room air. Breath sounds diminished. He is expectorating green-yellow sputum.

R: O_2 at 2 L/min via nasal cannula. Stat ECG. Repeat pulse oximetry.

CASE STUDY 21-3

You are just starting your morning shift in the adult ICU, and you have been assigned a 22-year-old woman with a history of acute asthma. The shift report to you is that she has been on q1h bronchodilator therapy with 2.5 mg albuterol in 3 mL normal saline for 18 hours; concurrently she has been receiving 50% via air-entrainment mask, with a "PRN ABG for SOB" order and with a continuous pulse oximeter and ECG. She has been alert and cooperative, and her SOB had diminished through the night shift. Her admission ABG levels on 50% F_IO_2 were pH, 7.46; Pa_{CO_2}, 30; Pa_{O_2}, 70; HCO_3^-, 22; BE, 1; Sa_{O_2}, 94%; Hb, 12.0; COHb, 0.7%.

When you arrive in the ICU, you note a slightly sleepy but easily aroused cooperative young adult. Her Sp_{O_2} is reading 94% on 50% O_2, heart rate is 126 beats/minute, and respiratory rate is 20 breaths/minute without accessory muscle use. Auscultation reveals that she has bilateral inspiratory and expiratory wheezing. Her chest radiograph report states that there is hyperinflation noted bilaterally, with patchy infiltrates and atelectasis in the right lung base. Her radial pulses are strong and unaffected by her respiratory pattern. Her stat morning electrolyte levels are all within normal limits; her CBC shows eosinophilia but otherwise is within normal limits. You start her treatment at 0700 and finish at 0715; vital signs and breath sounds are unchanged throughout the treatment. You finish your charting and go to your next patient.

At 0745, the nurse calls you and asks you to come see the same asthmatic patient. You immediately recognize that her ECG rate and respiratory rate have increased in the last 30 minutes, and her accessory muscle use has increased. She is becoming restless, pulling her air-entrainment mask off and complaining of increasing SOB. You cannot hear any breath sounds over her right lower lobe. With the nurse helping hold the patient's arm steady, you draw an arterial sample. Her Sp_{O_2} is now 89% on the air-entrainment mask

when she keeps it on. Before you go to analyze the ABG levels, you put her on a non-rebreather mask per physician orders. Her ABG levels are pH, 7.26, Pa_{CO_2}, 52 mm Hg; Pa_{O_2}, 50 mm Hg; HCO_3^-, 22; BE, 5; Sa_{O_2}, 87%; Hb, 12.0. On your return, the patient's physician is at the bedside, and she tells you the patient is going to be intubated and placed on a ventilator. The anesthesiologist is called to intubate as you leave to get the ventilator. The patient is successfully intubated and placed on the ventilator per physician initial orders. Before you start an in-line bronchodilator treatment, you note and report that her auto-PEEP is 12 cm H_2O at a respiratory rate of 14 breaths/minute with an I/E ratio of 1:2.5. After the in-line treatment, the breath sounds, peak pressures, and auto-PEEP are all unchanged, but the Sp_{O_2} has improved to 95%.

According to hospital policy, you now have to write an assessment in the medical record.

SOAP Format Example

Date: 2/27/12

Time: 0850

S: "I can't breathe!" "Help me!"

O: Increasing SOB, despite q1h bronchodilator treatments; increasing Pa_{CO_2} to 52 mm Hg with falling pH, Pa_{O_2} decreasing to 50 mm Hg concurrently, right lung sounds much more diminished than at start of shift. Patient was intubated and placed on a ventilator. Initial settings: respiratory rate of 14 breaths/min with an I/E ratio of 1:3.5; V_T, 700 mL; F_IO_2, 70%; Sp_{O_2}, 95%. Auto-PEEP is 12 cm H_2O initially on ventilator.

A:

1. Acute hypercapnia, respiratory acidosis
2. Hypoxemia despite O_2 therapy
3. Increased work of breathing with profound SOB
4. Greatly diminished breath sounds in RLL area

P:

1. Intubate and place on ventilator: done
2. Increase F_IO_2: done
3. Repeat ABG: pending
4. Continue bronchodilator therapy in-line, q1h: started
5. Monitor sedation needs and effectiveness
6. Monitor auto-PEEP
7. Check tube placement on chest radiograph
8. Adjust the ventilator settings, post-ABG, to new settings per physician orders

APIE Format Example

Date: 2/27/12

Time: 0850

A:

1. Acute hypercapnia and respiratory acidosis
2. Hypoxemia despite O_2 therapy
3. Increased work of breathing with profound SOB
4. Greatly diminished breath sounds in right lower lobe area

P:

1. Intubate and place on ventilator
2. Increase F_IO_2
3. Repeat ABGs

CASE STUDY—cont'd

4. Continue bronchodilator therapy in-line q1h
5. Monitor sedation needs and effectiveness
6. Monitor auto-PEEP
7. Check tube placement on chest radiograph
8. Adjust the ventilator settings, post-ABG, to new settings per physician orders

APIE Format Example

A.
1. Acute hypercapnia and respiratory acidosis
2. Hypoxemia despite O_2 therapy
3. Increased work of breathing with profound SOB
4. Greatly diminished breath sounds in right lower lobe area

P:
1. Intubate and place on ventilator
2. Increase F_IO_2
3. Repeat ABGs
4. Continue bronchodilator therapy in-line q1h
5. Monitor sedation needs and effectiveness
6. Monitor auto-PEEP
7. Check tube placement on chest radiograph
8. Adjust the ventilator settings, post-ABG, to new settings per physician orders

I:
1. Intubated and placed on ventilator with the following settings: respiratory rate of 14 breaths/min, with an I/E ratio of 1:2.5; V_T at 700 mL; F_IO_2, 70%
2. Increased F_IO_2: done
3. Continue bronchodilator therapy in-line q1h: done
4. Monitor auto-PEEP

E:
1. Patient is resting on ventilator, sedated
2. ABG: pending.
3. Spo_2 is 95% currently
4. Breath sounds unchanged

PIP Format Example

Date: 2/27/12
Time: 0850
P:
1. Acute hypercapnia and respiratory acidosis
2. Hypoxemia despite O_2 therapy
3. Increased work of breathing with profound SOB
4. Greatly diminished breath sounds in right lower lobe area

I:
1. Intubated and placed on ventilator
2. Increased F_IO_2
3. Repeat ABG: pending
4. Continue bronchodilator therapy in-line q1h: done

P:
1. Monitor sedation needs and effectiveness
2. Monitor auto-PEEP
3. Check tube placement on chest radiograph
4. Adjust the ventilator settings, post-ABG, to new settings per physician orders

CASE STUDY—cont'd

SBAR Format Example

Date: 2/27/12
Time: 0130
S: Increased shortness of breath and accessory muscle usage. Patient is restless.
B: History of asthma. Has been receiving bronchodilators q1h and is on 50% air-entrainment mask.
A: Pao_2 has decreased to 50 mm Hg on 50% air-entrainment mask. $Paco_2$ increased to 52 mm Hg, and pH is 7.26. Respiratory rate and heart rate are increased. Absent breath sounds over RLL.
R: Intubate patient
   Continue bronchodilators
   Repeat ABG
   Monitor auto-PEEP
   Check tube placement on chest radiograph

ASSESSMENT QUESTIONS

See Appendix for answers.

1. The patient's medical record is all of the following, *except*:
   a. A financial document
   b. A legal document
   c. An educational tool
   d. A contract
2. Which of the following influences what needs to be documented in a patient's medical record?
   a. TJC
   b. CMS
   c. Financial intermediary
   d. The patient's family
3. What is the primary goal of the TJC?
   a. Monitor financial reimbursement of hospitals
   b. Review HCOs to improve the quality of health care
   c. Provide health care workers with a safe work environment
   d. Monitor the ethical practice of medicine at HCOs
4. Which of the following statements is most appropriate for the RT to document in the assessment section of the SOAP documentation?
   a. Onset of asthma
   b. Viral pneumonia
   c. Hypoxemia on room air
   d. Diabetic ketoacidosis
5. Which of the following is *not* true regarding the legal definition of negligence?
   a. The defendant owed a duty of care to the plaintiff
   b. The defendant breached that duty
   c. The plaintiff suffered a legally recognizable injury
   d. The defendant's breach of duty of care did not cause the plaintiff's injury

6. Which of the following is *not* a type of medical record entry that the RT needs to perform in his/her daily routine?
   a. Treatment record
   b. History and physical examination
   c. Flowchart
   d. Test results

7. Your medical-legal duties to the patient are outlined by which of the following?
   a. TJC standards
   b. Your state's respiratory care practice act
   c. Your job description and employer's policies and procedures
   d. All of the above

8. All of the following are examples of "objective" data *except*:
   a. Laboratory results
   b. Observation of the patient's sleep apnea
   c. The patient's report of the amount of sputum he/she produces daily
   d. The physician's interpretation of the patient's ECG

9. What does the letter "I" stand for in the APIE method of documentation?
   a. Implementation
   b. Impact
   c. Inconsistencies
   d. None of the above

10. Which method of documentation is probably best for a clinician pressed for time?
    a. SOAP
    b. APIE
    c. PIP
    d. SBAR

References

1. Wood KJ. *Critical thinking: cases in respiratory care.* Philadelphia: FA Davis; 1998.
2. The Joint Commission. *Comprehensive accreditation manual for hospitals.* Oakbrook Terrace, IL: TJC; 2012.

Bibliography

Kettenback G. *Writing SOAP notes: with patient/client management formats.* Philadelphia: FA Davis; 2009.

Koch R. Therapist driven protocols: a look back and moving into the future. *Crit Care Clin* 2007;**23**:149.

Monroe M. SBAR: a structured human factors communication technique. *HealthBeat* 2006;**5**:1.

North SD, Serkes PC. Improving documentation of initial nursing assessment. *Nurs Manage* 1996;**27**:30.

Sebelius K. *Major progress in doctors, hospital use of health information technology.* Accessed from http://www.hhs.gov/news/press/2012pres/02/20120217a.html:March 9, 2012.

Sullivan D. *Guide to clinical documentation.* 2nd ed. Philadelphia: FA Davis; 2011.

Thomas JP. *Healthcare records: a practical legal guide.* Westchester, IL: Healthcare Financial Management Association; 1990.

Tietsort JA. Therapist driven protocols and newer models for patient care delivery. *Respir Care Clin North Am* 1996;**2**:147.

Assessment Questions Answer Key

Chapter 1: Preparing for the Patient Encounter

Answer Key

1. b	9. a
2. c	10. d
3. b	11. c
4. a	12. b
5. a	13. b
6. d	14. c
7. d	15. c
8. b	

Chapter 2: The Medical History and the Interview

Answer Key

1. T	9. d
2. b	10. a
3. b	11. c
4. d	12. d
5. d	13. b
6. b	14. b
7. a	15. c
8. c	

Chapter 3: Cardiopulmonary Symptoms

Answer Key

1. d	8. c
2. c	9. d
3. d	10. b
4. c	11. d
5. b	12. a
6. d	13. d
7. c	14. a

Chapter 4: Vital Signs

Answer Key

1. c	9. c
2. b	10. c
3. b	11. c
4. b	12. c
5. c	13. d
6. b	14. b
7. c	
8. c	

Chapter 5: Fundamentals of Physical Examination

Answer Key

1. d	16. a
2. b	17. c
3. c	18. b
4. a	19. a
5. c	20. a
6. c	21. b
7. b	22. d
8. b	23. c
9. b	24. d
10. b	25. c
11. b	26. c
12. b	27. a
13. d	28. c
14. b	29. c
15. b	30. d

Chapter 6: Neurologic Assessment

Answer Key

1. d	10. d
2. a	11. a
3. b	12. a
4. a	13. c
5. a	14. a
6. c	15. a
7. c	16. d
8. b	17. b
9. a	

Chapter 7: Clinical Laboratory Studies

Answer Key

1. b	17. b
2. b	18. b
3. c	19. b
4. c	20. a
5. a	21. d
6. c	22. d
7. a	23. c
8. c	24. d
9. a	25. d
10. b	26. a
11. d	27. c
12. c	28. a
13. d	29. b
14. c	30. b
15. d	31. b
16. d	

Chapter 8: Interpretation of Blood Gases

Answer Key

1. b	21. b
2. d	22. c
3. a	23. a
4. c	24. c
5. d	25. a
6. b	26. d
7. a	27. a
8. d	28. a
9. c	29. b
10. a	30. a
11. b	31. c
12. a	32. c
13. a	33. b
14. b	34. b
15. d	35. b
16. d	36. d
17. b	37. c
18. b	38. c
19. a	39. c
20. b	40. b

Chapter 9: Pulmonary Function Testing

Answer Key

1. b	16. d
2. a	17. b
3. a	18. b
4. a	19. c
5. c	20. b
6. b	21. a
7. c	22. b
8. a	23. a
9. b	24. a
10. c	25. b
11. d	26. c
12. b	27. d
13. c	28. c
14. c	29. b
15. a	30. b

Chapter 10: Chest Imaging

Answer Key

1. b	12. c
2. b	13. d
3. d	14. b
4. a	15. d
5. b	16. c
6. d	17. a
7. d	18. d
8. c	19. b
9. c	20. a
10. d	21. d
11. a	22. a

Chapter 11: Interpretation of Electrocardiogram Tracings

Answer Key

1. b	9. c
2. b	10. b
3. b	11. d
4. c	12. a
5. a	13. b
6. c	14. c
7. d	15. d
8. b	16. d

17. Rate: 80 beats/min
Rhythm: underlying rhythm is regular but irregular with PVCs
P wave: normal
PR interval: less than 0.2 second
QRS: less than 0.10 second
Interpretation: sinus rhythm with ST-segment elevation and multifocal PVCs
18. Rate: 60 beats/min

Rhythm: regular
P wave: absent
PR interval: absent
QRS: greater than 0.10 second
Interpretation: accelerated idioventricular rhythm
19. Rate: 180 beats/min
Rhythm: regular
P wave: normal, combined with T wave
PR interval: less than 0.2 second
QRS: less than 0.10 second
Interpretation: atrial tachycardia or supraventricular tachycardia
20. Rate: 80 beats/min
Rhythm: regular
P wave: normal
PR interval: less than 0.2 second
QRS: less than 0.10 second
Interpretation: normal sinus rhythm with ST-segment depression
21. Rate: 80 beats/min
Rhythm: regular
P wave: sawtooth, more than one per QRS complex, flutter waves
PR interval: not measurable
QRS: less than 0.10 second
Interpretation: atrial flutter
22. Rate: 80 beats/min
Rhythm: irregular
P wave: changing configuration, more than one per QRS complex, fibrillatory waves
PR interval: not measurable
QRS: less than 0.10 second
Interpretation: atrial fibrillation
23. Rate: not measurable
Rhythm: irregular
P wave: none
PR interval: none
QRS: chaotic, irregular waves
Interpretation: ventricular fibrillation
24. Rate: 160 beats/min
Rhythm: regular
P wave: none
PR interval: none
QRS: greater than 0.10 second
Interpretation: ventricular tachycardia
25. Rate: 80 beats/min
Rhythm: underlying rhythm is regular but irregular with PVCs
P wave: normal

PR interval: less than 0.2 second
QRS: less than 0.10 second
Interpretation: junctional rhythm with ST-segment elevation and unifocal PVCs
26. Rate: 60 beats/min
Rhythm: regular
P wave: normal
PR interval: greater than 0.2 second
QRS: less than 0.10 second
Interpretation: first-degree AV block with ST-segment depression

Chapter 12: Neonatal and Pediatric Assessment

Answer Key

1. c	16. c
2. a	17. b
3. b	18. a
4. d	19. d
5. d	20. b
6. d	21. d
7. a	22. a
8. c	23. c
9. a	24. b
10. b	25. b
11. d	26. b
12. c	27. c
13. a	28. a
14. a	29. c
15. a	30. c

Chapter 13: Older Patient Assessment

Answer Key

1. c	11. c
2. b	12. c
3. d	13. b
4. a	14. d
5. a	15. d
6. b	16. a
7. c	17. c
8. d	18. b
9. a	19. c
10. d	

Chapter 14: Respiratory Monitoring in Critical Care

Answer Key

1. c	15. c
2. c	16. c
3. a	17. d
4. b	18. b
5. c	19. c
6. a	20. b
7. b	21. c
8. a	22. d
9. c	23. d
10. d	24. d
11. c	25. a
12. d	26. b
13. d	27. b
14. a	28. c

Chapter 15: Vascular Pressure Monitoring

Answer Key

1. c	16. a
2. d	17. c
3. d	18. d
4. b	19. d
5. a	20. b
6. d	21. b
7. d	22. c
8. a	23. d
9. d	24. b
10. a	25. b
11. c	26. d
12. a	27. b
13. b	28. d
14. c	29. d
15. c	30. a

Chapter 16: Cardiac Output Measurement

Answer Key

1. a	11. d
2. b	12. a
3. b	13. d
4. a	14. b
5. a	15. b
6. c	16. a
7. d	17. b
8. c	18. c
9. a	19. a
10. d	

Chapter 17: Bronchoscopy

Answer Key

1. b	6. a
2. b	7. b
3. a	8. b
4. c	9. c
5. b	10. b

Chapter 18: Nutrition Assessment

Answers Key

1. b	11. d
2. c	12. a
3. a	13. c
4. b	14. d
5. c	15. b
6. b	16. a
7. b	17. d
8. a	18. d
9. d	19. d
10. b	20. b

Chapter 19: Sleep and Breathing Assessment

Answer Key

1. b	6. b
2. c	7. d
3. c	8. c
4. d	9. b
5. d	10. a

Chapter 20: Home Care Patient Assessment

Answer Key

1. c	8. d
2. d	9. d
3. d	10. a
4. c	11. d
5. b	12. d
6. a	13. b
7. d	

Chapter 21: Documentation

Answer Key

1. d	6. b
2. b	7. b
3. b	8. c
4. c	9. a
5. d	10. c

Glossary

A

abdominal paradox paradoxical movement of the abdomen during breathing, associated with diaphragm fatigue (Ch 5)

abortion termination of pregnancy, either spontaneous (natural interruption from abnormalities of the fetus, placenta, uterus, or mother) or therapeutic (induced interruption) (Ch 12)

acceptability as pertaining to pulmonary function tests, meeting prespecified criteria that assure the validity of the results, such as the FVC maneuver being free of artifacts (Ch 9)

accessory muscles muscles of the neck, back, and abdomen that may assist the diaphragm and the internal and external intercostal muscles in respiration, especially in some breathing disorders or during exercise (Ch 5)

acidemia as pertaining to arterial blood, an abnormally high hydrogen ion concentration, indicated by a pH less than 7.35 (Ch 8)

acidosis a respiratory or metabolic process causing acidemia or an abnormally decreased pH (Ch 8)

acrocyanosis a bluish discoloration of the extremities usually due to inadequate circulation; also known as peripheral cyanosis (Ch 5, 12)

action plan a written plan that involves patients in the goal-setting and self-care activities needed to help manage their disease process (Ch. 1)

action potential a brief reversal in the electrical potential difference across a nerve cell or muscle fiber membrane that occurs in response to a stimulus (Ch 10)

adenosine triphosphate (ATP) the body's energy currency molecules (Ch 18)

adventitious refers to adventitious lung sounds. Abnormal lung sounds superimposed on the basic underlying normal sounds (Ch 5)

afferent pertaining to nerves, those transporting impulses to the CNS (Ch 6)

afterload the resistance to blood flow out of a ventricle during systole (Ch 16)

ageism discrimination against older people (Ch 13)

air bronchogram abnormal radiographic finding that occurs when the air-filled bronchi are surrounded by consolidated alveoli (Ch 10)

airway hyperresponsiveness (AHR) state of airways that causes them to constrict abnormally in response to stress or insults (e.g., exercise, inhaled materials such as dust or allergens) (Ch 9)

airway resistance opposition to the movement of air in the respiratory tract; defined as pressure difference across the airway divided by the flow (the reciprocal of airway conductance) (Ch 9, 14)

alkalemia as pertaining to arterial blood, an abnormally low hydrogen ion concentration, indicated by a pH greater than 7.45 (Ch 8)

alkalosis a respiratory or metabolic process causing alkalemia or an abnormally elevated pH (Ch 8)

alveolar dead space alveoli that are ventilated but not perfused (Ch 14)

anabolism the constructive phase of metabolism in which more complex structures are made out of simple ones (Ch 18)

analyte a sample of blood or body fluids that undergoes chemical analysis (Ch 7)

analytic error error occurring during the analysis or measurement phase of a laboratory test (Ch 8)

anasarca widespread tissue edema (Ch 12)

anatomic dead space the volume of air in the trachea and other airways not in intimate contact with pulmonary capillaries (Ch 14)

anemia an abnormal decrease in the circulating red blood cells and/or hemoglobin (Ch 7, 8, 18)

anergy impaired reaction to antigens administered by skin test (Ch 7)

anaerobic threshold the point during incremental exercise at which blood lactate and CO_2 levels increase due to anaerobic metabolism occurring in the muscles (Ch 9)

angle of Louis slightly oblique angle where the manubrium articulates with the body of the sternum (Ch 5)

angina chest pain associated with inadequate coronary blood flow (Ch 3)

anion gap the difference between the measured cations and anions in serum, used to help differentiate among causes of metabolic acidosis (Ch 8)

anisocoria one pupil is larger than the other (Ch 6)

anterior fontanel the largest of the spaces between the bony plates of the skull in newborn infants, which close over the first few years of life (Ch 12)

anteroposterior (AP) view a chest radiograph in which the x-ray beam is directed from the front of the thorax, with the film or sensor placed at the back (Ch 10)

Apgar score a 10-point score used to evaluate the well-being of infants at birth and after delivery (Ch 12)

apical lordotic view a radiographic technique in which the patient is positioned at a 45-degree angle to better visualize the right middle lobe or the lung apices (Ch 10)

apnea the cessation of breathing; during sleep, the pause in breathing must be at least 10 seconds for apnea to be present (Ch 12)

apnea-hypopnea index the total number of apneas and/or episodes of reduced airflow occurring per hour of sleep (Ch 19)

arousal an abrupt change in sleep stage from a deeper level to a lighter one, typically accompanied by an increase in EMG activity (Ch 19)

arterial-to-alveolar tension ratio (Pao_2/PAo_2) the ratio of arterial oxygen partial pressure to the alveolar oxygen partial pressure; normally > 0.90 (Ch 14)

arterial-to-mixed venous oxygen content difference ($C[a-\bar{v}]o_2$) the difference between the oxygen content of the arterial blood and the oxygen content of the mixed venous sample; normally 3.5 to 5.0 mL/100 mL of blood (Ch 14)

ascites the accumulation of serous fluid in the abdominal cavity (Ch 5, 12)

ataxia loss of muscle coordination (Ch 6)

ataxic breathing an irregular and unpredictable breathing pattern that indicates that all brain function above the medulla is absent (Ch 6)

atelectasis   collapse of normally expanded lung tissue (Ch 10)

atrial kick   the added filling of the ventricles during diastole caused by atrial contraction (Ch 11)

attenuation   the decrease in the frequency range of sounds as they travel through lung tissue to the chest wall (Ch 5)

auscultation   the act of listening to bodily sounds, for example, heart or lung sounds (Ch 5)

automaticity   the ability of cardiac tissue to stimulate depolarization spontaneously (Ch 11)

auto-PEEP   positive pressure remaining in the alveoli after exhalation not associated with its therapeutic application; most often due to high expiratory airway resistance combined with inadequate expiratory times (Ch 14)

autotopagnosia   the inability to locate one's own body parts (Ch 6)

B

Babinski sign   dorsiflexion of the great toe with fanning of remaining toes during testing of the plantar reflex; a sign of neurologic disease (Ch 6)

back-extrapolated volume   a measure used to judge the validity of a forced expiratory volume (FEV) vs. time curve; equals the volume at time "0," which is defined as the point at which the tangent to the steepest portion of the FEV curve crosses the X-axis (Ch 9)

barrel chest   the abnormal increase in anteroposterior chest diameter (Ch 5)

barotrauma   physical injury sustained as a result of exposure to ambient pressures above normal, most commonly secondary to positive pressure ventilation (e.g., pneumothorax, pneumomediastinum) (Ch 14)

basal energy expenditure (BEE)   the measure obtained when a person is at absolute rest with no physical movement (Ch 18)

basal metabolic rate (BMR)   rate of oxygen consumption at rest (Ch 18)

basophilia   an abnormal elevation of the blood basophil count (Ch 7)

Berlin Questionnaire   a screening questionnaire used to identify the risk for sleep disordered breathing (Ch 19)

biologic control   as pertaining to pulmonary function testing, a healthy subject for whom quality control data is available (Ch 9)

Biot breathing   breathing characterized by irregular periods of apnea alternating with periods in which four or five breaths of identical depth are taken (Ch 5)

blasts   early cells that produce the formed elements in the blood (Ch 7)

body mass index (BMI)   one's weight in kg divided by the square of one's height in cm; the primary method for assessment of the appropriateness of weight for a given height (Ch 18)

brain death   irreversible cessation of all functions of the brain, including the brainstem (Ch 6)

bradycardia   a decrease in the heart rate below normal range (<60 beats/min in adults) (Ch 4, 12)

bradypnea   an abnormal decrease in the rate of breathing (Ch 4, 12)

breathing reserve   proportion of the maximum voluntary ventilation (MVV) that is unused after reaching maximum minute ventilation at peak exercise; typically exceeds 30% (Ch 9)

bronchial breath sounds   harsh breath sounds with an expiratory component equal to the inspiratory component (Ch 5)

bronchoalveolar lavage   the instillation of sterile fluid and its recollection from a portion of the lung via fiberoptic bronchoscopy, with the fluid analyzed by cytologic or microbiologic methods (Ch 17)

bronchophony   an increase in intensity and clarity of vocal resonance (Ch 5)

bronchoprovocation testing   a specialized pulmonary function test that uses substances such as methacholine or histamine to "provoke" the airways into contracting; a measure of airway hyperreactivity (Ch 9)

bronchopulmonary dysplasia (BPD)   chronic lung disease of newborns, usually premature (Ch 12)

bronchoscope   highly specialized medical devices that allows for examination of the patient's airways using a long tube with a fiberoptic light bundle and an open channel running its entire length; used for irrigating distal airways, suctioning, and obtaining specimens using brushes and biopsy forceps (Ch 17)

bronchoscopy   the procedure in which the patient's airways are examined with a bronchoscope (Ch 10, 17)

bruit   a cardiovascular term associated with the sound of blood passing through a site of obstruction (Ch 12)

bulging   the opposite movement of the skin between the ribs during exhalation (Ch 5)

C

cachectic   a state of poor health resulting from malnutrition (Ch 18)

calibration   exposing a measurement device to two or more known levels of measurement in order to confirm proper zeroing, gain, and linearity (Ch 8, 9)

capnography   monitoring the concentration of exhaled carbon dioxide using a graph (Ch 14)

capnometry   the general process of monitoring exhaled carbon dioxide (Ch 14)

carbon dioxide production   ($\dot{V}CO_2$) the amount of carbon dioxide produced by metabolism per minute (Ch 14)

cardiac index (CI)   the cardiac output indexed to a patient's body surface area (Ch 16)

cardiac output   the amount of blood pumped out of the left ventricle in 1 minute (Ch 16)

cardiac work   a measurement of the energy the heart uses to eject blood against the aortic or pulmonary pressures (resistance) (Ch 16)

cardiac work index   the work per minute per square meter of body surface area for each ventricle (Ch 16)

catabolism   the destructive phase of metabolism that breaks complex structures into simple ones (Ch 18)

Centers for Medicare and Medicaid Services (CMS)   a federal agency within the US Department of Health and Human Services that administers Medicare, Medicaid, the State Children's Health Insurance Program (SCHIP), and health insurance portability standards (Ch 20, 21)

central cyanosis   a bluish discoloration of the trunk or oral mucosa usually due to low arterial O_2 content and high proportions of deoxygenated hemoglobin (Ch 5)

central nervous system (CNS)   that part of the nervous system consisting of the brain and spinal cord (Ch 6)

central sleep apnea   pauses in breathing resulting from a temporary loss in the drive to breathe (Ch 19)

central venous pressure (CVP)   the pressure measured in the right atrium (Ch 15, 16)

cerebral perfusion pressure (CPP)   the pressure difference across the cerebral circulation; equals mean arterial pressure minus intracranial pressure (Ch 6)

Cheyne-Stokes respiration an abnormal breathing pattern that consists of phases of hyperpnea that regularly alternate with episodes of apnea; often caused by an intracranial lesion (Ch 6)

chest radiograph an x-ray image of the chest; a posteroanterior view and a lateral, or side, view are routinely obtained (Ch 10)

chest ultrasound a noninvasive procedure using transmission and reflection/detection of high-frequency sound waves to assess the organs and structures within the chest, such as the lungs, mediastinum, and pleural space (Ch 10)

chronologic age the age of an infant in days, weeks, months, or years from birth (Ch 12)

cholestasis the cessation or blockage of bile flow from the liver to the duodenum (Ch 12)

clubbing painless enlargement of the terminal phalanges of the fingers and toes (Ch 5)

coarctation of the aorta abnormal narrowing of the internal diameter of the aorta; usually around the ductus arteriosus (Ch 12)

compliance a measure of relative stiffness of the lung that is defined as volume change per unit change in pressure (Ch 9, 14)

computed tomography (CT) scanning a highly advanced means of imaging in which x-ray shadows are enhanced by using a computer (Ch 10)

confidentiality the ethical and legal obligation to maintain the privacy of protected health information except as allowed by the patient or as needed by other authorized persons (Ch 21)

content of consciousness the sum of cognitive and affective mental functions, including awareness of one's existence as well as memory and thinking processes (Ch 6)

contractility as pertaining to the heart, the force with which myocardial fibers shorten during systole (Ch 16)

corneal reflex used to test the afferent cranial nerve V and the efferent cranial nerve VII. The test is performed by lightly touching the cornea with a cotton swab. The normal response is that the patient should blink both eyes. (Ch 6)

cough a forceful expiratory maneuver designed to clear the larger airways; a common complaint of patients with lung disease (Ch 3)

crackles discontinuous adventitious lung sounds (Ch 5)

cranial sutures the open space between any two of the flat bones of the skull in the newborn and young infant (Ch 12)

creatine phosphate an energy reserve molecule in muscle (Ch 18)

creatinine a waste product of metabolism (Ch 18)

creatinine-height index (CHI) a predictor of muscle mass (Ch 18)

crepitus a grating or popping sound or sensation; when felt under the skin, indicates trapped air (subcutaneous emphysema), often a sign of pneumothorax (Ch 13)

critical congenital heart disease (CCHD) a category of heart defects present at birth that cause serious, life-threatening symptoms and typically require immediate intervention; includes hypoplastic left heart syndrome, tetralogy of Fallot, and transposition of the great arteries (Ch 12)

critical thinking the process of analyzing and/or evaluating empirically gathered information as a guide to action (Ch 21)

croup a disorder most often affecting small children that causes inflammation of the upper airway and trachea resulting from viral infection (Ch 12)

crying vital capacity (CVC) gas volume moved while an infant is crying; this is the closest measurement of vital capacity possible in infants (Ch 12)

culturally competent communication the application of general communication skills, self-awareness, situational awareness, and adaptability to identify and respond appropriately to the cultural cues affecting the clinical encounter (Ch 1)

Cushing triad an increasing systolic blood pressure with a widening pulse pressure, bradycardia, and bradypnea (Ch 6)

cyanosis a bluish cast to the skin that clinically may be difficult to detect, especially in a poorly lighted room and in patients with dark-pigmented skin (Ch 5)

cytology the study of cells of the body (Ch 7)

D

daytime somnolence an increased desire to sleep and associated lack of energy during the day as reported by a patient; a symptom of sleep-disordered breathing (Ch 3)

dead space-to-tidal volume ratio (V_D/V_T) the ratio of the dead space volume to the total amount of gas inhaled (Ch 14)

dead space ventilation ventilation that does not participate in gas exchange; includes both the volume of the conducting airways (anatomic dead space) and ventilated alveoli that are not perfused by the pulmonary circulation (physiologic dead space) (Ch 8)

decerebrate posture posture in which the upper extremity is in pronation and extension and the lower extremity is in extension (Ch 6)

decorticate posture a recognizable posture, caused by an upper motor neuron lesion, in which the patient's thumb is tucked under flexed fingers in a fisted position, with pronation of forearm and flexion at the elbow and the lower extremity in extension with foot inversion (Ch 6)

deep sulcus sign hyperlucency of the lateral costophrenic angle seen on chest x-ray of some patients in the supine position; suggests the presence of a pneumothorax (Ch 10)

deep tendon reflexes a physical examination test to evaluate spinal nerves; includes the triceps, biceps, brachioradialis, patellar, and Achilles tendon (Ch 6)

delirium an abnormal mental state characterized by confusion, incoherent speech, and hallucinations (Ch 6)

depolarization an electrical change in an excitable cell in which the inside becomes positive; associated with contraction of cardiac muscle cells (Ch 11)

diaphoresis excessive sweating (Ch 3, 5)

diastolic blood pressure the pressure in the arteries during relaxation of the ventricles (Ch 4)

dicrotic notch a secondary rise in the descending part of the arterial pulse pressure waveform that corresponds to closure of the aortic valve (Ch 15)

diet-induced thermogenesis the conversion of dietary calories in excess of those required to meet immediate metabolic needs into heat rather than being stored as fat (Ch 18)

diffusing capacity the ability of the lung to exchange oxygen between the alveoli and the pulmonary capillary blood; usually measured using low concentrations of carbon monoxide gas and expressed in mL/min/mm Hg (Ch 9)

diplopia blurred or double vision (Ch 5)

direct calorimetry measurement of metabolism by quantifying the total heat given off by the body when in an enclosed chamber (Ch 18)

doll's eyes reflex a neurologic test in which the physician turns the patient's head briskly from side to side; the eyes should turn to the left while the head is turned to the right, and vice versa. If this reflex is absent, there will be no eye movement when the patient's head is moved side to side. (Ch 6)

Do Not Resuscitate (DNR) order a physician's order based on a patient's legally authorized advance directive specifying that resuscitation should not be attempted in the event of a cardiorespiratory arrest; also called a *Do Not Attempt to Resuscitate (DNAR) order* (Ch 2)

dynamic compliance represents the total impedance to gas flow into the lungs (Ch 14)

dynamic hyperinflation a problem seen with severe airway obstruction in which mechanical breaths are stacked on one another (Ch 14)

dyshemoglobin any abnormal form of hemoglobin, such as carboxyhemoglobin or methemoglobin (Ch 8)

dyspnea shortness of breath as perceived by the patient (Ch 3)

dysrhythmia any deviation of the heart's normal sinus rhythm (Ch 11)

E

EEG arousal an abrupt shift in EEG frequency during sleep, usually lasting 3 seconds or more and commonly associated with the end of sleep-related obstructive events (Ch 19)

early inspiratory crackles abnormal high-pitched, discontinuous lung sounds heard early in inspiration and associated with obstructive airway diseases such as COPD and asthma (Ch 5)

ectopic impulse a heartbeat originating outside the SA node (Ch 11)

edema excessive fluid in tissue (Ch 3)

efferent as pertaining to nerves, those transporting impulses from the CNS to effector sites, such as muscle tissue (Ch 6)

ejection fraction (EF) the portion of the end-diastolic volume ejected during systole; normally about 60% to 70% (Ch 16)

electromagnetic navigation bronchoscopy an electromagnetic computerized procedure that tracks the position of a sensor incorporated into a flexible catheter advanced through a bronchoscope, used to reach and increase the biopsy yield from lesions in the smaller airways and mediastinum (Ch 17)

electronic health record (EHR) an electronically accessible and cumulative record of patient health information generated by the various encounters occurring across the spectrum of care delivery, also known as the *electronic medical record (EMR)* (Ch 2, 21)

electroencephalogram (EEG) the tracing of brain waves made by an electroencephalograph (Ch 6, 19)

encephalopathy a general term referring to any disorder or disease of the brain (Ch 6)

end-diastolic pressure (EDP) the pressure in a heart chamber at the end of diastole (Ch 16)

end-diastolic volume (EDV) the volume of blood in a heart chamber just before systole (Ch 16)

endoscopy a medical procedure in which a physician looks into the body of the patient using a scope (Ch 17)

end-tidal P_{CO_2} (P_{ETCO_2}) the partial pressure of CO_2 during the end-expiratory plateau phase of the capnogram (Ch 14)

eosinophilia an abnormal increase in the presence of eosinophils (Ch 7)

epiglottitis infection of the upper airway resulting from bacteria; most often seen in children (Ch 12)

Epworth Sleepiness Scale a short patient questionnaire used in diagnosing sleep disorders that assesses the magnitude of daytime somnolence (Ch 19)

escape beat a heartbeat that originates outside the sinus node after a period of SA node inactivity (Ch 11)

estimated date of confinement (EDC) estimated date of a term delivery of a pregnant woman (Ch 12)

excessive daytime sleepiness/somnolence (EDS) an abnormal increased desire to sleep during the day as reported by a patient; a symptom of sleep-disordered breathing (Ch 19)

expiratory reserve volume (ERV) the amount of gas that can be forcefully exhaled after a passive tidal exhalation (Ch 9)

expiratory view in chest radiography, an image taken during or after exhalation; the resulting reduction in lung volume can make small pneumothoraces more evident (Ch 10)

extremely low birthweight (ELBW) refers to newborns weighing less than 1000 g (Ch 12)

exudate when used to describe a pleural effusion, fluid with a high (>3 g/L) protein content (Ch 10)

F

F_ENO the fraction of expired nitric oxide in the exhaled breath, measured in parts per billion (ppb) (Ch 9)

fetal hemoglobin (HbF) hemoglobin present in the fetus in utero; has a higher affinity for oxygen than does adult hemoglobin; allows the fetus to survive and grow in the relatively low oxygen environment of the uterus (Ch 12)

fetid foul smelling (Ch 3)

fever an increase in body temperature above normal (Ch 3, 4)

fiberoptic bronchoscope a long, thin fexible tube consisting of a light-transmitting fiberoptic bundle and a channel used for examining a patient's airways; the channel allows the clinician to irrigate distal airways, suction fluids, and pass brushes or biopsy forceps to obtain tissue samples (Ch 17)

Fick principle a method for measuring cardiac output using oxygen consumption and the oxygen content difference between arterial and venous blood (Ch 14)

first-degree block a dysrhythmia in which the PR interval is prolonged, exceeding 200 msec; there are no missed beats, and the rhythm typically is regular (Ch 11)

flail chest the paradoxical motion seen as a sinking inward of the affected region with each spontaneous inspiratory effort and an outward movement with subsequent exhalation (Ch 5)

flow-volume loop a graphic plot of a patient's flow (Y-axis) vs. volume (X-axis) during a forced inspiratory and expiratory maneuver (Ch 9)

fluoroscopy the use of x-rays projected through the body onto a fluorescent screen to observe internal structures and their activity (such as swallowing) in the real time (Ch 10)

focus the site within the heart from which an ectopic impulse originates (Ch 11)

forced vital capacity (FVC) the maximum amount of air the patient exhales after a full, deep inspiration (Ch 9)

fractional saturation the amount of hemoglobin that is saturated compared with the total amount of hemoglobin present (Ch 14)

frothy descriptive term referring to a fluid with air bubbles (Ch 3)

fremitus internal vibrations sensed at the body surface with the flat of the hand (Ch 13)

functional lung volume lung volume in open communication with the airways (Ch 9)

functional residual capacity (FRC) the resting lung volume defined mechanically as the volume at which the expanding tendency of the chest wall is exactly counterbalanced by the contractile tendency of the lung; equals the sum of the residual and the expiratory reserve volumes (Ch 9, 14)

functional saturation the amount of hemoglobin that is saturated compared with the amount of hemoglobin that is capable of being saturated (Ch 14)

G

gag reflex a test performed by gently inserting a tongue depressor into the back of the throat; directly assesses the function of cranial nerve IX and more generally a patient's level of consciousness and upper airway protective reflexes (Ch 6)

gait the manner of walking (Ch 6)

gallop rhythm an abnormal condition in which a third or fourth heart sound is present (Ch 5)

gastroesophageal reflux abnormal movement of stomach contents into the esophagus or mouth; acid from the stomach may be aspirated into the lung and cause asthma-like symptoms (Ch 3)

gestational age the age of a fetus; estimated as the time in weeks from the last menses and typically measured using ultrasonic dimensions of the crown-to-rump length (up to 12 weeks' gestation) or the diameter of fetal head (after 12 weeks' gestation) (Ch 12)

Glasgow Coma Scale a clinical assessment scale used to quantify the degree of neurologic impairment (Ch 6)

gluconeogenesis converting protein (amino acids) to sugar (Ch 18)

glycosuria excessive sugar in the urine (Ch 7)

glycolysis process of converting glucose into pyruvic acid (Ch 18)

gravida number of prior pregnancies experienced by a woman (Ch 12)

grunting the sound heard when an infant exhales against a partially closed glottis; represents an effort to increase airway pressures and overcome the decrease in lung volumes associated with some neonatal respiratory disorders (Ch 12)

H

harsh breath sounds breath sounds with increased intensity (Ch 5)

heart block a category of dysrhythmias caused by defective transmission of the heart's electrical impulses through its conducting system (Ch 11)

heave a forceful, systolic thrust occurring during systole and felt over the precordium by the palpating hand (Ch 5)

hematemesis vomiting blood from the stomach (Ch 3)

hemoptysis coughing up blood from the lungs (Ch 3)

hemostasis the arrest of bleeding or stagnation of blood flow (Ch 7)

hepatomegaly enlargement of the liver (Ch 5, 12)

Holter monitor a portable device that continuously monitors and records the electrocardiogram, typically over an extended time period; used to assess for cardiac dysrhythmias (Ch 4)

home medical equipment (HME) devices designed for and used by patients whose care is being managed in the home by family members and/or nonprofessional caregivers; also called *durable medical equipment* (Ch 20)

Hoover's sign abnormal movement of the lateral chest wall during breathing in patients with chronic obstructive pulmonary disease with severe hyperinflation (Ch 5)

Hospital Consumer Assessment of Healthcare Providers and Systems (HCAHPS) a standardized survey instrument and data collection methodology for measuring patients' perspectives on hospital care (Ch 20)

HRmax the highest heart rate an individual can safely achieve at peak exercise capacity (Ch 9)

hyperbilirubinemia an excess of bilirubin in the blood (Ch 12)

hypercapnia abnormal elevation of $Paco_2$ (Ch 8)

hyperchloremia elevation of the chloride ion concentration in the blood plasma (Ch 7)

hyperdynamic precordium visible beating of the heart on the chest wall; usually indicates hypertrophy of the left or right ventricles (Ch 12)

hyperglycemia an abnormal elevation in blood glucose levels (Ch 7, 12)

hyperkalemia an abnormal elevation of plasma potassium (Ch 7)

hypernatremia an abnormal elevation of plasma sodium (Ch 7)

hyperoxemia the presence of excessive blood oxygen levels (Ch 8)

hyperresonant as compared with normal, a louder and lower-pitched sound heard when percussing the chest wall, typically indicating an increased volume of underlying air, as in hyperinflated states and pneumothorax (Ch 5)

hypertension an abnormal elevation of arterial blood pressure (Ch 4)

hyperthermia elevation of body temperature (Ch 12)

hypertrophy as applied to the heart, a pathologic increase in the bulk of the myocardial fibers, typically due to a chronic increase in afterload (Ch 11)

hyperventilation ventilation greater than necessary to meet metabolic needs; signified by a $Paco_2$ less than 35 mm Hg in the arterial blood (Ch 8)

hypoalbuminemia reduced blood protein levels (Ch 7)

hypocapnia presence of lower than normal amounts of CO_2 in the blood; as applied to arterial blood, a $Paco_2 < 35$ mm Hg (Ch 8)

hypochloremia an abnormal decrease in plasma chloride levels (Ch 7)

hypoglycemia reduced blood sugar levels (Ch 7, 12)

hypokalemia an abnormal decrease in serum potassium levels (Ch 7)

hyponatremia an abnormal decrease in serum sodium levels (Ch 7)

hypopnea generally refers to a reduction in the rate or depth of ventilation; as applied to diagnosis of sleep-disordered breathing, a 30% or more reduction in measured airflow lasting at least 10 seconds (Ch 19)

hypotension an abnormal decrease in arterial blood pressure (Ch 4)

hypothermia an abnormal decrease in body temperature (Ch 12)

hypotonia decreased muscle tone (Ch 12)

hypoventilation ventilation less than necessary to meet metabolic needs; signified by a Pa_{CO_2} greater than 45 mm Hg in the arterial blood (Ch 8)

hypoxemia an abnormal reduction in the partial pressure of oxygen in the arterial blood (Ch 8)

hypoxia a condition of in which oxygen levels in the tissues are inadequate to meet metabolic demands (Ch 8)

I

iatrogenic caused by treatment or diagnostic procedures (Ch 14)

iatrogenic alkalosis alkalosis caused by medical intervention; most often a respiratory alkalosis caused by overly aggressive mechanical ventilation (Ch 8)

ideal body weight the optimum weight of the patient as predicted from height and weight charts; also called *predicted body weight* (Ch 18)

immunosenescence the age-associated decline in the immune system (Ch 13)

impulse oscillometry noninvasive method to measure airway resistance by superimposing flow oscillations on the airways during spontaneous breathing; also called the forced oscillation technique (FOT) (Ch 12)

indirect calorimetry measurement of metabolic rate using inspired/expired gas analysis and computation of oxygen consumption ($\dot{V}_{O_2}$) and carbon dioxide production ($\dot{V}_{CO_2}$) (Ch 18)

inotropic agent a chemical agent that affects the contractility of the heart (Ch 15)

inspiratory capacity (IC) a physiologic unit of the lung defined as the sum of the tidal volume and the inspiratory reserve volume; the maximum amount of air that can be inhaled from resting FRC (Ch 9)

inspiratory reserve volume (IRV) a physiologic unit of the lung defined as the maximum volume of air that can be inhaled after a normal quiet inhalation (Ch 9)

intercostal referring to the muscle groups between the ribs (Ch 5)

interrupted aortic arch syndrome a developmental anomaly in which the aortic arch fails to completely form (Ch 12)

interstitial lung disease (ILD) respiratory disorder characterized by a dry, unproductive cough and dyspnea on exertion. X-rays usually show fibrotic infiltrates in the lung tissue, usually in the lower lobes. (Ch 9)

interventional radiology the use of imaging technologies to guide and gain access to vessels and organs for therapeutic purposes (Ch 10)

intracranial pressure (ICP) the level of pressure in the cranium (Ch 6)

intimate space the area around the patient within 18 inches (Ch 1)

intrapulmonary shunt ($\dot{Q}_s/\dot{Q}_t$) blood passing through the lung that is not exposed to ventilated alveoli (Ch 14)

intrauterine growth retardation (IGR) poor growth of a fetus in utero; exists when the estimated weight is below the 10th percentile for its gestational age (Ch 12)

intraventricular hemorrhage (IVH) bleeding in the lateral ventricles of the brain (grades I to III) or the tissue of the brain (grade IV) in premature infants (Ch 12)

isolated systolic hypertension (ISH) elevation of only the systolic pressure (Ch 13)

K

Kerley B lines a radiographic finding on a chest x-ray of a patient in congestive heart failure; the lines are short, parallel, and 1 mm thick and start at the lung base. They originate at the pleura and extend into the lung parenchyma 1 to 2 cm. They are caused by engorged pleural-based lymphatic vessels. (Ch 10)

kilocalories (kcal) the amount of energy it takes to raise the temperature of 1 kg of water 1° C (Ch 18)

kyphosis abnormal condition characterized by increased anteroposterior curvature of the spine (Ch 5)

kyphoscoliosis abnormal condition characterized by anteroposterior and lateral curvature of the spine (Ch 5)

L

lactic acid the product of anaerobic metabolism (Ch 18)

late inspiratory crackles abnormal, fine, and discontinuous breath sounds, heard at the latter part of inhalation over the dependent lung regions, often caused by sudden opening of peripheral airways (Ch 5)

last menstrual period (LMP) the date of the beginning of a woman's last menstrual period before pregnancy. This date can be used to calculate the estimated date of confinement. (Ch 12)

lateral decubitus view a radiographic technique used to demonstrate the presence of a free-flowing pleural effusion; the patient lies on the side with the hemithorax in question, allowing for gravity to act on the effusion and layering it out along the dependent lateral chest wall (Ch 10)

left shift a term used to indicate the presence of a high level of immature white cells in the circulating blood (Ch 7)

leukocytosis an abnormal increase in the circulating white blood cell count (Ch 7, 12)

leukopenia an abnormal decrease in the circulating white blood cell count (Ch 7, 12)

level of consciousness an assessment of the extent to which someone is alert and aware of their surroundings as well as their response to stimuli (Ch 6)

linearity (volume, flow) the extent to which a gas travels in a straight, unobstructed pattern (Ch 9)

loud P_2 increased intensity of S_2 as a result of more forceful closure of the pulmonic valve as occurs in pulmonary hypertension (Ch 5)

low birthweight (LBW) refers to infants of less than 2500 g, regardless of gestational age (Ch 12)

lower inflection point considered to be the minimal PEEP that should be applied to the lung as determined using a static pressure-volume curve (Ch 14)

lower motor neuron (LMN) motor neuron connecting the brainstem and spinal cord to muscle fibers (Ch 6)

lower/upper limit of normal (LLN/ULL) the upper and lower limits for predicted normal values of standardized tests results, such as pulmonary function tests and laboratory values (Ch 9)

lumbar puncture (LP) puncture of the lumbar region of the spinal cord to remove and test cerebral spinal fluid (Ch 6)

lymphadenopathy pertaining to a disease of the lymph nodes; refers also to the visualization of enlarged lymph nodes on radiographs (Ch 5)

lymphocytopenia an abnormal decrease in the number of circulating lymphocytes (Ch 7)

lymphocytosis an abnormal increase in the number of circulating lymphocytes (Ch 7)

M

macrocytic large cell size (Ch 7)

macrophage a monocyte that has left the circulation and entered tissue (Ch 7)

magnetic resonance imaging (MRI) a high-technology radiographic imaging technique (Ch 10)

maximum expiratory flow-volume curve (MEFV) the output graph showing the relationship between maximum expiratory flow and volume (Ch 9)

maximum inspiratory flow-volume (FEF$_{25-75\%}$) the output graph showing the relationship between maximum inspiratory flow and volume during the middle portion of the breath (Ch 9)

maximum inspiratory pressure (P$_I$max) a maximum pressure a patient can generate during a full inspiratory effort (Ch 14)

maximum voluntary ventilation (MVV) the volume of gas a patient can move in and out of the lung in 1 minute; value estimate based on patient performance for 15 seconds (Ch 9)

mean arterial pressure (MAP) the average pressure present in the arterial blood (Ch 15)

meconium the thick tarry stool that is present in the colon of a fetus in utero (Ch 12)

meconium aspiration syndrome (MAS) the inhalation of meconium passed into the amniotic fluid by the fetus in utero (Ch 12)

metabolic acidosis nonrespiratory processes resulting in acidemia (Ch 8)

metabolic alkalosis nonrespiratory processes resulting in alkalemia (Ch 8)

metabolic cart a computer-controlled unit composed of oxygen and carbon dioxide gas analyzers and flow transducers; used to measure indirect calorimetry (Ch 18)

metabolic equivalent of task (MET) the ratio of metabolic rate or rate of energy consumption during a specific physical activity to a reference metabolic rate (Ch 9)

metabolism the body's way of transferring energy from food to the body's energy currency molecules (adenosine triphosphate) (Ch 18)

microcytic small cell size (Ch 7)

micrognathia small lower jaw (Ch 19)

Mini-Mental State Examination (MMSE) a brief 30-point quantitative questionnaire used to assess cognition (Ch 6)

minute volume ($\dot{V}_E$) the volume of air inhaled or exhaled in 1 minute (Ch 9)

miosis small "pinpoint" pupils usually result from pontine hemorrhage or from ingestion of narcotics or organophosphates (Ch 5, 6)

mixed sleep apnea a condition characterized by a combination of both central and obstructive sleep apnea (Ch 19)

mixed venous oxygen saturation ($S\bar{v}O_2$) the percent saturation of mixed venous blood with oxygen; normally about 75% (Ch 14)

mixed venous oxygen tension ($S\bar{v}O_2$) the partial pressure of oxygen in the venous blood Sample obtained from the right atrium or pulmonary artery (Ch 14)

moderate sedation the administration of sedation to achieve a dreamlike, but arousable, state often used to facilitate selected procedures such as bronchoscopy (Ch 17)

monitoring the repeated or continuous observations or measurements of the patient, his/her physiologic function, and the function of life support equipment for the purpose of guiding management decisions (Ch 14)

monocytosis an abnormal increase in circulating monocytes (Ch 7)

montage (Ch 19)

mydriasis pupillary dilation that may be caused by serious brain injury or inadvertent exposure of the eyes to inhaled anticholinergics (Ch 5, 6)

N

nasal flaring the dilation of the ala nasi (the openings of the nose) during inspiration; this is an attempt by the infant to decrease airway resistance and increase tidal volume (Ch 12)

negative inotropic effect response of the heart in which the contractility is reduced (Ch 16)

negligence a legal term that refers to a health care professional acting outside the standards of care that causes harm to the patient (Ch 21)

neutropenia an abnormal decrease in the circulating neutrophils (Ch 7, 12)

neutrophilia an abnormal increase in the circulating neutrophils (Ch 7)

night sweats excessive diaphoresis during sleep (Ch 3)

nitric oxide (NO) a soluble gas that is normally produced in the body and serves as a powerful vasodilator (Ch 18)

nitrogen balance when the intake of nitrogen equals excretion of nitrogen (Ch 18)

nitrogen washout a technique used during pulmonary function testing to determine if there is maldistribution of ventilation of gas within the lung (Ch 9)

non–rapid eye movement (NREM) sleep a type of sleep composed of four stages: I, II, III, IV; this is the type of sleep in which the sleeper does not dream, and it makes up the majority of sleep time in the normal sleeper (Ch 19)

nonverbal communication means of communication that involves body positioning as well as facial and other expression and gestures, but that excludes verbal clues and language (Ch 1)

normoblasts immature nucleated red blood cells (Ch 7)

normocytic a form of anemia (low red blood cell count) that is somewhat common in elderly people, especially those older than 85 years (Ch 7)

nystagmus involuntary back and forth movement of the eyes (Ch 5, 6)

O

objective a desired result intended to be achieved and generally related to a broader goal (Ch 21)

objective data information about the patient that can be measured and is not a matter of opinion (Ch 2)

oblique views the patient is turned 45 degrees to either the right or left, with the anterolateral portion of the chest against the film (Ch 10)

obstructive sleep apnea intermittent pauses in breathing for more than 10 seconds resulting from upper airway blockage during sleep (Ch 3, 19)

obstructive ventilatory impairment a respiratory impairment characterized by a reduction or abnormally low inspiratory and or expiratory flow pattern (Ch 9)

oculocephalic reflex test of brainstem function in which the head is rotated side to side and eye movement is noted (Ch 6)

oculovestibular reflex also known as the ice caloric or cold caloric reflex. A physician instills at least 20 mL of ice water into the ear of a comatose patient. In patients with an intact brainstem, the eyes will move laterally toward the affected ear. (Ch 6)

oncotic pressure the pressure in the vascular space created by the presence of large protein molecules that draws fluid from outside the vessels into the vasculature (Ch 18)

orthodeoxia hypoxemia associated with sitting upright (Ch 3)

orthostatic hypotension a drop in blood pressure associated with standing or sitting up (Ch 3)

osteopenia of the premature a bone disease in premature infants that causes weak fragile bones; it is caused by inadequate phosphorus intake (Ch 12)

ototoxicity a drug that is toxic to the ear (Ch 13)

oxygen consumption the amount of oxygen consumed per minute by the body tissues (Ch 14)

oxygen content the amount of oxygen present in the blood; represents the oxygen combined with hemoglobin and dissolved in plasma; expressed as mL/100 mL of blood (Ch 14)

oxygen extraction ratio $(C[a - \bar{v}]_{O_2}/Ca_{O_2})$ the portion of oxygen content in the arterial blood extracted by the tissues (Ch 14)

O₂ pulse the ratio of oxygen consumption to heart rate (Ch 9)

oxygen transport the amount of oxygen moved by the blood per unit of time (Ch 14)

oxygen uptake the amount of oxygen used by the tissues per minute (Ch 18)

oxyhemoglobin dissociation curve (ODC) graphic depiction of the relationship between Pa_{O_2} and the oxygen content or hemoglobin saturation (Ch 14)

P

pack-years the number of packs of cigarettes smoked per day multiplied by the number of years smoked. Higher pack years are associated with greater risk for lung cancer and other lung diseases. (Ch 2)

palpation part of a physical examination in which an anatomic structure is felt to determine its size, shape, firmness, or location (Ch 5)

para the number of infants a woman has delivered (Ch 12)

paradoxical pulse an abnormally large decrease in systolic blood pressure during inspiration (Ch 4)

parenteral outside the gastrointestinal tract (Ch 18)

parenteral nutrition (PN) feeding a patient intravenously, bypassing the gastrointestinal tract (Ch 18)

paroxysmal nocturnal dyspnea the sudden onset of shortness of breath during sleep (Ch 3)

patellar reflex reflex tested by tapping on the patellar tendon with a reflex hammer while the patient's leg hangs loosely at a right angle with the thigh. Normally, the lower leg jerks forward when this reflex is intact. (Ch 6)

patent ductus arteriosus (PDA) the vessel that makes the anatomic connection between the pulmonary artery and the aorta during fetal life (Ch 12)

patient-centered care a model of care characterized by active involvement of patients and their families in the decision making and on-going care planning and implementation (Ch 1)

PC₂₀ the methacholine concentration at which a 20% decrease occurs in FEV_1 (Ch 9)

peak expiratory flow (PEF) the maximum flow rate achieved by the patient during the forced vital capacity maneuver (Ch 9)

peak inspiratory pressure the maximum pressure attained during the inspiratory phase of mechanical ventilation (Ch 14)

pectus carinatum a protrusion in the sternum (Ch 5)

pectus excavatum a depression or inward abnormality of the sternum (Ch 5)

pedal edema an accumulation of fluid in the subcutaneous tissues of the ankles (Ch 5)

percussion tapping on the skin surface to determine characteristics of the underlying anatomic structures (Ch 5)

periodic breathing an irregular breathing pattern in which periods of apnea are mixed in with periods of normal breathing (Ch 12)

peripheral cyanosis presence of cyanosis in the digits (Ch 5)

peripheral nervous system the nerves and ganglia outside of the brain and spinal cord (Ch 6)

PERRLA abbreviation often seen in the description of a physical examination finding that indicates the pupils are equal, round, and reactive to light and accommodation (Ch 6)

personal space the zone around the patient that can vary from 18 inches to 4 feet (Ch 1)

persistent vegetative state a condition in which a patient's eyes may be open but the patient is not able to be aroused (Ch 6)

pertinent negative a symptom related to the system in question but denied by the patient; for example, if the patient has lung disease but denies shortness of breath, dyspnea would be a pertinent negative (Ch 2)

pertinent positive a symptom the patient states is present that is related to the primary problem for which the patient is seeking help (Ch 2)

phlegm mucus from the tracheobronchial tree (Ch 3)

phlebostatic axis located at the fourth intercostal space and one half the anteroposterior (AP) diameter of the chest; approximates the location of the right atrium (Ch 15)

phrenic nerves the spinal nerves that pace the diaphragm (Ch 6)

physiologic dead space the conductive airways and alveolar units that are ventilated but not perfused (Ch 14)

phytochemicals naturally occurring chemical compounds that are responsible for color and other properties of organic substances (Ch 18)

plan of care outlines the diagnostic and therapeutic modalities for a patient aimed at achieving the goal of resolving a patient's disease, symptoms, and/or discomfort (Ch 20)

plantar reflex a superficial reflex that is commonly assessed in comatose patients and in those with suspected injury to the lumbar IV to V or sacral I to II areas of the spinal cord. It is tested by stroking the lateral plantar aspect of the foot with the handle of a reflex hammer or thumb nail. (Ch 6)

plateau pressure the pressure required to maintain a delivered tidal volume in a patient's lungs during a period of no gas flow (Ch 14)

platypnea shortness of breath in the upright position (Ch 3)

pleural friction rub an abnormal low-pitched, discontinuous breath sound characterized by grating of the pleural linings rubbing together (Ch 5)

pleurisy pain that comes from the pleural surface; usually a direct result of viral infections but has been generalized to any condition (e.g., pulmonary embolism) causing pleural pain; Synonymous with pleurodynia (Ch 5)

pneumoperitoneum air in the abdomen (Ch 12)

pneumothorax air in the pleural space (Ch 10)

point of maximal impulse the thrust of the contracting left ventricle; usually identified near the midclavicular line in the fifth intercostal space (Ch 5)

polycythemia an abnormal increase in the red blood cell count (Ch 7, 12)

polycythemia vera an uncontrolled proliferation of hematopoietic cells within the bone marrow (Ch 7)

polysomnogram (PSG) a sleep study used to diagnose sleep apnea and other sleep-related breathing disorders (Ch 19)

positive inotropic effect a medication or treatment that increases cardiac contractility (Ch 16)

positron emission tomography (PET) a high-technology radiographic technique used to determine whether a lesion seen on a standard x-ray contains cancer cells (Ch 10)

postanalytic error a problem occurring after sample analysis that alters the accuracy of blood gas results (Ch 8)

posteroanterior (PA) view a radiographic view of the chest in which the patient is placed in the upright position and turned so that the x-ray beam travels through the patient from his/her back (posterior) to front (anterior) before striking the x-ray film cassette (Ch 10)

postterm infants infants born later than 42 weeks' gestational age (Ch 12)

postural hypotension significant decrease in blood pressure associated with changes in position (Ch 4)

preanalytic error problem occurring before sample analysis that can alter the accuracy of blood gas results (Ch 8)

precordium chest wall overlying the heart (Ch 5)

preload the volume of blood in the ventricle just before systole (Ch 16)

presbycusis the progressive loss of hearing with age (Ch 13)

presbyopia the loss of the ability to focus on objects held near the eye with age (Ch 13)

pressure-volume loop a graph designed to display the relationship between the volume inhaled and the pressure generated (Ch 14)

preterm infants infants born younger than 37 weeks' gestational age (Ch 12)

privacy the ability to keep patients and their medical information inaccessible from public view (Ch 21)

proprioception one's sense of position of their body parts and strength while moving (Ch 6)

Protected Health Information (PHI) any information about health status, provision of health care, or payment for such services that can be linked to a specific patient and therefore must be kept private and secure (Ch 1)

protein-energy malnutrition loss of body protein (Ch 18)

pseudohypertension falsely high blood pressure in older adults because of arterial stiffness (Ch 13)

pseudoneutropenia a decrease in the neutrophil count associated with cells shifting from the circulatory pool to the marginated pool (Ch 7)

pseudoneutrophilia elevation of the neutrophil count that is the result of cells shifting from the marginated pool to the circulatory pool (Ch 7)

ptosis drooping of the upper eyelid (Ch 5)

pulmonary angiography a high-technology radiographic technique used to determine the presence of blood clots (embolisms) in the pulmonary circulation (Ch 10)

pulmonary capillary wedge pressure (PCWP) also known as *pulmonary artery occlusion pressure,* the pressure measured at the tip of the pulmonary artery catheter when the balloon is inflated; an estimate of left ventricular filling pressure (Ch 15, 16)

pulmonary interstitial emphysema (PIE) a diffuse form or lung injury found in neonates and infants exposed to mechanical ventilation for long time periods (Ch 12)

pulmonary vascular resistance (PVR) the resistance to blood flow through the pulmonary circulation (Ch 16)

pulse oximetry a monitoring technique used to estimate the oxygen saturation levels in the arterial blood (Ch 14)

pulse pressure the mathematical difference between the systolic and diastolic blood pressure measurements (Ch 4, 15, 16)

pupillary reflex contraction of the pupils when a light is directed at one eye (Ch 6)

Q

QRS complex central and most visually obvious part of an ECG tracing. It corresponds to the depolarization of the right and left ventricles of the human heart. (Ch 11)

QT interval time between the start of the Q wave and the end of the T wave in an ECG that represents electrical depolarization and repolarization of the left and right ventricles (Ch 11)

R

RR interval the time elapsing between two consecutive R waves in an ECG (Ch 11)

radiolucent a term used in describing the appearance of an x-ray film in which the x-ray beam has gone unimpeded through the patient and has turned that corresponding part of the resultant film black (Ch 10)

radionuclide lung scanning a technique in which a radioactive substance is introduced into the body to assess structure and function of tissues (Ch 10)

radiopaque a term used in describing the appearance of an x-ray film in which the x-ray beam has been absorbed, causing the corresponding part of the resultant film to be white (Ch 10)

rapid eye movement (REM) sleep the type of sleep in which dreaming is believed to occur (Ch 19)

rapid-shallow breathing index (RSBI) the ratio of respiratory frequency to tidal volume (Ch 14)

rate-pressure product obtained by multiplying the variables of heart rate and systolic blood pressure; used to assess the workload on the heart (Ch 16)

reference range sets the boundaries for any analyte (e.g., electrolyte, blood cell, protein, enzyme) that would likely be countered in healthy subjects. This range would encompass the variability reflected in the larger, presumably healthy, population. (Ch 9)

repeatability when the variation is smaller than some agreed limit for multiple measurements taken under the same conditions (Ch 9)

repolarization the return of a negative charge within the cell; occurs during relaxation of the myocardial cells (Ch 11)

residual volume (RV) a physiologic unit of the lung determined by pulmonary function testing, which describes the volume of gas remaining in the lung after maximal exhalation (Ch 9)

respiratory acidosis a decrease in pH resulting from elevation of the arterial P_{CO_2} (Ch 8)

respiratory alkalosis an increase in pH from a decrease in arterial P_{CO_2} (Ch 8)

respiratory alternans periods of breathing using only the chest wall muscles alternating with periods of breathing entirely by the diaphragm (Ch 5)

respiratory distress syndrome (RDS) a lung disease of premature infants characterized by inadequate amounts of lung surfactant (Ch 12)

respiratory effort–related arousal an arousal from sleep that follows a 10-second or longer sequence of breaths that are characterized by increasing respiratory effort, but that does not meet criteria for an apnea or hypopnea (Ch 19)

respiratory home care respiratory diagnostic and/or therapeutic modalities administered in a patient's home environment (Ch 20)

respiratory quotient (RQ) the ratio of carbon dioxide produced to oxygen consumed (Ch 18)

respirometer a device used to measure the volume and rate of breathing (Ch 9)

resting energy expenditure (REE) measure of oxygen uptake with the patient at rest (Ch 18)

restrictive ventilatory impairment an abnormal condition marked with the loss of lung volumes and capacities (Ch 9)

reticulocyte nucleated red blood cell (Ch 7)

retraction inward movement of the skin around the chest wall during inspiration; retractions are seen in any lung disease in which the compliance of the lung is less than the compliance of the chest wall (Ch 5, 12)

retrognathia a recessed or small lower jaw (Ch 19)

return demonstration after being instructed on a procedure, the patient and/or caregiver is observed by the clinician doing such procedure to help ensure they are competent (Ch 1, 20)

rhonchi low-pitched, discontinuous, abnormal breath sounds caused by air moving through airways with excessive secretions (Ch 5)

S

SBAR situation, background, assessment, and recommendation charting (Ch 1)

ST-elevation myocardial infarction (STEMI) a type of "heart attack" or myocardial infarction characterized by an elevation in the ST segment (Ch 11)

ST segment the interval between the end of the QRS complex and the T wave (Ch 11)

scalene referring to the three muscles arising from the cervical vertebrae, inserting into the first and second ribs; accessory muscles of ventilation (Ch 5)

scoliosis abnormal lateral curvature of the spine (Ch 5)

sensitivity the proportion of actual positives results that are correctly identified as such (e.g., the percentage of sick people who are correctly identified as having the condition) (Ch 7)

sensory dissociation one sensory system is affected, but the other one is not (Ch 6)

sensorium general term referring to the relative state of a patient's consciousness or alertness (Ch 4)

serum the watery fluid portion of the blood (Ch 7)

serum albumin the major protein fraction of blood (Ch 18)

serum transferrin the protein that transports iron in the body (Ch 18)

signs physical examination findings consistent with disease (Ch 2)

silhouette sign a radiographic finding that occurs when the edge of a well-established object (the heart) is obliterated because there is an infiltrate in anatomic contact (Ch 10)

sinus bradycardia an abnormal drop in heart rate with each beat originating in the SA node (Ch 12)

situation, background, assessment and recommendation charting (SBAR charting) a format of change-of-shift reporting that emphasizes selected elements of the patient's case (Ch 21)

six-MWD (6MWD) 6-minute walk distance used to help determine the degree of dyspnea and quality of life (Ch 9)

skinfold measurement a method for estimating the percent of body fat (Ch 18)

sleep apnea pauses in breathing of at least 10 seconds during sleep (Ch 19)

sleep architecture describes the structure and pattern of sleep and encompasses several variables (Ch 19)

sleep-disordered breathing periods of an absence of or insufficient breathing during sleep (Ch 3, 19)

slow vital capacity (SVC) a measure of the change in volume of gas in the lungs from complete inspiration to complete expiration or vice versa (Ch 9)

slow-wave sleep consists of stages 3 and 4 of non–rapid eye movement sleep (Ch 19)

snoring the hoarse or harsh sound that occurs when breathing is obstructed in some way during sleep (Ch 19)

social space the space of 4 to 12 feet from the patient (Ch 1)

Speak-Up initiative a national campaign to urge patients and their families to take a role in preventing health care errors by becoming active, involved, and informed participants on the health care team (Ch 1)

specific conductance (Gaw/TGV) a measure of how well water can conduct an electrical current (Ch 9)

specificity measures the proportion of negative test results that are correctly identified as such. For example, the percentage of healthy people who are correctly identified as not having the condition (Ch 7)

spirogram the tracing produced by a spirograph (Ch 9)

splenomegaly abnormal enlargement of the spleen (Ch 12)

spurious outwardly similar or corresponding to something without having its genuine qualities (Ch 7)

spurious polycythemia an increase in the red blood cell count resulting from a decrease in serum (as in dehydration) (Ch 7)

sputum secretions from the tracheobronchial tree that are expectorated through the mouth (Ch 3)

standard precautions guidelines recommended by the U.S. Centers for Disease Control and Prevention to reduce the risk for transmission of blood-borne and other pathogens in hospitals. Standard precautions apply to (1) blood; (2) all body fluids, secretions, and excretions, excluding sweat, regardless of whether they contain blood; (3) nonintact skin; and (4) mucous membranes. (Ch 1)

static compliance the lung volume change per unit of pressure during a period of no gas flow (Ch 14)

sternocleidomastoid a form of accessory muscles of breathing located in the anterior portion of the neck (Ch 5)

STOP-BANG analysis a measurement tool used to classify the severity of certain sleep disorders (Ch 19)

stridor continuous sound heard primarily over the larynx and trachea during inhalation when upper airway obstruction is present (Ch 5)

stroke volume (SV) the volume of blood ejected from the ventricle during systole (Ch 16)

subcutaneous emphysema a crackling sound and sensation when fine beads of air are palpated in the tissues (Ch 5)

subjective an individual's (such as a patient's) personal perspective, feelings, beliefs, desires, or discovery (Ch 21)

subjective data information obtained from the patient that cannot be confirmed with objective testing (Ch 2)

subjective, objective, assessment, and plan (SOAP) charting a format for obtaining and recording the major elements of a patient's assessment and care plan (Ch 21)

sudden infant death syndrome (SIDS) a condition of unexplained death of an infant. Usually seen in infants between 6 weeks and 6 months of age. The incidence of this disease is decreased by not letting the young infant sleep in a prone (face-down) position (Ch 12, 19)

switch-in error a specific type of error that can occur in pulmonary function tests (PFTs) (Ch 9)

symptoms subjective complaints by the patient (Ch 2)

syncope fainting or dizziness; often resulting from hypotension (Ch 3)

systemic vascular resistance (SVR) the amount of resistance experienced by the arterial blood as it passes through the peripheral vasculature (Ch 16)

systolic blood pressure the peak blood pressure in the arteries during ventricular contraction (Ch 4)

T

tachycardia an abnormal increase in the heart rate (Ch 4, 12)

tachypnea an abnormal increase in the rate of breathing (Ch 4, 12)

tactile fremitus vibrations that can be felt on a patient's chest wall and that are generally caused by air moving through secretions (Ch 5)

target a physical structure in the x-ray machine used to direct the x-ray beam (Ch 10)

teach-back method a way to confirm that the clinician has explained to the patient what he/she needs to know about a procedure in a manner that the patient understands (Ch 1)

telemetry monitoring patient data such as vital signs at a distance and generally using wireless technology (Ch 4)

tenacious tending to stick firmly and not easily removed (Ch 3)

term infant an infant born between 37 and 42 weeks' gestational age (Ch 12)

territoriality the patient's sense that items around his/her hospital bed belong to him/her while admitted (Ch 1)

The Joint Commission (TJC) an organization designed to survey and improve the quality of health care organizations (Ch 20, 21)

thoracentesis surgical perforation of the chest wall and pleural space with a needle for diagnostic or therapeutic purposes or for the removal of a specimen for biopsy (Ch 10)

thoracic gas volume (TGV) technique that measures lung volume (Ch 9)

thrombocytopenia an abnormal decrease in the circulating platelets (Ch 7, 12)

thrombocytosis an abnormal increase in the number of circulating blood platelets (Ch 7, 12)

tidal volume (V_T) a physiologic unit of the lung that is the amount of gas moved in and out of the lung during relaxed, at-rest breathing (Ch 9)

tinnitus an auditory perception not caused by external sounds that may be described as ringing, buzzing, roaring, or chirping (Ch 13)

total lung capacity (TLC) a physiologic unit of the lung determined during pulmonary function testing, which describes the total amount of gas in the lungs after maximum inspiration (Ch 9)

tracheal breath sound tubular, loud breath sounds normally heard over the trachea (Ch 5)

transient tachypnea of the newborn (TTN) a lung disease with increased lung water in infants born by cesarean delivery (Ch 12)

transmural pressure the net distending pressure within the ventricle; it provides a true estimation of left ventricular end-diastolic filling because the effect of pressure around the heart is considered (Ch 15)

transudate when used to describe a fluid associated with a pleural effusion, with a low (<3 g/L) protein content (Ch 10)

trepopnea better breathing associated with a certain position (Ch 3)

U

upper airway resistance syndrome (UARS) a common cause of sleep fragmentation in patients who snore (Ch 19)

upper inflection point the part of the curve on a static pressure-volume curve that indicates overdistention of the lung (Ch 14)

upper motor neuron motor neurons that originate in the motor region of the cerebral cortex or the brainstem (Ch 6)

V

venous return the amount of blood returned to the right side of the heart (Ch 16)

ventricular compliance the ability of the ventricle to expand as blood enters from the atrium (Ch 16)

ventricular function curves graphs demonstrating the various stroke volumes achieved at various degrees of filling pressure (Ch 16)

ventricular stroke work the amount of work performed by the left ventricle during systole (Ch 16)

very low birthweight (VLBW) describes a newborn who weights less than the 95th percentile of weight for newborns (Ch 12)

vesicular breath sound a soft, muffled sound heard during auscultation over the lung parenchyma of a healthy person (Ch 5)

vital capacity (VC) the maximum amount of air that can be expelled after a full inspiratory effort (Ch 9)

vocal fremitus vibration felt by a hand placed on the chest of an individual who is speaking (Ch 5)

volutrauma a lung injury that occurs from overdistention of the terminal respiratory units (Ch 14)

$\dot{V}O_2$max maximum oxygen consumption or uptake as measured by calorimetry (Ch 9)

volumeter an instrument used for measuring the volume of gas (Ch 9)

W

wheeze the musical sounds heard from the chest of the patient with intrathoracic airway obstruction (e.g., asthma) (Ch 5)

Index

A

a wave, in central venous pressure, 356, 357f
A_2, loud, 95, 95b
a/A ratio (arterial-to alveolar tension ratio), in critically ill patients, 335–336
Abdomen
    examination of, 96, 96f
    of infant
        auscultation of, 275
        palpation of, 274–275
    quadrants of, 96, 96f
Abdominal distention, 96
Abdominal paradox, 82, 82t
Abducens nerve, 112f, 113t
ABG analysis. *See* Arterial blood gas (ABG) analysis.
Abortion, 264–265
Absorptive phase, of metabolic process, 418, 419f
Accelerated idioventricular rhythm, 256
Acceptability, of forced vital capacity maneuver, 184, 185b
Accessory hemiazygos vein, 224f
Accessory muscles, of ventilation, 81–82
Accessory nerve, 112f, 113t
Acetylcoenzyme A (Acetyl CoA), in metabolism, 418, 419f
Achilles reflex, 116t
Acid group (COOH), 421
Acid-base balance
    assessment of, 162–164
        base excess in, 153t, 163
        Henderson-Hasselbalch equation in, 163–164
        partial pressure of carbon dioxide ($Paco_2$) in, 153t, 162–163, 163b
        pH in, 153t, 162
        plasma bicarbonate in, 153t, 163
        systematic, 170–173
    protein intake and, 421–422
Acid-base imbalances
    combined, 167
        metabolic and respiratory alkalosis as, 167
        respiratory and metabolic acidosis as, 167
    mixed, 167–168, 167b
        metabolic acidosis and respiratory alkalosis as, 168
        metabolic alkalosis and respiratory acidosis as, 168
    simple, 164–166, 166t
        metabolic acidosis as, 163, 165–166, 165b, 166t
        metabolic alkalosis as, 163, 166, 166b, 166t
        respiratory acidosis as, 163–165, 165b, 166t
        respiratory alkalosis as, 163, 165, 166t
Acidemia, 162
Acid-fast stain, 142
    of lung tissue, 144–145
Acidosis
    metabolic, 165–166, 166t

Acidosis (*Continued*)
    acute (uncompensated), 165, 165b
    anion gap in, 165
    defined, 163
    Kussmaul respirations in, 165
    and respiratory acidosis, 167
    and respiratory alkalosis, 168
    respiratory, 164–165, 166t
        acute (uncompensated), 164
        chronic, 164
        compensation for, 164, 166t
        defined, 163, 165b
        fully compensated, 164
        and metabolic acidosis, 167
        metabolic alkalosis and, 168
Acoustic nerve, 112f, 113t
Acquired immunodeficiency syndrome (AIDS), CT scan for, 227
Acrocyanosis, 97
    of newborn, 266
Action plans, 7, 8b
Action potential, 239
Activated partial thromboplastin time (APTT), 135, 135b
    in infants, 278, 278t
Activities of daily living (ADLs), 310
    in home care assessment, 460
    instrumental, 310
Adaptability, in culturally competent communication, 6
Adenosine triphosphate (ATP), 412, 413f
Admission note, 28
Adventitious breath sounds, 87–88, 88b
Afferent division, of peripheral nervous system, 103–104, 105f
Afterload, 380–382
    calculation of systemic and pulmonary vascular resistance for, 378f, 381–382, 381b
    conditions associated with alterations in, 384t–385t
    decreased, 381
    defined, 380
    increased, 381
    peripheral resistance in, 381
    ventricular wall stress in, 380–381
AFV (amniotic fluid volume), in biophysical profile, 268t
AGA (appropriate for gestational age), 268
Age
    chronologic, 264
    gestational, 264
        assessment of, 268–270, 269f
Ageism, 297
Age-related changes, 299–301
    in cardiovascular system, 300, 300b
    in pulmonary system, 300–301
Age-related sensory deficit, 298–299
    hearing impairment as, 298–299
        assessing for, 298
        compensating for, 298–299
    vision impairment as, 299
        assessing for, 299
        compensating for, 299, 299b

Aging, of organ systems, 299–302
    age-related changes in, 299–301
        in cardiovascular system, 300, 300b
        in pulmonary system, 300–301
    pulmonary defense mechanisms in, 301
        and immunity, 301
    and unusual presentation of illness, 301–302
        for asthma, 302, 302b
        for myocardial infarction and congestive heart failure, 302
        for pneumonia, 301–302
AHI (apnea-hypopnea index), 443, 445, 445b
AHR. *See* Airway hyperresponsiveness (AHR).
AIDS (acquired immunodeficiency syndrome), CT scan for, 227
Air
    in arterial blood gas sample, 169t
    on radiographs, 210
Air bronchogram, 214
Air hunger, 42t
Air leak, around endotracheal tube, in newborns, 282–283, 283f
Air trapping, in critically ill patients, 317
Airway hyperresponsiveness (AHR), 195–198
    bronchoprovocation testing for, 196, 196b, 197f
    exhaled nitric oxide (F_ENO) analysis for, 196–198, 197b–198b, 197f, 198t
Airway management problems, in SOAP charting, 474
Airway patency, of critically ill infant, 286–287
Airway pressure(s), in critically ill patients, 319–323
    auto-PEEP as, 322
    infants as, 286–287
    maximum inspiratory, 316t, 321–322, 322b
    mean, 320–321
    peak inspiratory, 319–320, 320b, 320f
    plateau, 320, 321f
Airway pressure release ventilation-assist (APRV), in newborns, 283
Airway resistance (Raw), 194–195, 195b
    in critically ill patients, 317, 323
    in newborns, 282
Alanine aminotransferase (ALT), 136t, 140
    in newborn, 278
Alanine transaminase (ALT). *See* Alanine aminotransferase (ALT).
Albumin, 139
    in newborn, 278, 278t
    in older patients, 309
    serum, 428, 428t
Alert and oriented times three, 109–110
A-line, 155–156, 156f, 156t
Alkalemia, 162
Alkaline phosphatase (ALP), 136t, 140
Alkalosis
    metabolic, 163, 166, 166b, 166t
        and respiratory acidosis, 168
        and respiratory alkalosis, 167
    respiratory, 163, 165, 166t
        metabolic acidosis and, 168
        metabolic alkalosis and, 167
    ventilator-induced (iatrogenic), 167

Page numbers followed by *f* refer to figures; *t*, tables; *b*, boxes.